Case Studies in Neurological Infections of Adults and Children

ERRATUM

Solomon et al.: *Case Studies in Neurological Infections of Adults and Children* 9781107634916

We regret omitting from Case 65 *Twitchy and Twitching* and the contributor list:

Dr Marc Boix Codony MD MSc FEBN,
Consultant Neurologist
The Walton Centre NHS Foundation Trust

Case Studies in Neurological Infections of Adults and Children

Edited by

Tom Solomon
Walton Centre NHS Foundation Trust, and
Institute of Infection and Global Health, University of Liverpool

Benedict D. Michael
Walton Centre NHS Foundation Trust, and
Institute of Infection and Global Health, University of Liverpool

Alastair Miller
Formerly Royal Liverpool University Hospital and Broadgreen NHS Trust, and
Institute of Infection and Global Health, University of Liverpool

Rachel Kneen
Alder Hey Children's NHS Foundation Trust, Liverpool

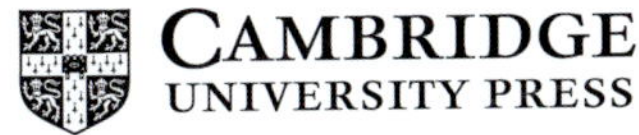

CAMBRIDGE
UNIVERSITY PRESS

University Printing House, Cambridge CB2 8BS, United Kingdom

One Liberty Plaza, 20th Floor, New York, NY 10006, USA

477 Williamstown Road, Port Melbourne, VIC 3207, Australia

314–321, 3rd Floor, Plot 3, Splendor Forum, Jasola District Centre, New Delhi – 110025, India

79 Anson Road, #06–04/06, Singapore 079906

Cambridge University Press is part of the University of Cambridge.

It furthers the University's mission by disseminating knowledge in the pursuit of education, learning, and research at the highest international levels of excellence.

www.cambridge.org
Information on this title: www.cambridge.org/9781107634916
DOI: 10.1017/9781139628839

First published 2019

Printed and bound in Great Britain by Clays, St Ives plc, Elcograf S.p.A.

A catalogue record for this publication is available from the British Library.

Library of Congress Cataloging-in-Publication Data
Names: Solomon, Tom, editor. | Michael, Benedict D., editor. | Miller, Alastair, editor. | Kneen, Rachel, editor.
Title: Case studies in neurological infections of adults and children / edited by Tom Solomon, Benedict D. Michael, Alastair Miller, Rachel Kneen.
Description: Cambridge, United Kingdm ; New York, NY : Cambridge University Press, 2019. | Includes bibliographical references.
Identifiers: LCCN 2018009857 | ISBN 9781107634916 (paperback)
Subjects: | MESH: Nervous System Diseases – diagnosis | Nervous System Diseases – therapy | Diagnosis, Differential | Case Reports
Classification: LCC RC346 | NLM WL 141 | DDC 616.8–dc23
LC record available at https://lccn.loc.gov/2018009857

ISBN 978-1-107-63491-6 Paperback

Contents

Contributors

Baba Aji MSc MRCP DipNeurol
The Walton Centre NHS Foundation Trust, Liverpool, UK

David Bargiela MRCP
Department of Neurology, Brigham and Women's Hospital, Boston, MA, USA

Nicholas J. Beeching MA FRCP FRACP FFTM RCPS (Glasg) FESCMID DCH DTM&H
Tropical and Infectious Disease Unit, Royal Liverpool University Hospital & Liverpool School of Tropical Medicine, Liverpool, UK

Laura A. Benjamin BSc MRCP PhD
Institute of Infection and Global Health, University of Liverpool, Liverpool, UK

Hema Bentur
Children, Young People, Paediatric & Neonatal Services, St Helens and Knowsley Teaching Hospitals NHS Trust, St Helens, UK

Michael Bonello MD MRCP MRes DTM&H
The Walton Centre NHS Foundation Trust, Liverpool, UK

Hannah E. Brindle MSc BSc MRCP MRes DTM&H
Institute of Infection and Global Health, University of Liverpool & Wellcome Trust Liverpool Glasgow Centre for Global Health Research, University of Liverpool, Liverpool, UK

Gemma Buxton MBBS MRCPCH DTM&H
Royal Hospital for Sick Children, Edinburgh, UK

Suresh Kumar Chhetri MD FRCP FHEA
Department of Neurology, Royal Preston Hospital, Preston, UK

Aleš Chrdle MUDr
Infectious Disease Department, České Budějovice Hospital, České Budějovice, Czech Republic & Tropical and Infectious Disease Unit, Royal Liverpool University Hospital, Liverpool, UK

Theresa Cole PhD MRCPCH
Department of Allergy and Immunology, Royal Children's Hospital, Melbourne, Australia

Sylviane Defres BMSc DO&G DRCOG MRCP MRCGP DTM&H
Institute of Infection and Global Health, University of Liverpool; Tropical and Infectious Disease Unit, Royal Liverpool University Hospital & Liverpool School of Tropical Medicine, Liverpool, UK

Katherine C. Dodd MRCP
Department of Neurology, Royal Preston Hospital, Preston, UK

Charlotte F. Dougan MD FRCP
The Walton Centre NHS Foundation Trust, Liverpool, UK

Richard J. B. Ellis MPhil MRCP
The Walton Centre NHS Foundation Trust, Liverpool, UK

Liene Elsone
The Walton Centre NHS Foundation Trust, Liverpool, UK

Hedley C. A. Emsley PhD FRCP
Department of Neurology, Royal Preston Hospital, Preston, UK

Claire Gall BSc MRCP
Department of Neurology, Royal Preston Hospital, Preston, UK

Mona Ghadiri-Sani
The Walton Centre NHS Foundation Trust, Liverpool, UK

Anu Goenka DTM&H PGDipPID MRCGP MRCPCH
Manchester Collaborative Centre for Inflammation Research, University of Manchester, Manchester, UK

Lynsey C. Goodwin BSc MRCP
Tropical and Infectious Disease Unit, Royal Liverpool University Hospital, Liverpool, UK

Karolina Griffiths MBChB MSc
Royal Liverpool and Broadgreen University Hospital NHS Trust, Liverpool, UK & La Timone University Hospital, Marseille, France

Michael Grosdenier CSCT DCH MRCPCH
Children's & Adolescent Services, Mid-Cheshire Hospitals NHS Trust, Crewe, UK

Heli Harvala MD MSc PhD FRCPath
Specialist Virology Centre, Edinburgh Royal Infirmary, NHS Lothian, Edinburgh, UK

Syed Hyder MRCPI
The Walton Centre NHS Foundation Trust, Liverpool, UK

Anand Iyer MD MRCPCH
Littlewood's Neurosciences Foundation, Alder Hey Children's NHS Foundation Trust, Liverpool, UK

Rachel Kneen BMedSci DCH FRCPCH
Littlewood's Neuroscience Foundation, Alder Hey Children's NHS Foundation Trust & Institute of Infection and Global Health, University of Liverpool, Liverpool, UK

Jennifer Lemon BM MSc MRCPCH
Institute of Infection and Global Health, University of Liverpool, Liverpool, UK

Fiona McGill MRCP
Institute of Infection and Global Health, University of Liverpool, Liverpool, UK

Benedict D. Michael MRCP PhD
The Walton Centre NHS Foundation Trust, & Institute of Infection and Global Health, and NIHR Health Protection Research Unit in Emerging and Zoonotic Infections, University of Liverpool, Liverpool, UK & Center for Immunology and Inflammatory Disease, Massachusetts General Hospital, Harvard Medical School, Boston, MA, USA

Alastair Miller MA FRCP FRCPEd DTM&H
North Cumbria University Hospitals Trust & Institute of Infection and Global Health, University of Liverpool, Liverpool, UK & Joint Royal Colleges of Physicians Training Board, London, UK

Sophie Miller MBChB
University of Liverpool and Wirral University Teaching Hospital NHS Foundation Trust, Liverpool, UK

Sam Nightingale MRCP PhD DTM&H
Institute of Infection and Global Health, University of Liverpool, Liverpool, UK

Jay Panicker MD MRCP
The Walton Centre NHS Foundation Trust, Liverpool, UK

Graham A. Powell MPhil MRCP
Institute of Translational Medicine, University of Liverpool & The Walton Centre NHS Foundation Trust, Liverpool, UK

Stephen Ray MPhil MRCPCH MRes DTM&H
Institute of Infection and Global Health, University of Liverpool & Wellcome Trust Liverpool Glasgow Centre for Global Health Research, University of Liverpool, Liverpool, UK

Katie Rose MPhil MRCPCH
Institute of Translational Medicine, University of Liverpool, Liverpool, UK

Derek J. Sloan PhD MRCP DTM&H
University of St Andrews, Scotland & Liverpool School of Tropical Medicine, Liverpool, UK

Tom Solomon BA DCH DTM&H PhD FRCP
The Walton Centre NHS Foundation Trust & Royal Liverpool University Hospital, Liverpool & Institute of Infection and Global Health and National Institute for Health Research (NIHR) Health Protection Research Unit in Emerging and Zoonotic Infections, University of Liverpool, Liverpool, UK

Lance Turtle BSc PhD MRCP DTM&H
Institute of Infection and Global Health, University of Liverpool & Tropical and Infectious Disease Unit, Royal Liverpool University Hospital, Liverpool, UK

Scott Williams MRCP BMedSci (Hons)
The Countess of Chester Hospital NHS Foundation Trust, Cheshire, UK

John Williamson
The Walton Centre NHS Foundation Trust, Liverpool, UK

Besa Ziso MRCP
The Walton Centre NHS Foundation Trust, Liverpool, UK

Preface

Introduction

Neurological infectious diseases provide some of the most fascinating and challenging cases faced by clinicians. The presenting syndromes are often elusive, establishing the causative organism can be problematic, and determining the best treatment difficult. Perhaps nothing better illustrates this than their regular appearance as case reports in the medical journals; nearly one-quarter of all the case reports in *The Lancet* were patients with neurological infections in one recent year.

The Book's Origins

Most of the cases presented in this book were seen initially in our neurological infectious diseases services in Liverpool, and many have been presented at the Liverpool Neurological Infectious Disease Course. The services were established in 2005 between colleagues at The Walton Centre NHS Foundation Trust, The Royal Liverpool University Hospital, Alder Hey Children's Hospital, Liverpool School of Tropical Medicine and the University of Liverpool. The Neurological Infectious Disease Course began two years later. What was intended initially to be a one-off occasion for local trainees rapidly became a popular annual event, oversubscribed each year, with attendees from across the UK, and around the world (more than 800 people from 30 countries in the first 10 years).

Who the Book is for

Just like the course, this book will appeal to those working in the many disciplines involved in the care of patients with neurological infections: primary care, general, internal and emergency medicine, paediatrics, foundation year and core medical training, intensive care, radiology, pathology, microbiology, virology, tropical and infectious diseases, genitourinary medicine, HIV, public health, neurosurgery and neurology. While the book is aimed at trainees in these specialties it is also suitable for medical students eager to learn more, and attending physicians and consultants who wish to refresh their memories and get up to date.

The Cases

The majority of cases are typical of those seen in Western industrialised countries, acquired locally or in returning travellers, but we couldn't resist including one or two cases from The Liverpool Brain Infections Group's research studies in Asia, Africa and Latin America. As well as adults and children with acute and chronic neurological infections, we have included some with post-infectious neurological diseases, and others whose final diagnoses were non-infectious immune conditions; these latter because of the similar presenting syndromes and shared differential diagnoses.

All of the cases presented are based on real patients; some details have been modified to protect identities, or for greater clarity or brevity. Many were seen initially in secondary care and transferred into one of our centres; we have tried not to become bogged down with details of what happened where, and are aware that viewed with hindsight from the ivory towers of tertiary care, things can look very different. Our focus has been to draw out the learning points from the case, to make them useful and informative. It's an eclectic collection of cases, and just like in real life, diseases may present more than once, in different forms.

How to Use the Book

The cases have cryptic titles, and are presented so that they can be worked through as learning exercises. After reading the history and examination the reader can decide on the preliminary differential diagnosis, before seeing the thoughts of those managing the patient. With the results of initial investigations, those usually available within a day or two of admission, the differential is refined, before the results of definitive investigations and the final diagnosis are given.

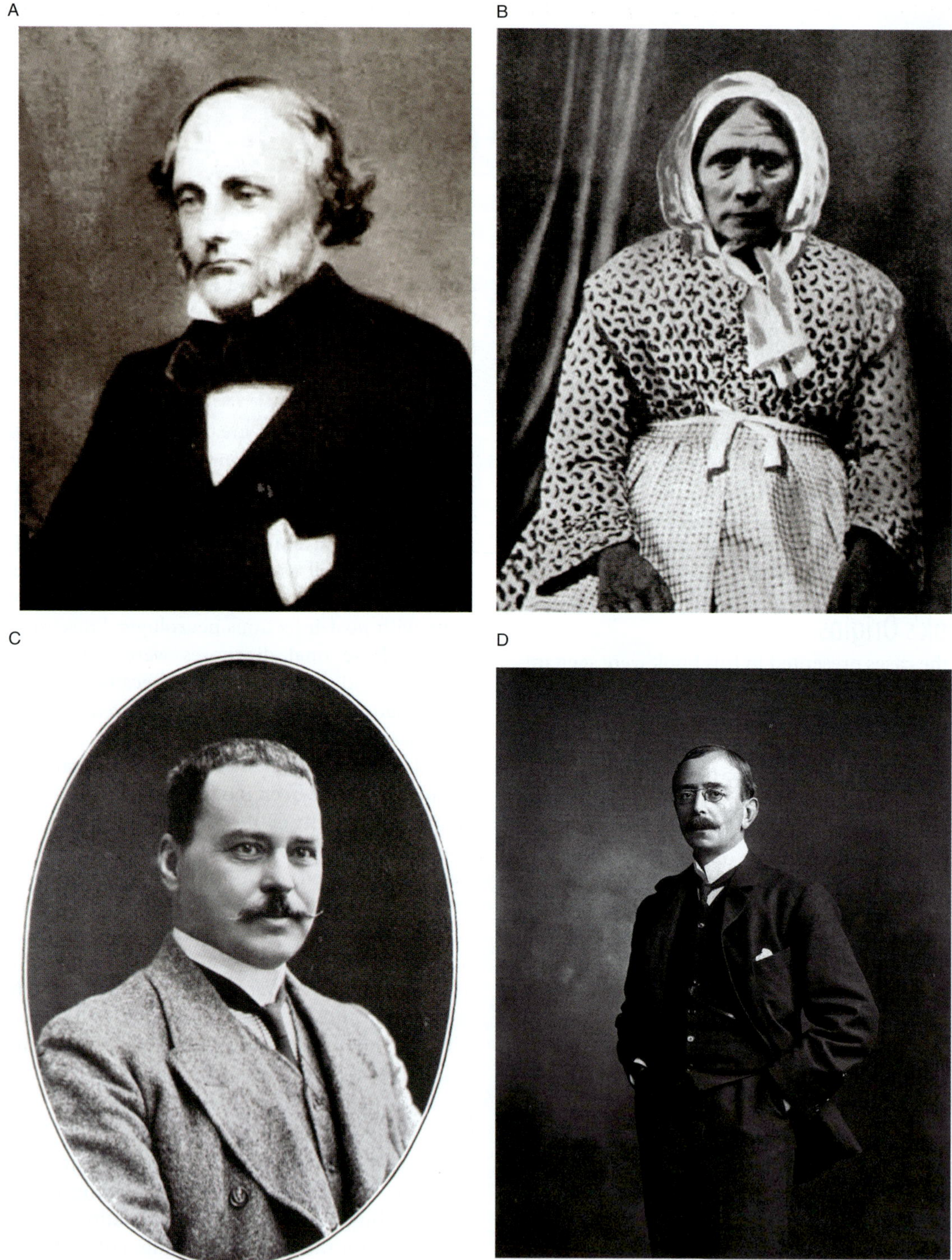

Figure 1 Liverpool's long tradition of excellence in infection and neuroscience. (A) William Henry Duncan (1805–1863), Britain's First Medical Officer of Health (artist unknown); (B) Kitty Wilkinson (1786–1860), who created Britain's first public wash houses and baths (photo courtesy of Centenary of Baths Committee, City of Liverpool); (C) Sir Ronald Ross (1857–1932), who won a Nobel Prize (1902) for his work showing that malaria is spread by mosquitoes (photo courtesy of National Institutes of Health, USA); (D) Sir Charles Sherrington (1857–1952), who won a Nobel Prize (1932) for his functional analysis of the muscle motor unit (photo courtesy of the National Library of Medicine).

Diagnostic images are presented along the way; the reader can consider what they show, before reading the legend to see what we thought. Essential elements of the management and any preventative measures are reviewed before a brief final discussion of the case and the disease. Each chapter concludes with the key learning points, plus historical gems and some intriguing observations to impress your friends at dinner parties, or on ward rounds. In an appendix all the cases are listed according to presenting syndrome for the reader who is looking for an example of a specific presentation.

We are grateful to our many colleagues who have shared their cases with us for use in this book. None more so than Dr Nick Beeching and Professor Enitan Carrol, who play a key role in both the clinical services and the course. All the author proceeds from this book will be used to support our work in Liverpool, including international scholarships for the Neurological Infectious Diseases course. If you enjoy the book we hope to see you on the course at some stage in the future.

Did You Know?

Liverpool's interest in neuroscience and infection is longstanding. Liverpool's Sir Charles Sherrington, the neuroscientist, and Sir Ronald Ross, the malariologist, both won Nobel prizes early in the twentieth century (**Figure 1**). However, even before that, in the middle of the nineteenth century, William Henry Duncan became Liverpool's Medical Officer for Health, the country's first public health doctor; he worked alongside local woman Kitty Wilkinson, who set up Britain's first public wash houses and baths, to control some devastating cholera outbreaks.

CASE 1

Occam's Razor through the Neuroaxis

Benedict D. Michael

History

A 68-year-old lady with a long history of rheumatoid arthritis presented with urinary incontinence. Her arthritis had been quiescent for many years on treatment with methotrexate, leflunomide and low-dose prednisolone. She developed a 4-week history of progressive urinary incontinence and urgency and for 2 weeks had been unaware of the need to defecate and thus had some faecal incontinence. On directed questioning she described saddle anaesthesia and her husband had noticed that her gait was unusual.

There was no history of back pain, radiating pain or trauma. However, she had a history of osteoporosis for which she was receiving alendronic acid and calcium/vitamin D3 supplementation. There was no history of weight loss, night sweats, rash or fever; and no travel history.

Examination

On examination she had reduced power (Medical Research Council power grade 4/5) in all groups of the lower limbs bilaterally, knee jerks were present, but ankle jerks were absent bilaterally. Planters were flexor bilaterally. There was reduced sensation to pinprick in the S2–S4 dermatomes; otherwise sensation was normal. There was faecal loading in the rectum with impaired anal tone.

Upper limb and cranial nerve examinations were normal. She was apyrexial and there were no skin changes. Lower limb pulses were normal.

Initial Differential Diagnosis

- Conus medullaris syndrome
  - Prolapsed disc
  - Spinal stenosis
  - Vascular (malformation or ischaemia)
  - Neoplasia (primary or secondary)
  - Infection (pyogenic and non-pyogenic)
- Other

Results of Initial Investigations

She had a mild, stable, normocytic anaemia, normal white cell and platelet counts, normal renal and liver function and a normal serum calcium level. A magnetic resonance imaging (MRI) scan was performed (**Figure 1.1**).

Progress and Further Investigations

During the first 4 days of her admission, while her lower limb and sphincter disturbance remained stable, she began to develop blurring of vision in the left eye, predominantly in the central field. There were no episodes suggestive of amaurosis fugax and no transient visual obscuration with valsalva manoeuvres or eye movements. The left pupil was slightly more dilated than the right and poorly reactive to light. Visual acuity was normal in the right eye, but in the left it was reduced to 18/6 and slit-lamp examination demonstrated changes (**Figure 1.2**).

Refined Differential Diagnosis

Acute retinal necrosis and conus medullaris syndrome.

- Viral infection
  - Herpes simplex virus
  - Varicella zoster virus
  - Cytomegalovirus
- Treponemal infection
  - Syphilis
- Autoimmune vasculitis

Figure 1.1. T2-weighted sagittal MRI in a 68-year-old lady with rheumatoid arthritis, who presented with urinary incontinence.

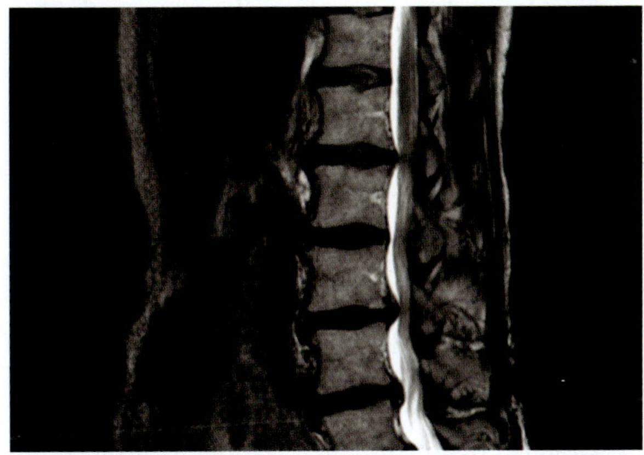

This demonstrates multiple-level intervertebral disk disease. However, cerebrospinal fluid is visible either side of the spinal cord and there is no significant cord compression or oedema; therefore, this is not the cause of the patient's conus medullaris symptoms and signs.

Figure 1.2. Funduscopy findings of the asymptomatic right eye (A) compared with the affected eye (B–F).

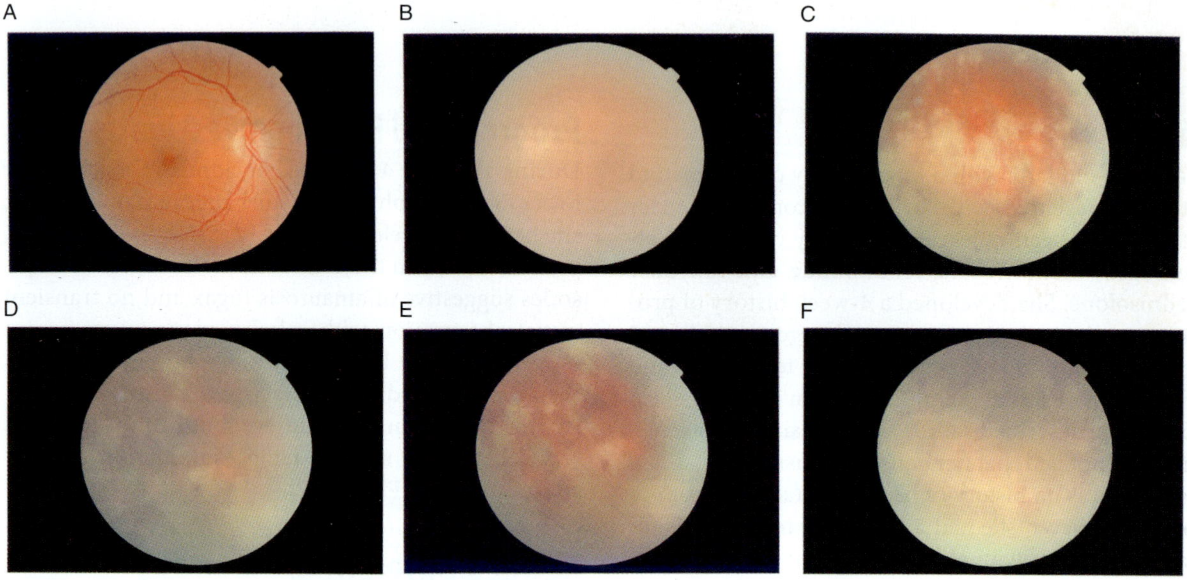

A B C D E F

This shows disk oedema and acute retinal necrosis in the left eye.

Definitive Investigation Results

She had a lumbar puncture (LP), which demonstrated an opening pressure of 16 cm H_2O of cerebrospinal fluid (CSF), white cell count (WCC) 16 per mm^3 (lymphocyte predominance), red cell count (RCC) 2 per mm^3, protein 0.61 g/l and glucose ratio 69%.* Microscopy, Gram stain and culture were negative. Polymerase chain reaction (PCR) of the CSF for herpes simplex virus and cytomegalovirus were negative, but PCR for varicella zoster virus (VZV) was positive.

She also underwent a tap of the vitreous fluid of the left eye and PCR analysis of this was also positive for VZV.

Diagnosis

Varicella zoster virus retinitis and conus medullaris infection.

Management and Outcome

Aciclovir was commenced under the advice of the regional virology unit. Her HIV antibody and antigen tests were both negative.

Despite treatment, her vision continued to deteriorate. Therefore, she was changed to intravenous ganciclovir and intraocular foscarnet. In addition, her rheumatological drugs were withheld because of the concern that immunosuppression had caused the VZV reactivation. The retinal necrosis gradually improved over a couple of weeks and her gait returned to normal. However, her vision remained impaired, she continued to have abnormal perianal sensation, and she remained under the care of the community continence team, requiring intermittent self-catheterisation. At follow up, her rheumatoid arthritis remained under control, requiring only intermittent pain relief with diclofenac.

Prevention

Patients on long-term immunosuppressive therapies are at increased risk of reactivation of latent viruses, particularly neurotropic viruses such as herpes viruses. In the USA, vaccination is given against VZV during childhood. However, because it is a live attenuated vaccine its use in people with immunocompromise is not straightforward. It is used in those with no evidence of pre-existing immunity against VZV under some circumstances.

Discussion

VZV (**Figure 1.3**) is an alpha herpes virus that can infect any part of the neuraxis. Primary infection with VZV causes chicken pox (varicella) in children. The virus then becomes latent in the nervous system,

* Reference ranges are given in Appendix B (pp. 297–300).

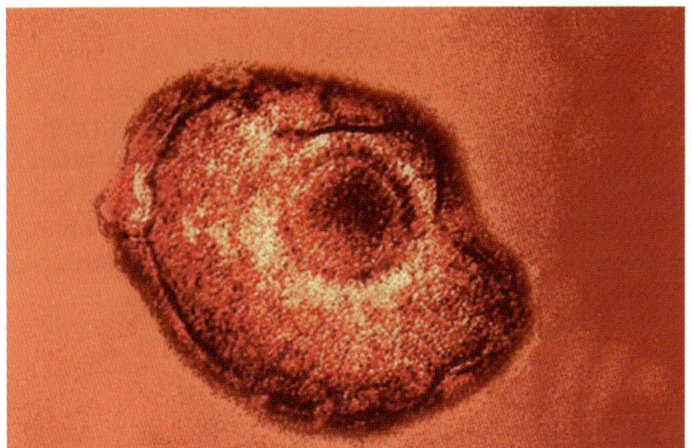

Figure 1.3. Electron micrograph of varicella zoster virus. (Photo courtesy of Cavallini James/BSIP)

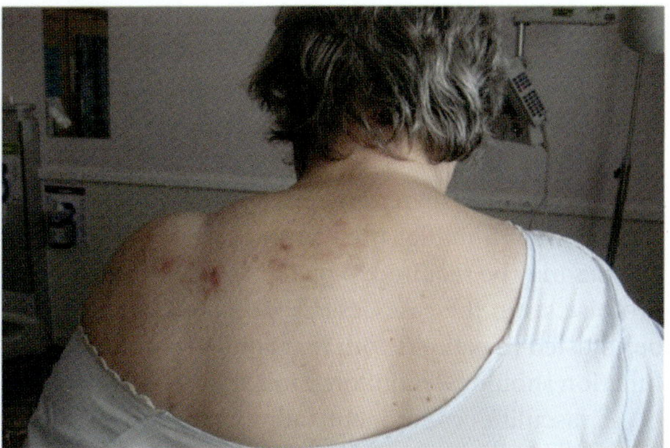

Figure 1.4. A different patient with a dermatomal vesicular eruption of varicella zoster virus.

but can reactivate years later to cause the dermatomal rash that characterises zoster (shingles; **Figure 1.4**). Following primary infection, VZV can cause a primarily immune-mediated, usually self-limiting demyelinating cerebellitis [1], or an encephalitis. There is a wide range of neurological syndromes associated with VZV reactivation (**Table 1.1**). They appear to be primarily caused by immune-mediated reactions to the virus, rather than viral replication itself.

In the case described here, VZV caused disease in the optic nerve and the conus medullaris. The virus accounts for around one-third of all viral central nervous system (CNS) infections. It is the second most commonly identified sporadic cause of encephalitis after herpes simplex virus type 1 [1–3]. VZV can also cause a vasculopathy, which may involve small or large vessels, or both, and can occur in a segmental or diffuse fashion [1]. This usually presents as an ischaemic stroke. Other vasculopathic complications of VZV include aneurysm development and sub-arachnoid haemorrhage.

Neurological complications of VZV reactivation can occur before, during or after the development of a rash. They may also occur in the absence of the any rash at all, so-called '*Zoster Sine Herpete*', as in the case described here [3]. This underscores the importance of investigating for VZV in patients in whom a viral CNS infection is suspected, even if there is no rash, and especially if they are immunocompromised.

In acute infection, CSF PCR will often be positive, as in the case described here. However, if the presentation is a post-infectious phenomenon, such as cerebellitis, or if testing is delayed due to a sub-acute presentation or the treatment is commenced prior to testing, the PCR may be negative. In such cases the detection of CSF antibodies is useful. However, this titre should be interpreted in the context of the serum antibody level and the CSF:serum albumin ratio [5]. Imaging changes at the grey/white matter interface, which are typically ischaemic although occasionally haemorrhagic, are suggestive of VZV. However, cortical and deep structure changes are also often seen [3]. As in this case, the spinal cord changes on neuroimaging may be subtle or absent (**Figure 1.3**).

Table 1.1 Neurological complications of varicella zoster virus. Reproduced with permission from reference [4].

Complications of acute infection (varicella)
Cerebellitis
Acute encephalitis
Complications of viral reactivation (zoster)
Cranial neuropathies
Ramsay Hunt syndrome
Herpes zoster ophthalmicus
Trigeminal neuronitis
Optic and oculomotor neuropathies/retinitis
Mononeuritis of other cranial nerves
Polyneuritis cranialis
Stroke syndromes
Herpes zoster ophthalmicus with delayed contralateral hemiparesis
Cervical zoster with posterior circulation infarcts
Granulomatous angiitis of the basilar artery
Encephalitis syndromes
Encephalitis
Diffuse small/medium vessel arteritis
Myelitis

Post-infectious VZV cerebellitis, which typically occurs in children, does not require any specific treatment, as the course is usually self-limiting [5]. However, neurological complications of VZV reactivation, as confirmed by PCR detection of the virus, should be treated with intravenous aciclovir. Acute VZV CNS infection is less responsive to aciclovir than herpes simplex virus and therefore some advocate higher doses, such as the 15 mg/kg used in the case [5]. Prolonged courses may be required in patients with immune compromise, as in the case described [2]. The dose should be adjusted in patients with renal impairment and renal function should be monitored in all. If there is evidence of a vasculitic component, adjunctive steroids may be useful [5].

Key Points

- Varicella zoster virus (VZV) can affect both the central and peripheral nervous system.
- Consider VZV infection in patients with a lymphocytic pleocytosis even when a rash is absent.
- VZV antibodies in the CSF should be analysed in the context of serum antibody levels and adjusted for the CSF:serum albumin ratio, to establish intrathecal production.

Looking Back

Although one of the most ancient neurotropic viruses, the discovery that VZV could cause a vasculopathy is a fairly recent discovery; 50 years ago, Cravioto and Faigin described a neurological granulomatous angiitis and 10 years later Rosenblum and Hadfield found this to be due to VZV in patients with lymphosarcoma [6,7]. VZV causing retinal vascular disease was only identified in the 1980s [8].

Did You Know?

Varicella and zoster were initially described as two distinct skin conditions. In the early twentieth century physicians began to realise that children often developed chickenpox soon after their parents had suffered shingles, and eventually they were shown to be caused by the same virus, hence the name varicella zoster virus.

References

1. Hausler M, Schaade L, Schaade L, et al. Encephalitis related to primary varicella-zoster virus infection in immunocompetent children. J Neurol Sci 2002;**195**:111e6.
2. De La Blanchardiere A, Rozenberg F, Caumes E, et al. Neurological complications of varicella-zoster virus infection in adults with human immuno-deficiency virus infection. Scand J Infect Dis 2000;**32**:263e9.
3. Gilden DH, Kleinschmidt-DeMasters BK, LaGuardia JJ, Mahalingam R, Cohrs RJ. Neurologic complications of the reactivation of varicella-zoster virus. N Engl J Med 2000;**342**:635e45.
4. Solomon T. Encephalitis, and infectious encephalopathies. In: Donaghy M, editor. *Brain's Diseases of the Nervous System*. 12th ed. Oxford: Oxford University Press; 2009: 1355–428.
5. Solomon T, Michael BD, Smith PE, et al. Management of suspected viral encephalitis in adults: Association of British Neurologists and British Infection Association National Guideline. J Infect 2012;**64**:347–73.
6. Cravioto H, Feigin I. Noninfectious granulomatous angiitis with a predilection for the nervous system. Neurology 1959;**9**:599–608.
7. Rosenblum WI, Hadfield MG. Granulomatous angiitis of the nervous system in cases of herpes zoster and lymphosarcoma. Neurology 1972;**22**:348–54.
8. Hall S, Carlin L, Roach ES, McLean WT Jr. Herpes zoster and central retinal artery occlusion. Ann Neurol 1983;**13**:217–18.

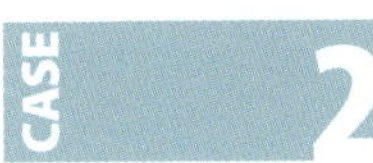

Between the Head and the Heart

Theresa Cole

History

A 2-year-old girl presented with a 3-week history of unsteadiness on her feet and concerns over her vision. Her parents explained she appeared to be turning her head to the left in order to see things that were directly in front of her. She had been vomiting intermittently over the preceding 5 weeks. There was no history of fever.

She had a past medical history of complex congenital heart disease requiring surgery at 4 days of age, but she still had a residual ventricular septal defect and pulmonary artery band *in situ*. Two months prior to admission she had a fever and was found to have a raised C-reactive protein (CRP) with no obvious cause. She had been treated with cefotaxime for 10 days and the fever settled. Two weeks prior to admission she was found to have a reduction in her oxygen saturation, which had fallen to 75–80% on air. Therefore, she underwent a cardiac assessment including an echocardiogram and cardiac catheterisation, although this did not show any new changes. She had one sibling who was fit and well and there was no other family history of note. There was no history of recent foreign travel.

Examination

On examination the child was miserable and was noted to be slightly tilting her head to the right throughout most of the examination. She had normal eye movements. Formal neurological examination was not possible, due to limited cooperation, but she walked with a normal gait. Her head circumference was 47 cm (50th centile). She was tachycardic with a heart rate of 140 beats per minute. Cardiovascular examination revealed a grade 3 systolic murmur. Systemic examination was otherwise unremarkable, in particular she was apyrexial.

Initial Differential Diagnosis

At the time it was felt that the ataxia may be explained by para- or post-infectious cause, such as cerebellitis.

However, given the suggestion of visual field disturbance a more extensive process was considered, such as a space-occupying lesion, which may have been infectious (e.g. a brain abscess) or neoplastic.

Results of Initial Investigations

Full blood count demonstrated a slight neutrophilia (neutrophil count 12.3×10^9/l), but was otherwise normal. CRP was mildly elevated at 35 mg/l.

A computer tomography (CT) head was performed (**Figure 2.1A** and **2.1B**) and subsequently a magnetic resonance imaging (MRI) brain scan was performed (**Figure 2.2**).

Results of Definitive Investigations

Due to uncertainty about whether this was a cystic malignant mass or an abscess, the patient underwent an initial burrhole aspiration of one of the lobules of the cyst.

This aspirated frank pus confirming the lesion was an abscess.

Diagnosis

Multi-loculated right-sided fronto-temporal–parietal brain abscess, presumed to be secondary to preceding infective endocarditis.

Management and Outcome

The neurosurgeons proceeded immediately to perform a craniotomy and aspiration of the abscess cavities. Two hundred millilitres of pus were drained. Intravenous (IV) cefotaxime and metronidazole were commenced. A repeat echocardiogram demonstrated no valve vegetations.

The following day she underwent a further MRI and was then transferred to theatre for insertion of an external ventricular drain and aspiration of further pus from the abscess cavities.

The child had a stormy post-operative course requiring a further craniotomy and drainage. She developed a left hemiplegia and also required a ventricular–peritoneal shunt insertion for hydrocephalus. She completed 8 weeks of intravenous antibiotics in total and a period of neurorehabilitation. At follow up, she has residual left-sided visual field loss, some difficulties with speech and a left hemiplegia.

Figure 2.1. Axial images from a non-contrast CT brain scan of a 2-year-old child presenting with ataxia and visual field loss.

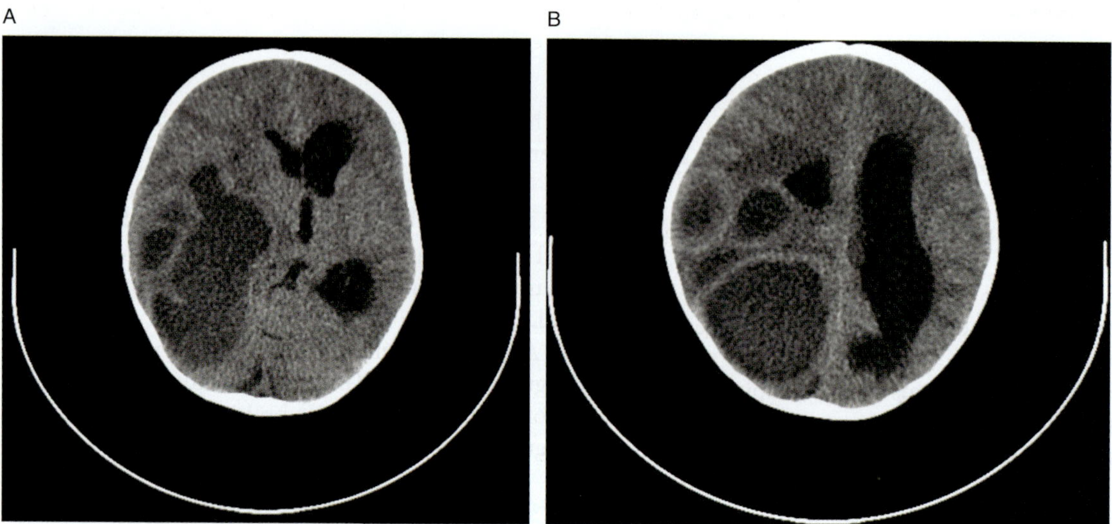

This shows an extensive multi-loculated lesion in the right hemisphere with midline shift and compression of the lateral ventricle.

Figure 2.2. Axial T2-weighted MRI from the same patient. This demonstrates more clearly the multi-loculated nature of the large lesion with surrounding oedema.

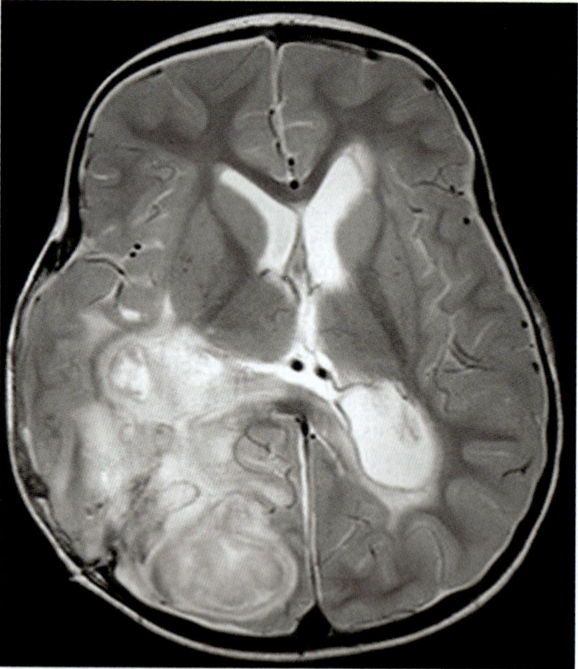

Figure 2.3. Post-mortem coronal brain slice of a patient who died from a brain abscess .

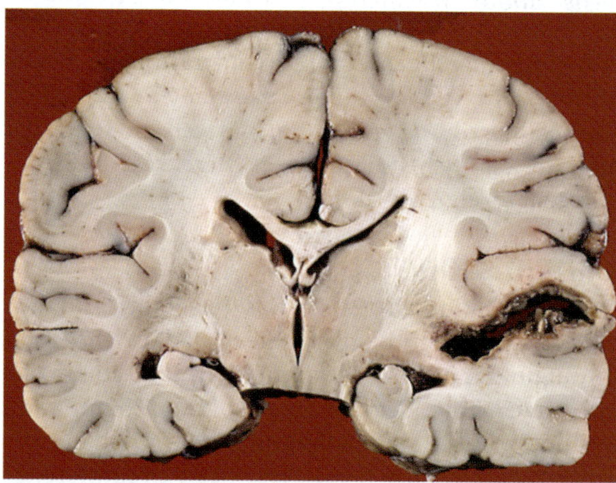

This demonstrates a left temporal brain abscess (http://neuropathology-web.org/chapter5/chapter5aSuppurative.html).

Discussion

Brain abscesses are uncommon CNS infections in childhood in the UK. They occur throughout the whole paediatric age range as well as in adults. They result from either haematogenous or direct spread of a pathogen from a contiguous site. They can also occur following penetrating head trauma or neurosurgery [1]. Predisposing factors for developing brain abscesses include congenital heart disease, immunocompromise and infections in contiguous sites, particularly the ears and sinuses [2–5]. Congenital heart disease has become a much less common predisposing factor over recent years [5]. In up to 30% of cases no predisposing factor is identified [4].

Common causative organisms are aerobic and anaerobic streptococci and staphylococci. Mixed organisms are found in many cases. Certain predisposing factors are associated with the more unusual organisms, for example, *Citrobacter* and *Enterobacter* in neonates, *Streptococcus viridians* in children with congenital heart disease and fungi in the immunocompromised [5].

The classical triad of fever, headache and vomiting occurs in 60–70% of patients at presentation [2,4]. However, the absence of fever does not rule out an abscess. In the neonate the only signs may be irritability and increasing head circumference. Altered conscious level is a common sign and focal neurological deficits relate to the location of the abscess [2,6].

Early surgical intervention is recommended to achieve the best outcome. Antibiotics are essential; as in this case a third-generation cephalosporin and metronidazole are often used as first-line therapy [3,7,8], with or without a penicillin for staphylococcal cover [1], or vancomycin if there are any concerns about methicillin-resistant *Staphylococcus aureus* [4,9]. However, antibiotic choice should be directed by local microbiological protocols, dependent on the patient's immune status and predisposing risk factors, and subsequently reviewed in light of the findings of microscopy, culture and sensitivity of aspirated pus.

Historically, long courses of IV antibiotics have been used. However, recent data have demonstrated that a good outcome may be possible with initial IV therapy but then a switch to oral agents [10], although in complicated cases, prolonged IV treatment may be needed followed by a course of oral antibiotics [1,3].

In 2000 the *Infection in Neurosurgery* working party of the British Society for Antimicrobial Chemotherapy published guidelines for the treatment of brain abscesses [11]. They recommended 4–6 weeks of treatment for abscesses that had been drained and 6–8 weeks (or longer) for those that were not drained. However, they also stated that shorter courses might be adequate for some. For example, 3–4 weeks of parenteral therapy might be adequate for those that had the abscess excised, 4–6 weeks for those that had the lesion aspirated and a minimum of 4 weeks for those that did not have surgical intervention. They recommended monitoring the CRP to assess the response to treatment rather than imaging, as radiological findings can lag behind the clinical response. The guidelines also recommended that, in addition to the suggested time frames above, conversion from IV to oral antibiotics should only be considered once the CRP had begun to fall.

Historically, brain abscesses had high levels of mortality (**Figure 2.3**). However, this has decreased over time and in recent series many of the patients that did not survive had serious underlying medical comorbidities [5]. Recent UK data have demonstrated an overall mortality of 6% with a 33% mortality in immunocompromised patients [10]. Neurological sequelae continue to be problematic, with approximately a third having ongoing problems [2,10]. Overall, mortality in adults has been reported as between 17% and 32%, and is reduced by early diagnosis and antimicrobial treatment, in addition to neurosurgical intervention, particularly for abscesses more than 2 cm in diameter [12].

Key Points

- Brain abscess are a rare but clinically significant infection in children and adults.
- Fever, vomiting and headache are the classical symptoms, although the fever may preceed presentation, as in this case.
- Surgical drainage of the abscess is usually required.
- Long courses of antibiotics are needed.
- There has been a move in recent years to complete antibiotic therapy with oral agents in patients who are responding well after a minimum period of IV treatment.

Looking Back

One of the first descriptions of successful surgery for a brain abscess was reported in 1872 by an American army surgeon, Dr J. F. Weeds. The patient had received a gunshot to the front of the head and developed meningitis, from which he recovered. However, approximately 10 days later he developed papilloedema, focal seizures and hemiparesis. The surgeon trephined the area of the gunshot, 'plunged his knife in the cerebral substance' and dark green pus flowed from the wound. Surprisingly, the soldier survived [13]!

Did You Know?

Most medics know the basic story of Phineas Gage, the American railroad worker whose frontal lobe was damaged by an explosive accident with a large iron rod. You may not know that after the accident he very nearly died from a cerebral abscess. Fortunately the doctor looking after him was one of the few at that time who had experience of draining cerebral abscesses. He laid open the wound and *"immediately there were discharged eight ounces of ill-conditioned pus, with blood, and excessively fetid."* Gage survived the procedure and began touring around New England like a living exhibit. He lived for nearly 12 years with the disinhibited personality for which he is remembered.

References

1. Saez-Llorens X. Brain abscess in children. Semin Pediatr Infect Dis 2003;**14**:108–14.
2. Leotta N, Chaseling R, Duncan G, Isaacs D. Intracranial suppuration. J Paediatr Child Health 2005;**41**:508–12.
3. Sheehan JP, Jane Jr JA, Ray DK, Goodkin HP. Brain abscess in children. Neurosurg Focus 2008;**24**:1–5.
4. Yogev R, Bar-Meir M. Management of brain abscesses in children. Pediatr Infect Dis J 2004;**23**:157–9.
5. Goodkin HP, Harper MB, Pomeroy SL. Intracerebral abscess in children: historical trends at Children's Hospital in Boston. Pediatrics 2004;**113**:1765–70.
6. Sharma R, Mohandas K, Cooke RPD. Intracranial abscesses: changes in epidemiology and management over five decades in Merseyside. Infection 2009;**37**:39–43.
7. Jansson AK, Enblad P, Sjolin J. Efficacy and safety of cefotaxime in combination with metronidazole for empirical treatment of brain abscesses in clinical practice: a retrospective study of 66 consecutive cases. Eur J Clin Microbiol Infect Dis 2004;**23**:7–14.
8. Bernardini GL. Diagnosis and management of brain abscess and subdural empyema. Curr Neurol Neurosci Rep 2004;**4**:448–56.
9. Bockova J, Rigamonti D. Intracranial empyema. Pediatr Infect Dis J 2000;**19**:735–7.
10. Felsenstein S, Williams B, Shingadia D, et al. Clinical and microbiologic features guiding treatment recommendations for brain abscesses in children. Pediatr Infect Dis J 2013;**32**:129–35.
11. de Louvois J, Brown EM, Bayston R, Lees PD, Pople IK. The rational use of antibiotics in the treatment of brain abscess: report by the 'Infection in Neurosurgery' working party of the British Society for Antimicrobial Chemotherapy. Br J Neurosurg 2000;**14**:525–30.
12. Muzumdar D, Jhawar S, Goel A. Brain abscess: an overview. Int J Surgery 2011:**9**;136–44.
13. Canale DJ. William Macewen and the treatment of brain abscesses: revisited after one hundred years. J Neurosurg 1996;**84**:133–42.

CASE 3 Thinking Laterally

Baba Aji

History

A 67-year-old woman with a previous history of migraine presented with a 4-day history of new-onset headache, dizziness and mild neck stiffness, one week after returning from Portugal. She was admitted to hospital and 2 days later she deteriorated with worsening headache, fever, increasing drowsiness and confusion. On day 3 of admission she developed numbness of the left jaw, unsteadiness and an inability to walk, which progressively worsened over 24 hours.

Examination

On examination she was febrile with confusion and neck stiffness. By day 2 of admission she had developed ataxia, dysarthria and left-sided facial hypoaesthesia and tongue deviation to the left with right-sided hemi-sensory loss of the arms, trunk, abdomen and leg.

Initial Differential Diagnosis

The presentation of a febrile illness, drowsiness and neck stiffness was suggestive of an acute central nervous system infection and clinically she had signs reflecting a left lateral medullary syndrome. The differential diagnosis included:

- meningoencephalitis, with brainstem involvement (rhombencephalitis)
  - likely viral infection
  - less likely parenchymal infection due to bacteria or mycobacteria

Or

- meningitis with a secondary vascular event due to
  - bacterial infection
  - tuberculosis
  - or possibly malignant meningitis.

Results of Initial Investigations

She had mild polymorphonuclear leucocytosis, normal red cell and platelet counts, and normal renal and liver function tests. A computer tomography brain scan was reported as normal. Lumbar puncture revealed a cerebrospinal fluid (CSF) white cell count of 350 cells/ml, of which 60% were lymphocytes. The CSF glucose was 0.3 mmol/l with a matched blood glucose of 5.0 mmol/l and the protein was 2.3 g/l.

Progress and Further Investigations

She was treated with fluid resuscitation, antibiotics (cefotaxime), antiviral (aciclovir), and antipyretic (IV paracetamol) drugs, and a short course of dexamethasone. There was no improvement over the following 48 hours and she continued to be drowsy. She had a magnetic resonance imaging (MRI) scan (**Figure 3.1**).

Definitive Investigation Result

The CSF culture grew highly motile Gram-positive rods within 24 hours, which were later confirmed to be *Listeria monocytogenes*.

Diagnosis

Rhomboencephalitis (brainstem encephalitis) caused by *Listeria monocytogenes*.

Figure 3.1. MRI scan similar to that performed in a patient presenting with fever, drowsiness and meningism, who was found to have hypoaesthesia of the face on the left and of the rest of the body on the right along with a left-sided tongue deviation.

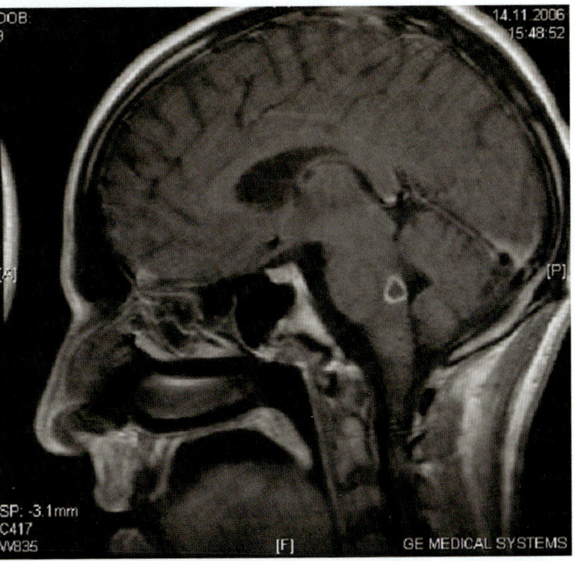

The T1-weighted axial MRI scan shows ring-enhancing brainstem lesions with gadolinium enhancement. With permission from [1].

Management and Outcome

When the Gram-positive rods were grown in the CSF, her antibiotics were promptly changed to IV ampicillin and gentamycin. She gradually started improving. Over the next few days her fever settled, her headache subsided, and both tongue movement and gait improved. A repeat MRI scan showed reduction in oedema and enhancement. She continued on ampicillin 2 g 4-hourly for 6 weeks. Her symptoms resolved completely apart from residual right-sided numbness. A repeat MRI at 4 months showed almost complete resolution of the abnormalities.

Discussion

Listeria monocytogenes (**Figure 3.2**) is an anaerobic Gram-positive bacillus which causes sporadic food-borne outbreaks and life-threatening infections primarily in immunocompromised hosts, neonates, pregnant women, or those over 60 [2–5]. Therefore, the British Infection Society and Association of British Neurologist guidelines recommend empirical IV amoxycillin is included in the initial treatment of suspected bacterial meningitis for anyone over 60 years [5]. If the guidelines had been followed for this patient, her empirical antibiotic treatment would have covered listeria from admission, because of her age. Listeria can also infect otherwise healthy adults. Infection can cause meningitis, meningoencephalitis or rhombencephalitis. There is a bimodal distribution of age at presentation. Patients typically complain of headache, fever and non-specific neurologic symptoms during the prodromal week. Patients may then develop symptoms and signs of brainstem involvement such as multiple cranial neuropathies, cerebellar ataxia and long-tract motor and sensory deficits. Some may develop cardiovascular and/or respiratory instability as well.

The CSF in listeria infection typically has a leucocytosis up to 1000 cells/mm^3, with lymphocytic predominance, although a predominance of polymorphonuclear cells is also sometimes seen. The protein is usually raised, and the CSF:plasma glucose ratio is often low, as it was in this patient. Therefore, think of listeria if the initial routine CSF results resemble those of tuberculosis (lymphocyte predominance, low glucose ratio) but the history is acute, especially in at-risk groups. The organism grows easily in culture, often within 24 hours, and being motile can be detected with a motility test. The MRI often shows changes of the ponto-medullary junction and cerebellum (**Figure 3.1**) [2].

Although relatively rare, listeriosis has an important impact in public health because of its highest morbidity and mortality among food-borne infections [6].

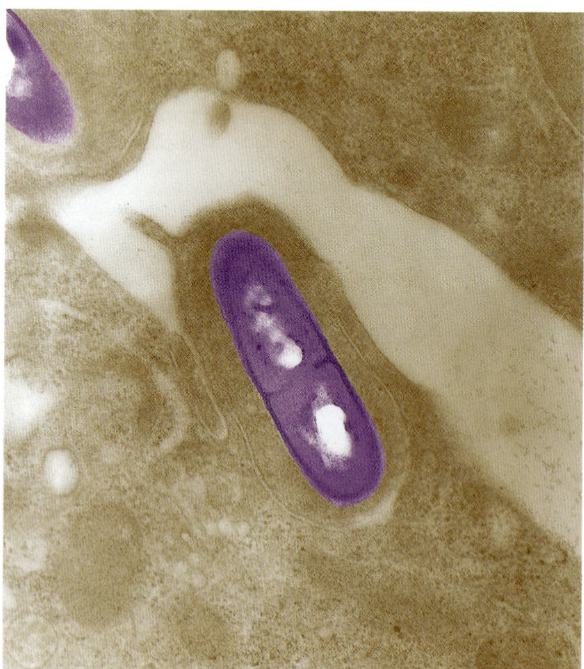

Figure 3.2. A transmission electron microscopic image of a listeria bacterium. Reproduced with permission from www.cdc.gov/listeria/

Key Points

- Listeria causes rhombencephalitis especially in the immunocompromised, elderly, neonates or pregnant women.
- Think of listeria in acute-onset progressive cranial neuropathies following headache and fever, or if the spinal fluid is reminiscent of tuberculosis but the presentation is acute.
- Current national UK guidelines recommend amoxicillin (or co-trimoxazole if the patient is allergic) for patients over 60 years with a bacterial meningitis picture, and in the immunocompromised, because cephalosporins do not give sufficient cover.

Looking Back

Listeria meningoencephalitis was first described in 1934 and rhombencephalitis was first described by Eck in 1957 [7,8].

Did You Know

Listeria was discovered by James Hunter Harvie Pirie, who named the organism in honour of the English pioneer of sterile surgery, Joseph Lister, even though Lister had no role in its discovery.

References

1. Kayaaslan BU, Akinci E, Bilen S, et al. Listerial rhombencephalitis in an immunocompetent young adult. Int J Infect Dis 2009;**13**:e65–7.
2. Alper G, Knepper L, Knaal E. MR findings in Listeria rhombencephalitis. Am J Neuroradiol 1996;**17**:593–6.
3. Mylonakis E, Hohmann EL, Calderwood SB. Central nervous system infection with *Listeria monocytogenes* 33 years' experience at a general hospital and review of 776 episodes from the literature. Medicine (Baltimore) 1998;**77**:313–36.
4. Abbs A, Nandakumar TP, Bose P, Mooraby D. Listeria rhombencephalitis. Pract Neurol 2012;**12**:131–2.
5. McGill F, Heyderman RS, Michael BD, et al. The UK joint specialist societies guideline on the diagnosis and management of acute meningitis and meningococcal sepsis in immunocompetent adults. J Infect 2016;**72**:405–38.
6. Oeuermann A, Zurbriggen A, Vanderelde M. Rhombencephalitis caused by *Listeria monocytogenes* in humans and ruminants: a zoonosis on the rise? Interdisc Perspect Infect Dis 2010;**632513**:22.
7. Burn CG. Unidentified Gram-positive bacillus associated with meningoencephalitis. Proc Soc Exper Biol Med 1934;**31**:1095–7.
8. Eck H. Encephalomyelitis listeriaca apostematosa. Schweiz Med Wochenschr 1957;**87**:210–14.

CASE 4

No Laughing Matter

Besa Ziso

History

A 39-year-old male presented with a 3-week history of productive cough, fever, drenching night sweats and generalised malaise. For the 5 days before admission he also reported numbness and weakness affecting his lower limbs. There was paraesthesia and numbness affecting his toes with associated weakness and myalgia in the lower limbs. It started gradually, but then worsened rapidly over the next few days. He felt that balance and walking were both impaired.

On direct questioning he denied any past history of back pain, sphincter disturbance, difficulties with speech or swallowing, or weight loss.

There was no history of foreign travel or recent vaccinations. The patient had a past history of syphilis and had received treatment 5 years earlier.

Examination

On examination he was apyrexial. Tone was reduced in the lower limbs with Medical Research Council power grade 3+/5 weakness and decreased deep tendon reflexes. Plantar reflexes were flexor. Sensory examination to pinprick and fine touch was normal. Vibration was impaired to the ankles bilaterally, but joint position sensation was normal. Examination of the cranial nerves and upper limbs was normal.

Initial Differential Diagnosis

Although there is a long differential for acute flaccid paralysis (**Table 4.1**), the symmetrical onset of symptoms which progressed up the lower limbs made Guillain–Barré syndrome the most likely.

Table 4.1. Differential diagnosis of acute flaccid paralysis (arranged anatomically).

- Spinal cord
  - Acute anterior poliomyelitis
  - Acute transverse myelitis
- Peripheral nerve disorders
  - Guillain–Barré syndromes
  - Diphtheritic neuropathy
  - Heavy metal poisoning
  - Acute intermittent porphyria
  - Vasculitic neuropathy
- Disorders of neuromuscular junction
  - Myasthenia gravis
  - Lambert–Eaton syndrome
  - Botulism
- Disorders of muscle
  - Inflammatory myopathy
  - Acute rhabdomyolysis
  - Trichinosis
  - Hypokalaemic/hyperkalaemic periodic paralyses

Results of Initial Investigations

Full blood count, renal, liver function and creatine kinase were all normal. C-reactive protein was slightly raised at 35 mg/l. Electrocardiogram (ECG) showed sinus rhythm with a rate of 86 beats per minute. Chest X-ray was normal.

A lumbar puncture was carried out which showed an opening pressure of 18 cm H_2O cerebrospinal fluid (CSF), red cell count 18/mm^3, white cell count of 26/mm^3 (95% lymphocytes), protein 0.72 g/l, glucose 3.4 mmol/l, with a serum glucose of 5.4 mmol/l. No organisms were seen and Gram stain and polymerase chain reaction for herpes simplex virus, varicella zoster virus and enterovirus were negative.

A magnetic resonance imaging scan of the brain and whole spine were also normal.

Progress and Further Investigations

During the first 2 days of admission the weakness progressed. The patient developed 4/5 weakness affecting his upper limbs, with reduced reflexes. Sensory examination remained unchanged. Lower limb power worsened to 2/5 proximally and 3/5 distally. He also developed bilateral lower motor neuron VII cranial nerve palsies. Eye movements were normal and there was no other cranial nerve deficit. The patient also complained of some shortness of breath. He was noted to have postural hypotension with a blood pressure of 140/80 mmHg lying dropping to 110/70 mmHg on standing.

Refined Differential Diagnosis

This progression of the weakness, with associated autonomic failure, made Guillain–Barré syndrome even more likely. The severe progression suggested it might be the acute motor axonal neuropathy form, rather than the more common acute inflammatory demyelinating polyneuropathy. However, the CSF pleocytosis was unusual for Guillain–Barré syndrome. Vasculitis neuropathy and porphyric neuropathy remained possible alternative diagnoses.

Results of Definitive Investigations

Because of the unusual features described above, particularly the CSF pleocytosis, the patient went on to have an HIV antibody test, which was positive. His HIV viral load was more than 100,000 copies/ml and CD4 count was 408 cells/mm^3.

Nerve conduction studies showed prolonged distal and F-wave latencies and reduced conduction velocities consistent with a generalised demyelinating neuropathy, as seen in Guillain–Barré syndrome.

Diagnosis

HIV-associated Guillain–Barré syndrome.

Management and Outcome

The patient was started on intravenous immunoglobulin 0.4 g/kg/day for 5 days. Careful monitoring of his forced vital capacity was carried out on the ward, and intensive care was not needed. He made a slow recovery and was transferred to a local rehabilitation unit.

Prevention

HIV in adults is prevented by avoiding unprotected sexual intercourse with someone who is infected, and by not sharing needles with people who may be infected.

Discussion

Guillain–Barré syndrome is a rare complication of HIV infection, first described in 1985. It most often occurs as part of a seroconversion illness, i.e. an illness which occurs in people newly infected with HIV as they start to develop antibodies to the infection, or 'seroconvert' [1–3]. This is most likely what happened in the patient described here, whose seroconversion illness included fever, sweats and malaise, and then Guillain–Barré syndrome. The fact that HIV virus load was high but CD4 count had not yet fallen is the clue that this is a seroconversion illness. Guillain–Barré syndrome is also sometimes seen in patients with much more advanced HIV disease, who have much lower CD4 counts if they are not on treatment.

Guillain–Barré syndrome is one of a range of neurological disorders, which can be part of a patient's seroconversion illness to HIV, including meningoencephalitis and myelitis. Several other neurological conditions, such as stroke and dementia, may be the presenting complaint for patients with unknown underlying HIV, but in them it is usually a sign of more advanced HIV disease. Hence any patient with an unexplained neurological problem should be tested for HIV.

The pathogenesis of Guillain–Barré syndrome in HIV is incompletely understood. Possible mechanisms include direct HIV neurotoxicity or autoimmunity [1,4,5]. The pathological picture of Guillain–Barré syndrome is that of multifocal mononuclear cell infiltration throughout the peripheral nervous system (**Figure 4.1**). The distribution of inflammation corresponds to the clinical deficit. Patients can present with pain, numbness, paraesthesia or weakness in the limbs. Weakness may be proximal, distal or a combination of both. Facial nerves and, less commonly, ocular and bulbar involvement are seen. Autonomic involvement has been described with sinus bradycardia, tachycardia, hypotension or hypertension and urinary retention. Around 30% of patients with Guillain–Barré syndrome may require ventilatory support, due to

Figure 4.1. Nerve fibre from patient with acute inflammatory demyelinating polyneuropathy.

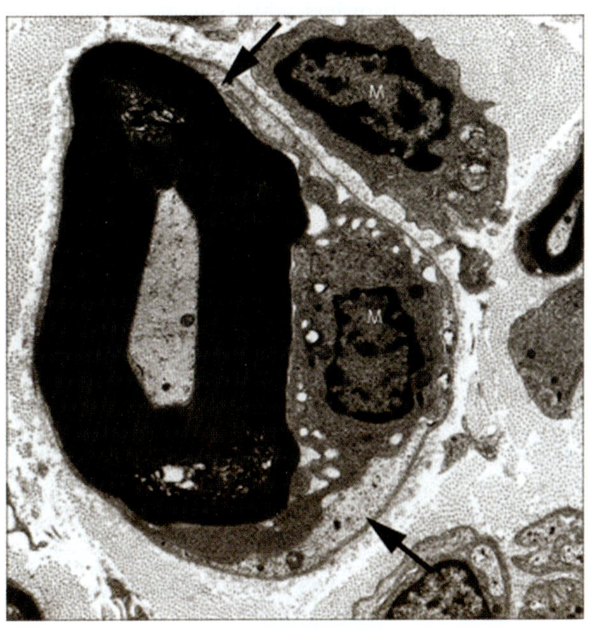

Electron micrograph shows a macrophage (M) has invaded Schwann cell basement membrane and stripped the axonal Schwann cell cytoplasm (arrows). Reproduced from Hughes et al. [6] with permission of Elsevier.

respiratory muscle weakness. Therefore, monitoring of respiratory function through forced vital capacity measurement is essential [6,7].

Raised CSF protein is seen in the majority of patients with Guillain–Barré syndrome and reflects the widespread inflammation of the nerve roots. However, CSF protein can be normal early in the course of the illness [6,8]. CSF pleocytosis is unusual in Guillain–Barré syndrome and may suggest it is due to HIV infection, other infections such as Lyme disease, or malignancy. However, lack of pleocytosis does not exclude HIV infection and so should be looked for in all patients with Guillain–Barré syndrome.

Treatment for Guillain–Barré syndrome includes plasma exchange and IVIG. Treatment with plasma exchange is usually most beneficial when given during the first 4 weeks of illness, with the greater benefit the earlier it is given. The usual regime is the exchange of five plasma volumes over the course of 2 weeks. Corticosteroids are ineffective in the treatment of Guillain–Barré syndrome [9].

Key Points

- CSF pleocytosis is unusual in Guillain–Barré syndrome and other causes such as HIV, other infections and malignancy should be considered.
- Guillain–Barré syndrome is one of a range of neurological disorders, which can be part of a patient's seroconversion illness to HIV.
- Other neurological conditions, such as stroke and dementia, may be the presenting complaint for patients with unknown underlying HIV. Hence, all patients with unexplained neurological problems should be tested for HIV.

Looking Back

First described in 1834 by Wardrop and Oliver, the clinical features were also described in Landry's report of 1859 as an acute, ascending motor paralysis seen among serfs. However, it was not until 1916 that Guillain, Barré and Strohl described the key CSF abnormality of an elevated protein with normal cell count 'albuminocytological dissociation' and the condition acquired its current name.

Did You Know?

Joseph Heller, author of *Catch-22*, was diagnosed with Guillain–Barré syndrome in 1981 and wrote a book about his illness and recovery entitled *No Laughing Matter.*

References

1. Brannagan TH, Zhou Y. HIV-associated Guillan–Barré syndrome. J Neurol Sci 2003;**208**:39–42.
2. Qureshi, A, Cook A, Mishu HP, Krendel DA. Guillan–Barré syndrome in immunocompromised patients: a report of three patients and review of the literature. Muscle Nerve 1997;**20**:1002–7.
3. Simpson DM, Tagliati M. Neurologic manifestations of HIV infection. Ann Intern Med 1994;**121**:769–85.
4. Parry O, Mielke J, Latif AS, et al. Peripheral neuropathy in individuals with HIV infection in Zimbabwe. Acta Neurol Scand 1997;**96**:218–22.
5. Howlett WP, Vedeler CA, Nyland H, Aarli JA. Guillain–Barré syndrome in northern Tanzania: a comparison of epidemiological and clinical findings with western Norway. Acta Neurol Scand 1996;**93**:44–9.
6. Hughes RAC, Cornblath DR. Guillan–Barré syndrome. Lancet 2005;**366**:1653–66.
7. Schleicher GK, Black A, Mochan A, Richards GA. Effect of human immunodeficiency virus on intensive care unit outcome of patients with Guillan–Barré syndrome. Crit Care Med 2003;**31**:1848–50.
8. Ropper AH. The Guillan–Barré syndrome. N Engl J Med 1992;**326**:1130–6.
9. French Cooperative Group on plasma exchange in Guillain–Barré syndrome. Appropriate number of plasma exchanges in Guillain–Barré syndrome. Ann Neurol 1997;**41**:298–306.

CASE 5

An Expanding Head

Hema Bentur and Rachel Kneen

History

A 14-day-old neonate presented to an Emergency Department with a 2-day history of fever and poor feeding. On the second day of her illness she had a seizure with jerking of all four limbs associated with apnoea. She was the second twin, born prematurely at 34+5 week's gestation after a normal pregnancy. Growth parameters were normal for gestational age. Her mother had a spontaneous onset of labour and a normal vaginal delivery. The infant only required brief resuscitation at birth and neither she nor her twin required an admission to a neonatal unit. She was discharged on day 5 and was feeding and growing well until day 12 of life.

Examination

On examination she was febrile with a temperature of 38.9°C but was in reasonable condition, handled well and had normal tone. Her respiratory rate was 40 breaths per minute with signs of mild respiratory distress. Oxygen saturation was 97% in air. Her heart rate was 145 beats per minute, blood pressure was 60/35 mmHg and the central capillary refill time was 2 seconds. Cardiac and chest auscultation were normal, as was abdominal palpation. Her anterior fontanelle was bulging. There was no rash noted or any signs of local skin infection. She had several infrequent periods of stiffening of all four limbs associated with apnoea, which were considered to be epileptic seizures and so she was treated with phenobarbitone. She required non-invasive positive pressure ventilation for the periods of seizure-related apnoea.

Initial Differential Diagnosis

- Late-onset neonatal sepsis, e.g. Group B streptococcus
- Meningoencephalitis
  - bacterial, e.g. *Escherichia coli*, listeria
  - viral, e.g. herpes simplex virus type 2
- Inborn error of metabolism, e.g. organic acidaemia
- Early infantile epileptic encephalopathy, e.g. Ohtahara syndrome
- Cerebral haemorrhage or venous sinus thrombosis and infarction

Investigations

Initial bloods were all normal except the C-reactive protein which was 146 mg/l.

Cerebrospinal fluid (CSF) examination revealed 569 white blood cells (WBC) cells/mm^3 (90% polymorphs), red blood cells (RBC) 8 cells/mm^3, glucose 0.5 mmol/l (plasma glucose was 4.6 mmol/l, giving a ratio of 10%), protein 2.6 g/l.

A chest X-ray and urinalysis were normal.

Further Progress and Investigations

A diagnosis of probable bacterial meningitis was made and she was treated with intravenous cefotaxime and amoxicillin as per the local neonatal antibiotic policy.

Over the next few days she developed an increasing head circumference. She also remained irritable with intermittent vomiting. A cranial ultrasound showed a grade 4 intraventricular haemorrhage and a computer tomography (CT) scan was taken shortly afterwards (**Figure 5.1**). She was transferred to a tertiary centre for neurosurgical intervention. An external ventricular drain was inserted on day 7. CSF examination revealed

Figure 5.1. Axial CT head of neonate with poor feeding, fever and seizures.

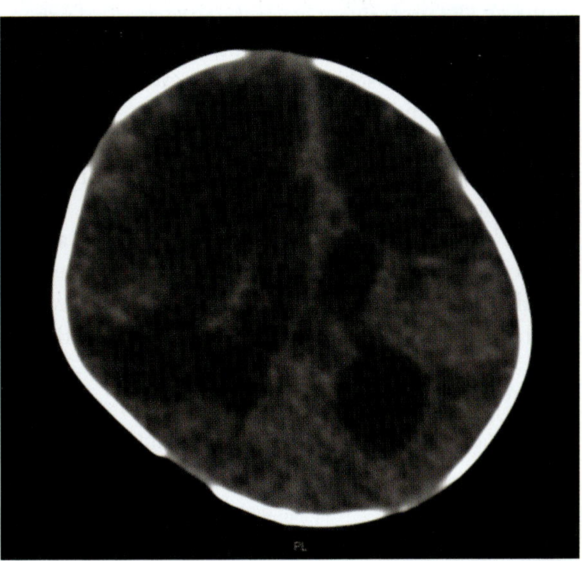

This shows multiple hypodense lesions bilaterally with moderate ventriculomegaly and mass effect from the right with midline shift, consistent with multiple brain abscesses.

Figure 5.2. T2-weighted axial and coronal view MRI of the same patient.

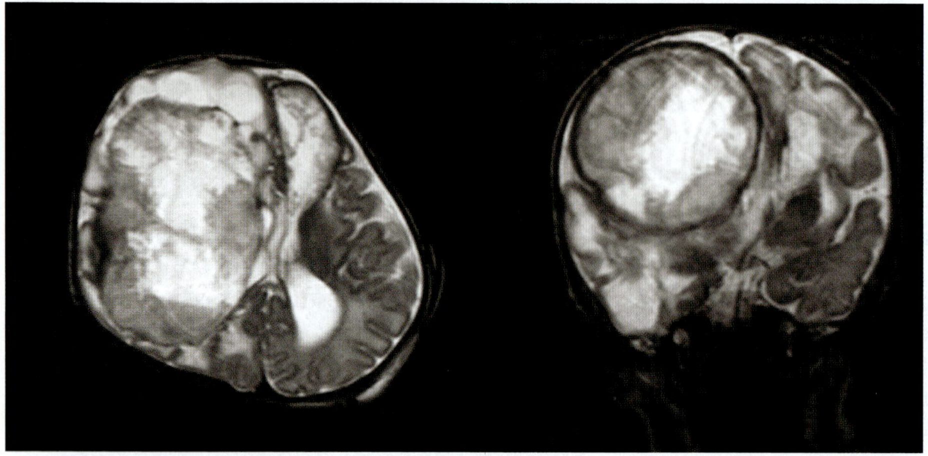

This demonstrates a large right-sided abscess with multiple small fluid-filled cysts surrounding the lesion (satellite abscesses or cystic encephalomalacia) and a smaller abscess in the left frontal lobe.

7444 WBC cells/mm^3 (95% polymorphs). The culture of the initial CSF was negative but the second sample grew *Citrobacter koseri*; this was sensitive to cefotaxime, aminoglycosides, ciprofloxacillin and meropenem. Magnetic resonance imaging was performed on day 14 of the illness (**Figure 5.2**).

Subsequent Management

The intravenous antibiotics were changed to cefotaxime and ciprofloxacillin and then meropenem and ciprofloxacillin, after *Citrobacter koseri* had been cultured. She underwent several neurosurgical procedures to drain the abscesses through external ventricular drains. She subsequently had surgical excision of the abscesses, and insertion of a ventriculo-peritoneal shunt for obstructive hydrocephalus. After 8 weeks of intravenous antibiotics she was given oral ciprofloxacillin for a further 6 weeks.

She subsequently developed a four-limb asymmetrical quadriplegic cerebral palsy. Follow-up at 20 months of age revealed a significant global developmental delay. She also developed a multifocal epilepsy.

Diagnosis

Meningoencephalitis, caused by *Citrobacter koseri*.

Discussion

Citrobacter koseri is an uncommon cause of fulminant central nervous system (CNS) infection in neonates. Affected infants may appear surprisingly well initially; therefore, a high index of suspicion and early imaging are needed to detect brain abscesses.

Citrobacter is a Gram-negative bacillus of the family Enterobacteriaceae. The genus *Citrobacter* consists of three species, namely *C. freundii, C. amalonaticus* and *C. koseri* [1,2]. It may exist as non-pathogenic bacteria in the gastrointestinal or female genitourinary tract. Both vertical acquisition from the mother and horizontal acquisition from the environment are possible sources of infection [2,3]. *C. koseri* is a particularly devastating and rare cause of neonatal meningitis with a high incidence of brain abscesses (75%). Other complications include cerebral oedema, diffuse necrotising meningoencephalitis, ventriculitis, cerebritis, empyema, pneumatocephalus, cerebral infarction, hydrocephalus and severe neurological impairment (50% of cases) [1,4]. Seizures occur in 75% of cases [1]. The mortality rate is high (30%), with the surviving infants frequently having severe neurological sequelae [3].

Once *C. koseri* gains host entry, it primarily resides within macrophages, neutrophils and brain microvascular endothelial cells. This infiltration of macrophages allows invasion into the CNS where the bacteria replicate within the membrane-enclosed phagosomes [5,6]. All of this occurs without killing the host macrophage cells, explaining the tendencies of the bacteria to form expansive brain abscesses and to persist despite seemingly appropriate antibiotic therapy [5]. Several instances of epidemic, sporadic and nosocomial neonatal sepsis by this organism have been reported [6]. Most are sensitive to aminoglycosides and third-generation cephalosporins and resistant to ampicillin [2]. Ciprofloxacin and meropenem are recommended in neonates, based on both macrophages and the CNS

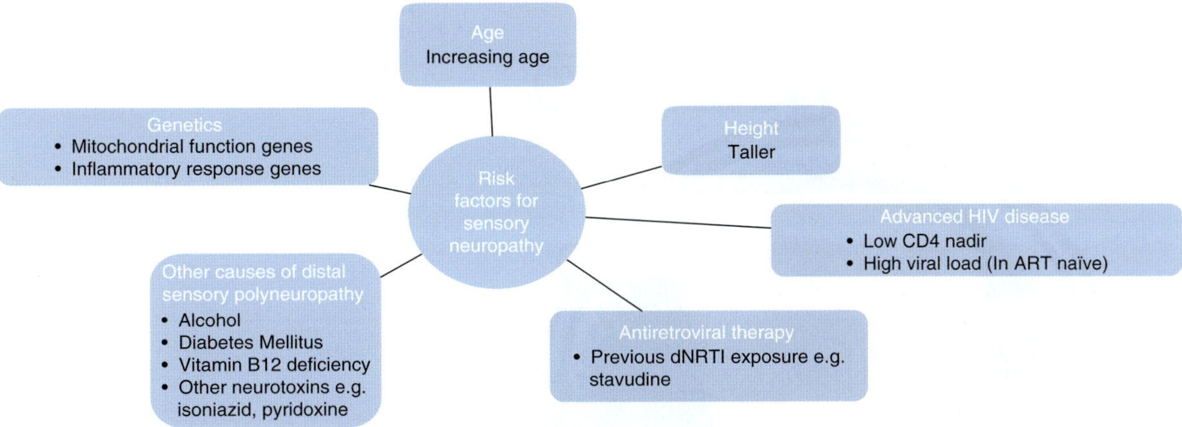

Figure 6.1. Risk factors for HIV-associated sensory neuropathy.

post-cART era [1]. It consists of two clinically indistinguishable subtypes, a distal sensory polyneuropathy due to the HIV virion itself (**Figure 6.2**) and a toxic neuropathy caused by the antiretroviral drugs used to treat the infection (**Figure 6.3**). Nucleoside reverse transcriptase inhibitors (especially stavudine, didanosine, zalcitabine) carry the highest risk. In particular, stavudine, frequently used as the backbone of older antiretroviral regimens, is often responsible for neurotoxic damage. Additional contributing risk factors include increasing age, height, advanced HIV disease (including a low nadir CD4+ cell count) and a more recently elucidated genetic predisposition in some [2–4]. HIV-associated sensory neuropathy is associated with intra-epidermal nerve fibre swelling and macrophage infiltration of large sensory neurons.

As for the patient described here, the diagnosis is suggested by history and examination findings in an HIV-positive patient after other common causes of neuropathy have been excluded. A frequently used tool to define HIV-associated sensory neuropathy in a research setting is the AIDS Clinical Trials Group Peripheral Neuropathy Screen [5]. Neuropathy typically presents with hypoaesthesia, paraesthesia and burning pains which begin in the feet and slowly spread proximally and, once they have reached the knee, progress to involve the hands. Usually pin-prick sensation is lost first. However, once established additional signs may include reduced/absent ankle reflexes and reduced vibration perception. Nerve conduction studies can reveal a pattern of distal axonal loss affecting sensory nerves. However, it has more value in excluding other causes of polyneuropathy and it is not uncommon to find a normal result, as was the case in this patient [6].

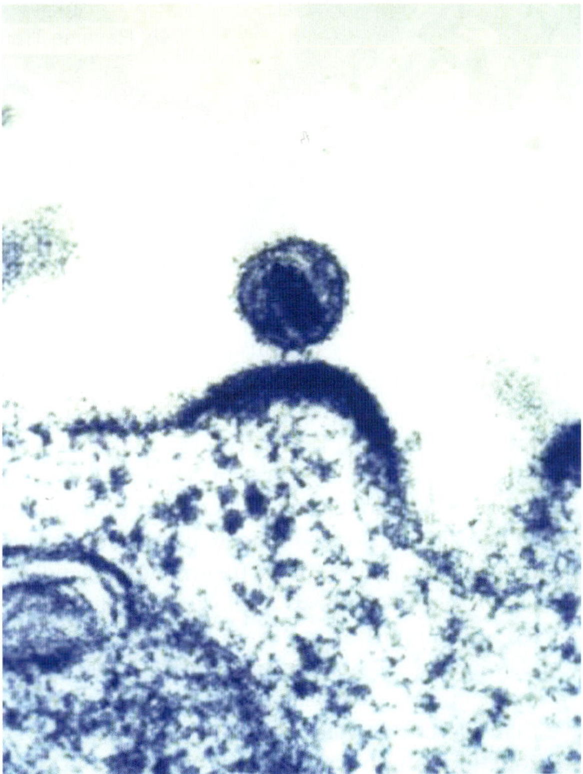

Figure 6.2. This digitally colourized transmission electron microscopic image depicts a single HIV particle, as it was budding from a human leucocyte, which the virus infects, and within which the HIV virus replicates itself. (Image courtesy of the National Institute of Allergy and Infectious Diseases (NIAID).)

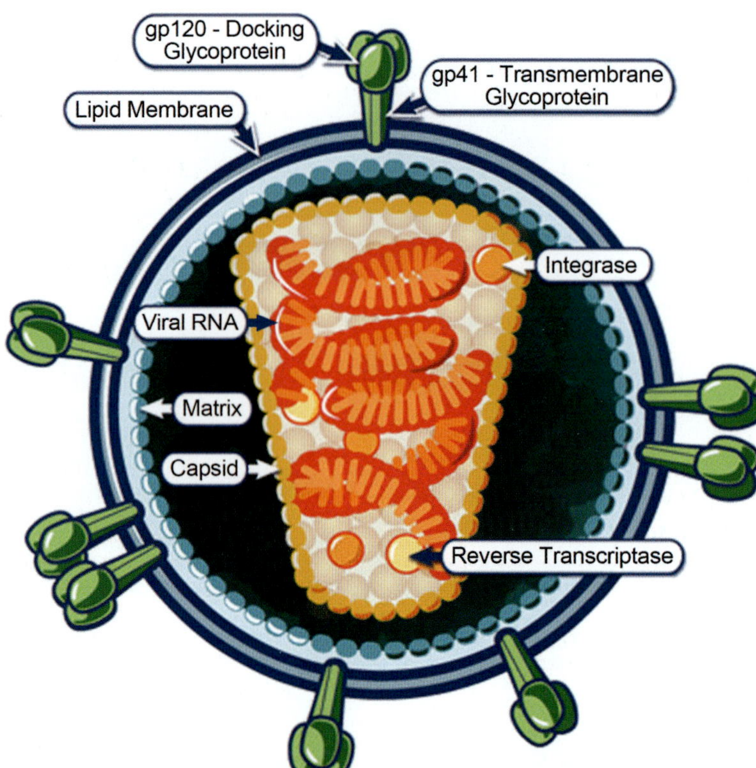

Figure 6.3. The ultrastructural morphology of HIV and some sites of action of antiretroviral drugs. (Image courtesy of the National Institute of Allergy and Infectious Diseases (NIAID).)

Treatment involves optimisation of HIV care by effective viral suppression and cessation or substitution of neurotoxic drugs in exchange for newer, less-neurotoxic regimens. Furthermore, avoidance of peripheral nerve insults (e.g. from vitamin B12 deficiency or poorly controlled diabetes) to avoid additional damage is also recommended. As neuropathic pain is common, symptomatic treatment with analgesic agents that target this is a priority, despite limited evidence to support their efficacy [7]. High-dose topical capsaicin, recombinant nerve growth factor and smoked cannabis have been shown to be more effective than placebo in treating HIV-associated sensory neuropathic pain in a recent meta-analysis, but their use currently remains limited due to financial or legal reasons [7].

Key Points

- HIV-associated sensory neuropathy is relatively common in patients with HIV, particularly in those with poorly controlled infection, and on certain drugs.
- Nucleoside reverse transcriptase inhibitors (especially stavudine, didanosine, zalcitabine) carry the highest risk.
- The diagnosis is clinical, made in the presence of symptoms and/or signs of a length-dependent small-fibre neuropathy even in the absence of changes on nerve conduction studies, after excluding other causes.
- Treatment involves effective management of HIV with non-neurotoxic ART, avoidance of other peripheral nerve insults and symptomatic management with particular attention to effective neuropathic analgesia.

Looking Back

Andreas Vesalius' book *De humani corporis fabrica* published in 1543 included some of the earliest detailed images of the peripheral nerves, along with key aspects of the central nervous system.

Did You Know?

Neuropathic symptoms can paradoxically worsen for a short period after the offending neurotoxic antiretroviral drug has been stopped – this is known as the 'coasting' phenomenon and is also seen in other toxic neuropathies such as chemotherapy-induced neuropathy.

References

1. Brew BJ. The peripheral nerve complications of human immunodeficiency virus (HIV) infection. Muscle Nerve 2003;**28**:542–52.
2. Cherry CL, Affandi JS, Imran D, et al. Age and height predict neuropathy risk in patients with HIV prescribed stavudine. Neurology 2009; **73**:315.
3. Nakamoto BK, McMurtray A, Davis J, et al. Incident neuropathy in HIV-infected patients on HAART. AIDS Res Hum Retroviruses **26**:759–65.
4. Kamerman PR, Wadley AL, Cherry CL. HIV-associated sensory neuropathy: risk factors and genetics. Curr Pain Headache Rep 2012;**16**:226–36.
5. Cherry CL, Wesselingh SL, Lal L, McArthur JC. Evaluation of a clinical screening tool for HIV-associated sensory neuropathies. Neurology 2005;**65**:1778.
6. Keswani SC, Pardo CA, Cherry CL, Hoke A, McArthur JC. HIV-associated sensory neuropathies. AIDS 2002;**16**:2105–17.
7. Phillips TJ, Cherry CL, Cox S, Marshall SJ, Rice AS. Pharmacological treatment of painful HIV-associated sensory neuropathy: a systematic review and meta-analysis of randomised controlled trials. PLoS ONE 2010;**5**:e14433.

CASE 7

The Masquerader

Laura A. Benjamin

History

A previously well 37-year-old female, originally from Uganda, presented to a district hospital in the UK with sudden-onset right arm and leg weakness and associated hemi-sensory loss. There was no associated speech or visual disturbance and there was no history of headache, vomiting, vertigo or recent physical trauma. There were no associated symptoms to suggest a seizure or other alteration in consciousness. She did not report any preceding or concomitant fever, night sweats, weight loss or other constitutional symptoms. She was married with two children, aged 5 and 7 years, and worked in a local supermarket. She had no past medical history and there were no neurological disorders in the family. She did not take prescribed medications, such as the oral contraceptive, and denied illicit drug use. She did not smoke or drink alcohol.

Examination

She was alert, orientated and afebrile. Her facial examination was abnormal (**Figure 7.1**), otherwise cranial nerve examination was unremarkable. She had a right-sided spastic hemiparesis, with increased tone, a pyramidal distribution of weakness, hyper-reflexia and an extensor plantar. Also on the right she had complete hemi-sensory loss to pinprick, temperature, joint position and vibration sense. There was no muscle wasting or fasciculations. Cardiovascular, respiratory and abdominal examination was unremarkable. Specifically her blood pressure was normal, she was clinically in sinus rhythm and there were no murmurs. There were also no stigmata of infective endocarditis or track-marks of intravenous drug use. Her modified Rankin score was 3 (i.e. she had moderate disability, required some help, but was able to walk unassisted).

Figure 7.1. Image of the forehead of a 37-year-old female from Uganda who presented with an acute right hemiparesis and hemi-sensory loss.

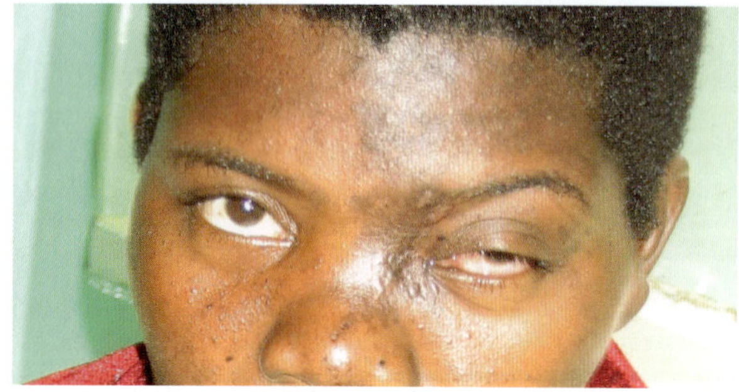

The patient had scars on the left side of her forehead, ptosis and an injected left conjunctiva.

Working Diagnosis

Clinically she had presented with a cerebrovascular accident, for which there might be a number of underlying aetiologies

- Haemorrhagic
  - Aneurysmal
  - Clotting disturbance
- Ischaemic
  - Atherosclerotic
  - Dissection
  - Cardioembolic (including infective endocarditis)
  - Vasculitis
    - Autoimmune
    - Infection-related

Investigations

The full blood count showed a white cell count of 4×10^9/l, haemoglobin 120 g/l and platelet 267×10^9/l. Serum cholesterol was 3.4 mmol/l and random blood glucose 9.0 mmol/l. Blood venereal disease reference laboratory (VDRL) and rapid plasma reagin (RPR) testing was negative.

An electrocardiogram was normal with sinus rhythm and transthoracic echocardiogram showed normal valves, with no thrombus or evidence of vegetation. In addition, carotid doppler ultrasound did not find any evidence of carotid stenosis.

A magnetic resonance imaging (MRI) scan was performed (**Figure 7.2**).

A lumbar puncture demonstrated a cerebrospinal fluid (CSF) white cell count of 0 cells/mm^3, red cell count of 0 cells/mm^3, glucose 2.65 mmol/l and protein 3.5 g/l.

Results of Definitive Investigations

Serology was positive for HIV and the CD4 count was 134 cells/mm^3.

Figure 7.2. T2-weighted axial MRI in a 37-year-old female from Uganda with an acute right hemiparesis and hemi-sensory loss.

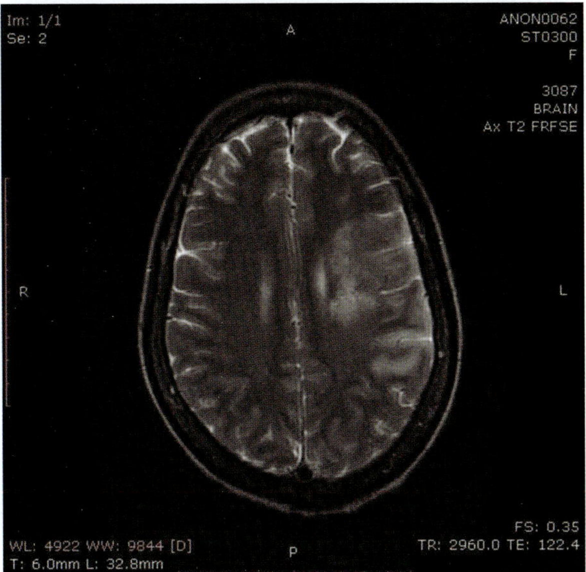

This shows increased intensity in the left fronto-parietal lobe, consistent with a left middle cerebral artery infarct.

Testing of her serum and CSF for antibody against varicella zoster virus (VZV) showed there was production of intrathecal IgG antibody.

Diagnosis

She had a stroke, most likely caused by varicella zoster virus vasculopathy, secondary to HIV infection.

Management and Outcome

She was started on high-dose intravenous aciclovir for 10 days. At discharge her modified Rankin score had improved to 2 (slight disability, able to look after her own affairs but unable to carry out all of her previous activities). She was referred to the HIV clinic to commence combined antiretroviral treatment as an outpatient. At 3-month follow-up, her modified Rankin score had improved from 0 (i.e. no deficit).

Prevention

Two live attenuated VZV vaccines are licensed in the UK currently. Vaccination is recommended for targeted groups only, e.g. for susceptible healthcare workers at risk of varicella exposure [1]. The vaccine is contraindicated in HIV-infected individuals, because it is a live vaccine [1].

Discussion

VZV is ubiquitous and highly infectious. Primary infection usually occurs in childhood resulting in acute varicella or 'chickenpox'. After initial infection, the virus remains dormant for life in the cranial nerves and dorsal root ganglia. It can reactivate years to decades later. This commonly results in herpes zoster (shingles), but occasionally in more severe neurological manifestations; these include Ramsay Hunt syndrome (shingles affecting the ear), associated with a facial nerve lesion, myelopathy, mononeuropathies, plexopathies and vasculopathy.

VZV vasculopathy produces stroke secondary to viral infection of cerebral arteries [2]. It is often the large vessels that are involved and it can be unifocal or multifocal. Classically there is a delayed contralateral hemiparesis, weeks, or even months, after herpes zoster ophthalmicus – shingles affecting the eye, and upper part of the face, as seen in the case described here. However, up to one-third of patients have no dermatological manifestation of viral re-activation [3]. It is seen typically in the elderly or immunocompromised. The clinical features and imaging, angiographic and CSF findings or VZV vasculopathy are similar to those of other causes of vasculopathy.

Confirming the diagnosis of VZV as a cause of stroke is not straightforward. Most laboratories limit the diagnosis of this infection to detection of viral DNA in CSF, which is negative in most cases of varicella zoster virus vasculopathy; this is because the virus has cleared from the CSF by the time patients present with stroke. Although a positive polymerase chain reaction (PCR) is helpful, a negative PCR result does not exclude the diagnosis. The detection of immunoglobulin (Ig) G antibody in CSF is the best test [4]. CSF abnormality (i.e. pleocytosis) may be a clue but it is not completely reliable either, as it is absent in one-third of patients with VZV vasculopathy [4]. If antibody screening had not been done, the diagnosis of stroke caused by VZV vasculopathy would have been missed in 10 (71%) of 14 patients in one cohort study [4].

In a patient with a recent varicella rash, especially in the first division of the trigeminal nerve, who presents with hemiparesis, and has leucocytes in the CSF, the diagnosis is likely, and it is worth encouraging the virology laboratory to send samples for antibody testing. In stroke patients with no rash and no CSF pleocytosis, convincing virologists to test for VZV can be a challenge; however, in stroke patients with

HIV or other severe immunosuppression, VZV vasculopathy is a strong possibility, and testing should be pursued [5].

The optimal treatment for VZV vasculopathy, for example dosing, type and duration of antiviral treatment, and concurrent steroid use is still uncertain [4,6]. However, VZV vasculopathy is caused by productive viral infection in arteries and thus all patients are typically treated with intravenous aciclovir. A study of 30 patients did not show any advantage of using aciclovir alone versus aciclovir and steroids, but many clinicians feel its use is warranted [4].

Key Points

- VZV classically causes a hemiparesis several weeks after herpes zoster ophthalmicus in the immunocompromised or elderly, although in up to one-third of patients the skin lesions are absent.
- Look for underlying immunocompromise in patients presenting with this syndrome.
- In patients with known immunocompromise who present with stroke, investigate for VZV, even if there are no skin lesions.
- Detection of IgG antibody in the CSF is the most useful test, although PCR is sometimes positive as well.

Looking Back

The earliest recorded description of VZV vasculopathy was in 1959 when Cravioto and Feigin described "a non-infectious granulomatous angiitis with a predilection for the nervous system, characterized by thrombosis in cerebral arteries" with a characteristic inflammatory response, of histiocytes, mononuclear cells and multinucleated giant cells. Just over a decade later, Rosenblum and Hadfield linked the same granulomatous angiitis of the nervous system to herpes zoster.

Did You Know?

The name of the viral family 'herpesviridae', which includes varicella zoster virus, is derived from the Greek word *herpein* ('to creep'), referring to recurring infections typical for this group of viruses.

Zoster comes from Greek *zōstēr*, meaning 'belt' or 'girdle', after the characteristic belt-like dermatomal rash.

The Nobel laureate Thomas Huckle Weller was the first person to isolate VZV in cell cultures in 1953.

References

1. UK Health Protection Agency (Prevention section). www.hpa.org.uk.
2. Gilden D, Cohrs RJ, Mahalingam R, Nagel MA. Varicella zoster virus vasculopathies: diverse clinical manifestations, laboratory features, pathogenesis, and treatment. Lancet Neurol 2009;**8**(8):731–40.
3. Nagel MA, Cohrs RJ, Mahalingam R, et al. The varicella zoster virus vasculopathies: clinical, CSF, imaging, and virologic features. Neurology 2008;**70**(11):853–60.
4. Nagel MA, Forghani B, Mahalingam R, et al. The value of detecting anti-VZV IgG antibody in CSF to diagnose VZV vasculopathy. Neurology 2007;**68**(13):1069–73.
5. Benjamin LA, Bryer A, Emsley HC, Khoo S, Solomon T, Connor MD. HIV infection and stroke: current perspectives and future directions. Lancet Neurol 2012;**11**:878–90.
6. Solomon T, Michael BD, Smith PE, et al. Management of suspected viral encephalitis in adults: Association of British Neurologists and British Infection Association National Guideline. J Infect 2012;**64**(4):374–77.

An Old Enemy

Michael Bonello and Tom Solomon

History

A 17-year-old male was transferred to a tertiary regional neurological centre from a psychiatric hospital. This followed a 4-month history in which he gradually developed depression, strange behaviour and suicidal ideation; he had also complained of a blurred vision, being unable to sign for his dole payment at the post office. In the psychiatric hospital his vision continued to deteriorate and he became incontinent of urine. His admission to the neurology hospital was precipitated by a generalised tonic–clonic seizure.

He'd had a normal birth and his development was normal. He had a past history of asthma, measles aged 3, and chickenpox aged 4, respectively. He had been vaccinated against diphtheria, tetanus and polio at 3 months. There was no relevant family history.

Examination

On examination he had diminished visual acuity of 6/36 in both eyes. He had left-sided pyramidal weakness, cerebellar ataxia, dressing apraxia and myoclonic jerks in his left arm. Deep tendon reflexes were brisk on the right, and more so on the left, with extensor plantars on both sides. The sensory examination was normal.

Initial Differential Diagnosis

- Diffuse sub-acute encephalitis
  - Autoimmune
  - Infective (**Table 8.1**)
- Rapidly evolving dementia, such as prion disease
- Metabolic white matter disease, such as mitochondrial encephalopathy with lactic acidosis and stroke-like episodes (MELAS)
- X-linked adrenoleukodystrophy
- Progressive myoclonic epilepsies
  - Lafora body disease
  - Sialidosis
  - Others

Table 8.1 Sub-acute and chronic central nervous system presentations – microbiological causes, modified from [1].

Viruses	
	In immunocompromised patients
	Measles virus (inclusion body encephalitis)
	Varicella zoster virus (causes a multifocal leukoencephalopathy)
	Cytomegalovirus
	Herpes simplex virus (especially HSV-2)
	Human herpes virus 6
	Enteroviruses
	JC/BK* virus (progressive multifocal leukoencephalopathy)
	HIV (dementia)
	In immunocompetent patients
	JC/BK* virus (progressive multifocal leukoencephalopathy)
	Measles virus (sub-acute sclerosing panencephalitis, years after primary infection)
Bacteria	
	Mycobacterium tuberculosis
	Treponema pallidum (syphilis)
	Borrelia burgdorferi (Lyme neuroborreliosis)
	Tropheryma whipplei (Whipple's Disease)
Fungi	
	Cryptococcus neoformans
Parasites	
	Trypanosoma brucei (African trypanosomiasis)
	Toxoplasma gondii (toxoplasmosis)
Prions	
	Creutzfeldt–Jakob disease

* JC and BK viruses are named after the initials of the patients from whom they were first isolated.

Results of Initial Investigations

Initial investigations including full blood count, urea, electrolytes, liver and thyroid function tests were normal. The cerebrospinal fluid (CSF) was clear and colourless, with no cells; CSF glucose was 3.4 mmol/l (serum glucose of 4.9 mmol/l) and CSF protein was slightly elevated at 0.5 g/l. CSF immunoglobulin (Ig)

G was elevated at 0.13 g/l (range: < 0.035 g/l) and CSF IgG:albumin index was 2.46 (range: 0.3–0.7).

A T2-weighted magnetic resonance imaging (MRI) scan was performed (**Figure 8.1**), followed by a single photon emission computed tomographic (SPECT) scan (**Figure 8.2A**) and an electroencephalogram (EEG) (**Figure 8.3**).

Results of Definitive Investigations

The CSF and serum measles titres came back from the laboratory, and were raised at 1/64 and 1/640, respectively.

Diagnosis

Sub-acute sclerosing panencephalitis (SSPE).

Management and Outcome

The patient continued to deteriorate over the next 4 weeks, becoming bed-bound. Because SSPE is almost always fatal, and there is no established treatment, experimental treatment was initiated. An Ommaya reservoir was inserted and the patient treated with intraventricular interferon-alpha, ribavirin (intravenously for 2 months, and then orally) and oral inosiplex.

He improved gradually over the next 10 weeks, with improved visual acuity, increased power on the left, and a reduction in the severity and frequency of myoclonus, and he was no longer bed-bound. Neuropsychological testing showed improvement in his attention and concentration, verbal performance and full-scale IQ, and general memory score. Both

Figure 8.1. T2-weighted MRI in a 17-year-old male presenting with 4 months of altered behaviour.

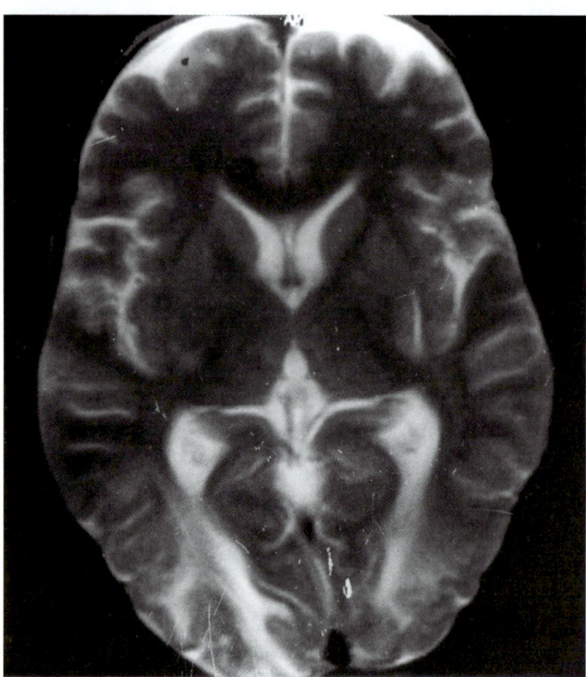

This shows high signal intensity in the occipital regions.

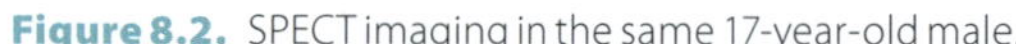

Figure 8.2. SPECT imaging in the same 17-year-old male.

A

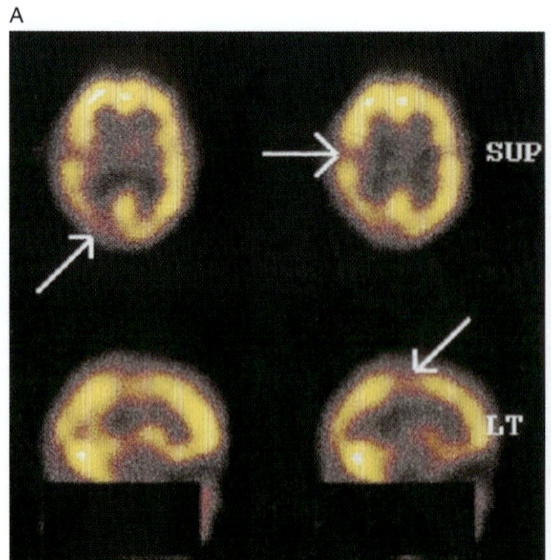

B

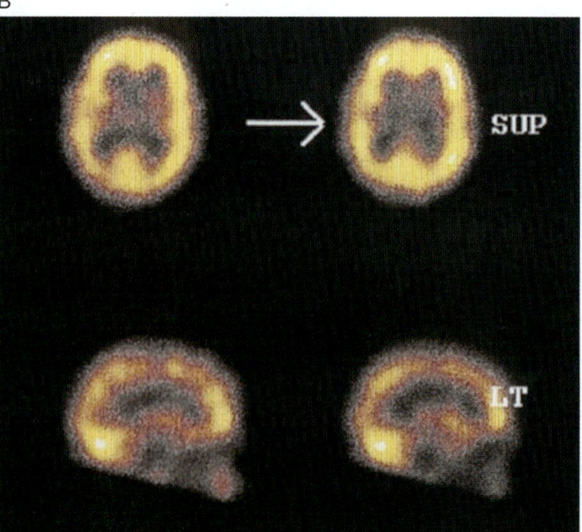

This shows perfusion defects in the right parietal and occipital regions before treatment (arrows; A) which have largely resolved 8 weeks into treatment (arrow; B) [2].

Figure 8.3. Electroencephalogram in the same 17-year-old.

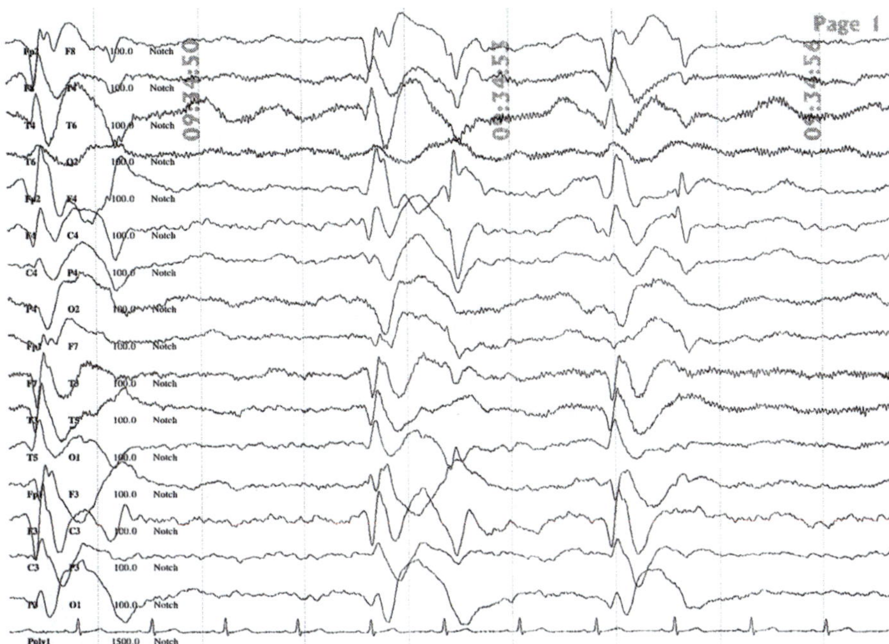

This shows widespread large amplitude rhythmic slow waves every 3 seconds on a low-amplitude background.

the MRI scan and the SPECT scan showed improvement in the white matter changes (**Figure 8.2B**).

Unfortunately, the Omaya reservoir became infected with coagulase-negative staphylococcal infection, which persisted despite prolonged intraventricular treatment with vancomycin. The reservoir was therefore removed at 10 weeks, and the intraventricular interferon-alpha stopped. Oral treatment continued with ribavirin and oral inosiplex, and there was continuing improvement, until 10 months after treatment when he deteriorated suddenly and died.

Prevention

The introduction of the measles vaccine in the 1950s has reduced the incidence of measles infection quite dramatically. Measles, mumps and rubella (MMR) vaccination introduction in the UK national vaccination programme decreased the incidence further (**Figure 8.4**).

Discussion

SSPE is a persistent and chronic encephalitis secondary to measles virus infection that causes widespread demyelination of the central nervous system (CNS). The prognosis is very poor with a fatal outcome in 95% of affected individuals.

SSPE is a rare complication of measles infection occurring in about 4–11 per 100,000 cases of measles; acquiring measles at a young age is a risk factor for subsequently developing SSPE. The incidence of SSPE is inversely related to measles vaccination coverage. In the developed world, SSPE has declined steadily since the introduction of the measles virus vaccine in the 1960s and there is strong evidence that this condition could be eliminated if complete herd immunity were achieved for this virus [3].

Measles can cause two other types of encephalitis: an acute encephalitis, which occurs during convalescence from acute measles infection, and a subacute encephalitis which occurs in immunocompromised hosts several months after the original infection.

The onset of symptoms in SSPE is variable, but usually occurs about 6 years after measles infection. The age at presentation is usually between 8 and 11 years old, thus the patient described above developed the disease relatively late. Initial symptoms include poor school performance with progressive intellectual decline, personality changes and behavioural abnormalities. This is usually associated with visual symptoms, including visuo-spatial disorientation. Motor features are often prominent, beginning with myoclonic jerks which progress to hypertonia. The cognitive decline and prominent myoclonus are similar to those seen in Creutzfeldt–Jakob Disease, and this is often the main differential. Seizures can be a feature. SSPE usually progresses relentlessly until death [4].

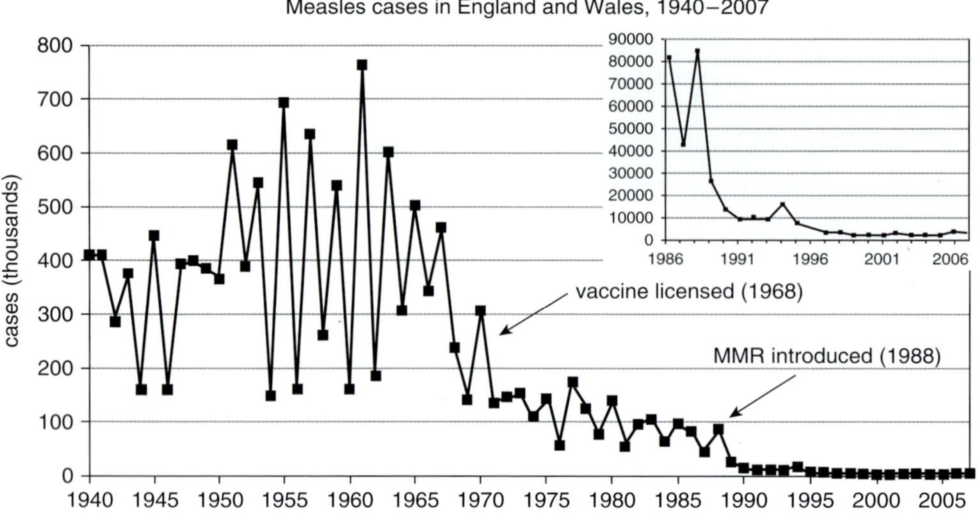

Figure 8.4. Number of cases and death reports secondary to measles from 1940 to 2006. Data from reference [5].

The clinical presentation with intellectual deterioration and myoclonus, as seen in the patient described here, is very characteristic; diagnosis is confirmed by the detection of measles IgG antibody in the CSF. CSF analysis shows pleocytosis, increased gamma globulins, normal glucose and a normal or elevated total protein. IgG against measles virus in the CSF is normally raised to a higher degree than the serum measles IgG, confirming intrathecal production of antibody.

MRI may be normal initially, but will typically progress to show cortical and subcortical hyper-intensities on T2-weighted sequences more prominent in the posterior CNS, as seen in this patient. The thalamus, corpus callosum and basal ganglia can also be affected [6]. On EEG, SSPE is characterised by bilaterally symmetrical and synchronous generalised high-amplitude slow waves recurring at regular intervals of typically 5–15 s [7]; in the patient described above, they occurred every 3 seconds. In contrast, in Creutzfelt Jacob Disease, large-amplitude periodic complexes are seen at a rate of approximately 1 per second. If there is still diagnostic uncertainty then brain biopsy is the gold standard for diagnosis (**Table 8.2**).

Although untreated SSPE is considered almost universally fatal, the course is often variable; slowing of the progression and stabilisation of the disease was seen in 35% of patients following treatment with inosiplex alone, or inosiplex and intraventricular interferon alpha in one series, which compared favourably with historical untreated controls [8]. Ribavirin has been used in case reports [2] as well as amantadine, steroids, cimetidine and plasmapherisis. Anti-epileptic drugs may reduce the myoclonus. Vaccination against measles in early life remains the best way to reduce the incidence of this severe condition.

Table 8.2 Diagnostic criteria for SSPE. Adapted from reference [6].

Major	
1.	Elevated CSF measles antibody titres
2.	Typical or atypical clinical history
Minor	
3.	Typical EEG changes
4.	Increased cerebrospinal fluid IgG
5.	Brain biopsy
6.	Special tests: molecular diagnostic test to identify measles virus mutated genome

Usually two major criteria plus one minor criterion are required; the more atypical the history the more the minor criteria are needed for diagnosis

Key Points

- SSPE is a late complication of measles infection which presents years after the original disease.
- Consider it in a child or young adult with cognitive decline, visual impairment and myoclonus.
- Globally, SSPE causes significant morbidity and mortality and, although rare in the UK, is still common in countries where a national vaccination programme is not undertaken.

Looking Back

SSPE was described first by Dawson in 1934, in an individual with rapidly progressive encephalitis. Later, in 1945, van Bogaert described another individual with the same clinical presentation but in whom the disease exhibited a more gradual course.

Did You Know?

In the UK in the late 1990s use of the measles, mumps and rubella (MMR) vaccine declined, and there was a resurgence of measles, when the vaccine was controversially and falsely linked to autism in a *Lancet* publication which subsequently was withdrawn. The UK General Medical Council subsequently removed the medical licence of lead author Dr Andrew Wakefield, after he was charged with fraud and undeclared conflicts of interest.

References

1. Campbell C, Levin S, Humphreys P, Walop W, Brannan R. Subacute sclerosing panencephalitis: results of the Canadian Paediatric Surveillance Program and review of the literature. BMC Pediatrics 2005;**5**:47.
2. Solomon T, Hart CA, Vinjamuri S, et al. Treatment of subacute sclerosing panencephalitis with interferon-alpha, ribavirin, and inosiplex. J Child Neurol 2002;**17**:703–5.
3. Campbell H, Andrews N, Brown KE, Miller E. Review of the effect of measles vaccination on the epidemiology of SSPE. Int J Epidemiol 2007;**36**:1334–48.
4. Gutierrez J, Issacson RS, Koppel BS. Subacute sclerosing panencephalitis: an update. Dev Med Child Neurol 2010;**52**:901–7.
5. Public Health England, Epidemiological data on measles. www.hpa.org.uk/Topics/InfectiousDiseases/InfectionsAZ/Measles/EpidemiologicalData/ (accessed May 30, 2013).
6. Tuncay R, Akman-Demir G, Gökyigit A, et al. MRI in subacute sclerosing panencephalitis. Neuroradiology 1996;**38**:636–40.
7. Praveen-kumar S, Sinha S, Taly AB, et al. Electroencephalographic and imaging profile in a subacute sclerosing panencephalitis (SSPE) cohort: a correlative study. Clin Neurophysiol 2007;**118**:1947–54.
8. Gascon GG. Randomized treatment study of inosiplex versus combined inosiplex and intraventricular interferon in subacute sclerosing panencephalitis (SSPE): international multicenter study. J Child Neurol 2003;**18**:819–27.

CASE 9

Floppy and Falling

Hannah E. Brindle and Benedict D. Michael

History

A 6-year-old girl presented to her local hospital in rural Vietnam with a 3-day history of fever, vomiting and headache. This was followed by rapid development of difficulty walking due to weakness and pain of her left leg. She also complained that she had been unable to pass urine over the preceding 24 hours. There were no periods of loss or alteration in consciousness and no skin lesions or visual symptoms.

She had been well recently with no preceding gastrointestinal symptoms and otherwise had no past medical history and took no regular medications. She had not had contact with any animals prior to this presentation. She had the polio vaccine as part of her routine childhood immunisations, but had received no recent vaccinations. There was no significant family history and no other family members or other contacts had been unwell. She had not recently travelled outside of her village.

Examination

On examination her temperature was 38.7°C, heart rate and respiratory rate were within the normal range. There was some neck stiffness. Neurological examination of the cranial nerves, including funduscopy, and of the upper limbs, including tone, power and reflexes, was normal.

Tone, power and reflexes were also normal in the right lower limb. However, in the left lower limb the tone was reduced, power was markedly reduced to Medical Research Council grade 1–2 out of 5, and the knee and ankle reflexes were absent. Both plantars were flexor. Sensation to pin-prick, temperature, proprioception, and vibration was normal. There were no cerebellar signs.

Investigations

A lumbar puncture was performed and the opening pressure was 30 cm H_2O. The cerebrospinal fluid (CSF) showed a white cell count of 160 cells/mm^3 (70% lymphocytes, 30% neutrophils), red cell count < 5 cells/mm^3, protein 0.48 g/l, glucose 3.6 mmol/l (no serum measurement); Gram stain and culture were negative.

Differential Diagnosis

- Inflammation of the anterior horn cells of the spinal cord (myelitis)
    - Poliomyelitis
    - Japanese encephalitis virus (JEV)
    - Other arbovirus
    - Non-polio enteroviruses (e.g. coxsackie virus, enterovirus-71 and echovirus)
- Lesion of the nerve root/peripheral nerve
    - Guillain–Barré syndrome
    - Acute motor axonal neuropathy
    - Infection (e.g. varicella zoster virus (VZV), HIV)
    - Lead poisoning
    - Porphyria

(The latter four diagnoses are less likely in the context of a CSF pleocytosis.)

Results of Definitive Investigations

A stool sample was sent for isolation of poliovirus; however, none was detected. The CSF was positive for anti-JEV IgM antibodies.

Diagnosis

Myelitis caused by Japanese encephalitis virus.

Management and Outcome

Three days after admission, the patient developed pneumonia. She had worsening respiratory function and required a period of ventilation. Despite this, she made a good recovery over the next month. Nevertheless, there was ongoing wasting and weakness in the affected limb (**Figure 9.1**).

Prevention

General measures to prevent mosquito bites include wearing long-sleeved clothing and using insect repellent [1,2].

A vaccination for Japanese encephalitis (JE) has been increasingly available across Asia since the 1990s, and since its uptake there have been significant reductions in cases. In wealthier parts of Asia, where there have been long-standing high-quality vaccination programmes, such as Japan and Taiwan, the current incidence is 0.003/100,000/year, whereas in poorer countries where

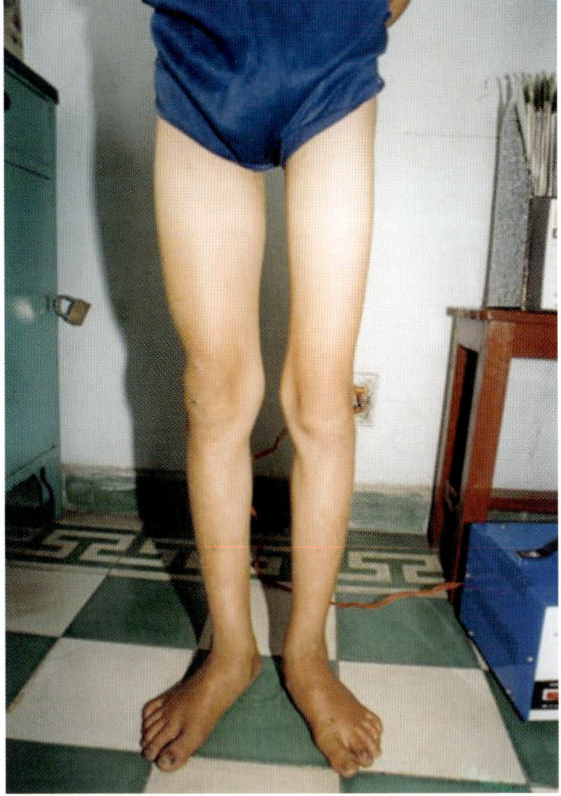

Figure 9.1. Wasting of the left lower limb one year after presentation in a similar child with an acute flaccid paralysis secondary to JEV infection. (Photo: Tom Solomon, reproduced with permission from [9].)

there has been nascent or no vaccination programmes, the incidence is up to 10.6/100,000/year [3,4].

Travellers to areas where JEV circulates are advised to get vaccinated, if their stay may be prolonged (e.g. several weeks) or they are at increased risk of exposure to the disease (e.g. staying in or around rice-growing areas) (**Figure 9.2**) [5]. Vaccination may also be considered for those with frequent shorter trips to endemic areas.

Discussion

Japanese encephalitis virus is a flavivirus, endemic in South and South-East Asia. It is a zoonotic disease transmitted from animals, the natural hosts, to humans following the bite of an infected mosquito, typically *Culex* spp. (**Figure 9.3**) [6]. In highly endemic areas of rural Asia almost everyone is infected during childhood. Most infections are asymptomatic or cause a mild febrile illness, but an important minority result in disease. Symptoms range from fever and headache to encephalitis with coma and, in 10–30% of cases, death [7]. Approximately 50% of children with Japanese encephalitis are left with severe neuropsychiatric sequelae [8].

Although the differential diagnosis of flaccid paralysis is broad (**Figure 9.4**), clinical features can help establish distinguish direct viral infection from an immune-mediated process, such as Guillain–Barré syndrome (**Table 9.1**). Other enteroviruses, particularly enterovirus 71, and paralytic rabies are important causes of myelitis [9].

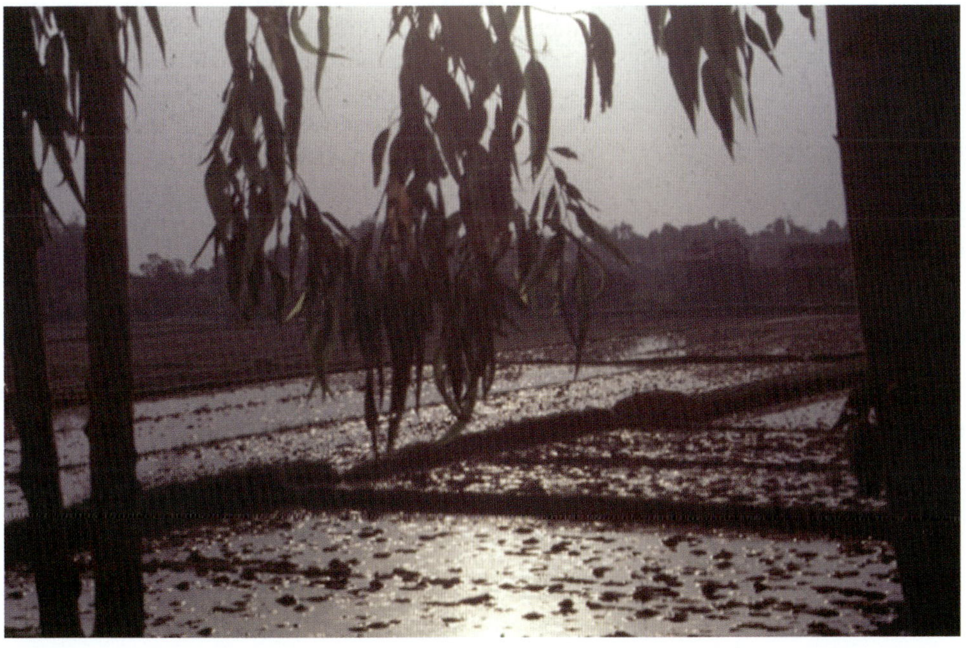

Figure 9.2. Rice paddy fields, a common breeding ground for *Culex* mosquitos. (Photo: Tom Solomon.)

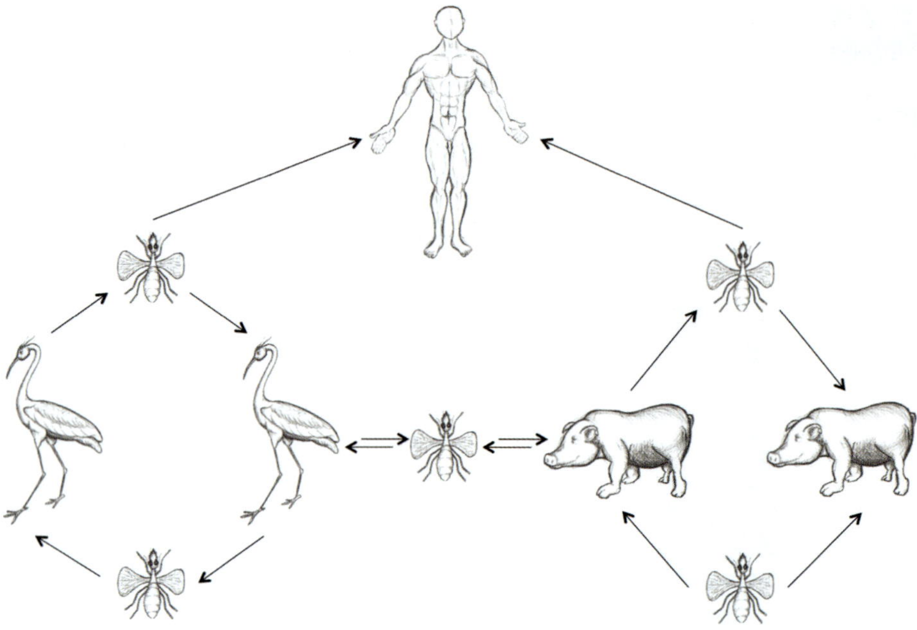

Figure 9.3. Enzoonotic transmission of Japanese encephalitis virus. Figure: Benedict D. Michael.

Table 9.1 Causes of acute flaccid paralysis. Adapted from reference [9] with permission of Elsevier.

	Direct viral damage of anterior horn cell (e.g. JEV)	Immune-mediated damage of nerve roots/ peripheral nerves (e.g. GBS)
Onset	During/shortly after febrile illness	Several weeks after febrile illness
Pattern	Asymmetrical	Symmetrical
Time to maximum weakness	2–3 days	7–14 days
Sensory	Not involved	Often (excluding AMAN)
Pain	Often muscular pain	Often back pain
Cerebrospinal fluid	Lymphocytosis	Albuminocytologic disassociation

AMAN, acute motor axonal neuropathy; GBS, Guillain–Barré syndrome; JEV, Japanese encephalitis virus.

In the patient described here there was no predisposing gastrointestinal illness, which might occur in campylobacter infection preceeding Guillain–Barré syndrome, and there was no contact with a potentially rabid animal.

Similar to poliovirus infection, children with JEV myelitis may have symptoms of vomiting, headache and fever prior to developing an asymmetrical acute flaccid paralysis of the lower limbs, which is due to anterior horn cell damage. However, unlike poliovirus infection, those children with JEV infection are more likely to have symptoms of encephalitis, urinary retention and extrapyramidal signs. Some may develop respiratory failure due to paralysis of the respiratory muscles. Other flaviviruses that cause myelitis include West Nile virus, Murray Valley encephalitis virus and St. Louis encephalitis virus, and Zika virus [9,10,13].

Key Points

- Think of JEV myelitis in those presenting with acute flaccid paralysis in countries in which JEV is endemic.
- The differential includes poliomyelitis, other enteroviruses, other flaviviruses, rabies virus, and Guillain–Barré syndrome.

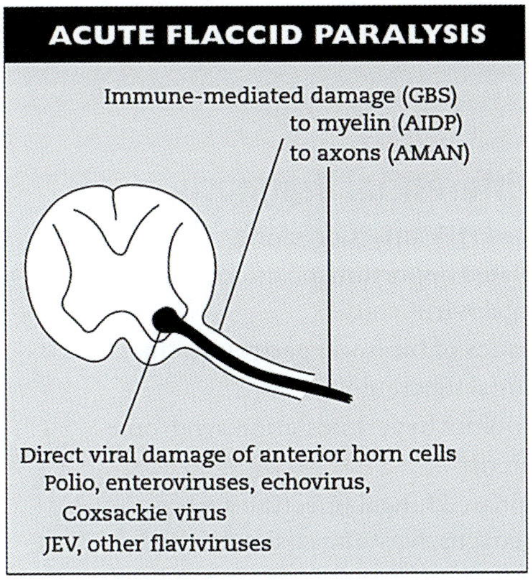

ACUTE FLACCID PARALYSIS

Immune-mediated damage (GBS)
to myelin (AIDP)
to axons (AMAN)

Direct viral damage of anterior horn cells
Polio, enteroviruses, echovirus,
Coxsackie virus
JEV, other flaviviruses

Figure 9.4. Immune-mediated Guillain–Barré syndrome (GBS) occurs in two forms: in acute inflammatory demyelinating polyneuropathy (AIDP) the myelin is damaged; in acute motor axonal neuropathy (AMAN) the motor axons are targeted. Viruses such as poliovirus and Japanese encephalitis virus cause paralysis by directly attacking the lower motor neurones (the anterior horn cells); the latter virus also occasionally causes GBS. (Reproduced from [14] with permission of John Wiley & Sons, Inc.)

Looking Back

Japanese encephalitis was first described in Japan in the 1870s, but the virus is thought to have originated in the Malay archipelago several thousand years ago. It has spread across Asia since then, reaching Australia in 1995 [11].

Did You Know?

Encephalitis has long been recognised in the medical literature. As far back as the Mesopotamian medical texts of approximately 2000 BC 'Brain Fever' was described [12]:

'Headache roameth over the desert, blowing like the wind……
It standeth hostile against the wayfarer, scorching him like the day
This man it hath struck and
Like the one with heart disease he staggereth,
Like the one bereft of reason he is broken.'

References

1. Centers for Disease Control and Prevention, USA. Japanese Encephalitis. 2012. www.cdc.gov/japaneseencephalitis/prevention/index.html (accessed May 21, 2018).
2. World Health Organisation. Japanese encephalitis vaccines. Wkly Epidem Rec 2006;**81**:325–80.
3. Solomon T, Dung NM, Kneen R, et al. Neurological aspects of tropical diseases: Japanese encephalitis. J Neurol Neurosurg Psych 2000;**68**:405–15.
4. National Travel Health Network and Centre. Health Professionals, Travel Health Information Sheets – Japanese Encephalitis. 2010. https://travelhealthpro.org.uk/factsheet/55/japanese-encephalitis (accessed May 21, 2018).
5. Campbell GL, Hills SL, Fischer M, et al. Estimated global incidence of Japanese encephalitis: a systematic review. Bull WHO 2011;**89**:766–74E.
6. Solomon T. Control of Japanese encephalitis – within our grasp? N Engl J Med 2006;**355**:869–71.
7. Solomon T, Vaughan DW. Pathogenesis and clinical features of Japanese encephalitis and West Nile virus infections. Curr Top Microbiol Immunol 2002;**267**:171–94.
8. Kumar R, Mathur A, Singh KB, et al. Clinical sequelae of Japanese encephalitis in children. Indian J Med Res 1993;**97**:9–13.
9. Solomon T, Ooi MH, Mallewa M. Viral infections of lower motor neurons. In: Eisen AE, Shaw PJ, editors. *Handbook of Clinical Neurology*, vol. 82: *Motor Neuron Disorders and Related Diseases*. Amsterdam: Elsevier; 2007: 179–206.
10. Solomon T, Kneen R, Dung NM, et al. Poliomyelitis-like illness due to Japanese encephalitis virus. Lancet 1998;**351**:1094–7.
11. Erlanger T, Weiss S, Keiser J, Utzinger J, Wiedenmayer K. Past, present, and future of Japanese encephalitis. Emerg Infect Dis 2009;**15**:1–7.
12. Johnson RT. *Viral Infections of the Nervous System*. Philadelphia: Lippincott-Raven; 1998.
13. Mehta R, Soares CN, Medialdea-Carrera R, et al. The spectrum of neurological disease associated with Zika and chikungunya viruses in adults in Rio de Janeiro, Brazil: A case series. PLoS Negl Trop Dis 2018;**12**: e0006212.
14. Solomon T, Kneen R. Acute flaccid paralysis. In: Gill GV, Beeching NJ, Gill G, eds. *Tropical Medicine (Lecture Notes)*. 7th ed. London: Wiley-Blackwell; 2004: 248–50.

CASE 10

Disseminated in Time and Space

Aleš Chrdle

History

A 27-year-old informatics student from Sub-Saharan Africa was referred from a walk-in centre with fever of 38.5°C, weight loss of more than one stone in the last 6 months, and blood in the stool for several days. There was no significant previous medical history.

He had never been tested for HIV and denied any high-risk sexual contacts in the past. He had not travelled abroad since his arrival to the UK 2 years earlier.

He was not aware of any fever until it was detected in the walk-in centre. Communication with him was somewhat difficult because of his vagueness and slow responses, rather than any poor understanding of English. He reported little cough in the past, and was not sure about night sweats. His main problem was repeat occurrence of fresh blood in the stool over the last couple of days. He reported normal appetite, no nausea or diarrhoea, and no problems passing urine.

Examination

The young man appeared exhausted, feverish and restless. He was cooperative, and orientated, although he took time to think before he replied to questions about his health. Weight loss was apparent from his baggy clothes, which showed at least 10 cm loss of waist circumference; he weighed 52 kg.

There was no apparent lymphadenopathy, no skin lesions, and tongue and throat appeared unremarkable. Chest was clear and during examination, he did not cough, and was not able to bring up any phlegm when asked to do so. Abdominal examination revealed some mild periumbilical tenderness with no organomegaly, and rectal digital examination showed a non-tender bean-sized mass in the anterior rectum with no blood visible on glove.

Neurological examination revealed normal cranial nerves, no cerebellar signs and normal power, tone and sensation in all four limbs. There was no nystagmus, no neck stiffness, no photophobia or phonophobia. Reflexes appeared to be overall rather brisk, probably reflecting his anxiety and inability to relax. Plantars were down-going in both legs. There was no tremor, and finger–nose coordination was slightly imprecise, but with no overshooting. His heel–shin testing was slightly imprecise. He was slightly unstable when standing up or walking.

Initial Differential Diagnosis

- Advanced HIV infection alone
- HIV-related opportunistic infection, such as cytomegalovirus colitis
- Malignancy of the lower gastrointestinal tract
- Abdominal tuberculosis (TB)
- Strongyloides hyperinfestation syndrome
- Cysticercosis
- Disseminated fungal infection such as Cryptococcus, blastomycosis, etc.
- Vasculitis or other autoimmune condition
- Inflammatory bowel disease
- Haematological malignancy
- Disseminated *Mycobacterium avium intracellulare* complex infection
- Other

Results of Initial Investigations

Body mass index (BMI) 17 kg/m^2, weight loss 16%.

Blood count: haemoglobin 96 g/l, platelets 63 × 10^9/l, white blood cells 6.3 × 10^9/l, neutrophils 5.4 × 10^9/l, lymphocytes 0.5 × 10^9/l.

Serum: urea 3.5 mmol/l, creatinine 77 µmol/l, Na 123 mmol/l, K 4.4 mmol/l, Cl 91 mmol/l.

Liver function tests: bilirubin 12 µmol/l, alaninaminotransferase 182 U/l, gamma-glutaryltransferase activated partial thromboplastin time 147 U/l, alkaline phosphatase 129 U/l, albumin 29 g/l, total protein 63 g/l.

Clotting: prothrombin time 16.4 s, activated partial thromboplastin time 30.9 s.

Other: glucose 5.9 mmol/l, C-reactive protein 36 mg/l, blood-borne viruses: HIV test negative, hepatitis B core Ab, surface Ag neg, and hepatitis C Ab negative.

Chest radiograph was performed (**Figure 10.1**).

Progress and Further Investigations

Over the first few days of admission, he needed to be repeatedly reminded of the severity of his condition and he kept expressing a desire to be discharged. He spiked daily fevers up to 40°C. Central nervous system (CNS) involvement was suspected and lumbar puncture was performed. Cerebrospinal fluid (CSF) was clear and colourless, with opening pressure 17 cm H_2O, white cell count 4 cells/mm^3, red cell count

Figure 10.1. Chest X-ray in 27-year-old student from sub-Saharan Africa presenting with fevers, weight loss and bloody stools.

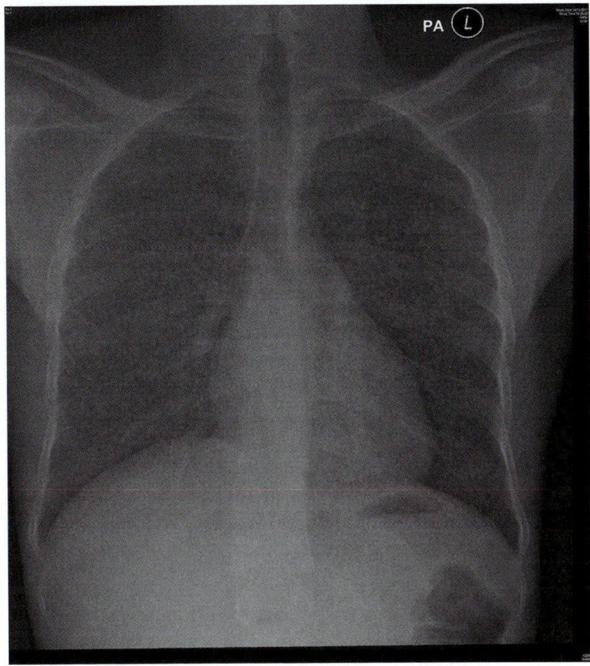

This shows a miliary pattern of disseminated tuberculosis.

14 cells/mm^3, protein 3.1 mg/l, CSF glucose 2.4 mmol/l, serum glucose 6.4 mmol/l (CSF/serum ratio 0.375). Funduscopy revealed multiple choroideal granulomas. Based on observation that he was not able to use his mobile phone and his laptop, Mini-Mental State Examination (MMSE) was checked and scored 23/30. Brain imaging was performed (**Figure 10.2**).

Refined Differential Diagnosis

- Miliary TB with CNS involvement
- Disseminated fungal infection
- Carcinomatosis

Results of Definitive Investigations

Induced sputum was positive on Ziehl–Neelsen stain, as was his early morning urine, and *Mycobacterium tuberculosis* was cultured from sputum, CSF, blood and urine (**Table 10.1**).

Diagnosis

Disseminated miliary tuberculosis in an immunocompetent individual with involvement of the lungs, central nervous system (tuberculomas), eyes, spleen, large intestine and genitourinary tract.

Table 10.1 Mycobacterial culture results in miliary tuberculosis case.

Sample	Ziehl–Neelsen stain	Culture positive	PCR FastTrack
Sputum	+/–	6 days	
Induced sputum	+	9 days	Negative
Early morning urine	+	11 days	
CSF	–	23 days	
Blood	n/a	38 days	

CSF, cerebrospinal fluid; PCR, polymerase chain reaction.

Management and Outcome

The patient was promptly started on a conventional regimen of four first-line anti-tuberculous drugs, with isoniazid, rifampicin, pyrazinamide and streptomycin, which he tolerated well. His fevers settled within a week and general condition gradually improved. His liver enzymes normalised about 3 weeks into anti-tuberculous treatment. He was discharged home after 20 days. His CSF TB culture came back positive one week after his discharge, and because he was remarkably improved at that time, a decision was made not to start corticosteroids. After 2 weeks at home, he was briefly readmitted with thrombocytopaenia of 24 × 10^9/l and left-sided epididymitis, which was thought to be a paradoxical reaction and resolved on non-steroidal anti-inflammatory drug treatment. His platelets slowly normalised. His mental condition improved remarkably and he was able to resume his studies two months after his first admission. After one year of treatment his chest X-ray showed complete resolution, he was well and his weight was back to his normal 64 kg.

Prevention

The only approved vaccine so far is the classical viable whole-cell based Bacille–Calmette–Guerin (BCG) [1]. This has protective effect against miliary or meningeal TB, but inconsistent protection level against other forms of TB. Since the late 1990s, there have been other vaccines in development, some of which are in stage II clinical testing. These first-generation vaccines are neither designed to prevent infection nor to achieve sterile eradication, but rather to better prime and/or boost infection control [2].

Figure 10.2. T1-weighted magnetic resonance images of the brain post-intravenous gadolinium in the same young man.

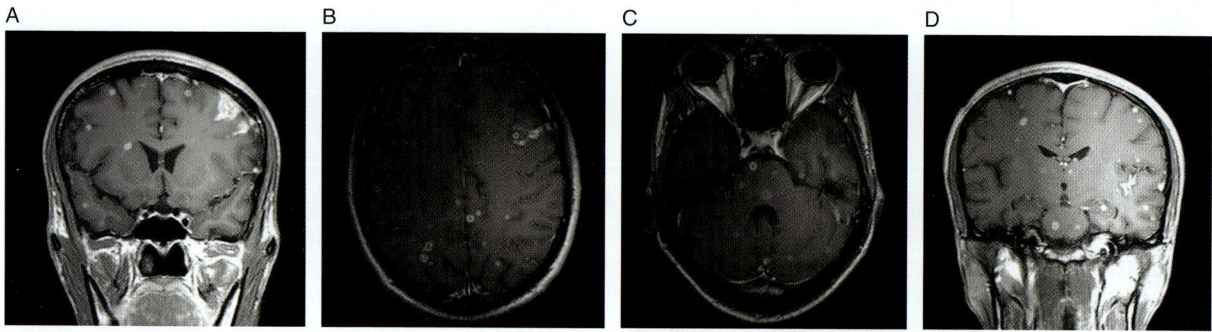

This shows multiple small-ring post-contrast enhancing lesions throughout the brain including the thalamus, brain stem and cerebellum consistent with tuberculomas. A confluent area of nodular change is seen anterolaterally in the left frontal lobe (A).

Discussion

In this young man from Sub-Saharan Africa, with marked weight loss and fever, HIV was initially at the top of the differential, but the HIV test proved negative. The challenge was then to establish which other infections might be contributing to his clinical condition. The vagueness and slow responses indicated possible CNS disease. Despite the lack of a CSF pleocytosis, the low glucose ratio was consistent with TB in the CNS, and microscopy and culture confirmed this.

Approximately 5–10% of the two billion people who are infected with TB worldwide develop active disease at some time during their life. In the UK, the incidence of TB in 2011 in the UK-born people was 4.1/100,000 population, while in people born abroad the incidence rate was 83.6/100,000 population. In the non-UK-born patients, half of TB cases develop within 5 years after immigration. In active TB cases, about half have extra-pulmonary involvement, and a miliary/cryptic form has been reported in 3%, TB meningitis in 2.1% and other CNS TB in 1.0% of cases [3]. About 100 cases of tuberculous meningitis (TBM) occur annually in the UK [3].

TBM develops when subependymal or subpial tubercules (Rich foci) resulting from *Mycobacterium tuberculosis* bacteraemic seeding during disseminated disease or primary infection, rupture into the subarachnoid space [4]. Alternatively, TB granulomas can coalesce to form tuberculomas or TB abscesses. In the case presented here, the imaging findings and lack of a CSF pleocytosis indicate tuberculomas and abscess, rather than meningitis [5]. On imaging (CT or MRI), tuberculomas appear as contrast-enhancing ring lesions with surrounding oedema. Differentiation from other focal CNS infections or neoplasia may not be possible without biopsy [6,7].

Table 10.2 Severity of meningitis grading and mortality improvement on anti-tuberculous therapy with adjunctive corticosteroids.

Grade [11]	GCS	Focal neurological deficit	Mortality on ATT [8]	Mortality on ATT + DXM [8]
I	15	Absent	30%	17%
II	15	Present	40%	31%
	10–14	Absent or present		
III	< 10	Absent or present	60%	55%

Adapted from references [8,9].
ATT, antituberculous therapy; DXM, dexamethasone.

Tuberculosis of the CNS is associated with very high mortality and morbidity. Based on severity of initial presentation and time to initiating treatment, mortality ranges from 15% to 60% and significant neurological disability is noted in 50% of survivors (**Table 10.2**) [8].

Clinical presentation is usually sub-acute, and duration of symptoms for more than 5–6 days is one of the parameters used in differentiating it from bacterial meningitis. TBM does not classically have typical signs of a bacterial meningitis, such as stiff neck or photophobia. In mild cases, only subtle changes in personality, vomiting or malaise may be present [6,7,10]. Retinal examination finds tuberculomas in 5–18% of immunosuppressed patients with disseminated TB, as it did in this case [11].

Investigation of extra-meningeal sites is especially useful for diagnosing CNS TB. Extra-meningeal disease can be found in up to three-quarters of such patients, and enables easier and safer acquisition of proper microbiological and histological samples. Chest X-ray is pathological in about half of TBM cases [6,9].

Table 10.3 Results of cerebrospinal fluid investigations in this case and in typical tuberculous meningitis.

	Diagnostic criteria TBM [8]	This case
Opening pressure	> 25 cm H_2O	17 cm H_2O
White cells	5–1000 cells/µl	4 cells/µl
Lymphocytes	30–90%	n/a
Protein	> 4.5 mg/l	3.1 mg/l
Glucose	< 2.2 mmol/l	2.4 mmol/l
Serum glucose	–	6.4 mmol/l
CSF/serum glucose	< 0.5	0.375
Ziehl–Neelsen stain	+	–
TB culture	+	+

TBM, tuberculous meningitis; CSF, cerebrospinal fluid.

Findings in the CSF may only partially meet the triad of lymphocytic pleocytosis, elevated protein and low glucose (**Table 10.3**), but occasionally may be completely normal [6,7,10].

The chance of detecting mycobacterium increases with volume of CSF; at least 6 ml should be taken if TBM is suspected. Culture takes several weeks and has low sensitivity (40–80%). Nucleic acid amplification helps with rapid detection of resistant strains. Repeat samples of large volumes CSF increase microbiological yield [6,7,10].

TBM is a medical emergency and treatment should be initiated empirically if a high level of suspicion is present, before culture results are available. Treatment of fully sensitive TBM should last 12 months, with isoniazid, rifampicin, pyrazinamide and streptomycin or ethambutol administered daily for the first 2 months, and then isoniazid and rifampicin daily for the rest of treatment duration. Some use pyrazinamide for the whole time of treatment. There is no good evidence on the best treatment for multi-drug resistant (MDR) TBM, and so management recommendations are extrapolated from pulmonary MDR-TB (**Table 10.4**) [6–8,10].

Steroids reduce mortality in adults and HIV-negative children with TBM [8]. There are only limited data on the use of steroids in tuberculomas without meningitis.

Complications of TBM include hydrocephalus, vasculitic stroke, cranial neuropathies, tuberculous abscess, haemorrhage or seizures (especially in children). Another complication of TBM is hyponatraemia, presumably from the syndrome of inadequate antidiuretic hormone secretion (SIADH) [6–8,10].

Table 10.4 Pharmacodynamic activity and CSF penetration of anti-TB drugs.

Anti-TB drug	Activity	CSF penetration
1st-line drugs		
Isoniazid	Cidal	90–95%
Rifampin	Cidal	5–25%
Pyrazinamide	Cidal	95–100%
Streptomycin	Static	20–25%
Ethambutol	Static	10–50%
Ciprofloxacin	Cidal	15–35%
Levofloxacin	Cidal	60–80%
Moxifloxacin	Cidal	70–80%
2nd-line drugs		
Ethionamide	Cidal	80–95%
Cycloserine	Static	40–70%
Amikacin	Cidal	10–25%
Streptomycin	Cidal	10–20%
Capreomycin	Static	Unknown
Para-aminosalicylic acid	Static	Unknown
Thioacetazone	Static	Unknown
Linezolid	Cidal	80–100%
New agents		
Bedaquiline (TMC207)	Cidal	Unknown
Delamanid (OPC-67683)	Cidal	Unknown

Key Points

- TBM is the most severe form of TB with high mortality and morbidity. It usually develops subacutely. The majority of cases have another, usually pulmonary, site of active TB.
- Characteristic CSF findings of TB in the CNS include a lymphocytic-predominant pleiocytosis, elevated protein and low glucose, but these features may not be always present.

- Treatment of TB in the CNS is a medical emergency; the treatment course should be prolonged to 12 months in cases of fully sensitive strains, and longer in cases of resistant TB.
- Adjunctive corticosteroids improve the outcome of TBM.
- Underlying immunocompromise, especially HIV, increases the risk of disseminated TB, including TBM.

Looking Back

Tuberculosis, known as consumption (from the Latin) or phthisis (from the Greek) or the white plague (old English), has been one of the leading killers throughout human history. TBM and tuberculomas were first described by Robert Whytt in 1768 [12]. It was not until the advent of streptomycin in 1940s, that TBM became treatable [9].

Did You Know?

In nineteenth-century Europe, 'consumption' was considered a romantic disease; its sufferers looked pale and it was thought to bestow heightened sensitivity on them. Lord Byron, the most notorious of the Romantic poets, joked that the disease would have ladies saying: 'See that poor Byron – how interesting he looks in dying.' It features in much literature from the time, including *Les Miserables* by Victor Hugo.

References

1. Calmette A, Guérin C, Boquet A, Négre L. *La vaccination préventive contre la tuberculose par le "BCG"*. Masson; 1927.
2. Ottenhoff T, Kaufmann S. Vaccines against tuberculosis: where are we and where do we need to go? PLoS Pathog. 2012;**8**(5):e1002607.
3. UK Enhanced Tuberculosis Surveillance Data. http://webarchive.nationalarchives.gov.uk/20140714073824/http://www.hpa.org.uk/Topics/InfectiousDiseases/InfectionsAZ/Tuberculosis/TBUKSurveillanceData/EnhancedTuberculosisSurveillance/ (all accessed May 30, 2018).
4. Rich AR, McCordock HA. The pathogenesis of tuberculous meningitis. Bull Johns Hopkins Hosp 1933;**52**:5–37.
5. Thwaites GE, Tran TH. Tuberculous meningitis: many questions, too few answers. *Lancet Neurol* 2005;**4**:160–70.
6. Marx GE, Chan ED. Tuberculous meningitis: diagnosis and treatment overview. Tuberc Res Treat 2011;**2011**:798764.
7. Thwaites G, Fisher M, Hemingway C, et al. British Infection Society guidelines for the diagnosis and treatment of tuberculosis of the central nervous system in adults and children. J Infect 2009;**59**:167–87.
8. Thwaites GE, Nguyen DB, Nguyen HD, et al. Dexamethasone for the treatment of tuberculous meningitis in adolescents and adults. N Engl J Med 2004;**351**:1741e51.
9. British Medical Research Council. Streptomycin treatment of tuberculous meningitis. BMJ 1948;**1**:582–97.
10. Fitzgerald DW, Sterling TR, Haas DW. *Mycobacterium* tuberculosis. Extrapulmonary tuberculosis. In: *Mandell, Douglas, and Bennett's Principles and Practice of Infectious Diseases*. 7th ed. Philadelphia, PA: Elsevier; 2010: 3151–3.
11. Saranchuk P, Bedelu M, Heiden D. Retinal examination can help identify disseminated tuberculosis in patients with HIV/AIDS. Clin Infect Dis 2013;**56**:310–12.
12. Whytt R. Observations on the Dropsy in the Brain. Edinburgh: J. Balfour, 1768.

CASE 11

Double Trouble

Michael Bonello

History

A 19-year-old, right-handed female presented to a district hospital following a prodrome of 4 weeks of headaches, retro-orbital pain, chest pain and lethargy. Four days prior to admission, she developed double vision on looking to the extremes of gaze bilaterally, and impaired left facial sensation. Two days before admission she deteriorated, becoming unsteady with weakness and numbness in both lower limbs.

She had no preceding history of diarrhoea or swallowing problems. There was no history of trauma or involvement of her bowel or bladder. However, she did complain of intermittent palpitations. She lived with her parents, and was a non-smoker who did not take any illicit substances. She had received contraceptive implants over the preceding 2 years.

Examination

She had a regular tachycardia with normal heart sounds. Chest examination was normal. Her other vital signs were normal, in particular she was apyrexial.

On neurological examination, she had a complex ophthalmoplegia with impairment of sensation in the first and second divisions of the left trigeminal nerve. In addition she had a left-sided lower motor neuron facial nerve palsy. She had asymmetrical mild arm weakness and mild bilateral symmetrical leg weakness. All her reflexes were absent bilaterally and there was mild impairment of sensation. Marked incoordination of all extremities was also noted.

Initial Differential Diagnosis

A variant of Guillain–Barré syndrome was considered probable, with Miller Fisher syndrome being the most likely. Other possibilities included:

- Brainstem lesions, although that would not explain the bilateral lower motor neuron signs
- Infectious causes that can affect the brainstem/cranial nerves, including neuroborreliosis, diphtheria
- Neuromuscular junction disorders, such as myasthenia gravis or botulism, although this would not explain the sensory features
- Thiamine deficiency causing Wernicke's encephalopathy, although this would not explain the extensive bilateral lower motor neuron signs.

Results of Initial Investigations

Routine bloods, inflammatory markers and an autoimmune profile were normal. Viral serology was consistent with a recent cytomegalovirus infection. Both Cytomegalovirus (CMV) IgG and IgM were detected on enzyme-linked immunosorbent assay testing. CMV IgG avidity was low, which suggested a primary CMV infection had occurred within the 3 months prior to the sample being tested. Serology for HIV was negative.

Cerebrospinal fluid (CSF) studies demonstrated an opening pressure of 16 cm H_2O and the CSF white cell count was 1/mm^3, red cell count 0/mm^3, protein 1 g/l and CSF glucose was 3.3 mmol/l.

A magnetic resonance imaging head scan was normal.

Nerve conduction studies were undertaken 4 weeks after the onset of symptoms (**Table 11.1**). These were consistent with patchy demyelination, mainly in the form of conduction block, involving the left median and ulnar nerves. The distal latencies and conduction velocities were only very mildly abnormal. The responses in the lower limbs showed very patchy demyelination, particularly in the left peroneal nerve more proximally. The motor amplitudes were within normal limits, apart from the responses recorded from the foot. The facial responses showed reduced amplitudes, but normal conduction. There was also evidence of proximal demyelination in the F waves in both upper and lower limbs with absent/increased F-wave latencies. These neurophysiological results were consistent with a demyelinating Guillain–Barré syndrome such as Miller Fisher syndrome.

Results of Definitive Investigations

A panel of anti-ganglioside antibodies were analysed in serum and anti-GQ1b was positive.

Diagnosis

Miller Fisher syndrome, following cytomegalovirus infections.

Table 11.1 Findings from nerve conduction studies undertaken 4 weeks after the onset of symptoms.

Median motor conduction (APB to axilla)	**Right**	**Left**	**Unit**	**Normal range**
Latency APB–wrist	4.7	4.3	ms	2.0–4.4
Amplitude APB–wrist	7.5	**10.2**	mV	4.2–20.0
Amplitude APB–C fossa	7.4	**5.1**	mV	4.2–20.0
Velocity (Med L1–med L2)	58	48		
Amplitude APB–axillae	7.6	6.9	ms	
Velocity (Med L2–med L3)	48	48		
F-wave latency ApB	**35.8**	**40.7**	ms	20.0–31.0
Ulnar ADM motor conduction to axilla	**Right**	**Left**	**Unit**	**Normal range**
Latency ADM–wrist	–xxx–	3.3	ms	2.0–3.5
Amplitude ADM–wrist	–xxx–	**10.2**	mV	5.6–25.0
Amplitude ADM–below epi	–xxx–	**9.0**	mV	5.6–25.0
Velocity (ULN L1–ULN L2)	–xxx–	57		
Amplitude ADM–above epi	–xxx–	**5.6**	mV	5.6–25.0
Velocity (ULN L2–ULN L3)	–xxx–	43		
Amplitude ADM–axilla	–xxx–	**5.1**	mV	5.6–25.0
Velocity (ULN L3–ULN L4)	–xxx–	50		
F-wave latency ADM	–xxx–	**0.0**	ms	30.0–56.0
Peroneal EDB motor conduction	**Right**	**Left**	**Unit**	**Normal range**
Latency EDB–ankle	–xxx–	4.4	ms	3.0–5.7
Amplitude EDB–ankle	–xxx–	**1.8**	mV	2.2–10.0
Amplitude EDB–head of fibula	–xxx–	**1.0**	mV	2.2–10.0
Velocity (Per L1–Per L2)	–xxx–	42		
Amplitude EDB–pop. fossa	–xxx–	**0.9**	mV	2.2–10.0
Velocity (Per L2–Per L3)	–xxx–	33		
F-wave latency EDB	–xxx–	**0.0**	ms	30.0–56.0
Peroneal tib. anterior motor conduction	**Right**	**Left**	**Unit**	**Normal range**
Latency tib. ant–head of fibula	–xxx–	2.7	ms	
Amplitude tib. ant–head of fibula	–xxx–	3.6	mV	
Amplitude tib. ant–pop. fossa	–xxx–	3.3	mV	
Velocity (Per TA L1–PER TA L2)	–xxx–	71		
Tibial abductor hallucis motor conduction	**Right**	**Left**	**Unit**	**Normal range**
Latency abductor hallucis–ankle	–xxx–	3.8	ms	3.0–5.7
Amplitude abductor hallucis–ankle	–xxx–	5.9	mV	2.6–30.0
Amplitude abductor hallucis–pop. fossa	–xxx–	5.1	mV	2.6–30.0
Velocity (Tib L1–Tib L2)	–xxx–	44		
F-wave latency AH	–xxx–	**0.0**	Ms	30.0–56.0
Facial motor conduction	**Right**	**Left**	**Unit**	**Normal range**
Latency orbicularis oculi	–xxx–	3.3	ms	–
Median sensory conduction palm–wrist	**Right**	**Left**	**Unit**	**Normal range**
Latency wrist–palm	1.9	1.7	ms	1.5–2.2
Amplitude wrist–palm	52.6	57.8	µV	40.0–120.0
Ulnar sensory conduction palm–wrist	**Right**	**Left**	**Unit**	**Normal range**

Table 11.1 (cont.)

Median motor conduction (APB to axilla)	Right	Left	Unit	Normal range
Latency wrist–palm	1.9	2.0	ms	1.5–2.2
Amplitude wrist–palm	19.8	20.1	μV	15.0–50.0
Radial sensory conduction	**Right**	**Left**	**Unit**	**Normal range**
Latency superficial radial sensory	–xxx–	2.5	Ms	
Amplitude superficial radial sensory	–xxx–	25.2	μV	
Sural sensory conduction	**Right**	**Left**	**Unit**	**Normal range**
Latency Sural Sensory	–xxx–	2.8	ms	2.0–4.2
Amplitude Sural Sensory	–xxx–	19.0	μV	5.0–40.0
Superficial peroneal sensory conduction	**Right**	**Left**	**Unit**	**Normal range**
Latency sup. peroneal	–xxx–	2.8	ms	2.0–3.4
Amplitude sup. peroneal	–xxx–	13.3	μV	5.0–35.0

Management and Outcome

The patient was commenced on a 5-day course of intravenous immunoglobulin (IVIG), given prophylaxis against deep venous thrombosis, and observed on a cardiac monitor. Two days after starting IVIG she became more fatigued, with bilateral facial weakness and required further intensive monitoring on the high-dependency unit. She started making spontaneous recovery soon after. She commenced physiotherapy and occupational therapy and was discharged to a rehabilitation bed, and ultimately home.

Discussion

Miller Fisher syndrome is a variant of Guillain–Barré syndrome, which presents with the clinical triad of an acute external ophthalmoplegia, ataxia and areflexia, as seen in this patient [1]. It accounts for about 5% of patients with Guillain–Barré syndrome, and has an incidence of about 1 per million.

Like Guillain–Barré syndrome, Miller Fisher syndrome is an autoimmune disease that may follow infectious or neoplastic disorders, or may be a primary autoimmune condition associated with other autoimmune diseases. Infectious associations with Miller Fisher syndrome include *Campylobacter jejuni, Haemophilus influenza, Staphylococcus aureus, Mycoplasma pneumonia, Coxiella burnetii*, Epstein–Barr virus, varicella zoster virus, mumps virus and, as in this case, CMV [2]. Antibodies generated against the pathogen are thought to also react against ganglioside lipid molecules on the surface of neurons, through the process of 'molecular mimicry' – i.e. a similarity between the molecular structures (**Figure 11.1**). The role of anti-ganglioside antibodies in the pathogenesis of Miller Fisher syndrome was recognised in the early 1990s [3] and more than 80% of patients have anti-GQ1b antibodies [4]. Antibodies to GQ1b also cross-react to lipopolysaccharides found on microorganisms such as *Campylobacter jejuni* [5]. The GQ1b ganglioside is present on the surface of Schwann cells on cranial nerves, especially the oculomotor nerves, and the presynaptic terminals of the neuromuscular junctions.

Albuminocytological dissociation of the CSF (i.e. elevated CSF protein with a relatively normal CSF white cell count) is a typical feature in Miller Fisher syndrome and other forms of Guillain–Barré syndrome, such as acute demyelinating encephalomyelitis and Bickerstaff's brainstem encephalitis. However, in the hyper-acute phase of the disease CSF may be normal. Nevertheless, anti-GQ1b antibodies may still be positive early on during the disease.

The interpretation of the findings from nerve conduction studies in Miller Fisher syndrome are not as straightforward as in Guillain–Barré syndrome [6]. The consensus in the literature is that sensory changes predominate with significant loss of amplitudes, only mild motor and sensory conduction velocity slowing and reduction or loss of facial motor responses with evidence of denervation in cranial muscles on electromyography [7].

As in a number of other rare neurological conditions there are no randomised controlled trials evaluating treatment in Miller Fisher syndrome. IVIG or plasma exchange, which are effective in Guillain–Barré syndrome, are reported to hasten recovery in a number of case reports, although a large retrospective study found that neither influenced patients' outcomes [8], and the disease usually runs

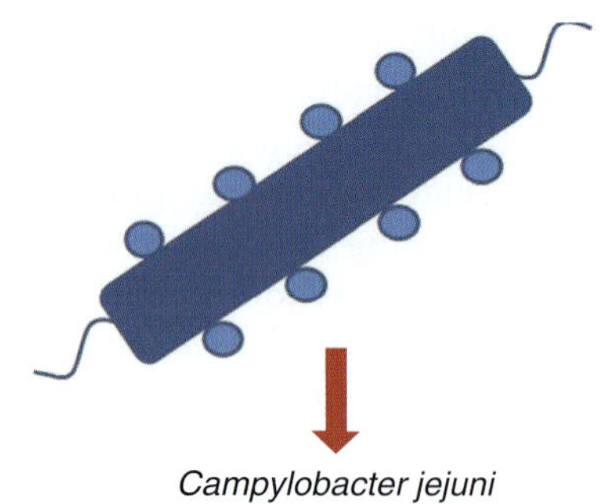

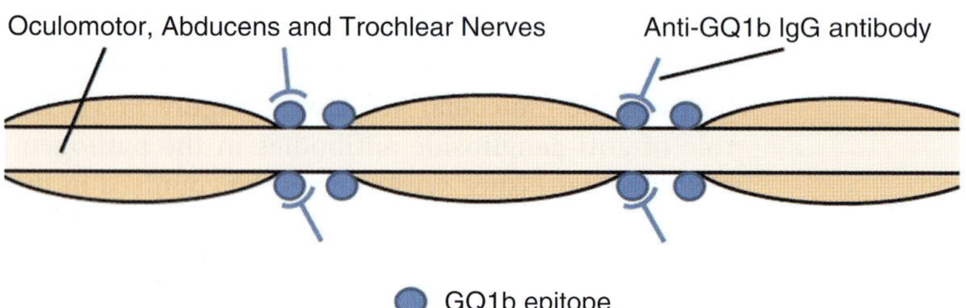

Figure 11.1. Postulated pathogenesis of Miller Fisher syndrome. An infecting organism (here *C. jejuni*) which has GQ1b-like lipopolysaccharide on its surface triggers the production of anti-GQ1b antibodies; these target the invading pathogen but also attack the GQ1b on the oculomotor nerves and result in the clinical presentation of Miller Fisher syndrome. (Adapted from [5] with permission of John Wiley and Sons, Inc.)

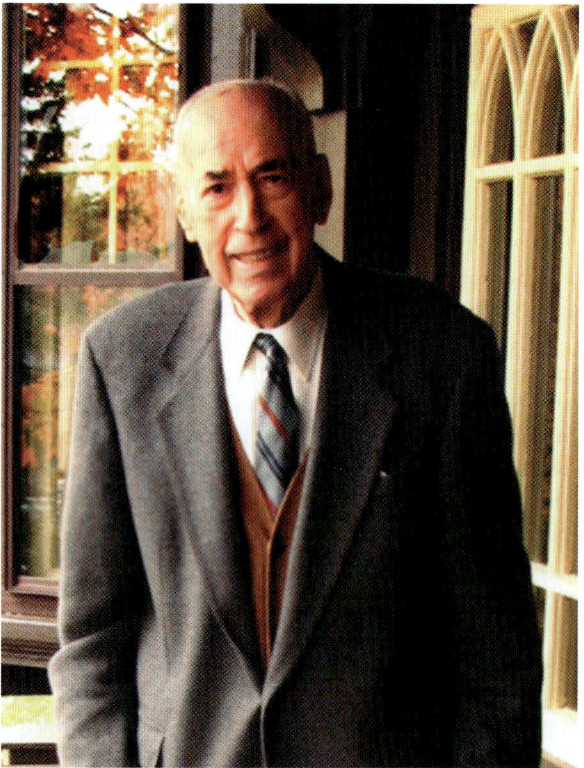

Figure 11.2. Dr C. Miller Fisher on the occasion of his 93rd birthday.

a benign course, as recognised by Dr Miller Fisher in his original report:

> the presenting symptoms and signs were most alarming for the attending physician on each occasion – unnecessarily so, since the course of the illness appears to be benign (Dr Miller Fisher, **Figure 11.2**, [1]).

Key Points

- Miller Fisher syndrome is a variant of Guillain–Barré syndrome, which presents with the clinical triad of an acute external ophthalmoplegia, ataxia and areflexia
- CSF and nerve conduction studies may be normal, especially in the acute phase, so they should be repeated if there is a strong suspicion and the diagnosis is still uncertain.
- Finding anti-GQ1b antibodies in the serum confirms the diagnosis.
- The disease generally runs a benign course with proper supportive care, including early involvement of critical care teams.

Looking Back

The disease is named after Dr Charles Miller Fisher, a canadian neurologist who was working at Massachusetts General Hospital and Harvard University Boston when he described three cases of 'An Unusual Variant of Acute Idiopathic Polyneuritis (Syndrome of Ophthalmoplegia, Ataxia and Areflexia)' in the *New England Journal of Medicine* in 1956.

Did You Know?

Although Dr Miller Fisher is well known for his eponymous disease, by far his biggest contribution to neurology was in the area of stroke medicine, where he was the first to describe transient ischaemic attacks, and prove the link between atrial fibrillation, clot formation in the heart and subsequent stroke.

References

1. Fisher M. An unusual variant of acute idiopathic polyneuritis (syndrome of ophthalmoplegia, ataxia and areflexia). New Engl J Med 1956;**255**:57–65.
2. Yuki N. Infectious origins of, and molecular mimicry in, Guillain–Barré and Fisher syndromes. Lancet Infect Dis 2001;**1**:29–37.
3. Willison HJ, Veitch J, Paterson G, Kennedy PG. Miller Fisher syndrome is associated with serum antibodies to GQ1b ganglioside. J Neurol Neurosurg Psychiatry 1993;**56**:204–6.
4. Nishimoto Y, Odaka M, Hirata K, Yuki N. Usefulness of anti-GQ1b IgG antibody testing in Fisher syndrome compared with cerebrospinal fluid examination. J Neuroimmunol 2004;**148**:200–5.
5. Yuki N, Taki T, Takahashi M, et al. Molecular mimicry between GQ1b ganglioside and lipopolysaccharides of Campylobacter jejuni isolated from patients with Fishers syndrome. Ann Neurol 1994; **36**: 791–3. Fross RD, Daube JR.
6. Fross RD, Daube JR. Neuropathy in the Miller Fisher syndrome: clinical and electrophysiologic findings. Neurology 1987;**37**:1493.
7. Mori M, Kuwabara S, Yuki N. Fisher syndrome: clinical features, immunopathogenesis and management. Expert Rev Neurother 2012;**12**:39–51.
8. Ackerman RH. Celebrating the life of C. Miller Fisher. Int J Stroke 2012;**7**:444–6.

CASE 12

Hiking into Danger

Aleš Chrdle

History

A 19-year-old, previously fit and well, young woman presented to hospital with fever, myalgia, headache and vomiting.

She had been seen by her family doctor a week earlier and had just finished a 7-day course of oral penicillin for presumed streptococcal throat infection. The referral letter stated that she had first presented with fever, sore throat, general fatigue and myalgia, which all settled within 3 days of starting oral penicillin.

For the 2 days before hospital admission she reported fevers over 38.5°C and severe headache, which did not respond to paracetamol and ibuprofen. She also complained of pain in her right arm and shoulder.

She had recently returned from her summer holidays touring the Czech Republic, Austria and Hungary, where she did some camping, hiking and horse riding with her friends. She did not recall any tick bite or skin rash. She denied any new sexual contact. She was a non-smoker and drank socially. She denied recent use of any illegal drugs.

Review of bloods done by her family doctor a week earlier revealed: white blood cells (WBC) 3.6 × 10^9/l (neutrophils 2.0 × 10^9/l, lymphocytes 1.5 × 10^9/l), platelets 113 × 10^9/l, alanine aminotransferase (ALT) 198 IU/l, C-reactive protein (CRP) 26 mg/l. Infectious mononucleosis monospot test negative.

Examination

The young lady was visibly unwell. Her rate of speech was slightly slow with some delay before answering questions, but no signs of dysphasia or confusion.

Although her throat looked sore, her tonsils were not enlarged and there was no exudate. There was no apparent lymphadenopathy. There was mild neck stiffness.

Her chest and abdominal examination were unremarkable. There were no rashes or other skin lesions.

Overall, she was clammy and shaky, had photophobia and appeared hypersensitive to noise. There was fine tremor of her fingers and marked past-pointing. Her heel–shin coordination test was grossly abnormal. She was unstable when standing and walking. The cranial nerves were intact. She had no nystagmus.

Brisk reflexes were elicited in her right-sided limbs, while tone, power and sensation were symmetrical and normal on all four limbs. Both her plantars were down-going.

Initial Differential Diagnosis

- Viral encephalitis, due to herpes simplex virus (HSV), tick-borne encephalitis virus (TBEV), West Nile virus (WNV), HIV seroconversion illness, other
- Bacterial meningitis/brain abscess
- Vasculitis/venous sinus thrombosis
- Leptospirosis
- Lyme disease
- Alcohol/drug withdrawal or intoxication

Results of Initial Investigations

White blood count 12.6 × 10^9/l, haemoglobin 156 mg/l, platelets 265 × 10^9/l. Serum urea, creatinine and electrolytes were unremarkable, alanine aminotransferase 76 IU/l, bilirubin and other liver enzymes were normal. The C-reactive protein was 45 mg/l.

Non-enhanced computer tomography (CT) of the brain did not show any abnormalities and a lumbar puncture (LP) was performed: cerebrospinal fluid (CSF) was clear and colourless, opening pressure 24 cm H_2O; lymphocytes 86 cells/μl, neutrophils 26 cells/μl, red cells 36 cells/μl, protein 9.5 mg/l, CSF/serum glucose ratio 0.5 and CSF lactate 2.0 mmol/l (serum lactate 1.2 mmol/l).

Progress and Further Investigations

Over the next 3 days her headache, nausea and vomiting seemed to improve with aciclovir and symptomatic treatment; however, she remained pyrexial. She developed a cough after drinking or eating, and weakness in her right arm. Neurological examination revealed poor swallowing and reduced power in the right arm, specifically Medical Research Council power score 2/5 for abduction, adduction, extension and flexion of her right shoulder, 3/5 in her right biceps muscle and 4/5 of her triceps, with normal power in her forearm and fingers. Her right biceps tendon reflex was reduced, while her triceps reflex was equivocal and distally the reflexes were normal.

Reflexes, power and tone in the remaining three limbs were normal. Sensation was normal in all four limbs.

Refined Differential Diagnosis

At this stage the clinical progression suggested involvement of the brain stem and right cervical spinal cord, which thus altered the differential diagnosis:

- Poliomyelitis-like syndrome, due to TBEV, WNV, or vaccine-associated paralytic poliomyelitis
- Pyogenic lesion of the cervical spine/ retropharyngeal abscess extending to the brachial plexus
- Brain stem lesion such as tumour/abscess/ vasculitis/stroke
- Rabies
- Acute disseminated encephalomyelitis
- Transverse myelitis
- Limbic encephalitis/paraneoplastic meningoencephalitis
- Hashimoto encephalopathy

Results of Definitive Investigations

Magnetic resonance imaging of her head/cervical spine was unremarkable. Chest X-ray showed an elevated right diaphragm. The results of her repeat LP on day 4 of admission are summarised in **Table 12.1**.

Polymerase chain reaction (PCR) of both samples of her CSF was negative for HSV1, HSV2, varicella zoster virus, Epstein–Barr virus, adenoviruses and enteroviruses. Serology for TBEV, WNV, Lyme disease, leptospirosis, HIV antibody and syphilis *Treponema pallidum* particle agglutination assay (TPPA) taken the first day of her admission were all negative. HIV was also negative by PCR.

Table 12.1 Summary of CSF studies.

CSF studies	Day 1	Day 4
Opening pressure (cm H_2O)	24	20
Appearance	Clear, colourless	Clear, colourless
Lymphocytes (cells/μl)	86	102
Neutrophils (cells/μl)	26	2
Red blood cells (cells/μl)	36	524
Protein (mg/l)	9.5	12
Glucose CSF/serum	0.5	0.6
Lactate (mmol/l)	2.0	1.2
Viruses PCR	Negative	Negative

Repeat serology taken 1 week into her admission showed strongly positive Immunoglobulin (Ig) M and positive IgG for TBEV.

Diagnosis

Meningoencephalomyelitis caused by tick-borne encephalitis virus, affecting the brainstem, cerebellum and anterior horns C2–6 resulting in weakness of the pharyngeal muscles, phrenic muscle, muscles of the shoulder, biceps and triceps muscles.

Management and Outcome

The patient was transferred to a high-dependency unit, a nasogastric tube was inserted for enteral feeding due to the risk of aspiration, and intensive respiratory physiotherapy commenced. Symptomatic and supportive management included pain relief, intravenous fluids and electrolytes; dexamethasone 8 mg 6-hourly was added for 4 days with subsequent tapering over the next 2 weeks. Her fever rapidly resolved and over the following days she did not develop any further neurological features; in fact, the extent of her previous cognitive impairment and ataxia became apparent as her slow rate of speech and delay in responses, seen in the first week of her stay, resolved and she became much brighter. Gradually her swallowing improved as did movement in the right shoulder and arm. She was discharged after 27 days in hospital, to continue with outpatient physiotherapy. During follow-up, neurological deficit improved so that after 6 months she was able to comb her hair with her right hand. She missed nearly half a year of school due to poor concentration, headaches when stressed and fatigue, as well as her residual right arm proximal weakness (**Figure 12.1**).

Prevention

TBEV is prevalent over large parts of Europe and Asia (**Figure 12.2**).

The disease is prevented by vaccination, avoiding tick bites by wearing appropriate clothing when venturing outdoors in endemic areas, and promptly removing any ticks discovered on the skin (**Box 12.1**).

Box 12.1. Tick Removal.

The use of blunt, medium-tipped, angled forceps offers the best results. Following tick removal, the bite area should be inspected carefully for any retained mouthparts, which should be excised. The area is then cleaned with antiseptic solution, and the patient is instructed to monitor for signs of local or systemic illness.

Figure 12.1. Six months after admission, the patient has been asked to put both arms above her head (A), and to leave them resting (B).

A

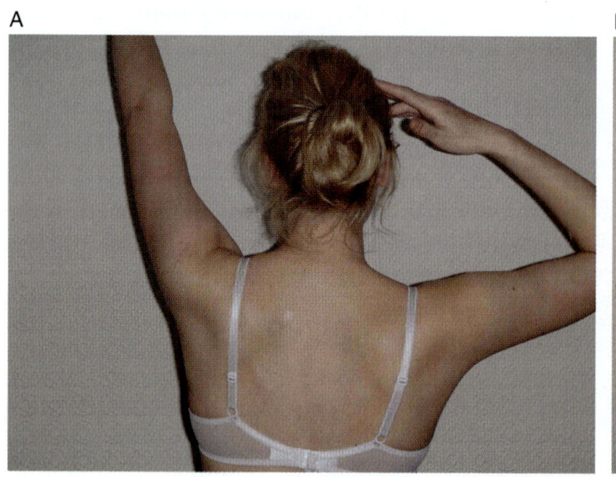

B

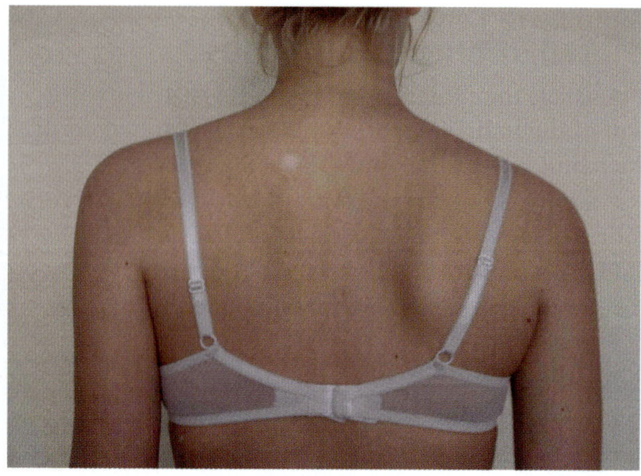

There is residual inability of upward rotation of the right scapula, limiting her ability to raise her arms (A). With the arms at rest, there is residual right shoulder weakness with prominence (winging) of the right scapula (B). (Photos: Aleš Chrdle, with patient's permission.)

Table 12.2 Vaccination schedule.

Name	FSME-Immun*	Encepur	TBE Moscow	EnceVir
Manufacturer	Pfizer, Inc., Austria	GlaxoSmithKline, Germany	Chumakov Institute, Moscow, Russia	Microgen, Tomsk, Russia
Year of approval	1976	1994	1982	2001
Standard regimen (3 doses)	0/1–3/9–12 months	0/1–3/9–12 months	0/1–7/12 months	0/5–7/16–18 months
Rapid/accelerated regimen	0/day 14/month 5–12	0/day 7/day 21/month 12–18	n/a	0/day 21–35***/day 42–70***/month 5–12
Paediatric use	1–15 years**	1–12 years	From 3 years of age	From 3 years of age
Paediatric formulation	FSME-Immun Junior (half of adult dose)	Encepur-Children (half of adult dose)	Same dose as adults	n/a, recommended to half the adult dose
Availability	EU including the UK, Russia, Canada	EU, Russia, not available in the UK	Russia, Ukraine, Kazakhstan, Belarus	Russia, Ukraine, Kazakhstan, Belarus
Booster	Every 5 years	Every 5 years	Every 3 years	Every 3 years
Booster in > 60 years of age	Every 3 years	Every 3 years	Every 3 years	Every 3 years

* FSME is *Fruhsommer meningoenzephalitis,* German for early summer meningoencephalitis, a pseudonym for tick-borne encephalitis. The Austrian FSME-Immun vaccine is marketed as 'TicoVac' in the UK.

** From 6 months of age in high-risk areas (off label).

*** Double dose.

Vaccination is recommended for all those who will engage in outdoor activities in the endemic areas (**Table 12.2**) [1]. The vaccination schedules require three jabs with boosters thereafter. The manufacturers offer conventional regimens, as well as rapid/accelerated vaccination regimens suitable for travellers. Vaccination covers all subtypes of TBEV. The vaccines are highly effective (95–99%) and safe.

All four vaccines are cell-cultured, inactivated TBEV, adjuvanted with aluminium hydroxide, administered by intramuscular injection.

Rapid or accelerated schedules for travellers: depending on the choice of TBE vaccine, the manufacturers recommend either an accelerated schedule of immunisation on day 0, day 14 and month 5–7, or a rapid schedule of immunisation on days 0, 7 and 21. The effectiveness after two doses of the Western vaccines is estimated over 90% in rapid/accelerated schedule and nearly 100% after three doses with rapid decline in titres requiring finishing full vaccination regimen. Adapted from [2].

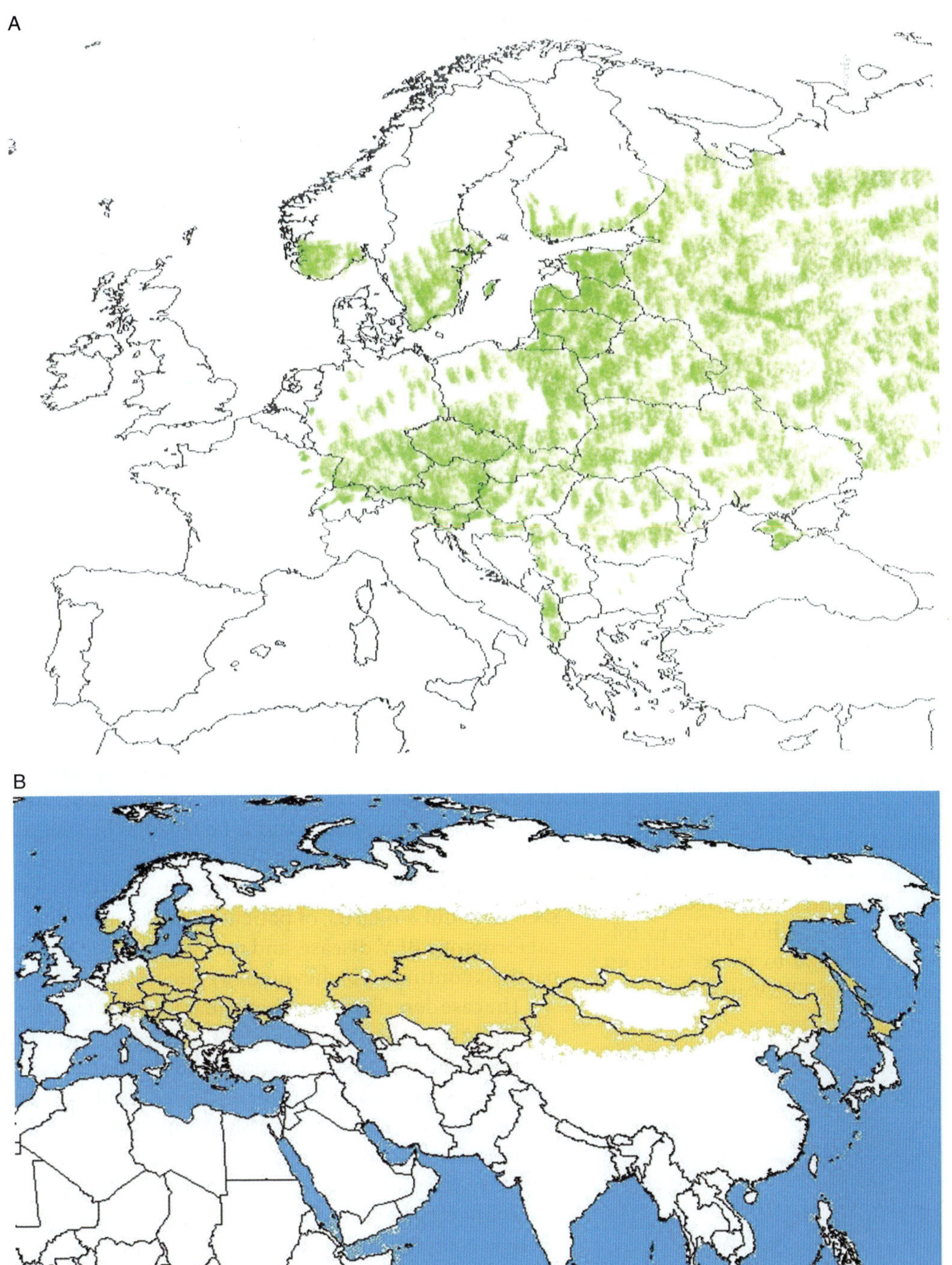

Figure 12.2. Tick-borne encephalitis in Europe/Eurasia. (A) Endemic areas for TBEV in ticks in Europe. Adapted from [2]. (B) Areas of known occurrence of TBEV across Europe and Asia. Adapted with permission from [2].

At one stage post-exposure vaccination (i.e. giving people a vaccination after a tick bite before they develop symptoms), or post-exposure treatment with specific immunoglobulin were considered potentially useful, but they are no longer recommended.

Discussion

Tick borne encephalitis (TBE) is an acute febrile illness with neurological involvement that is caused by the flavivirus, TBEV. Other flaviviruses include the mosquito-borne West Nile and Japanese encephalitis viruses. There are three subtypes of the TBEV – European/Western, Siberian and Far Eastern. The distribution of the virus in ticks and endemic areas of human disease (in Europe and Asia) are shown on the map in **Figure 12.2**. Closely related tick-borne flaviviruses include Loupin Ill, which affects sheep in the Scottish highlands, and occasionally humans, and Powassan virus, which causes a similar disease in North America.

Humans become infected with TBEV following the bite of an infected tick. Occasionally humans develop the disease after drinking unpasteurized milk and dairy products from cows, sheep or goats which are infected with the virus; this used to be known as biphasic milk fever. There is a theoretical risk of inter-human transmission via blood transfusion or breastfeeding from a viraemic individual, but these have never been documented. The vector as well as a reservoir for the virus is the sheep tick (also known as the castor bean tick *Ixodes ricinus*) in Central/Eastern Europe (**Figure 12.3**) and the taiga tick (*Ixodes persulcatus*) in Siberian and Far Eastern regions; both species of tick overlap in Northern Europe and the European part of Russia. The circulation of the virus in tick populations in forested areas of moderate climate is maintained by co-feeding on small vertebrates and game deer, who appear to tolerate persistent viraemia for days to weeks without major illness. The prevalence of TBEV in ticks in the endemic areas ranges from 0.5% to 30%. The risk of TBE infection after a single tick bite is estimated to be less than 1:100 [2,3].

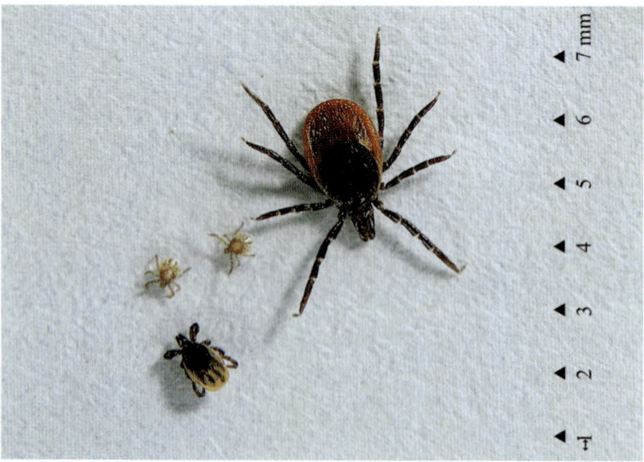

Figure 12.3. Unengorged *Ixodes ricinus* ticks in different developmental stages. From top anticlockwise: one adult female, two larvae, and one nymph. Reproduced with permission from [3].

There are about 10,000 cases of TBE reported annually worldwide, Russia alone accounting for nearly half of this number. In Europe, Austria, southern Germany, the Czech Republic and Slovenia, along with Baltic States and southern parts of Scandinavia are the most affected regions. Depending on the climate, there is a seasonal pattern of TBE, spanning from March to November, with one or two peaks [2,4].

The clinical presentation of the disease depends on whether the meninges, brain and/or spinal cord are predominantly affected; meningitis accounts for about 50% of cases, meningoencephalitis 40%, and meningo-encephalomyelitis 10%. Mortality ranges from 1–2% in central Europe to 5–20% in the Far East. Long-term morbidity is significant, especially in the encephalitic and encephalomyelitic forms, and may last from months to years, ranging from post-encephalitic syndrome (cognitive impairment, poor concentration, headaches, fatigue, ataxia, neuropsychiatric disorders and mood disorders) to permanent palsies and seizures [5]. Disease severity and long-term disability increases with the patient's age, although a small subgroup of paediatric patients may have significant long-term sequelae [6]. A 'chronic form' of TBE has been described in Russia, and is believed to be caused only by the Siberian subtype of the virus. Spontaneous regular contractions (myoclonic jerks) of the limbs are seen in about a quarter of patients with all neurological forms of TBEV disease, and may persist as epilepsia partialis continua (Kozhevnikov's epilepsy).

The case described here shows many typical features of TBE [2–8]. About a third of patients with TBE will not notice a tick bite. Mere exposure to the outdoors in the endemic area within the incubation period of 7–28 days is sufficient to consider TBE. About two-thirds of cases have a bi-phasic illness: initially there is a non-specific viraemic illness that may include leukopaenia, thrombocytopaenia and elevated transaminases; then there is complete resolution of symptoms from a few days to a couple of weeks before fever recurs, this time with neurological impairment (**Figure 12.4**). At the onset of the second phase, leukocytes and CRP may be elevated, as they were in this case; diagnostic serology changes may lag behind the clinical manifestations. Serology shows cross-reactions with other flaviviruses, especially in the IgG class. Initial CSF studies may reveal a predominance of lymphocytes or neutrophils with

Figure 12.4. Biphasic course of tick-borne encephalitis – temperature chart.

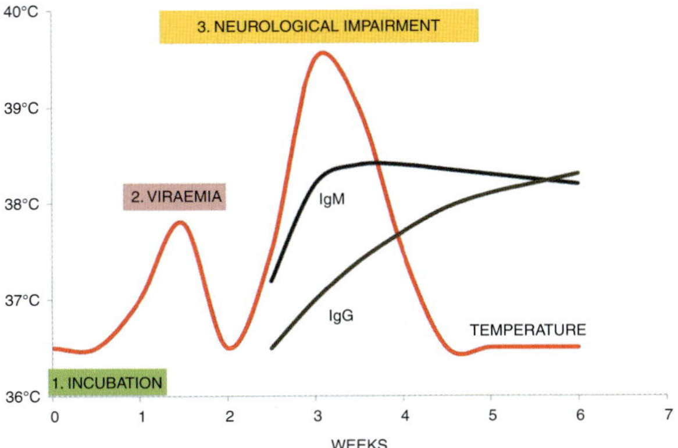

After 7–14 days' incubation there is 2–4 days of viraemia with non-specific flu-like symptoms (fever, myalgia, headache), thrombopaenia, leukopaenia and transaminitis. This is followed by a symptom-free interval usually less than 1 week, but up to 30 days. The second phase manifests with high fever, severe headache and neurological impairment. Serum TBEV-specific antibodies develop usually at the onset of the second phase.

a borderline elevation of lactate. The brain regions mostly affected by the virus include the basal ganglia, caudate nucleus, brainstem, cerebellum and thalamus; hence, ataxia including fine tremor with impaired balance and reduced level of consciousness are the main symptoms of encephalitis. The anterior horns of the spinal cord may be affected in the myelitic form resulting in polio-like disease; this predominantly affects the proximal parts of the upper limbs. Imaging is usually unremarkable; however, T2 and turbo FLAIR sequences may show non-specific lesions in these regions. The diagnosis is confirmed by either positive IgM or a significant raise in IgG titres of TBE-specific antibodies. Treatment for TBE is only symptomatic and supportive. The use of corticosteroids, although widespread in some highly endemic countries, is controversial; there have been no randomised controlled trials, and one observational study did not find any benefit [9].

Key Points

- Tick-borne encephalitis should be considered in any person with fever, headache and/or neurological symptoms who recently travelled to Central and Eastern Europe, Scandinavia, Russia, northern China and northern Japan, especially if they were hiking or camping in forest areas.
- About one-third of patients are not aware of a tick bite.
- Treatment of this flavivirus infection is supportive and symptomatic.
- Pre-exposure vaccination is safe and highly effective, and should be offered to any person living or travelling to the above regions who might be engaging in outdoor activities.

Looking Back

Although first clinically reported in 1931 by H. Schneider in Austria, it was Soviet scientist L. Zilber in 1939 who demonstrated that the viral illness is transmitted to humans by ticks.

Austria developed the first successful vaccine and using extensive health promotion campaigns from the 1980s achieved over 85% vaccination coverage in the Austrian population with a reduction of TBE incidence rate from 5.7 to 0.9/100,000 [10].

Did You Know?

The risk of acquiring tick-borne encephalitis in endemic regions of Europe and Asia is comparable to the risk of acquiring *Plasmodium vivax* malaria or typhoid fever in endemic regions of India [11]. In the 1960s, because of the observation that TBEV can cause chronic progressive inflammation of motor neurons, it was postulated that a virus may be the cause of motor neuron disease (amyotrophic lateral sclerosis), but the theory was subsequently discounted.

References

1. Chrdle A, Chmelik V, Ruzek D. Tick-borne encephalitis: what travellers should know when visiting an endemic country. Hum Vaccin Immunother. 2016; 12:2694–99. doi: 10.1080/21645515.2016.1218098.
2. Kollaritsch H, Krasilnikov V, Holzmann H, et al. Background Document on Vaccines and Vaccination

against Tick-borne Encephalitis (TBE) WHO Position Paper. www.who.int/immunization/sage/6_TBE_backgr_18_Mar_net_apr_2011.pdf (accessed May 30, 2018).

3. Lindquist L, Vapalahti O. Tick-borne encephalitis. Lancet 2008;**371**:1861–71.
4. Růžek D, Dobler G, Donoso Mantke O. Tick-borne encephalitis: pathogenesis and clinical implications. Travel Med Infect Dis 2010;**8**:223–32.
5. Kaiser R. Tick-borne encephalitis: clinical findings and prognosis in adults. Wien Med Wochenschr 2012;**162**:239–43.
6. Rostasy K. Tick-borne encephalitis in children. Wien Med Wochenschr 2012;**162**:244–7.
7. Studahl M, Lindquist L, Eriksson BM, et al. Acute viral infections of the central nervous system in immunocompetent adults: diagnosis and management. Drugs 2013;**73**:131–58.
8. Mansfield KL, Johnson N, Phipps LP, et al. Tick-borne encephalitis virus – a review of an emerging zoonosis. J Gen Virol 2009;**90**:1781–94.
9. Mickiene A, Laiskonis A, Günther G, et al. Tick-borne encephalitis in an area of high endemicity in Lithuania: disease severity and long-term prognosis. Clin Infect Dis 2002;**35**:650–8.
10. Heinz FX, Stiasny K, Holzmann H, et al. Vaccination and tick-borne encephalitis, central Europe. Emerg Infect Dis 2013;**19**:69–76.
11. Rendi-Wagner P. Risk and prevention of tick-borne encephalitis in travelers. J Travel Med 2004;**11**:307–12.

CASE 13

A Runny Nose, Running into Trouble

Theresa Cole

History

An 11-year-old boy presented to hospital with a 10-day history of being unwell with headache, fever and vomiting. Two weeks earlier he had been seen by his general practitioner and diagnosed with a viral upper respiratory tract infection, having presented with low-grade fever, nasal discharge and sinus pain. He had continued to worsen following this, complaining of constant headache, becoming more lethargic and vomiting multiple times per day. Over the 24 hours preceding admission he had become unsteady on his feet.

Examination

On examination he had a temperature of 39°C. He was tachycardic with a heart rate of 130 beats per minute and his capillary refill time was normal. He was drowsy, with a Glasgow coma score of 13/15: he was opening his eyes to speech, following commands, but was obviously confused when speaking. Neurological examination of the limbs demonstrated increased tone and moderately reduced power in his right arm and right leg. The deep tendon reflexes were exaggerated on the right side and the plantar response on the right was extensor.

Initial Differential Diagnosis

Infectious causes:

- Meningoencephalitis
- Subdural empyema with cerebritis
- Brain abscess

Other (non-infectious/para-infectious) causes:

- Venous sinus thrombosis with venous infarction
- Acute disseminated encephalomyelitis

Results of Initial Investigations

Initial bloods showed a white cell count of 29×10^9/l (neutrophils 26) and the C-reactive protein (CRP) was 282 mg/l. Electrolytes were normal.

A CT head scan was performed (**Figure 13.1**).

Diagnosis

Subdural empyema secondary to bacterial maxillary sinusitis.

Management and Outcome

The neurosurgeons performed a craniotomy and washout of the subdural empyema. He also had a washout of his left maxillary and ethmoid sinuses performed by ear, nose and throat surgeons. Pus from the subdural empyema was sent to the microbiology laboratory and grew *Streptococcus intermedius*.

Following surgery the patient was admitted to the intensive care unit for intracranial pressure monitoring.

On weaning off sedation he had a generalised tonic–clonic seizure, which required treatment with intravenous lorazepam. A follow-up computer tomography (CT) scan was performed urgently (**Figure 13.2**).

This revealed a venous sinus thrombosis in the sagittal sinus and he was anticoagulated with low molecular weight heparin.

He made a good recovery in terms of motor function of his right side and was independent with minimal residual weakness on discharge from hospital.

Discussion

Subdural empyema is a relatively uncommon but serious infection, which historically had very high mortality. There is a bi-modal distribution with a peak in infancy and a larger peak in adolescence and young adults, with 70% occurring in the second or third decade [1].

Sinusitis is the most common predisposing factor for subdural empyema, as it was in this case, and in particular frontal sinusitis is most often implicated. Subdural empyema can also occur following mastoiditis, otitis media and meningitis, particularly in infants [2]. The causative organisms depend on the predisposing factors, with organisms from the *Streptococcus milleri* group the most common [1]. However, *Neisseria meningitidis, Streptococcus pneumoniae* and, now rarely, *Haemophilus influenza* can cause a subdural empyema following meningitis [3]. Also, staphylococcal infection can result from surgery or trauma [4]. Other organisms including *Pseudomonas aeruginosa* and clostridia have been implicated in subdural empyema after neurosurgery [1]. Anaerobes are difficult to culture but can also sometimes be isolated [5].

Figure 13.1. (A) Contrast-enhanced coronal CT image and (B) axial contrast-enhanced CT image of an 11-year-old boy presenting with fever, confusion and right-sided pyramidal weakness.

A

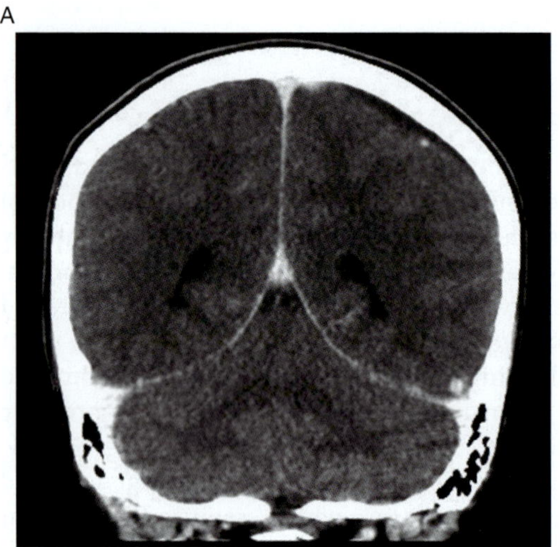

B

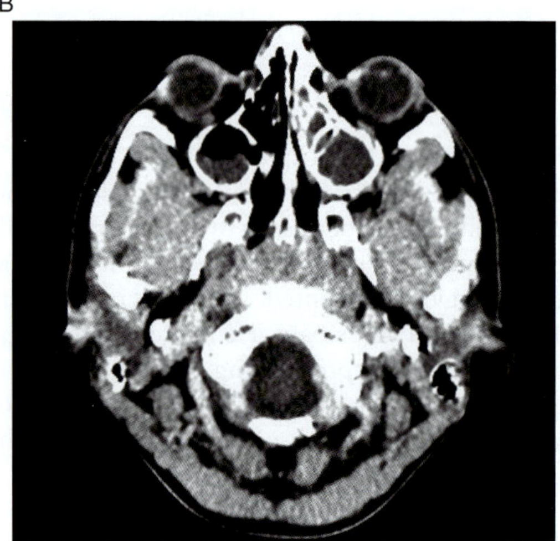

These demonstrate a left-sided subdural empyema (A) and maxillary sinusitis (B).

Figure 13.2. A follow-up coronal CT scan in the same patient who developed a generalised seizure despite antibiotic therapy.

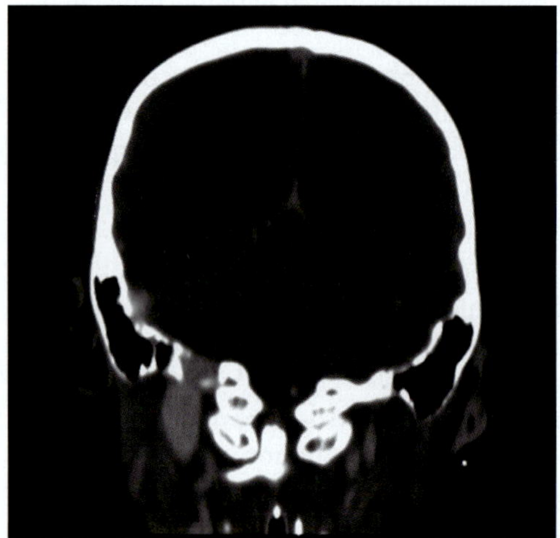

This demonstrates a sagittal venous sinus thrombosis as a complication of a subdural empyema.

The clinical presentation of subdural empyema is influenced by a number of factors, including the site of the collection and the patient's age and immune status. Common presenting symptoms include fever, headache and vomiting, as seen here [6]. Neuroimaging is crucial for diagnosing a subdural empyema. Magnetic resonance imaging (MRI) with gadolinium is the preferred option, but CT with contrast is usually performed first in the UK due to easier availability. A non-contrast CT has poor sensitivity and may appear normal; therefore, contrast should be used if an empyema is suspected [7].

Laboratory tests such as full blood count and inflammatory markers are non-specific and may be normal, and blood cultures may be negative.

A subdural empyema can be drained via a burr hole or craniotomy. In addition, surgical drainage of the locus of primary infection is also recommended where possible, for example drainage of the sinuses, as performed here, has been shown to reduce the need for repeated neurosurgical exploration and reduce the duration of hospitalisation [8].

Antibiotics are the mainstay of medical treatment, usually for a number of weeks. There have been no randomised controlled trials regarding empirical antibiotics, so recommendations are based on the known common causative organisms and their antibiotic susceptibilities. Antibiotics with anaerobic activity are recommended even when anaerobic organisms have not been isolated as they may have been present, but are difficult to culture [1].

Complications of a subdural empyema include cerebritis and, as seen in this case, a venous sinus thrombosis; if severe, the latter may lead to an infarct. Both of these may lead to motor deficits, acute symptomatic seizures and focal symptomatic epilepsy in the longer term [5,6]. The mortality from appropriately treated subdural empyema is now low at approximately 3% [1].

Key Points

- A subdural empyema is an uncommon but serious infection, most commonly found in adolescents and young adults.

- Sinusitis is an important predisposing factor.
- The most common causative organisms are streptococci.
- Diagnosis requires cranial imaging, with MRI being most sensitive. If a CT is performed, contrast should be given whenever possible.
- In most cases surgery will be required to drain the empyema and if possible drain the source of infection (e.g. sinuses).
- Medical management involves long courses of antibiotics.

Looking Back

A subdural empyema was first described in the late nineteenth century [9]; however, in the absence of intracranial imaging there was very little to distinguish it from a brain abscess or meningitis. Many of the early cases were diagnosed at post-mortem, as, without antibiotics, outlook was poor, even if surgery was undertaken.

Did You Know?

Even in the era of antibiotics, the significant mortality associated with subdural empyema lead Le Beau and colleagues to call it 'the most imperative of neurosurgical emergencies' in 1973 [10].

References

1. Greenlee JE. Subdural empyema. Curr Treat Option Neurol 2003;**5**:13–22.
2. Legrand M, Roujeau T, Meyer P, et al. Paediatric intracranial empyema: differences according to age. Eur J Pediatr 2009;**168**:1235–41.
3. Cole TS, Clark ME, Jenkins AJ, Clark JE. Pediatric focal intracranial suppuration: a UK single-centre experience. Childs Nerv Syst 2012;**28**:2109–14.
4. Bockova J, Rigamonti D. Intracranial empyema. Pediatr Infect Dis J 2000;**19**:735–7.
5. Kombogiorgas D, Seth R, Athwal R, Modha J, Singh J. Suppurative intracranial complications of sinusitis in adolescence. Single institute experience and review of literature. Br J Neurosurg 2007;**21**:603–9.
6. Leong SC, Waugh LK, Sinha A, De S. Clinical outcomes of sinogenic intracranial suppuration: the Alder Hey experience. Ann Otol Rhinol Laryngol 2011;**120**:320–5.
7. Adame N, Hedlund G, Byington CL. Sinogenic intracranial empyema in children. Pediatrics 2005;**116**:e461–7.
8. Hoyt DJ, Fischer SR. Otolaryngologic management of patients with subdural empyema. The Laryngoscope 1991;**101**:20–4.
9. Kubik CS, Adams RD. Subdural empyema. Brain 1943;**66**:18–42.
10. Le Beau J, Creissard P, Harispe L, Redondo A. Surgical treatment of brain abscess and subdural empyema. J Neurosurg 1973;**38**:198–203.

CASE 14

An Undulating Fever

Derek J. Sloan and Nicholas J. Beeching

History

A 48-year-old Syrian man presented with a 6-week history of intermittent fever with chills, rigors and night sweats and intermittent headache. For 1 week he had also experienced double vision, nausea and vomiting. His headache was unusual; it varied in severity and was associated with periods of photophobia. He had no history of migraine.

He also reported hip pain for several months, but had background osteoarthritis. Otherwise he had no prior illnesses or comorbidities.

Examination

On admission, he had low-grade fever (37.8°C). Neurological examination revealed an abducens (VI) nerve palsy affecting the right eye. He did not have neck stiffness or rash. Kernig's and Brudzinski's tests for meningism were negative. He had blurred disc margins on funduscopy, but it was difficult to confirm papilloedema. Examination of other systems was normal, apart from a palpable spleen tip below the left costal margin.

Initial Differential Diagnosis

The long history of headache and fever suggested chronic meningoencephalitis, rather than acute bacterial meningitis, including:

- Tuberculous meningitis
- Cryptococcal meningitis (more likely if there was concurrent evidence of immunosuppression)
- Neuroborreliosis (especially if there had been a history of 'tick' or 'insect' bite).

The presence of abducens nerve palsy, vomiting and possible papilloedema suggested raised intracranial pressure ± space-occupying lesions, including:

- An infective mass (e.g. tuberculoma)
- Primary or metastatic brain tumour.

Non-infective inflammatory causes were also considered, including:

- Central nervous system (CNS) vasculitis
- Neurosarcoidosis
- Neuro-Behçet's disease (which may occur without systemic features, and has increased incidence in the Middle East).

Results of Initial Investigations

Blood tests were unremarkable; white cell count (WCC): 6.2 × 10^9cells/l, erythrocyte sedimentation rate: 45 mm/h, C-reactive protein: 0.46 g/l. Serum biochemistry was normal. Immunological markers including antinuclear antibodies, immunoglobulins, C3, C4 and serum angiotensin-converting enzyme were normal. Routine blood cultures were negative.

Serological tests for HIV and syphilis were negative.

Chest X-ray and brain magnetic resonance imaging (MRI) were normal. Abdominal ultrasound scan confirmed mild splenomegaly. Pelvic X-rays and hip ultrasound confirmed degenerative disease only.

LP showed slightly raised opening pressure (25 cm H_2O). Cerebrospinal fluid (CSF) biochemistry showed an elevated protein (1.2 g/l) and reduced glucose (2.4 mmol/l compared to a serum level of 6.4 mmol/l). The CSF WCC was 201 cells/mm^3 (95% lymphocytes). Gram stain, Ziehl–Neelsen stain and cryptococcal antigen test were all negative. Blood and fungal cultures were negative. Mycobacterial cultures were set up and reported as negative 8 weeks later.

Progress and Further Investigations

He was admitted to hospital and an undulating fever was observed (temperature fluctuation from 36.5°C to 38.7°C). He had a single grand mal seizure on the fourth day. Further interrogation of his background revealed that his family were goat farmers in a rural community in Syria.

Brucella IgG antibodies were detected on enzyme-linked immunosorbent assay (ELISA) at a titre of 1:2560 in serum and 1:640 in CSF. A diagnosis of neurobrucellosis was made. Repeat blood and CSF cultures remained negative.

Diagnosis

Neurobrucellosis.

Management and Outcome

Treatment was commenced with intravenous ceftriaxone 2 g twice daily, oral doxycycline 100 mg twice daily and oral rifampicin 600 mg once daily. Parenteral therapy was discontinued at 1 month but oral therapy was continued for 6 months before stopping completely. He did not receive corticosteroids.

His fever settled completely on the 12th day of therapy and he had no more seizures. His headache and double vision improved gradually over 6 months. He remained well over the next 2 years of follow-up.

Prevention

Brucellosis may be prevented by vaccination of domestic livestock. Pasteurisation of milk prevents transmission of infection to humans by dairy products.

Although human-to-human transmission of brucellosis is extremely rare, in endemic regions there is a family history of brucellosis in up to 50% of cases, so screening of household members may allow early detection of unrecognised cases.

There is no vaccine to prevent human brucellosis. Agricultural or slaughterhouse workers and medical laboratory staff exposed to bacterial isolates may be at risk. Samples from patients with suspected brucellosis should be handled in a Biosafety Level 3 facility. Accidental laboratory exposure should prompt serological screening and prophylactic therapy.

Discussion

Brucellosis is one of the most important and widespread zoonotic infections worldwide. Six species are commonly recognised within the genus *Brucella* and four, from different animal hosts, cause human disease: *B. melitensis* (sheep, goats and camels), *B. abortus* (cattle), *B. suis* (swine) and *B. canis* (dogs). *B. melitensis* is responsible for the majority of human infections. Infected animals transmit the organism by excreting it in urine, semen, milk, blood and birth products (including the placenta).

Brucellae are small (0.5–0.7 μm diameter), non-motile, aerobic, Gram-negative coccobacilli. They survive for 2 days in milk at 8°C, for 3 weeks in frozen meat and for up to 3 months in goat cheese. However, they are killed by heat, ionising radiation, disinfectants and pasteurisation.

Brucellae are ingested by polymorphonuclear cells or macrophages and undergo intracellular replication. Organisms within host cells are killed by cell-mediated immunity, but may avoid this response to set up persistent infection. Non-caseating granulomas may be recognised if histological samples are obtained in any affected organ.

The global epidemiology of brucellosis is shown in **Figure 14.1** [1]. Except for a small number of cattle-associated *B. abortus* cases in Northern Ireland, the UK has been brucellosis-free since 1991, but from 2001 to 2008, three human neurobrucellosis cases were detected serologically at the national Brucellosis Reference Unit in Liverpool [2]. All were imported from the Middle East. A careful travel history is essential when considering brucellosis in the differential diagnosis of neurological illness.

Brucellosis usually presents after incubation of 1–4 weeks, although time to onset of symptoms is variable. The pattern of illness may be sub-acute or chronic. Common features are insidious fever, night sweats, arthralgia, myalgia and non-specific weakness or fatigue. Focal infection occurs in 30% of cases; most commonly with sacroileitis or large joint involvement in the lower limbs, which may be the explanation for the hip pain in this case. Paravertebral, epidural and psoas abscesses may complicate brucellar spondylitis. Multi-system involvement includes skin rashes (10%), genitourinary complications (2–20%), pulmonary features (7%) and hepatitis (3–6%). Endocarditis is rare (1–2%), but is an important cause of death. Brucellosis in pregnancy is associated with spontaneous abortion, premature delivery and intrauterine death.

From endemic settings in Turkey and Kuwait neurobrucellosis is seen in 7% and 8% of cases, respectively. Non-neurological features may coexist or be absent. The spectrum of neurological presentation is wide, and overlaps with many other conditions, especially tuberculosis. Features may be syndromically classified as shown in **Figure 14.2**. Meningoencephalitis is common, but classical signs of meningism are often absent (neck stiffness in only 37%). Cranial nerve palsies, commonly of the abducens and vestibulocochlear nerve, may be important clues. Seizures are reported in 8%. Space-occupying abscesses are relatively rare. Psychiatric disturbance may be under-reported [3].

Diagnostic confirmation is difficult. Cultures require enriched media and hazardous sample manipulation in the laboratory. Modern automated systems are more reliable than the traditional bi-phasic culture technique of Ruiz-Castaneda, but < 30% of neurobrucellosis patients have positive blood cultures and < 15% have organisms grown from CSF. Cranial imaging excludes alternative pathologies, identifies abscesses and ensures the safety of lumbar puncture, but computed tomography or MRI scans are normal in > 70% of neurobrucellosis patients [4]. A recent study reported

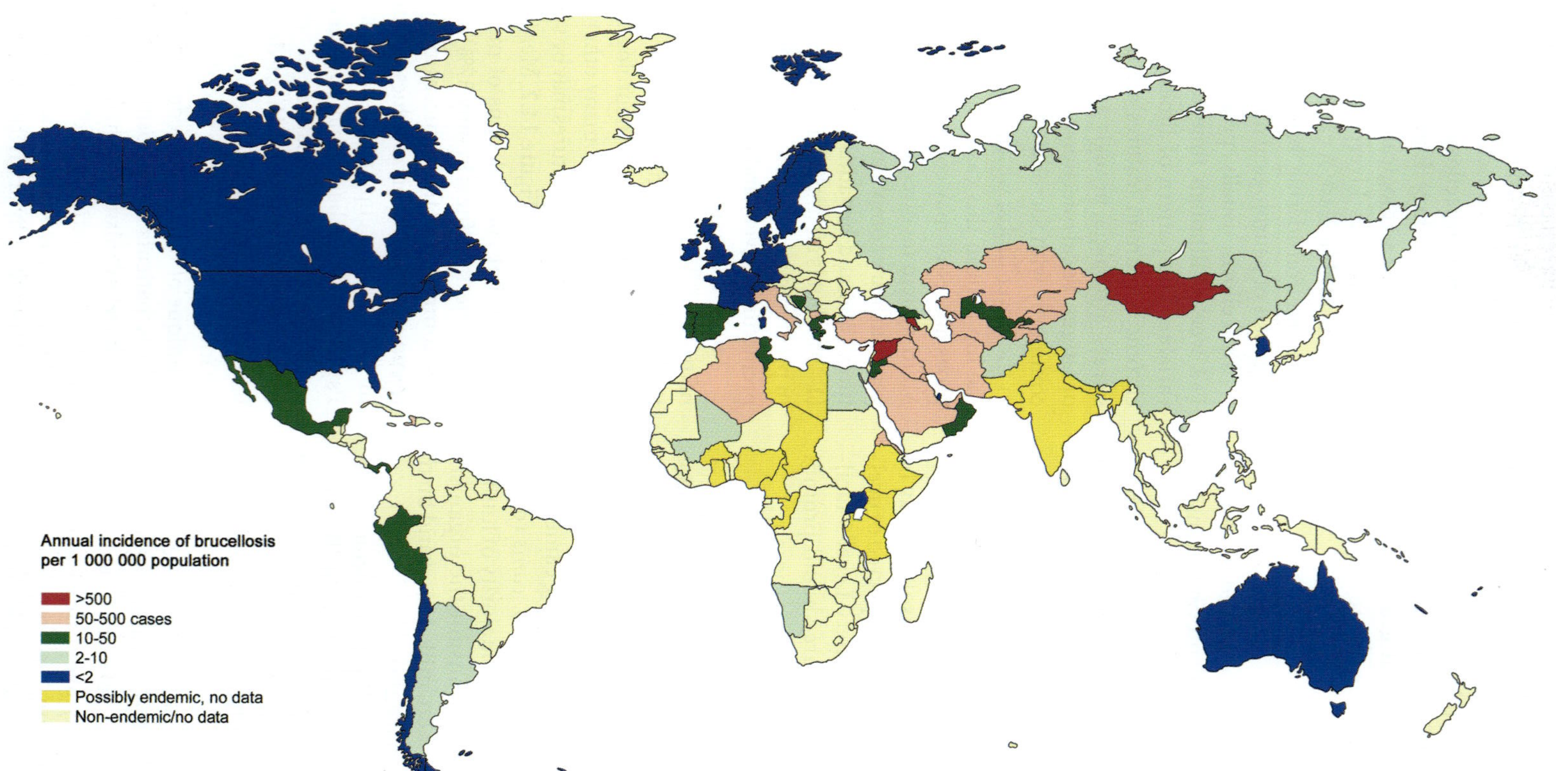

Figure 14.1. Global epidemiology of brucellosis (reproduced with permission from [1]). Brucellosis is non-endemic in most developed countries, but remains an important zoonosis in the Middle East and Asia.

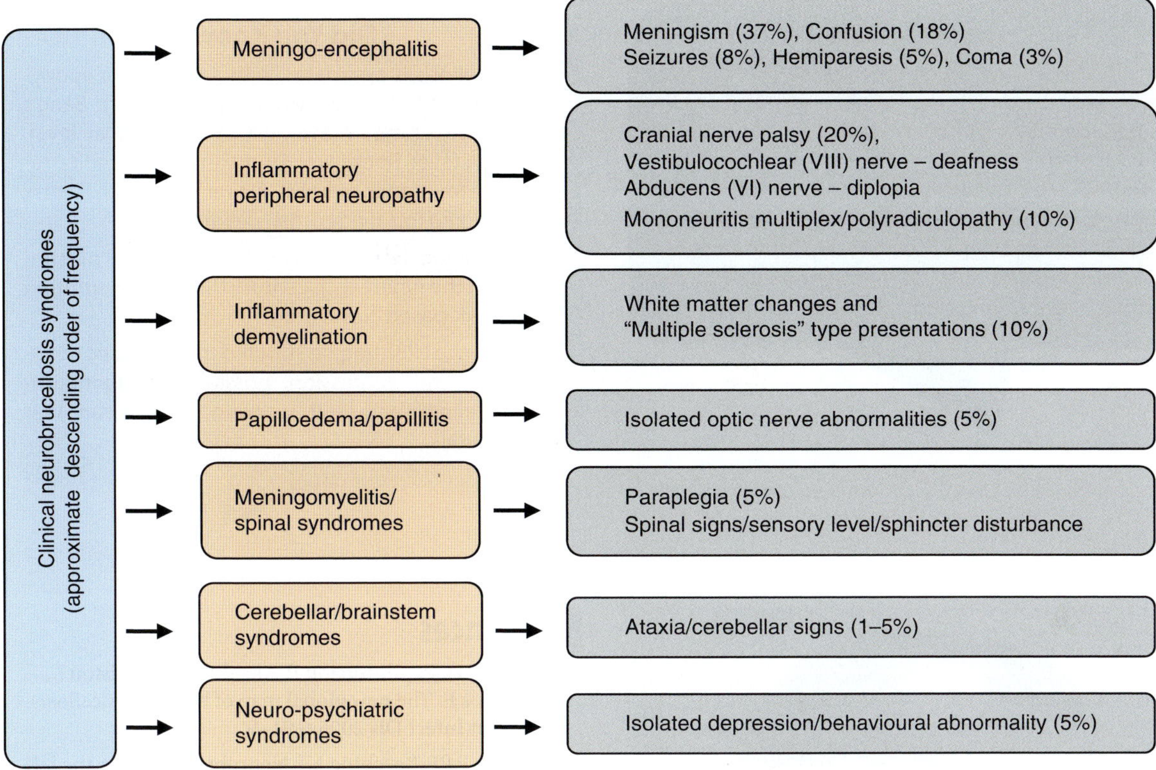

Figure 14.2. Clinical presentations of neurobrucellosis.

leptomeningeal enhancement in 17% of cases, nodular lesions in 8% and granulomatous lesions in only 4%. CSF typically shows moderate inflammation (raised protein, low glucose) with lymphocytosis. Elevated levels of adenosine deaminase in the CSF are suggestive of neurobrucellosis or tuberculous meningitis.

Serology is often the key investigation and a range of immunological tests are available including tube agglutination tests, the Rose Bengal test and IgM/IgG ELISAs [5]. Serological tests must be performed on serum and CSF when neurological disease is suspected. Real-time polymerase chain reaction assays have been developed, but are not in routine clinical use.

Treatment is not standardised but involves prolonged use of three drugs which effectively cross the blood–brain barrier. Neuropenetrative regimens include doxycycline, rifampicin and either ceftriaxone or trimethoprim-sulfamethoxazole. Ceftriaxone-based regimens are preferred and allow shorter overall duration of therapy [6]. The role of corticosteroids is controversial; although not routinely recommended, they are sometimes used in disease complicated by oedematous space-occupying lesions, ocular disease and cranial nerve palsies [7]. They were not used in this case, where there was a high CSF opening pressure, and a VI cranial nerve lesion, which was presumably a false localising lesion related to raised pressure.

With appropriate antimicrobial therapy, mortality from brucellosis is less than 1%. Long-term neurological sequelae may occur in up to 40% of cases and 5–15% of treated cases may relapse due to incomplete eradication of intracellular organisms, necessitating prolonged follow-up [8].

Key Points

- Neurobrucellosis has a range of acute and chronic clinical presentations. Features may resemble tuberculous meningitis, which is an important differential.
- Only three cases have been described in the UK since 2001, all of which were imported from endemic regions. An accurate travel and occupational history is essential.
- Diagnosis is normally based on serological tests and requires analysis of serum and CSF.
- Treatment involves prolonged combination therapy with ceftriaxone, doxycycline and rifampicin. The role of corticosteroids is unclear.

Looking Back

Brucellosis was first recognised by British medical officers in Malta during the Crimean War. The organism was identified by Major-General Sir David Bruce from autopsy examinations in 1887 (**Figure 14.3**); *B. abortus* was microbiologically isolated by the Danish veterinarian Bang in 1897. In 1905, the Maltese doctor and archeologist Themistocles Zammit identified unpasteurised milk as the major source of the pathogen; he was knighted for this discovery in 1930.

Did You Know?

Brucellosis is associated with a long list of eponymous and descriptive names, including: Bang's disease, Crimean fever, fist of mercy, goat fever, Malta fever, Rock fever, Undulant fever, Mediterranean fever, milk sickness, Neapolitan fever, Satan's fever and (oddly) Scottish delight!

A high incidence was seen in British naval personnel in the nineteenth century due to consumption of milk-based 'Naval grog'.

Florence Nightingale suffered from chronic headaches and depression, possibly due to neurobrucellosis acquired working in Crimean War hospitals.

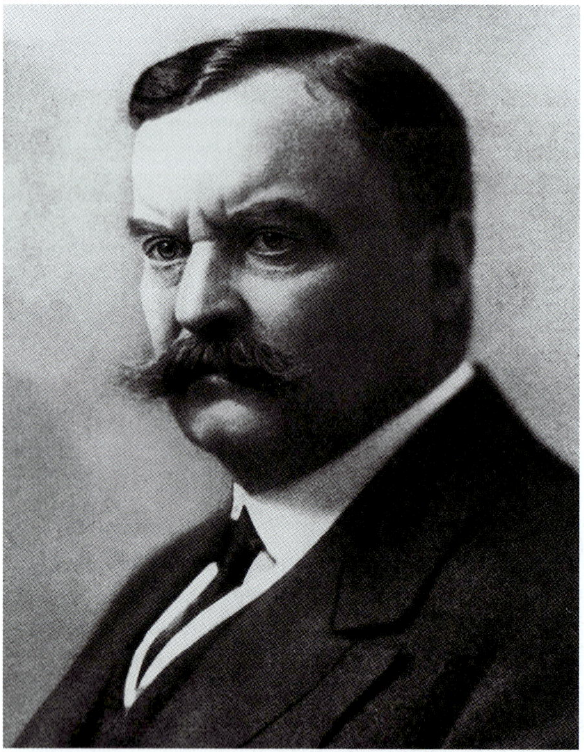

Figure 14.3. Major-General Sir David Bruce, who identified the trypanosome protozoan parasite as the cause of sleeping sickness, and after whom 'Brucellosis' is also named. (Photo courtesy of the Library & Archives Service, London School of Hygiene & Tropical Medicine.)

References

1. Pappas G, Papdimitriou P, Akridites N, Christou L, Tsianos E. The new global map of human brucellosis. Lancet Infect Dis 2006;**6**:91–9.
2. Cooke RPF, Beeching NJ. Neurobrucellosis in the UK. J Infect 2009;**58**:88–9.
3. Gul HC, Erdem H, Bak S. Overview of neurobrucellosis: a pooled analysis of 187 cases. Int J Infect Dis 2009;**13**:e339–43.
4. Guven T, Ugurlu K, Ergonul O, et al. Neurobrucellosis: clinical and diagnostic features. Clin Infect Dis 2013;**56**:1407–12.
5. Erdem H, Kilic S, Sener B, et al. Diagnosis of chronic brucellar meningitis and meningoencephalitis: the results of the Istanbul-2 study. Clin Microbiol Infect 2012;**19**:E80–6.
6. Erdem H, Ulu-Kilic A, Kilic S, et al. Efficacy and tolerability of antibiotic combinations in neurobrucellosis: results of the Istanbul Study. Antimicrob Agents Chemother 2012;**56**:1523–8.
7. Pappas G, Akriditis N, Bosilkovski M, Tsianos E. Brucellosis. N Engl J Med 2005;**352**:2325–6.
8. Beeching NJ, Gerada A, Thomas S. Brucellosis. BMJ Best Practice 2017: http://bestpractice.bmj.com/best-practice/monograph/911.html

CASE 15

Safari Headache

Hannah E. Brindle and Tom Solomon

History

A 34-year-old man presented with a 1-week history of intermittent fever, headache, breathlessness and myalgia. He had returned from a holiday in Zambia 3 weeks previously where he spent time camping and on safari walking through the bush. He had also noticed a lesion on his right foot and a rash over his arms, legs and abdomen. He had no past medical history. His only medication was mefloquine, which he had been taking as prophylaxis against malaria.

He had received all recommended travel vaccinations and had no other travel history.

Examination

On admission the patient had a pyrexia of 38.2°C, and tachycardia of 105 beats per minute, but blood pressure and oxygen saturation were unremarkable. Auscultation of his chest was clear and heart sounds were normal. There was evidence of hepatosplenomegaly and palpable enlarged axillary lymph nodes.

He had a rash on his arms, legs and abdomen and a tender area on his right arm (**Figure 15.1**).

Initial Differential Diagnosis

- Malaria, a possibility despite the antimalarial drugs
- Rickettsial infection
- Human African trypanosomiasis, due to the chancre
- HIV seroconversion illness, to be considered in anyone with febrile illness and rash
- Lymphoma, due to the hepatosplenomgaly and lymphadenopathy

Results of Initial Investigations

Initial blood results showed: haemoglobin 102 g/l, white cells 12.3 × 10^9/l and platelets 85 × 10^9/l. The other results were: urea 10.2 mmol/l, creatinine 223 μmol/l, bilirubin 32 μmol/l and C-reactive protein 140 mg/l.

Blood cultures and HIV antibody test were negative, and a chest X-ray, electrocardiogram (ECG) and computer tomography scan of his head were normal.

Giemsa-stained thick and thin blood films were examined for malaria parasites and were negative.

Definitive Investigation

The Giemsa-stained thin blood film showed the presence of *Trypanosoma brucei rhodesiense* (**Figure 15.2**).

Diagnosis

Human African trypanosomiasis, 'sleeping sickness', caused by *Trypanosoma brucei rhodesiense.*

Figure 15.1. A rash similar to that seen in a 34-year-old gentleman who presented 3 weeks after returning from a safari in Zambia.

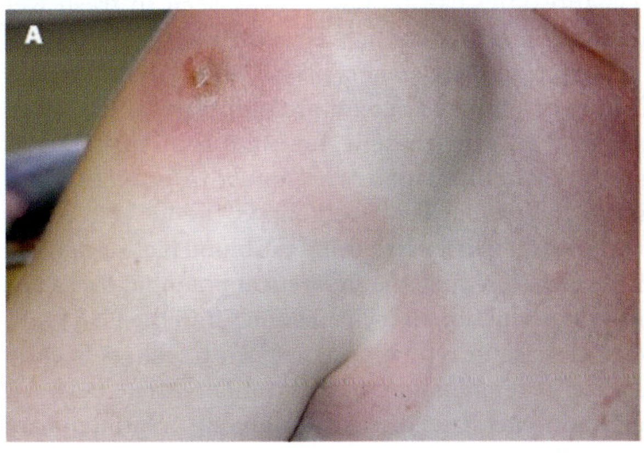

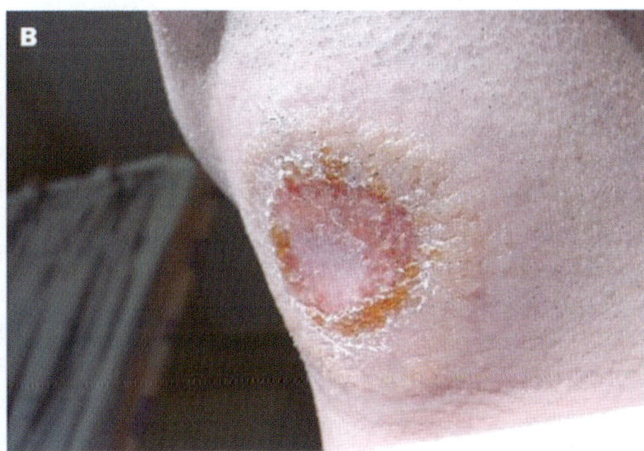

This shows an indurated purplish lesion – a chancre. Reproduced with permission from [1].

Figure 15.2. A thin blood film similar to that seen in our patient.

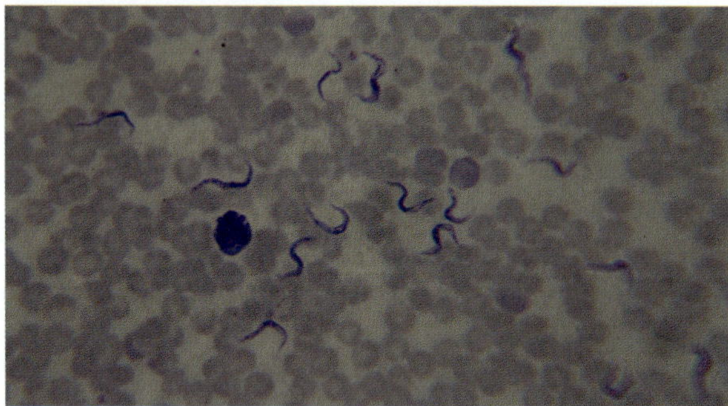

This demonstrates several *Trypanosoma brucei rhodesiense*. (Photo courtesy of Dr Russell Stothard, Liverpool School of Tropical Medicine.)

Management and Outcome

The patient was given a test dose of intravenous suramin with no evidence of a hypersensitivity reaction. Therefore a total of five doses of suramin were given on days 1, 3 , 7, 14 and 21.

A lumbar puncture (LP) was performed on day 5, once the repeat blood film was negative for trypanosomes. This is due to the theoretical risk that a traumatic LP could introduce trypanosomes into the cerebrospinal fluid (CSF). The analysis of the CSF did not identify an abnormal white cell count, protein, or glucose ratio and microscopy and culture were normal. This confirmed the patient had early stage disease.

He made a good recovery without any complications. The chancre disappeared within 5 days and his blood results returned to normal.

Prevention

Despite there being no drug or vaccine prophylaxis against human African trypanosomiasis, measures can be taken to prevent tsetse fly bites. Wearing long-sleeved clothing and avoiding areas of the bush where tsetse flies may be found are advised. Using insect repellent is also recommended, although not proven to be effective against tsetse flies [2]. Control programmes to reduce the disease reservoir of *T. b. rhodesiense* largely comprise vector-control measures including traps, screens and insecticides [2].

Discussion

Human African trypanosomiaisis is caused by *T. b. rhodesiense*, which occurs in East and Southern Africa, and *T. b. gambiense*, which occurs in West and Central Africa [3]. *T. b. rhodesiense* is a zoonotic disease with livestock often being the hosts. Humans acquire the disease via the bite of an infected tsetse fly (**Figure 15.3**) [4,5].

Symptoms in travellers tend to be different to those from endemic countries [3]. Following the bite, a chancre may develop. This lesion tends to increase in size before resolving after a few weeks [3]. Fever and headache are also common in travellers. A macular 'trypanosomal' rash, which differs from a chancre, may also be seen [3]. As the trypanosomes enter the central nervous system (CNS), neurological features including behavioural change, sleep disturbance and other symptoms of meningoencephalitis, may occur. However, these late changes are less common in those from non-endemic countries [3]. ECG changes including heart block and supraventricular tachycardia may be secondary to myopericarditis [3].

Impaired renal function, raised liver enzymes, thrombocytopaenia and raised inflammatory markers, as seen in this case, are not uncommon in those from non-endemic areas [3,6]. Findings on magnetic resonance imaging of the brain have been described by a few case reports and include demyelination, cerebral oedema, focal lesions and cerebral atrophy [3,7,8].

The suspicion of the diagnosis is based on the clinical symptoms and signs in patients with the appropriate travel history. In the patient described here, the recent return from an endemic area of Africa, where he had been camping in the bush, and history of febrile illness initially prompted examination of the Giemsa-stained blood film for malaria parasites; although they were not seen, trypanosomes were. Trypanosomes can be more easily seen in fresh wet preparations, because of their motility [1].

Detection of trypanosomes in the CSF and raised CSF white blood cell count are indicative of late-stage disease. However, these features are less sensitive and new markers for diagnosis are under investigation [3]. As for the patient described above, the LP is deferred until treatment has started and the blood is clear of trypanosomes to reduce the theoretical potential for iatrogenic introduction of trypanosomes into the CSF [1,3]. Most disease in returning European travellers is early disease. It remains important to differentiate between early and late-stage disease as different treatments are required.

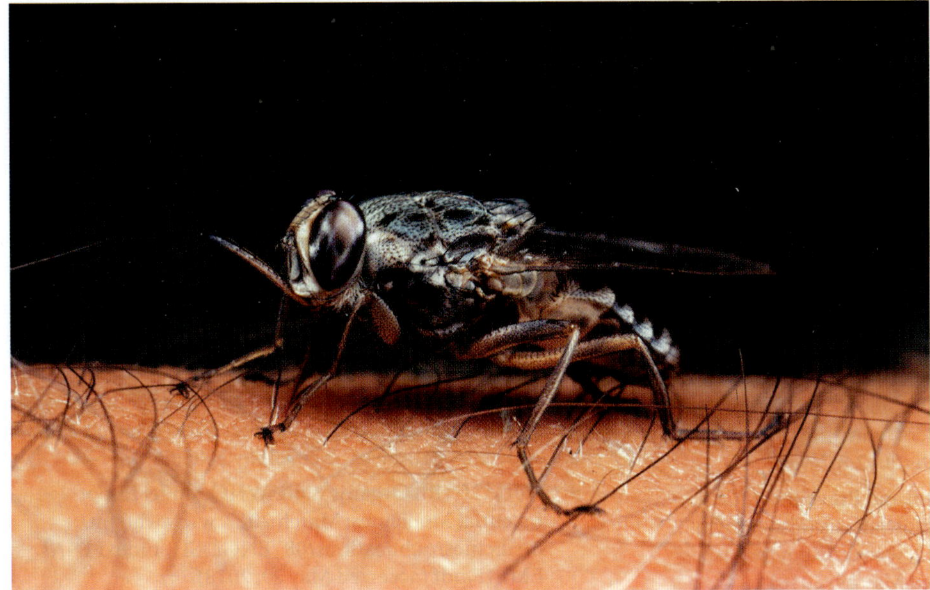

Figure 15.3. Tsetse fly feeding on a human arm. (Image Anthony Bannister / Getty Images.)

In early stage disease, the treatment choice is intravenous suramin as recommended by the World Health Organisation [9]. As with the patient described here, a test dose is given to assess for an anaphylactic reaction [1]. Melarsoprol is used for late-stage disease with CNS infection. However, this may be associated with severe side effects including encephalopathy, which can be fatal [3]. Following treatment, patients should be monitored for success of treatment by repeated analysis of the CSF.

Key Points

- With increasing numbers of travellers going on safari, the prevalence of human African trypanosomiasis in returning travellers may increase.
- Clinicians should remember to consider human African trypanosomiasis in the differential diagnosis for those returning from Africa with fever, especially if they were in the bush, and have a chancre or rash.
- Given the few cases and difficulty obtaining the appropriate drugs, the early involvement of a specialist tropical diseases centre is recommended [8].

Looking Back

Reports of sleeping sickness date back to the Middle Ages [10]. The first suggestion that tsetse fly bites caused the animal form for trypanosomiasis, which is also termed 'nagana', was made by the explorer David Livingstone (**Figure 15.4**). However, it wasn't until 1895 that David Bruce (**Figure 14.3**) first discovered that trypanosomes were the cause of nagana and then in 1901 that Michael Forde discovered these in human blood.

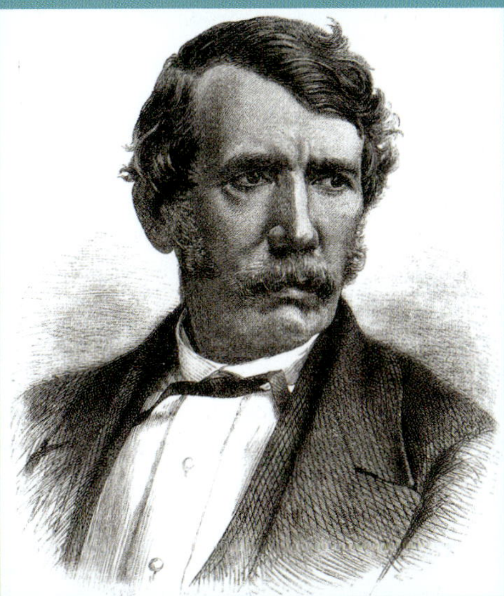

Figure 15.4. Portrait of Dr David Livingstone, 1866. (Image courtesy of Getty Images.)

Did You Know?

The term nagana which relates to the animal form of sleeping sickness is derived from the Zulu meaning 'to be depressed' [11].

References

1. Moore DAJ, Edwards M, Escombe R, et al. African trypanosomiasis in travelers returning to the United Kingdom. Emerg Infect Dis 2002;**8**:74–6.
2. Centers for Disease Control and Prevention, USA. Parasites – African Trypanosomiasis (also known as Sleeping Sickness). 2012. www.cdc.gov/parasites/sleepingsickness/ (accessed May 29, 2018)
3. Blum JA, Neumayr AL, Hatz CF. Human African trypanosomiasis in endemic populations and travellers. Eur J Clin Microbiol Infect Dis 2012;**31**:905–13.
4. Welburn SC, Picozzi K, Fèvre EM, et al. Identification of human-infective trypanosomes in animal reservoir of sleeping sickness in Uganda by means of serum-resistance-associated gene. Lancet 2001;**358**:2017–19.
5. Reto B, Johannes B, Francois C, Christian B. Seminar: human African trypanosomiasis. Lancet 2010;**375**:148–59.
6. Clerinx J, Vlieghe E, Asselman V, et al. Human African trypanosomiasis in a Belgian traveller returning from the Masai Mara area, Kenya. Eurosurveillance 2012;**17**:pii=20111.
7. Sabbah P, Brosset C, Imbert P, et al. Human African trypanosomiasis: MRI. Neuroradiology 1997;**39**: 708–10.
8. Braakman H, Boerman D, Van De Molengraft F, Hubert W. Lethal African trypanosomiasis in a traveler: MRI and neuropathology. Neurology 2006;**66**:1094–6.
9. World Health Organisation. WHO Model List of Essential Medicines; March 2017. www.who.int/medicines/publications/08_ENGLISH_indexFINAL_EML15.pdf (accessed May 29, 2018).
10. Steverding DD. The history of African trypanosomiasis. Parasites Vectors 2008;**1**(1).
11. World Health Organisation. Trypanosomiasis – Human African (Sleeping Sickness). 2018. www.who.int/mediacentre/factsheets/fs259/en/ (accessed May 20, 2018).

CASE 16

A Pain in the Ear

Liene Elsone, Mona Ghadiri-Sani and Tom Solomon

History

A 28-year-old female PhD student, who was normally fit and well, presented to an Accident and Emergency department with a 3-day history of feeling generally unwell with coryzal symptoms, and severe earache on the right. She was given simple analgesia and sent home. A week later she suddenly became unwell with deterioration in her consciousness level and agitation; she was admitted to hospital and transferred to the intensive care unit.

She had undergone some dental work a few months prior to this admission but had no other past medical or family history of note. There was no significant travel history, she had no pets and she had had no contacts with anyone who was unwell. Her family stated that she had had the standard childhood vaccinations, although no formal record was available. She had a 12-year history of smoking approximately 20 cigarettes per day but drank little alcohol.

Examination

On arrival in intensive care the patient was febrile (38°C) and agitated and there was blood-stained pus discharging from the right ear. Her Glasgow coma score (GCS) was 10/15, in that she was opening her eyes to pain, uttering inappropriate words and localising painful stimuli. She had a fixed dilated left pupil with partial ptosis and complete right lower motor neuron facial palsy. There was evidence of nuchal rigidity; however, limb muscle tone was normal. Plantar response was extensor bilaterally. Funduscopy revealed early changes of papilloedema. There were no rashes.

Initial Differential Diagnosis

- Bacterial meningitis

Given the history of a febrile illness with earache, a bloody discharge from the ear, nuchal rigidity and an acute reduction in consciousness, bacterial meningitis following otitis media was felt to be the most likely diagnosis. The protracted presentation and rapid decline in GCS suggested a complication secondary to meningitis may have developed, including:

- cerebritis,
- cerebral infarction,
- cerebral abscess,
- venous sinus thrombosis,
- hyponatraemia
- non-convulsive status epilepticus.

Additional differentials to consider included:

- other central nervous system infections, such as encephalitis,
- endocrine dysfunction, such as Addison's disease and hypothyroidism,
- other vascular diseases, such as subarachnoid haemorrhage,
- toxic encephalopathy.

Although many bacteria can cause meningitis (**Table 16.1**), given the purulent otitis, *Streptococcus pneumoniae* was suspected.

Results of Initial Investigations

The initial full blood count revealed an elevated white cell count (38×10^9/l with a neutrophilia); there was a raised C-reactive protein (360 mg/l). Renal and liver functions tests were normal and HIV serology and antigen testing were negative.

Table 16.1 Common causes of meningitis.

Type of meningitis	Common aetiological organisms
Bacterial meningitis	*Streptococcus pneumonia*
	Neisseria menigitidis
	Haemophilus influenza type B
	Listeria monocytogenes
	Enterobacteriaceae (*Escherichia coli*, *Klebsiella* spp., etc.)
	Staphylococcus aureus
	Borrelia burgdorferi
Viral meningitis	Enteroviruses
	Herpesviruses (HSV types 1&2, EBV, VZV, CMV, HHV6)
	Arboviruses (West Nile virus)
	Other viruses (mumps, rabies, influenza, HIV)
Tuberculous meningitis	Mycobacteria
Fungal meningitis	Candida, Cryptococcus, Histoplasma
Parasitic meningitis	Schistosoma
Non-infectious meningitis	Sarcoidosis, drugs, systemic lupus erythematosus

CMV, cytomegalovirus; EBV, Epstein–Barr virus; HHV6, human herpes virus type 6; HSV, herpes simplex virus; VZV, varicella zoster virus.

A computer tomography (CT) scan of the brain was performed before considering a lumbar puncture (LP) because of the papilloedema, focal neurological signs and low Glasgow coma score (**Figure 16.1**).

Subsequently, magnetic resonance imaging (MRI) was performed (**Figure 16.2**).

Results of Definitive Investigations

Both cultures of blood and the pus from the right ear were positive for *Streptococcus pneumoniae*, which was sensitive to penicillin and clarithromycin.

Diagnosis

Streptococcus pneumoniae meningitis with associated transverse sinus thrombosis and cerebral oedema.

Management and Outcome

LP was not carried out because of the severe cerebral oedema with tight basal cisterns identified on CT brain imaging. It could have been considered subsequently, but by this stage there was a microbiological diagnosis. The patient was treated empirically with ceftriaxone and dexamethasone for presumed pneumococcal meningitis. She was given ciprofloxacin eardrops for the otitis. The transverse sinus thrombosis was treated with intravenous heparin and then warfarin. She remained in intensive care for a week. She was then transferred to the ward at which time she made significant improvement both clinically and in terms of her inflammatory markers. She was apyrexial, alert and orientated. On neurological examination at this stage, tone and power were normal with flexor plantars.

She completed 14 days of antibiotics and the dexamethasone was weaned down slowly. The warfarin continued for 6 months. At 6-month follow-up, she had slight residual weakness on eye closure but no obvious asymmetry at rest. The rest of the neurological examination was normal.

Prevention

The introduction of the vaccine for *Streptococcus pneumoniae* has reduced the frequency of pneumococcal meningitis. In the UK, this vaccine is offered to all children under the age of 2 years, those over 65 years, and those with specified pre-existing medical conditions.

Figure 16.1. CT brain images of a 28-year-old patient presenting with a coryzal illness and earache progressing to deterioration in consciousness.

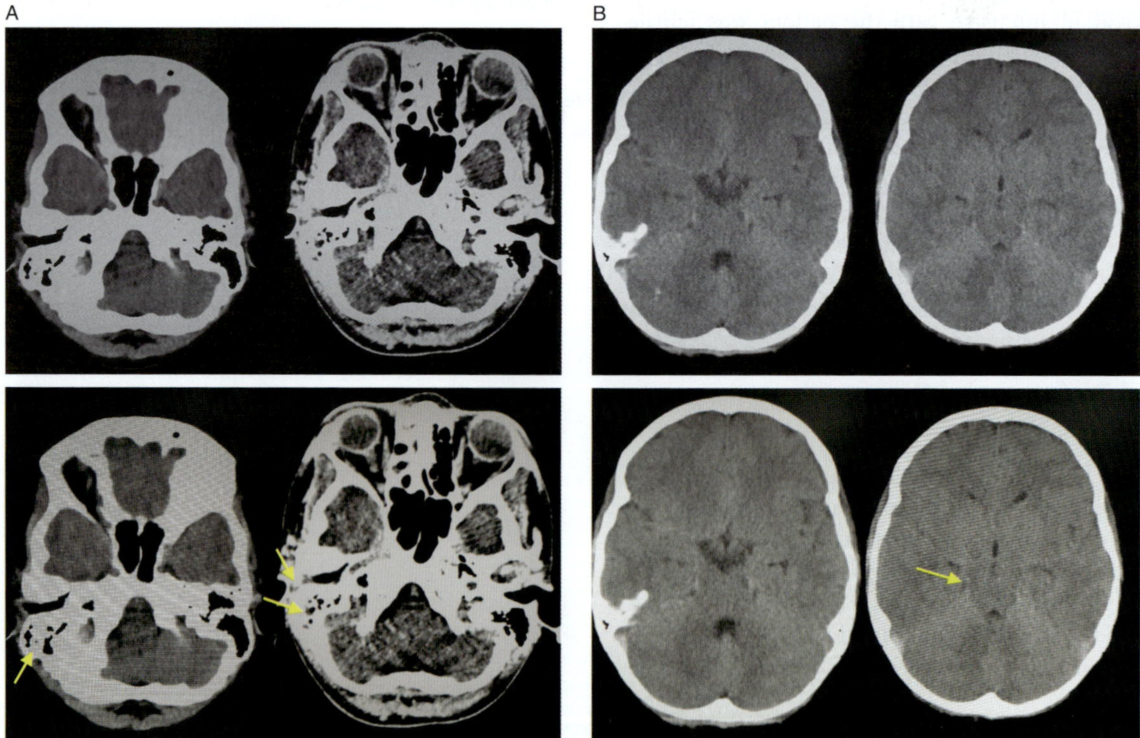

This shows (A) pus in the right ear, and mastoiditis and on the right (arrows on the lower image indicate where), and (B) diffuse cerebral oedema and tight basal cisterns (arrows on the lower image indicate where).

Figure 16.2. A T2 FLAIR MRI brain scan in the same patient.

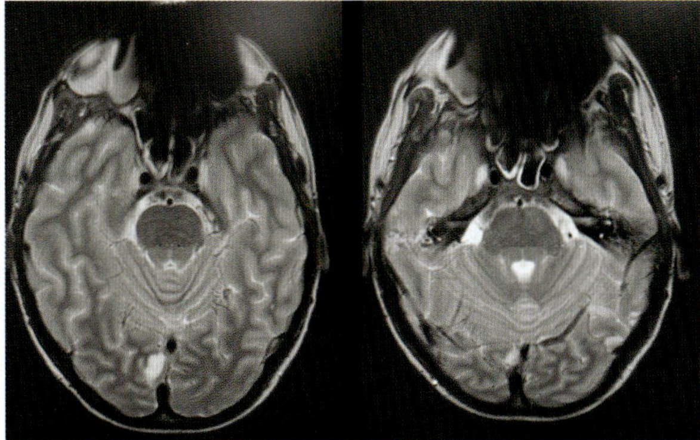

This shows high signal intensity in the right posterior occipital lobe, and a right transverse sinus thrombosis (arrows on the lower image indicate where).

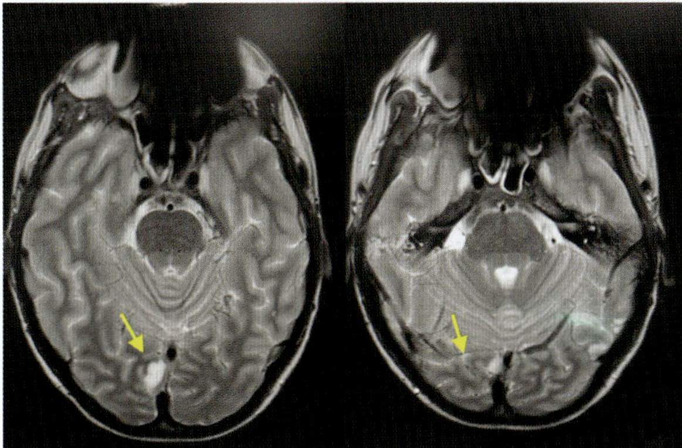

Discussion

Acute bacterial meningitis is inflammation of the meninges and the subarachnoid space caused by bacteria. The most common route of bacterial spread is through the bloodstream from an infection locus in the head (sinusitis or ear infection) or other part of the body. Although a wide range of bacteria can cause meningitis (**Table 16.1**), in Western settings *Streptococcus pneumoniae* or *Neisseria meningitidis* are the most common organisms in adults and children, respectively. *Hemophilus* is rare since vaccination was introduced. National UK guidelines recommend that *Listeria monocytogenes* should also be considered in patients over 60 years of age and immunocompromised patients.

There are many conditions which increase the risk of developing bacterial meningitis; therefore, careful history can aid earlier diagnosis. Risks are higher in unvaccinated children, adults aged > 60 years, immunocompromised patients (including those with HIV or on immunosuppressive drugs), those with underlying chronic disease (including renal failure, lung disease, leukaemia, diabetes, malignancy, and alcoholism), pregnancy, skull fracture, invasive neurosurgical procedure, cerebrospinal fluid (CSF) rhinorrhoea and mucosal epithelial damage caused by smoking, and recent viral illness.

Meningitis typically presents with fever, headache, vomiting, nausea, reduced conscious level and meningeal irritation such as nuchal rigidity and photophobia [1]. There may also be seizures, focal neurological deficits, rash, diarrhoea, lymphadenopathy and pharyngitis.

All patients should be investigated with bloods, imaging and, where possible, CSF studies [2].

Meningitis is a medical emergency and must be treated as soon as possible. National UK guidelines recommend that empirical iv antibiotic treatment should always be started within 30 minutes of admission [3]. Often this will mean that the patient has commenced treatment while awaiting investigations [4,5]. Nevertheless LP is still required, where possible, to identify the causative organism. This should be done urgently because delays in performing the LP after commencing intravenous antibiotics are associated with a reduced likelihood of identifying the pathogen by CSF culture. In one study, delays of 4 hours resulted in a significant reduction in CSF culture positivity rates, and beyond 8 hours all were negative by culture [6]. However, at later time points, polymerase chain reaction of the CSF may still be useful in identifying a cause, although sensitivity data will not be available.

Table 16.2 Deterioration in a patient with bacterial meningitis – possible causes, and action needed.

- Venous sinus thrombosis
  - Imaging, MRI, including magnetic resonance venogram
- Seizures including subtle motor seizures
  - Electroencephalogram
- Raised intracranial pressure and herniation syndromes
  - MRI, consider mannitol, steroids, pressure monitoring
- Infarct
  - MRI
- Septic shock
  - Ionotropic support
- Subdural empyema
  - Imaging, drain if large pressure effect
- Aspiration pneumonia
  - Chest X-ray antibiotics
- Hyponatraemia/syndrome of inappropriate antidiuretic hormone secretion
  - Renal function

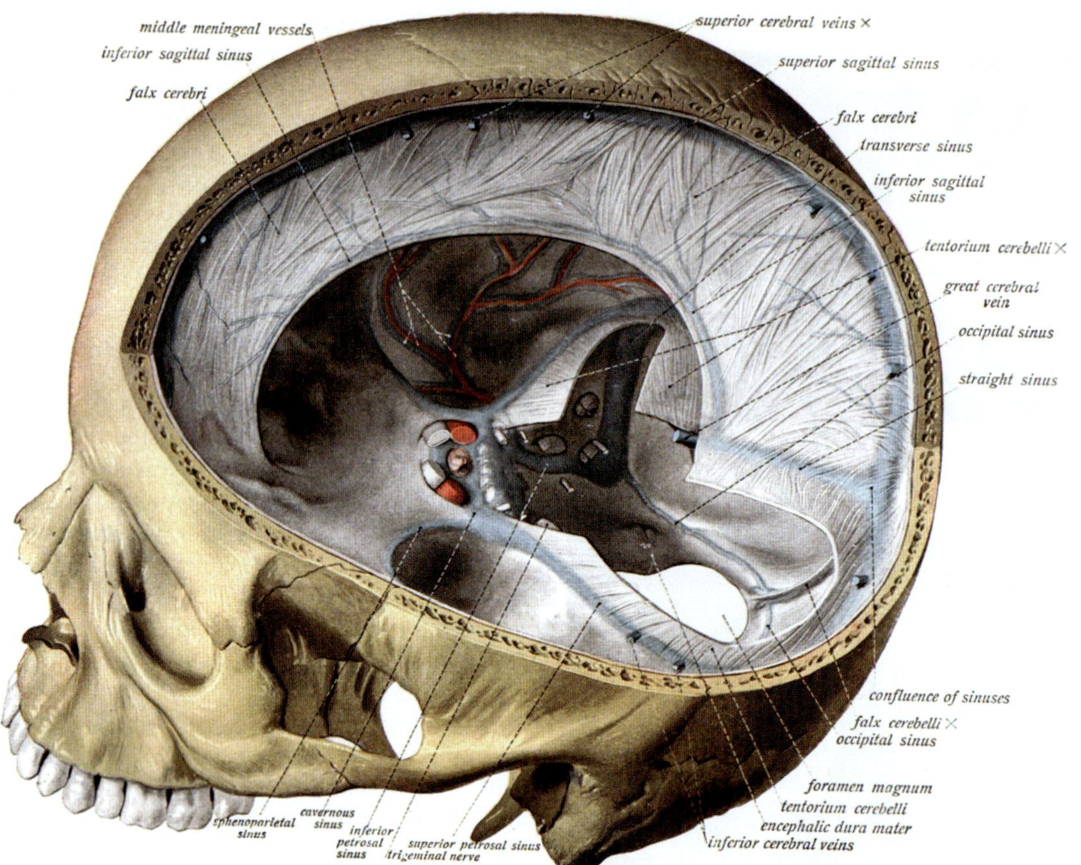

Figure 16.3. Cerebral venous sinuses.
(An anatomical illustration from Sobotta's *Human Anatomy* 1908.)

Complications of acute bacterial meningitis include seizures, focal neurological deficits, blindness and sensorineural deafness, cerebritis and venous sinus thrombosis, as in this case (**Table 16.2**) [1].

Venous sinus thrombosis can occur anywhere within the cerebral venous system (**Figure 16.3**). Suggestive clinical features of venous sinus thrombosis include a deterioration of consciousness, bilateral papilloedema and raised CSF opening pressure on LP. In severe cases Cushing's reflex (increased blood pressure with a reduction in heart rate) may be seen, indicating imminent brainstem herniation. In the patient described here the dilated pupil and ptosis suggest a partial 3rd cranial nerve lesion consistent with early uncal herniation.

Venous sinus thrombosis is treated with anticoagulation. The use of dexamethasone in bacterial meningitis remains controversial, although the data suggest it is useful for adults with pneumococcal meningitis [7].

Overall, the prognosis of bacterial meningitis is dependent on early diagnosis and prompt treatment. Mortality in recent studies has been reported up to 10% and increases with age. Hypotension, seizures and altered mental status are associated with worse outcomes in bacterial meningitis [8].

Key Points

- Bacterial meningitis is a medical emergency.
- Immediate empirical antibacterial treatment should be initiated; however, investigations should still be conducted urgently.
- Blood cultures should be taken immediately before giving antibiotics, and LP performed as soon as possible.
- Earache with purulent discharge suggests a bacterial aetiology, in the UK usually *Streptococcus pneuomiae*, especially if there is radiological evidence of mastoiditis.

- When a patient with bacterial meningitis has a rapid deterioration in their clinical condition, look for venous sinus thrombosis, cerebral infarction, hyponatraemia or cerebral herniation.
- In a comatose patient a unilateral fixed pupil with ptosis may be due to herniation of the temporal lobe uncus causing compression of cranial nerve III.

Looking Back

Although descriptions of symptoms consistent with bacterial meningitis date back as far as the Hippocratic writings, it is the seventeenth-century English Physician, Thomas Willis (**Figure 16.4**, eponymously associated with the Circle of Willis), who recognised the clinico-pathological correlation in his description 'Of the Phrensy', noting 'The *Phrensy* is defin'd: That it is a continual raving, or a deprivation of the chief faculties of the brain, arising from an inflammation of the meninges with a continual fever' [9]. This ancient sense of a hyperactive and at times almost maniacal state, used by Willis to describe some patients with bacterial meningitis, is preserved in our modern word 'frenzy'.

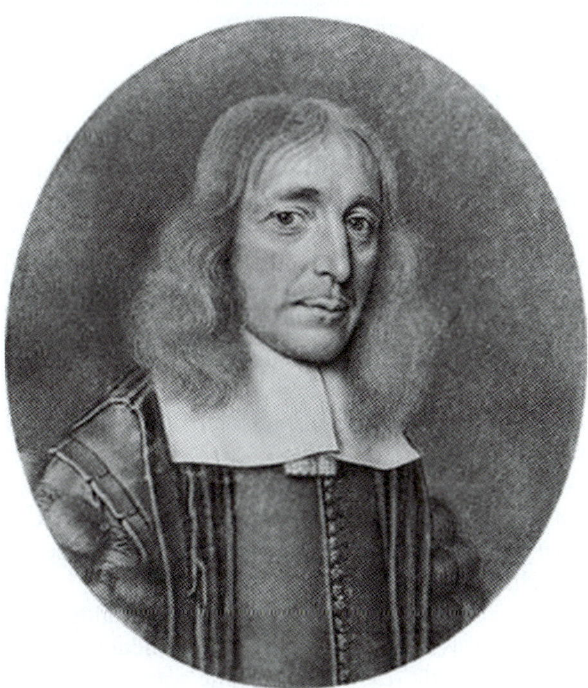

Figure 16.4. Thomas Willis (1621–1675), who gave one of the earliest clinico-pathological descriptions of bacterial meningitis.

Did You Know?

One rather intriguing study reports that people with dark eyes are less likely to suffer from deafness following bacterial meningitis than people with light-coloured eyes [10].

References

1. Durand ML, Calderwood SB, Weber DJ, et al. Acute bacterial meningitis in adults. A review of 493 episodes. N Engl J Med. 1993;**328**:21.
2. Chaudhuri A, Martinez-Martin P, Kennedy PG, et al. EFNS guideline on the management of community-acquired bacterial meningitis: report of an EFNS Task Force on acute bacterial meningitis in older children and adults. Eur J Neurol 2008;**15**:649–59.
3. McGill F, Heyderman RS, Michael BD, et al. The UK joint specialist societies guideline on the diagnosis and management of acute meningitis and meningococcal sepsis in immunocompetent adults. J Infect 2016;**72**:405–38.
4. Prasad K, Kumar A, Gupta PK, et al. Third generation cephalosporins versus conventional antibiotics for treating acute bacterial meningitis. Cochrane Database Syst Rev 2007;**17**:CD001832.
5. Tunkel AR, Hartman BJ, Kaplan SL, et al. Practice guidelines for the management of bacterial meningitis. Clin Infect Dis 2004;**39**:1267–84.
6. Michael BD, Menezes BF, Cunniffe J, et al. The effect of delayed lumbar punctures on the diagnosis of acute bacterial meningitis in adults. Emerg Med J 2010;**27**: 433–8.
7. Brouwer MC, McIntyre P, de Gans J, et al. Corticosteroids for acute bacterial meningitis. Cochrane Database Syst Rev 2010;**8**:CD004405.
8. Aronin SI, Peduzzi P, Quagliarello VJ. Community-acquired bacterial meningitis: risk stratification for adverse clinical outcome and effect of antibiotic timing. Ann Intern Med 1998;**129**:862–9.
9. Tyler KL. A history of bacterial meningitis. In: Vinken PJ, Bruyn, GW, editors. *Handbook of Clinical Neurology*. Amsterdam: Elsevier;2010;**95**:417–33.
10. Cullington HE. Light eye colour linked to deafness after meningitis. BMJ 2001;322.

CASE 17

Relapsing Infection and a Spelling Bug

Suresh Kumar Chhetri, Claire Gall and Hedley C.A. Emsley

History

A 53-year-old mechanic was referred to a neurology clinic with an 8-month history of progressive decline in memory. His family reported that he was repetitively telephoning his father and was not looking after himself or his flat properly. He was no longer able to manage his garage business, which he had been running for years. His family also stated that his driving had become dangerous. A month prior to presentation he developed intermittent brief rhythmic jerky movements of his left shoulder and upper limb, without alteration of consciousness. There were no symptoms suggestive of seizures.

Past medical history was significant for severe eczema and previous myocardial infarction. Enquiry also revealed that he had presented 2 years earlier with painful swollen joints, diarrhoea, weight loss, night sweats and conjunctivitis. A duodenal biopsy was performed at this time (**Figure 17.1**). He was treated with 2 weeks of intravenous ceftriaxone and, subsequently, co-trimoxazole for a further year. His systemic symptoms all improved and neurological examination was recorded at this point to be normal.

Medications included simvastatin, bisoprolol and aspirin. He was a smoker of approximately 3 cigarettes a day and drank alcohol socially. He had no pets or unusual hobbies, and did not have any significant travel history. Also, there was no family history of note.

Examination

Systemic examination of the skin of the palms and soles revealed several abnormalities (**Figure 17.2**). There was no lymphadenopathy. Examination of the abdomen, respiratory and cardiovascular system was unremarkable.

Neurological examination revealed complete restriction of voluntary vertical eye movements that could be overcome with passive neck flexion and extension performed by the examiner. Horizontal gaze to the left was also restricted. He had intermittent rhythmic jerking movements of the left shoulder and thoracic region, which was in keeping with segmental myoclonus. Cognitive assessment revealed deficits in attention, memory, and fluency. The rest of the neurological examination was unremarkable. Eye examination, performed by the ophthalmologists, revealed no signs of uveitis.

Initial Differential Diagnosis

The history of cognitive decline dominated by amnesia and impairment of attention was suggestive of encephalopathy or dementia. His limb jerks were due to segmental myoclonus. The restriction of eye movements, which could be overcome, indicated a supranuclear gaze palsy.

The differential diagnosis included Wernicke's encephalopathy as a result of his malabsorptive state; however, this possibility did not provide an explanation for the segmental myoclonus. Thyroid encephalopathy, prion disease and in a younger patient, subacute sclerosing panencephalitis, are causes of cognitive decline and myoclonus.

The previous history of systemic disease (malabsorption, arthritis) and PAS-positive macrophages on duodenal biopsy was suggestive of a possible previous *Tropheryma* infection.

Results of Initial Investigations

Full blood count showed normocytic anaemia of 122 g/l. Serum iron was slightly low at 8 μmol/l with a low iron saturation of 14% and normal serum ferritin, consistent with a pattern of chronic disease. Serum white cell count was 12.9 cells/mm^3 with a neutrophil count of 9.93 cells/mm^3.

The following were either normal or negative: C-reactive protein, erythrocyte sedimentation rate, HIV, treponemal serology, *N*-methyl-D-aspartate receptor antibodies, serum folate, B12, calcium, liver function tests and thyroid.

Cerebrospinal fluid (CSF) analysis showed a white cell count of $< 1 \times 10^9$ white cells/ml, RCC 1×10^9 white cells/ml, protein 0.37 g/l and glucose 3.2 mmol/l.

The electroencephalogram was encephalopathic, but there was no correlate with the segmental twitching. A magnetic resonance imaging scan of the brain was unremarkable, allowing for some motion artefact.

Figure 17.1. Duodenal biopsy samples in a 53-year-old man with progressive cognitive decline and abnormal jerky movements.

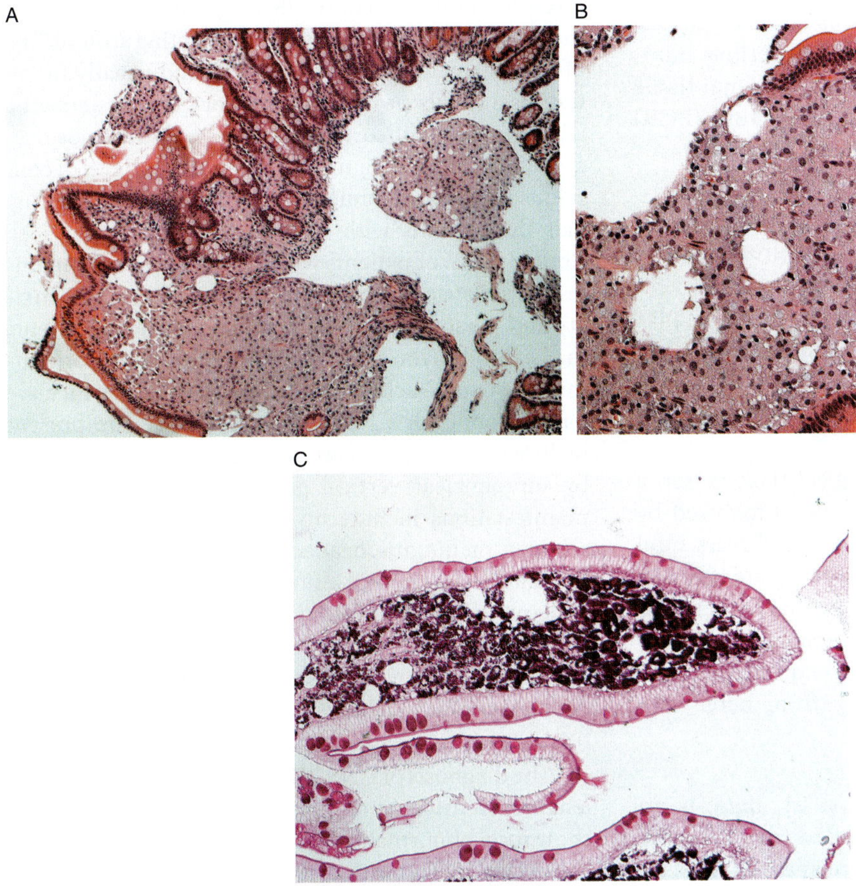

A B

C

These show: (A) Duodenal mucosa with infiltration of lamina propria by sheets of histiocytes (H&E, × 100); (B) higher magnification showing histiocytes in the lamina propria (H&E, × 200); (C) histiocytes laden with periodic acid–Schiff-positive and diastase-resistant organisms consistent with *T. whipplei* (PAS-D, × 100) .

Figure 17.2. Examination findings of the palms (A) and soles (B) of the same patient.

A B

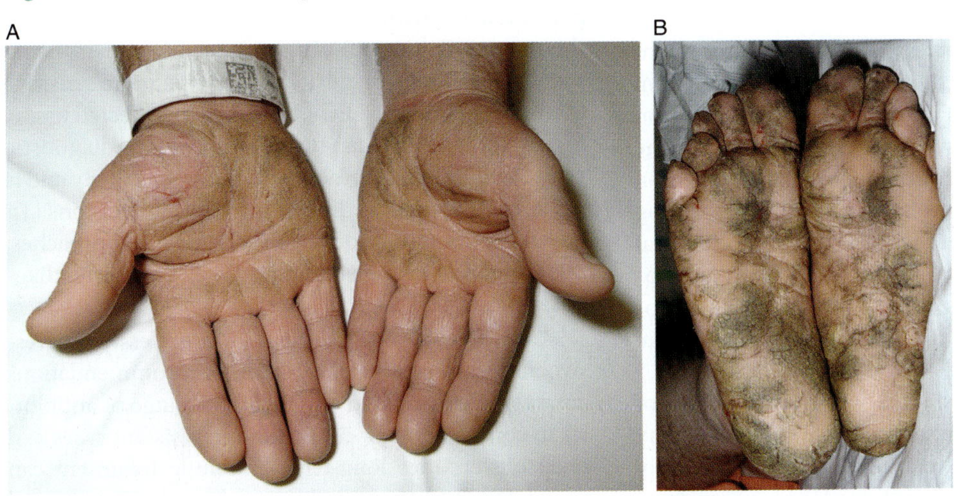

This shows discoloured, cracked and fissured skin on the palms and soles with patchy skin changes of the feet. A diagnosis of chronic eczema was made by the dermatologists following skin biopsy.

Results of Definitive Investigations

Polymerase chain reaction for *Tropheryma whipplei* performed on the CSF showed a borderline number of copies. Therefore, the original duodenal tissue was obtained and polymerase chain reaction (PCR) revealed a very heavy load of the bacteria.

Diagnosis

Given the highly suggestive clinical picture (cognitive decline, segmental myoclonus and supranuclear gaze palsy) and the PCR confirmation of systemic Whipple's disease a central nervous system (CNS) relapse of *Tropheryma whipplei* infection was diagnosed.

Management and Outcome

He was treated with intravenous ceftriaxone for a month (longer than the original course) followed by oral co-trimoxazole, to be taken for at least 2 years. Oral folic acid was given to counteract the antifolate effects of co-trimoxazole. Within a month of treatment there was some improvement in his attention span and ability to navigate around the ward. He was subsequently repatriated to his local hospital for discharge from there.

Prevention

Due to the paucity of confirmed cases, there is no clear trial evidence on the best way to treat systemic Whipple's disease to prevent CNS relapse. There is no evidence that Whipple's disease can be transmitted from human to human, but it is more common in those exposed to soil and animals.

Discussion

Whipple's disease is a rare, chronic, multi-system infectious disorder caused by a rod-shaped bacterium *Tropheryma whipplei* (**Figure 17.1**). The condition mainly affects middle-aged Caucasian men [1,2]. The onset is insidious and clinical picture variable; common manifestations include weight loss, non-deforming arthritis, diarrhoea, malabsorption and abdominal pain. Other features may include fever, lymphadenopathy, valvular heart disease, culture-negative endocarditis, polyseritis anaemia, and hyperpigmentation, as seen in this case [1–3].

Neurological manifestations occur in 10–40% of patients and irreversible neurological damage may persist despite adequate treatment [1]. Approximately 50% of patients may show infection of the CNS, as demonstrated by PCR analysis of the CSF, even in the absence of neurological features [1,2]. Whipple's disease may rarely be confined to the CNS. Cognitive impairment is the most common manifestation, affecting around 70% of patients with CNS involvement, and usually manifests as a slowly progressive memory loss or dementia with a frontal–subcortical pattern [1,2]. The most frequent neurological signs include an altered level of consciousness and supranuclear ophthalmoplegia affecting half the patients with CNS Whipple's disease [3,4]. Roughly 40% of patients with CNS involvement manifest psychiatric symptoms including depression, anxiety and personality changes, and a quarter of patients may exhibit myoclonus. Oculomasticatory myorhythmia and oculo-facial–skeletal myorhythmia, which are pathognomic for CNS Whipple's disease, are present in 20% of patients and are almost always accompanied by supranuclear vertical gaze palsy [4]. Other CNS manifestations include myoclonus, cerebellar ataxia, seizures, meningitis, headache, hypothalamic dysfunction and focal cerebral lesions [1–4]. It is important to recognise that only around 15% of patients with CNS Whipple's disease manifest the classical triad of dementia, supranuclear gaze palsy and myoclonus [4]. Other ocular signs may include uveitis, retinitis, vitritis, keratitis, optic neuritis and papilloedema [1,2].

The diagnosis of CNS Whipple's disease can be challenging. Neuroimaging may be unremarkable or may show focal abnormalities including enhancing or non-enhancing lesions with or without mass effect [4]. CSF examination may show raised protein and leucocytosis [4]. Small intestinal endoscopy may show lymphangiitis and histological examination of biopsy tissue, most often duodenal, may reveal foamy macrophages containing periodic acid–Schiff (PAS)-positive material, as seen for this patient (**Figure 17.3**). Immunohistochemistry using specific antibodies against *T. whipplei* is more sensitive than PAS staining [1]. PCR testing of the affected tissue, for instance the CSF, can further improve the diagnostic yield [1]. *T. whipplei* serology has a low specificity and is not recommended for informing clinical decisions [1]. Given the limitations of various diagnostic approaches, a combination of PAS staining and PCR is a useful diagnostic strategy [1,2].

Untreated, Whipple's disease is relentlessly progressive and ultimately fatal. Treatment recommendations are not evidence-based and include a range of antibiotics in combination [1–5]. Antibiotic-resistant cases and relapse even after long-term antibiotic treatment can occur. The mean time to clinical relapse is 4.2 years and is usually characterised by neurological involvement [5].

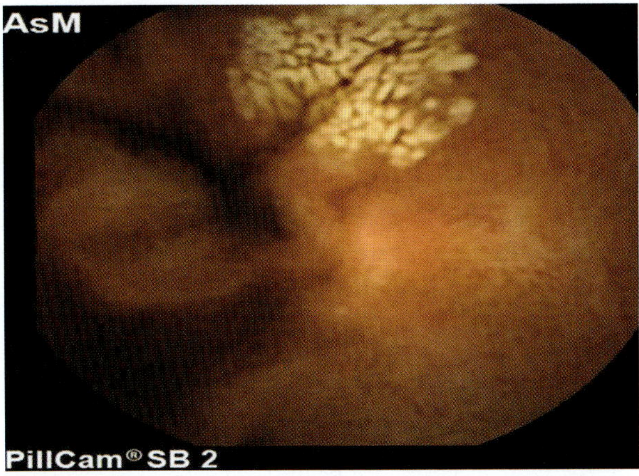

Figure 17.3. Capsule endoscopy showing lymphangiitis of the jejunum in a patient with *T. whipplei* infection confirmed on PCR. Reproduced with permission from [6].

Key Points

- Whipple's disease is a rare, chronic, multi-system infectious disorder caused by a rod-shaped bacterium *Tropheryma whipplei.*
- CNS Whipple's disease classically presents with the triad of dementia, supranuclear gaze palsy and myoclonus, although this combination is only seen in about 15% of patients.
- Most patients also have manifestations of systemic disease, which may include weight loss, diarrhoea, malabsorption and abdominal pain, non-deforming arthritis, fever, lymphadenopathy, anaemia and cardiac disease.
- Diagnosis is difficult, but periodic acid–Schiff staining of duodenal biopsy tissue and PCR of that tissue and CSF is a useful diagnostic strategy.
- In patients with systemic Whipple's disease, evidence for CNS infection should be sought, because even in the absence of overt neurological disease incomplete treatment of CNS infection can result in late relapse and the prognosis in these cases may be poor.

Looking Back

In 1907, George H. Whipple termed the disease 'intestinal lipodystrophy' [7]. The causative organism *T. whipplei* was successfully cultured nearly a century later in 2000 [8].

Did You Know?

Although the condition was described for a long time, the name of the causative organism was first proposed in 1992 as *Tropheryma whippelii* from the Greek word *trophe* (nourishment) and *eryma* (barrier) as it causes malabsorption, and from the name of G.H. Whipple [9]. For reasons that are not clear, his name was used with an uncommon spelling. The name was subsequently changed to *Tropheryma whipplei* in 2001 [10].

References

1. Schneider T, Moos V, Loddenkemper C, et al. Whipple's disease: new aspects of pathogenesis and treatment. Lancet Infect Dis 2008;**8**:179–90.
2. Fenollar F, Puéchal X, Raoult D. Whipple's disease. N Engl J Med 2007;**4**(356):55–66.
3. Ratnaike RN. Whipple's disease. Postgrad Med J 2000;**76**:760–6.
4. Louis ED, Lynch T, Kaufmann P, Fahn S, Odel J. Diagnostic guidelines in central nervous system Whipple's disease. Ann Neurol 1996;**40**:561–8.
5. Keinath RD, Merrell DE, Vlietstra R, Dobbins WO III. Antibiotic treatment and relapse in Whipple's disease: long term follow-up of 88 patients. Gastroenterology 1985;**88**:1867–73.
6. Ferreira F, Cardosa H, Albuqueque A, Magro F, Macedo G. Whipple's disease and giardiasis, an uncommon association. J Port Gastroenterol 2012:**19**:217–18.
7. Whipple GH. A hitherto undescribed disease characterized anatomically by deposits of fat and fatty acids in the intestinal and mesenteric lymphatic tissues. Bull Johns Hopkins Hosp 1907;**18**:382–91.
8. Raoult D, Birg M, La Scola B, et al. Cultivation of the bacillus of Whipple's disease. N Engl J Med 2000;**342**:620–5.
9. Relman DA, Schmidt TM, MacDermott RP, Falkow S. Identification of the uncultured bacillus of Whipple's disease. N Engl J Med 1992;**327**:293–301.
10. La Scola B, Fenollar F, Fournier PE, et al. Descriptionof *Tropheryma whipplei* gen. nov., sp. nov., the Whipple's disease bacillus. Int J Syst Evol Microbiol 2001;**51**:1471–9.

CASE 18

Scratching the Surface

Sylviane Defres

History

A 30-year-old butcher presented to the medical admissions unit with a 4-day history of bi-frontal headache, which started after he came home from work one day. It was accompanied by vomiting, fever and night sweats. He denied any neck stiffness, photophobia, rash or gastrointestinal symptoms. He was usually fit and healthy and was only admitted once before, 2 years prior, for what he was told was a viral illness. He had presented with spots in his mouth and genital area at that time.

Five days into hospitalisation the nurses reported that he had been agitated overnight and he had been found staggering in the corridor the following morning.

Examination

Examination on admission was essentially unremarkable except for a temperature of 38.6°C and a 2 cm epitrochlear lymph node; in addition, he had an area of inflammation on his right 5th digit, which he confirmed as being the site of an altercation with a stray cat 3 weeks earlier. Of note, there were no focal neurological signs and Kernig's and Brudzinki's signs were negative.

On day 5 of hospitalisation, neurological examination revealed a profound gait and limb ataxia, left facial weakness, left sensorineural hearing loss and a left 6th nerve palsy. This was followed by urinary retention and sleep disturbance, and a progressive decline in his speech and swallowing.

Initial Differential Diagnosis

After the neurological deterioration on day 5, the differential list included:

- Brainstem encephalitis (rhombencephalitis)
  - Infective causes include herpes simplex virus (HSV) 1&2, Epstein–Barr virus (EBV), mumps virus, Enterovirus 71, *Bartonella henselae* and *Listeria monocytogenes*
  - Bickerstaff's encephalitis
  - Paraneoplastic syndromes, e.g. lymphoma

Results of Initial Investigations

The peripheral white cell count on admission was 10.5 $\times 10^9$ cells/l, of which 8.0 $\times 10^9$ cells/l were neutrophils and 1.5 $\times 10^9$ cells/l lymphocytes. Urea was 8.2 mmol/l and creatinine was 110 µmol/l. Liver function tests were normal and C-reactive protein was < 3 mg/l.

At lumbar puncture the opening pressure was 32 cm of cerebrospinal fluid (CSF), protein was 0.77 g/l, glucose was 3.6 mmol/l (serum glucose 6.3 mmol/l); there were 2495 red blood cells/mm^3 and 194 white cells/mm^3, 100% of which were lymphocytes.

Computed tomography head was normal; therefore, a subsequent magnetic resonance imaging (MRI) was performed (**Figure 18.1**).

Autoantibodies, including ANA, ANCA, IgA antigliadin, IgA antiendomyosin, Anti GM1, GM2, GM3, GA1, GD1a, GD1b, GT1b, GQ1b, GD3 antibodies, antisulpatide, antigloboside antibodies all came back as negative.

Results of Definitive Investigations

Serological testing, including HIV, Cytomegalovirus, *Toxoplasma gondii, Brucella* spp., *Borrelia burgdorferi,*

Figure 18.1. A coronal FLAIR MRI image in a 30-year-old male with headache, encephalopathy seizures and cranial nerve palsies.

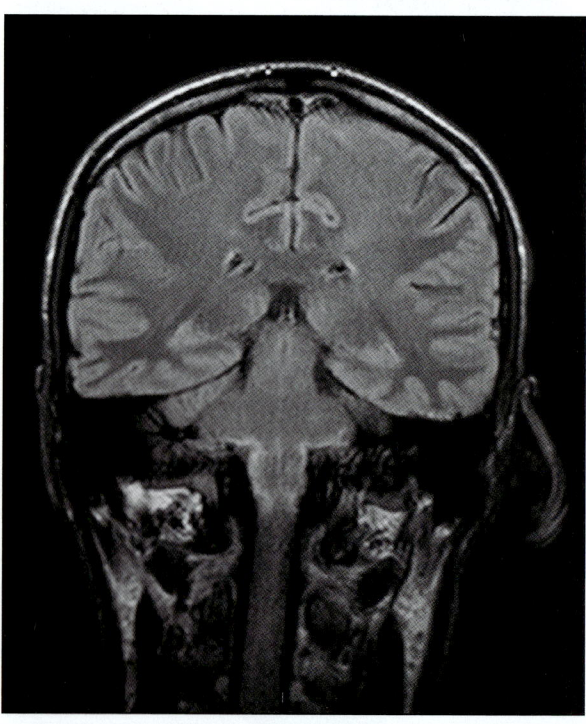

This shows subtle hyperintensity at the surfaces of the basal medulla and pons.

Figure 18.2. H&E-stained section of lymph node at low (×4) (left) and high (×20) (right) in the same patient.

A B

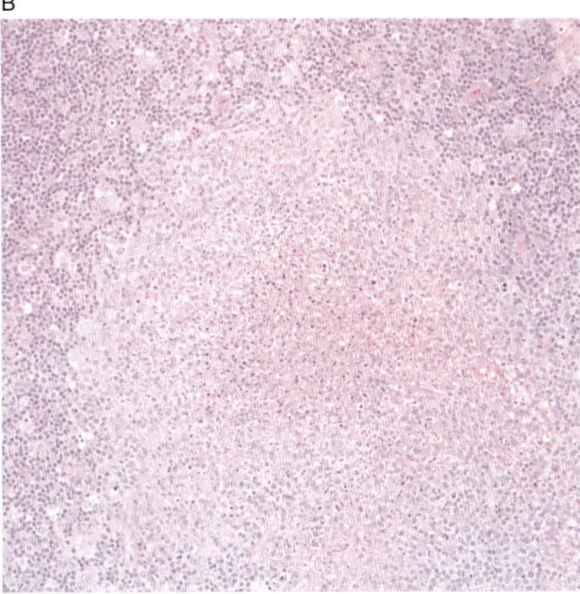

This shows reactive follicles with numerous areas of necrotic change occasionally containing giant cells. There was no evidence of vasculitis or caseation. Histological appearance and genetic studies showed no evidence of a lymphoproliferative disorder. Special stains for infectious agents were carried out, but no organisms were seen.

Coxiella burnetti, Chlamydia and *Mycoplasma* spp., was negative. EBV serology showed past infection.

A lymph node biopsy was performed (**Figure 18.2**).

Serological investigations: IgM and IgG *Bartonella* antibody titres confirmed a recent *Bartonella* infection. *Bartonella henselae* was detected by polymerase chain reaction (PCR) of the biopsy material, and speciation confirmed by DNA sequencing (**Figure 18.3**).

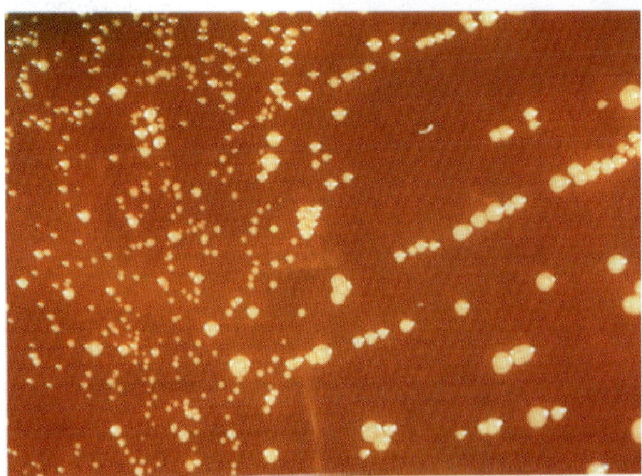

Figure 18.3. *Bartonella henselae* showing variable colony morphology on blood agar after 5 days of incubation in 5% CO_2 at 37°C. (Image from [1] with permission of Elsevier and courtesy of Dr T. H. Koh, Royal London Hospital.)

Diagnosis

Brainstem encephalitis secondary to *Bartonella henselae* infection (cat scratch disease).

Management and Outcome

After the initial assessment, the patient was empirically started on azithromycin to treat a presumptive diagnosis of cat scratch disease. After the neurological deterioration this was changed to aciclovir, amoxicillin, doxycycline and rifampicin, to treat other possible causes of brain infection, pending the results of investigations.

When he subsequently became more ataxic and encephalopathic and developed autonomic features (urinary retention and sleep disturbance) with speech and swallow involvement, he was commenced on intravenous immunoglobulin due to the possibility of Bickerstaff's encephalitis.

In total he received 4 weeks of doxycycline and rifampicin. Aciclovir and amoxicillin were stopped when HSV 1&2 and varicella zoster virus PCRs and culture for *Listeria monocytogenes* were all negative.

He progressed steadily with physiotherapy and occupational therapy and was discharged home after approximately 1 month; at that stage he was walking with the aid of crutches. At follow-up in clinic 6 weeks later he was entirely back to normal.

Prevention

The United States Centers for Disease Control and Prevention advise the avoidance of 'rough play' with cats, especially kittens, which may lead the cat to scratch or bite. If someone does get scratched or bitten, they should wash the area immediately and thoroughly with soap and water. People with open wounds should not allow cats to lick them, and control of cat fleas is also advised [2].

Discussion

Cat scratch disease is caused by the Gram-negative bacillus *Bartonella henselae*. Most cases are seen in young children. In approximately 90% of cases there is a primary cutaneous lesion that develops 3–7 days after the animal contact scratch or bite; this is usually a cat or kitten (**Figure 18.4**), but may be a dog with cat fleas or may be just contact with the fleas directly [3]. The skin lesion may remain for 1–3 weeks. Regional lymphadenopathy on the ipsilateral side is the most common presentation. In the majority of cases this is a single node, but around 20% may have multiple nodes at one site and a third of patients have nodes at multiple sites. However, widespread lymphadenopathy does not usually occur. Node enlargement usually persists for 2–4 months. Approximately 30–60% of individuals will have a low-grade fever, 25% have fatigue, 10% have a headache or sore throat and 10% a transient rash [4,5].

Atypical presentation of cat scratch disease occurs in approximately 10% of cases. About half of these are due to Parinaud's oculoglandular syndrome, a self-limiting granulomatous conjunctivitis with ipsilateral preauricular lymphadenitis. Other atypical presentations include self-limiting granulomatous hepatitis or splenitis, atypical pneumonitis and a range of neurological syndromes, mainly encephalopathy and neuroretinitis (Box 18.1) [6,7]. In immunocompromised individuals *B. henselae* can cause angiomatosis and peliosis (a type of vascular hepatitis).

Encephalopathy occurs in 2–4% of all cat scratch disease, usually following lymphadenopathy. Generalised headache and restlessness are common and nearly 50% of patients develop seizures. Any neurological deficits, such as aphasia, cranial nerve palsy, hemiplegia or ataxia, tend to be self-limiting, resolving in weeks to months. CSF findings are non-specific but help exclude other aetiologies. Protein and white cell count are raised in about a third with lymphocytes predominating. Only a minority have abnormalities on neuroimaging [6]. The pathogenesis of the neurological syndromes in cat scratch disease is uncertain, but may be due to direct invasion of the central nervous system by *B. henselae* or other mechanisms, such as vasculitis [6].

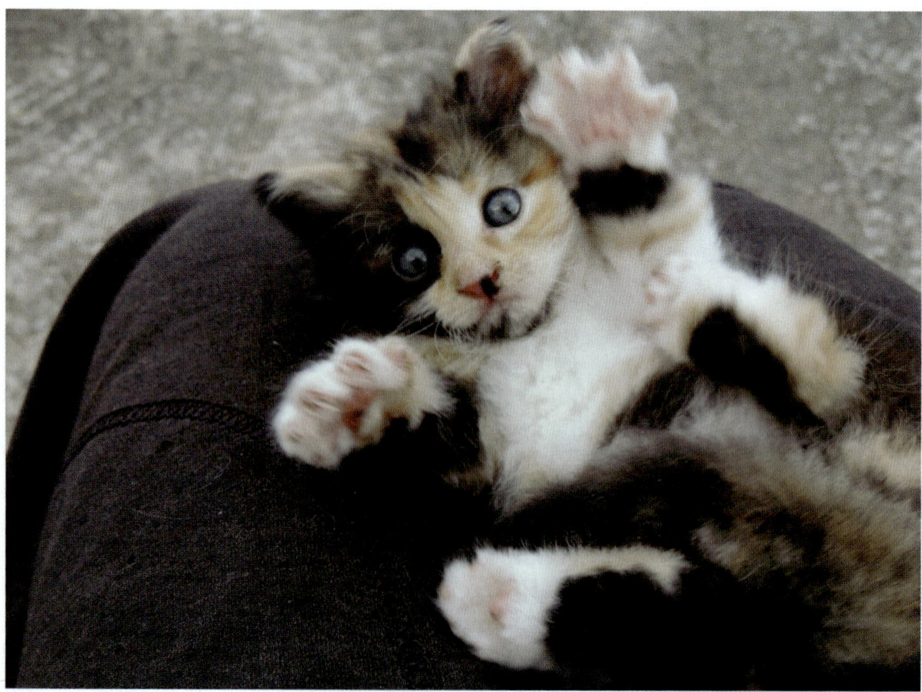

Figure 18.4. Cute, but potentially dangerous. (Photo © Loukas Loukopoulos / EyeEm.)

Box 18.1. Recognised Neurological Complications of Cat Scratch Disease.

Encephalopathy
Neuroretinitis
Myelitis
Cranial neuropathies
Isolated ataxia
Dysphasia
Polyneuropathy
Acute hemiplegia
Epilepsia partialis continua
Movement disorders*

* Includes: chorea, athetosis and tremor

Cat scratch disease is usually diagnosed clinically. However, a lymph node biopsy may be performed to exclude lymphoma, as it was in the case described here. The typical histopathology of an affected lymph node shows non-specific inflammatory reactions including granulomata and stellate necrosis, as was seen here. The bacilli of *B. henselae* are best demonstrated by silver staining with Warthin Starry stain [8]. Serological confirmation can be helpful [9].

Only azithromycin has been demonstrated to accelerate the resolution of typical cat scratch disease. It remains debatable whether treatment is necessary at all in a self-limiting condition. There is no evidence that antibiotics alter the course of most atypical presentations of cat scratch disease, especially neurological manifestations. However, reports suggest a more rapid resolution of treated neuroretinitis. Also, a combination of two agents has been suggested, and some have favoured erythromycin or doxycycline combined with rifampicin [10].

Key Points

- Cat scratch disease, a febrile illness with rash and lymphadenopathy due to infection with *Bartonella henselae*, is fairly common, especially among children, and is usually self-limiting
- Neurological complications occur in 2–4% of cases, the most common being encephalopathy, often with seziures
- Without seeking a history of contact with a cat (or occasionally a dog) and careful examination for lymphadenopathy and/or the site of inoculation, the diagnosis can be missed
- In brainstem encephalitis, as seen in this patient, a thorough exclusion of other causes is needed.
- The treatment of neurological cat scratch disease remains uncertain, but at present treatment with doxycycline ± rifampicin is suggested.

Looking Back

Cat scratch disease was defined as a syndrome in 1950 by Debre et al., but it took more than 30 years for the infectious agent *Bartonella henselae* to be recognised. Nearly 100 years earlier in 1889 Parinaud had described the oculoglandular syndrome which bears his name and is now known also to be due to *Bartonella henselae*.

Did You Know?

The Warthin Starry technique, which uses silver nitrate to stain organisms, was first used to detect spirochaetes in 1920, when introduced by Aldred Scott Warthin and Allen Chronister Starry. It stains organisms brown to black and the background is light golden brown/golden yellow.

American rockabilly band, Stray Cats, have no known link whatsoever to Cat Scratch Fever, but played some quite cool music in the 1980s (**Figure 18.5**).

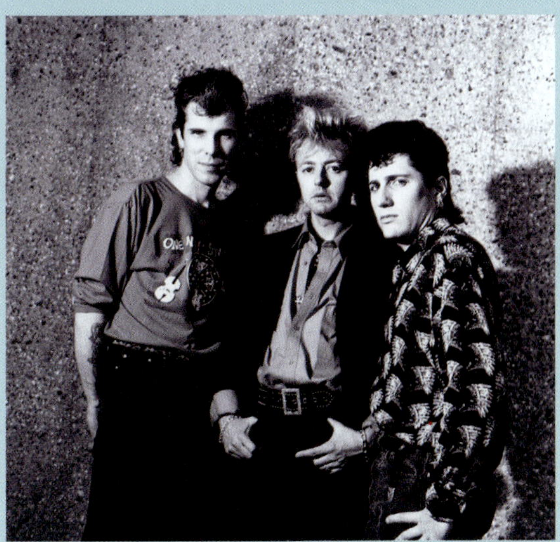

Figure 18.5. Stray Cats in Japan. (Photo courtesy of Masao Nakagami, reproduced under CC BY-SA 2.0.)

References

1. Stewart BA. Human infection with *Bartonella* species. Clin Microbiol Infect 1997;**3**:677–89.
2. www.cdc.gov/bartonella/prevention/index.html (accessed May 10, 2018).
3. Wear DJ, Margileth AM, Hadfield TL, et al. Cat scratch disease: a bacterial infection. Science 1983;**221**:1403.
4. Carithers HA. Cat scratch disease: an overview based on a study of 1200 patients. Am J Dis Child 1985;**139**:1124.
5. Moriarty RA, Margileth AM. Cat scratch disease. Infect Dis Clin Noth Am 1987;**1**:575.
6. Marra CM. Neurologic complications of *Bartonella henselae* infection. Curr Opin Neurol 1995;**8**:164.
7. Baylor P, Garoufi A, Karpathios T, et al. Transverse myelitis in 2 patients with *Bartonella henselae* infection (cat scratch disease). Clin Infect Dis 2007;**45**:e42.
8. Rolain JM, Lepidi H, Zanaret M, et al. Lymph node biopsy specimens and diagnosis of cat-scratch disease. Emerg Infect Dis 2006;**12**:1338.
9. Szelc-Kelly CM, Goral S, Perez-Perez GI, et al. Serologic responses to *Bartonella* and *Afipia* antigens in patients with cat scratch disease. Pediatrics 1995;**96**:1137.
10. Bass JW, Freitas BC, Freitas AD. Prospective randomized double-blind placebo controlled evaluation of azithromycin for treatment of cat scratch disease. Pediatr Infect Dis J 1998;**17**:447.

CASE 19

Cytokine Storm

Anu Goenka and Rachel Kneen

History

A 10-month-old girl presented with a 1-day history of fever, diarrhoea, coryzal illness and a brief generalised tonic–clonic seizure. Her older brother had been suffering with a diarrhoeal illness for the preceding week. Her father had returned from a trip to India 6 weeks previously, although she had not travelled outside of the UK. She had no previous history of febrile seizures or unprovoked seizures. She had been given paracetamol at home and there was no history of aspirin exposure. Her neurological development and growth were normal. Her immunisations were up to date and there was no other relevant past medical history.

Examination

On examination she was unwell, drowsy and floppy. Her airway was patent. Her respiratory rate was 40 breaths per minute and she had oxygen saturations of 99% while receiving 10 l/minute of oxygen. Her heart rate was 175 beats per minute, blood pressure 68/45 mmHg and capillary refill was 4 seconds centrally. Her Glasgow coma score (GCS) was 11/15 (eyes 2, verbal 4, motor 5) and her pupils were 3 mm bilaterally and reactive to light. The optic fundi were not visualised. Deep tendon reflexes were present and her plantar responses were equivocal. Her axillary temperature was 40.3°C. No rash or meningism was noted. Her mucous membranes were normal and the systemic examination was otherwise unremarkable.

Initial Differential Diagnosis

- Sepsis
- Meningitis
- Encephalopathy
  - Viral encephalitis
  - Para-/post-infectious, e.g. acute disseminated encephalomyelitis
  - Metabolic, e.g. Reye syndrome, mitochondrial disorder
- Toxic shock syndrome
- Haemolytic uraemic syndrome

Results of Initial Investigations

Her capillary blood glucose was 9.7 mmol/l and her venous blood gas demonstrated severe lactic acidosis. The full blood count showed a mildly raised neutrophil count and low platelets, although her C-reactive protein was normal. A blood film demonstrated schistocytes and Burr cells and clotting studies found a raised prothrombin time and low fibrinogen. Her renal and liver function tests showed significant impairment, with a markedly raised alanine aminotransferase. The blood creatinine kinase was also markedly elevated and the plasma ammonia was normal. A chest X-ray was unremarkable. An immediate lumbar puncture was contraindicated due to the condition of the patient; therefore, a computer tomography (CT) brain scan was performed (**Figure 19.1**).

Management and Outcome

Her circulatory shock responded to resuscitation with an intravenous fluid bolus. Initial antimicrobial treatment included ceftriaxone. Within 2 hours, she

Figure 19.1. Axial CT head in a 10-month-old girl presenting with a coryzal illness, fever, reduced consciousness and a seizure.

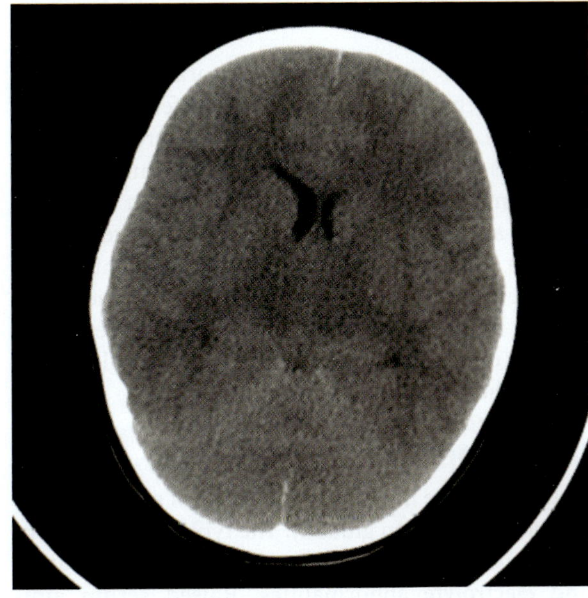

This shows that the brain is tight and swollen with effacement of the sulci due to cerebral oedema.

became more unresponsive and her GCS dropped to 8/15 (eyes 2, verbal 2, motor 4). She also had clinical signs of subtle motor seizures (rhythmical twitching of the right thumb and rapid flickering of the eyelids). During rapid sequence intubation she became bradycardic and required 3 minutes of cardiopulmonary resuscitation. Soon after this she received mannitol and hydrocortisone. Before transfer to intensive care, antimicrobial cover was broadened to include aciclovir and oseltamivir.

Twelve hours after initial presentation her clinical condition had failed to improve. Her liver function derangement, coagulopathy, metabolic acidosis and thrombocytopaenia had all deteriorated further. She had fixed and dilated pupils, bilateral retinal haemorrhages and absent brainstem reflexes. After consultation with her parents, intensive care support was withdrawn. A post-mortem was not performed.

Results of Definitive Investigations

A few days later the results of her blood, urine and throat cultures from admission were all found to be negative, as well as polymerase chain reaction (PCR) of her respiratory secretions. However, PCR of a faeces sample was positive for rotavirus.

Diagnosis

Haemorrhagic shock and encephalopathy syndrome in association with rotavirus.

Prevention

Rotavirus is transmitted faeco-orally; therefore, hand hygiene is critical to reduce infection risk. In 2009, the WHO recommended the introduction of rotavirus vaccines into all national immunisation programmes [1]. Two vaccines have been shown to be safe and efficacious: (a) a monovalent ressortant vaccine (Rotarix) and (b) an oral quintavalent bovine vaccine (RotaTeq) [1]. These vaccines provide protection for over 90% of the most common serotypes causing disease in the USA and Europe, but less than 70% of those in sub-Saharan Africa [1].

Discussion

Rotavirus is the most common cause of severe gastroenteritis in children globally. The typical symptoms of gastroenteritis can be accompanied by dehydration and electrolyte abnormalities. Raised serum aminotransferases are also a common finding. Rotavirus is associated with various neurological manifestations including febrile seizures and encephalopathic syndromes, such as haemorrhagic shock and encephalopathy syndrome. Rotavirus is not normally neurotropic; i.e. it does not usually invade the central nervous system (CNS). However, unlike influenza-related encephalopathy, several reports have described the presence of viral RNA in the cerebrospinal fluid [2]. It is not known by what route rotavirus may arrive in the CNS, although rotavirus has also been found in various other extra-intestinal sites, including the kidney and the liver [2]. The role of rotavirus in the pathogenesis of encephalopathy may be similar to that reported for influenza infection, with viral infection providing a trigger for an exaggerated proinflammatory host response [3].

Haemorrhagic shock and encephalopathy syndrome was first described by Levin in 1983 as a high-mortality condition characteristically affecting infants with a minor viral infection [4]. The clinical presentation includes hyperpyrexia, encephalopathy, diarrhoea, circulatory shock and multi-system dysfunction, such as renal and liver dysfunction, accompanied by coagulopathy, as was seen here. The term 'haemorrhagic shock' can be misleading, as circulatory shock usually precedes coagulopathy and bleeding [5]. A CT scan of the brain typically demonstrates cerebral oedema and a magnetic resonance imaging scan may delineate the extent of haemorrhagic brain injury [6]. Haemorrhagic shock and encephalopathy syndrome has been described in association with several viral infections, the most common being influenza (**Table 19.1**) [7]. The precise pathophysiological mechanism underlying the syndrome has not been elucidated. Proposed theories include the role of hyperpyrexia and elevated proinflammatory cytokines resulting in a 'cytokine storm' [8,9].

Modified diagnostic criteria for haemorrhagic shock and encephalopathy syndrome were suggested by Mizaguchi and colleagues in 2007 [10] (**Table 19.2**). It is important that relevant differential diagnoses are considered and appropriate investigations performed. For example, admission blood cultures are important to exclude sepsis. In addition, as in this case, normal or an only mildly elevated ammonia makes Reye's syndrome unlikely and negative stool cultures in the presence of diarrhoea make haemolytic uraemic syndrome less likely also. In this case, toxic shock syndrome was improbable given the absence of rash, mucosal involvement and failure to isolate

Table 19.1 Aetiology of reported cases of haemorrhagic shock and encephalopathy syndrome in the published literature (1983–2013 inclusive).

Organism Publication	No pathogen	Influenza	Parainfluenza	Rhinovirus	Adenovirus	RSV	Rotavirus	Norovirus	HHV-6	CMV	Polio
Levin et al. (1983) [4]	4		1	1						1	2
Weibley et al. (1989) [14]	2	1									
Rotbart (1996) [15]							2				
Takahashi et al. (2000) [16]		1									
Ince et al. (2000) [17]						1	1				
Gooskens et al. (2007) [18]		2									
Rinka et al. (2003) [9]	4	1			1		1	1			
Gefen et al. (2008) [19]					2						
Lung et al. (2011) [20]		1									
Hoshino et al. (2012) [7]		3				1		1	2		
Total	**10**	**9**	**1**	**1**	**3**	**2**	**4**	**2**	**2**	**1**	**2**

Table 19.2 Diagnostic criteria for haemorrhagic shock and encephalopathy syndrome (adapted from reference [10]).

- Age at onset during infancy (usually 2–10 months)
- Acute encephalopathy
- Fever
- Shock
- Disseminated intravascular coagulation
- Hepatic dysfunction
- Renal dysfunction
- Normal blood ammonia values
- Exclusion of similar infantile conditions (e.g. septic shock, toxic shock syndrome, Reye syndrome, and haemolytic–uraemic syndrome)

Staphylococcus aureus or group A streptococcus. The prognosis of haemorrhagic shock and encephalopathy syndrome is poor, with 50% mortality and 30% left with significant neurodisability [11]. Typical post-mortem findings include intravascular microthrombi and haemorrhages, plus centrilobular hepatic necrosis and cerebral oedema [8].

Key Points

- Haemorrhagic shock and encephalopathy syndrome is characterised by hyperpyrexia, encephalopathy, diarrhoea, circulatory shock and multi-system dysfunction.
- It is associated with several viral infections, including rotavirus and especially influenza.
- The mechanisms is thought to be a proinflammatory 'cytokine storm'.
- Rotavirus is also associated with other neurological manifestations including a milder encephalopathy.
- Treatment for haemorrhagic shock and encephalopathy syndrome is supportive and the prognosis is poor.

Looking Back

Rotavirus was discovered in 1973 by Bishop et al. and was named because of its characteristic wheel-like structure seen on electron microscopy (**Figure 19.2**) [12].

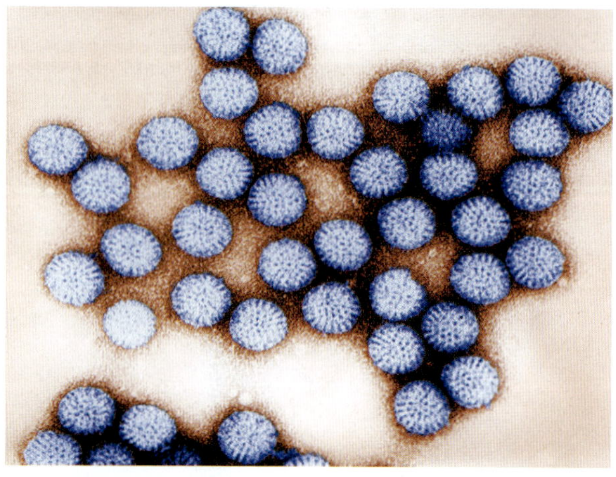

Figure 19.2. Transmission electron micrograph revealing ultrastructural morphology of rotavirus showing double-shelled particles (Courtesy of Centers for Disease Control and Prevention, USA).

Did You Know?

Experienced nurses may be able to identify rotavirus in stool by smell alone [13].

References

1. Vesikari T. Rotavirus vaccination: a concise review. Clin Microbiol Infect 2012;**18**:57–63.
2. Lynch M, Lee B, Azimi P, et al. Rotavirus and central nervous system symptoms: cause or contaminant? Case reports and review. Clin Infect Dis 2001;**33**:932–8.
3. İncecik F, Herguner M, Altunbasak S, Solgun H. Acute encephalopathy associated rotavirus gastroenteritis. J Pediatr Neurosci 2009;**4**:141.
4. Levin M, Hjelm M, Kay JD, et al. Haemorrhagic shock and encephalopathy: a new syndrome with a high mortality in young children. Lancet 1983;**2**:64–7.
5. Bacon CJ, Hall SM. Haemorrhagic shock encephalopathy syndrome in the British Isles. Arch Dis Child 1992;**67**:985–93.
6. Glauser TA, Pachter LM, Zimmerman RA. Abnormal magnetic resonance images in hemorrhagic shock and encephalopathy syndrome. J Child Neurol 1992;7:371–4.

7. Hoshino A, Saitoh M, Oka A, et al. Epidemiology of acute encephalopathy in Japan, with emphasis on the association of viruses and syndromes. Brain Dev 2012;**34**:337–43.
8. Bacon CJ, Bell SA, Gaventa JM, Greenwood DC. Case control study of thermal environment preceding haemorrhagic shock encephalopathy syndrome. Arch Dis Child 1999;**81**:155–8.
9. Rinka H, Yoshida T, Kubota T, et al. Hemorrhagic shock and encephalopathy syndrome – the markers for an early HSES diagnosis. BMC Pediatr 2008;**8**:43.
10. Mizuguchi M, Yamanouchi H, Ichiyama T, Shiomi M. Acute encephalopathy associated with influenza and other viral infections. Acta Neurol Scand 2007;**115**:45–56.
11. Thébaud B, Husson B, Navelet Y, et al. Haemorrhagic shock and encephalopathy syndrome: neurological course and predictors of outcome. Intensive Care Med 1999;**25**:293–9.
12. Bishop R. Discovery of rotavirus: implications for child health. J Gastroenterol Hepatol 2009;**24**:S81–5.
13. Poulton J, Tarlow MJ. Diagnosis of rotavirus gastroenteritis by smell. Arch Dis Childhood 1987;**62**:851–2.
14. Weibley RE, Pimentel B, Ackerman NB. Hemorrhagic shock and encephalopathy syndrome of infants and children. Crit Care Med 1989;**17**:335–8.
15. Rotbart HA. Rotavirus-associated hemorrhagic shock and encephalopathy. Clin Infect Dis 1996;**23**:1334.
16. Takahashi M, Yamada T, Nakashita Y, et al. Influenza virus-induced encephalopathy: clinicopathologic study of an autopsied case. Pediatr Int 2000;**42**: 204–14.
17. Ince E, Kuloglu Z, Akinci Z. Hemorrhagic shock and encephalopathy syndrome: neurologic features. Pediatr Emerg Care 2000;**16**:260–4.
18. Gooskens J, Kuiken T, Claas EC, et al. Severe influenza resembling hemorrhagic shock and encephalopathy syndrome. J Clin Virol 2007;**39**:136–40.
19. Gefen R, Eshel G, Abu-Kishk I, et al. Hemorrhagic shock and encephalopathy syndrome: clinical course and neurological outcome. J Child Neurol 2008;**23**:589–92.
20. Lung DC, Lui WYS, Ng HL, Lam DSY, Que TL. Hemorrhagic shock and encephalopathy syndrome in a child with pandemic H1N1 2009 influenza virus. Pediatr Infect Dis J 2011;**30**:998–9.

CASE 20

Ter-wit-ter-woo!

Sylviane Defres

History

A 38-year-old bisexual man presented to an Accident and Emergency department with a 3-day history of progressively worsening headache, light-headedness and increasing lethargy. In the 2 days prior to admission his partner stated that he had noticed the patient was having short-term memory problems, appeared to be having difficulty finding words and had been confused at home; he did not know the day of the week and was forgetting names of various family members. His partner also thought that his face looked 'puffy' on one side, and mentioned that the patient was due to see the optician for some bilateral blurred vision that he had been experiencing over the previous couple of weeks.

His past medical history included hospitalisation for pneumonia 2 years earlier and an episode of shingles about 4 months prior to this admission.

Examination

On admission, he had a temperature of 38.7°C and was lethargic but rousable. He was disorientated to time and place and was only able to follow simple one-step commands. Cranial nerve examination revealed a left facial nerve weakness affecting the whole side of his face, but the remainder of the cranial nerves were intact. Power and deep tendon reflexes were normal throughout, but Babinski's sign was equivocal. Evaluation for cerebellar signs was difficult because of poor cooperation from the patient.

Funduscopy was performed (**Figure 20.1**).

Initial Differential Diagnosis

- HIV infection with complicating opportunistic infection
  - Viral encephalitis including herpes simplex virus (HSV), varicella zoster virus (VZV), Cytomegalovirus (CMV)
  - Toxoplasma encephalitis
- The associated retinitis made VZV or CMV most likely

Results of Initial Investigations

Blood results were generally unremarkable apart from his sodium, which was 130 mmol/l; he had a slightly low creatinine (probably reflecting low muscle bulk) and a low peripheral white cell count of 3.0×10^6/ml.

He tested positive for HIV antibody and his CD4 count was 30 cells/µl with HIV viral load awaited.

A lumbar puncture was performed and the cerebrospinal fluid (CSF) showed 116 white cells, with 75% lymphocytes and 25% neutrophils, CSF glucose was 2.8 mmol/l (simultaneous serum glucose was 5.8 mmol/l) and protein was 1.39 g/l. Bacterial, mycobacterial and fungal stains were negative and CSF was negative for all cultures at 48 hours.

CSF polymerase chain reaction (PCR) for HSV 1&2, VZV, parechovirus and enterovirus was negative. Cryptococcal antigen was negative.

A magnetic resonance imaging (MRI) brain scan was performed at this stage (**Figure 20.2**).

Results of Definitive Investigations

CMV PCR of the CSF was positive.

Diagnosis

Advanced human immunodeficiency disease with Cytomegalovirus (CMV) ventriculoencephalitis and CMV retinitis.

Management and Outcome

He was given a combination of intravenous ganciclovir and foscarnet to treat the CMV infection. He had an unsteady course, as do many newly diagnosed HIV-positive individuals who are profoundly immunosuppressed at presentation. His hospitalisation was complicated by an episode of *Pneumocystic jirovecii* pneumonia and a period in intensive care due predominantly to the deterioration in his conscious level. He developed anaemia, thrombocytopaenia and renal dysfunction, all secondary to ganciclovir and foscarnet.

After discharge from intensive care he had a slow improvement and was eventually discharged on

Figure 20.1. Funduscopic images similar to those seen in a 38-year-old bisexual man presenting with progressive blurring of vision, headache and cognitive impairment.

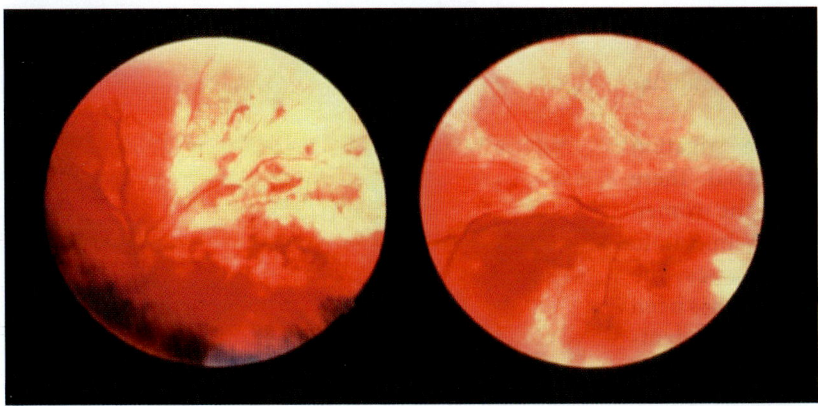

This demonstrates retinitis with a 'cottage cheese and ketchup' appearance. (Photo courtesy of Dr Mas Chaponda.)

Figure 20.2. Axial T2 FLAIR MRI brain scans for the same patient.

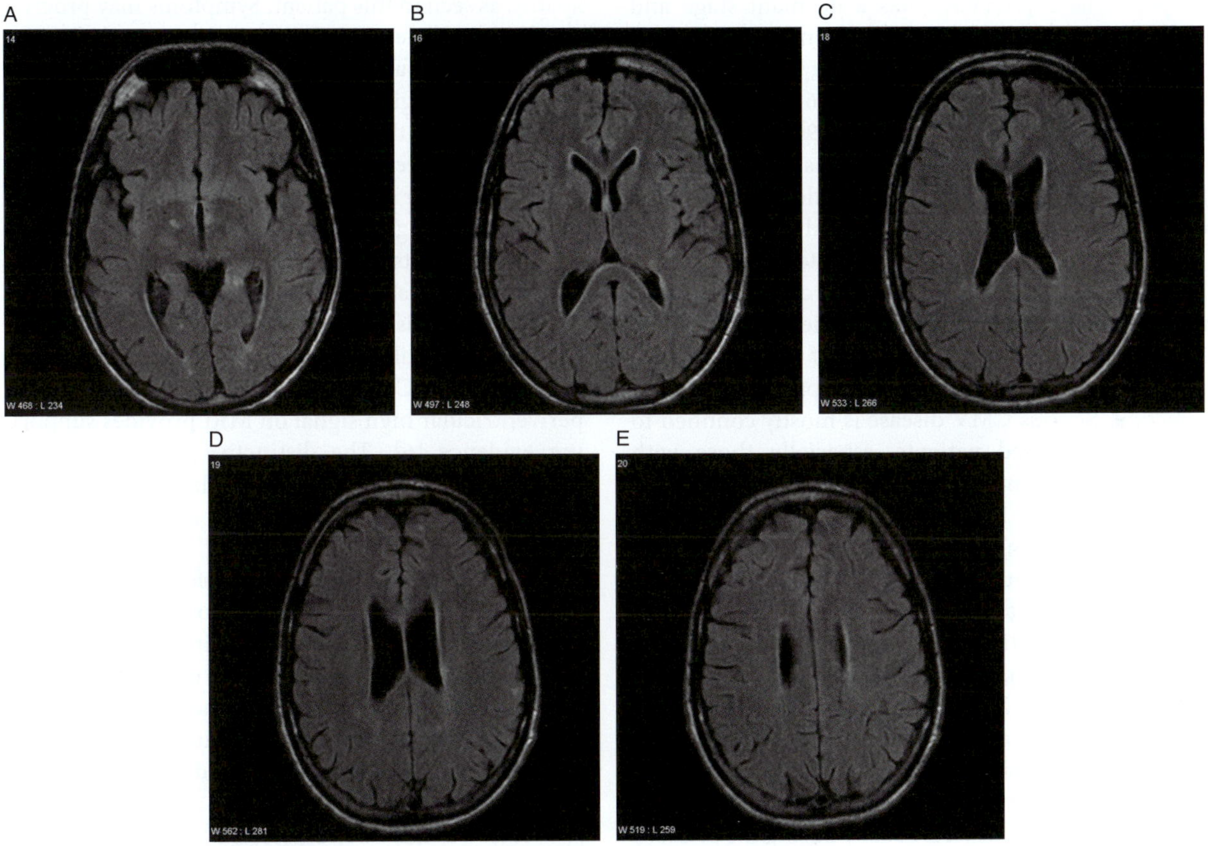

A B C D E

These demonstrate high signal surrounding the ventricles bilaterally.

combination antiretroviral therapy, prophylactic co-trimoxazole and maintenance oral valganciclovir for CMV. He continued to have problems with his memory and his vision remained disturbed.

Prevention

There is no vaccine at present for CMV. Nevertheless, when a transfusion is required, the risk of CMV infection in immunocompromised patients, such as those with HIV, who are CMV-negative can be minimised by the use of CMV antibody-negative blood components [1]. CMV intravenous immunoglobulin may be used for the prophylaxis of CMV disease associated with solid organ transplantation either alone or in combination with an antiviral agent.

A few potential vaccines are under investigation and one has been evaluated in a clinical trial. There was a reduction in the CMV infections in the women studied and a reduction in congenital CMV infection. However, the study was underpowered to assess the latter adequately [2]. Finding a CMV vaccine has been given a high priority because of the severity of congenital CMV infection.

Discussion

Like all herpes viruses, CMV (also known as human herpes virus 5 [HHV5]), has a dormant stage and may reactivate if the immune system becomes compromised [3]. CMV is thought to lie latent in T lymphocytes. Approximately 60% of 6-year-olds have been infected with CMV, rising to 90% by 80 years. Transmission occurs sexually, in breast milk, via organ transplants, blood transfusions and close contact with other body fluids, including urine and saliva.

Initial infection is usually asymptomatic or a self-limiting 'mononucleosis-like' syndrome with fever, malaise and sweating. A third of patients will develop hepatitis, but there are lower rates of pharyngitis and cervical lymphadenopathy than in Epstein–Barr virus infection. Serious CMV disease is mostly confined to immunosuppressed patients, especially those with HIV infection, and transplant and chemotherapy patients. It is rare in the otherwise healthy individuals. Active CMV infection after a transplant resembles infectious mononucleosis with evolution to involve specific organs, resulting in pneumonitis, hepatitis, colitis, oesophagitis, gastritis, adrenalitis and rarely encephalitis. Often, the organ affected is that which has been transplanted. In patients with profound immunosuppression, such as those with advanced HIV infection or stem cell transplants, multiple organs are often involved. When CMV encephalitis occurs in immunocompetent individuals, it is usually during the primary infection as part of the systemic illness.

Patients present with headache, fever, lethargy, seizures and focal weakness, which is typical for any viral encephalitis. In patients with advanced HIV infection, CMV encephalitis tends to present more indolently, with confusion and disorientation, lethargy, withdrawal and apathy, as seen in this patient. Symptoms may progress to affect multiple cranial nerves, for example causing nystagmus and facial palsy, and patients typically have a ventriculitis, giving periventricular high signal on MRI, as seen for this patient. The prognosis is generally poor, but has been improved with the use of combination ganciclovir and foscarnet therapy, and treatment of the underlying HIV, if that was the cause [4]. There have been reports of suspected immune reconstitution syndrome unmasking CMV ventriculitis. [5]

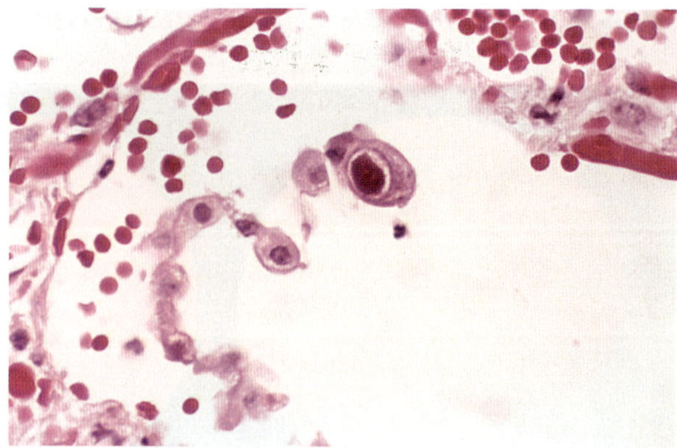

Figure 20.3. Neurohistopathological specimen demonstrating CMV inclusion bodies, described as an 'Owl's eye appearance'. (From: https://en.wikipedia.org/wiki/Cytomegalovirus#/media/File:Cytomegalovirus_01.jpg)

The diagnosis of CMV encephalitis is made on the basis of a compatible clinical picture and demonstration of CMV in the CSF by PCR; seeing the characteristic periventricular high signal on MRI provides supporting evidence [6]. The distinctive histopathological feature of CMV infection is the enlarged infected cell with inclusion bodies, described as an 'Owl's eyes appearance' (**Figure 20.3**).

Ganciclovir, foscarnet and cidofovir are all active against CMV. These have been shown to treat CMV retinitis in patients with HIV and their use in encephalitis has been extrapolated from this. The use of combination therapy with gangiclovir and foscarnet is probably more effective, although not ultimately curative. Both drugs are rather toxic and the patient needs to be monitored closely for bone marrow suppression and nephrotoxicity, as occurred in this case. Cidofovir has unreliable central nervous system penetration and is not recommended [7].

Key Points

- CMV, like other herpes viruses, remains latent after primary infection and can reactivate when the immune system becomes compromised.

- CMV infection can cause the full spectrum of neurological syndromes. It most commonly causes a retinitis and can also cause a ventriculitis, seen as periventricular high signal on FLAIR MRI.
- Combination therapy with ganciclovir and foscarnet, along with treatment of the underlying immune condition, is beneficial, although the prognosis remains poor.
- After CMV ventriculitis, patients with HIV should remain on prophylactic CMV therapy where possible [7].

Looking Back

In 1881 Ribbert discovered characteristic cytomegalovirus cells, but interpreted them as protozoal. Later, researchers found these cells in salivary glands, prompting the term 'salivary gland virus'. It was then in 1950 that Wyatt coined the term 'generalized cytomegalic inclusion disease'.

Did You Know?

Cytomegalovirus comes from the Greek: cyto, 'cell' and megalo, 'large'.

The term 'Owl's eyes appearance' is not exclusive to CMV infection (**Figure 20.4**). It also refers to nucleoli of Reed–Sternberg cells seen in Hodgkin's lymphoma and some radiological appearances.

The characteristic description of CMV retinitis is 'cottage cheese and tomato ketchup'.

CMV is one of several pathogens investigated for as part of the TORCH screen of neonates for vertically transmitted infections; being the 'C'; the 'T' is for Toxoplasma, the 'R' for Rubella, the 'H' for Herpes simplex virus, and the 'O' for a long list of others. Many neonatologists no longer like the term because it fails to highlight other important infections, such as HIV.

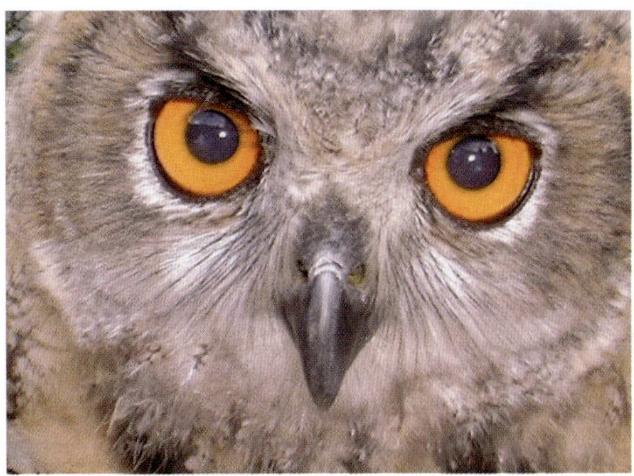

Figure 20.4. Owl's eyes. (From: www.owlpages.com/articles.php?section=owl+physiology&title=vision)

References

1. www.transfusionguidelines.org.uk/?Publication=HTM&Section=9&pageid=1135 (accessed May 10, 2018).
2. Pass RF, Zhang C, Evans A, et al. Vaccine prevention of maternal cytomegalovirus infection. N Engl J Med 2009;**360**:1191–9.
3. Tselis A. Epstein Barr virus and cytomegalovirus infections. In: *Birkhäuser Advances in Infectious Diseases: Viral Infections of the Human Nervous System*. New York, NY: Springer Books; 2013: 23–46.
4. Anduze-Fafri B, Fillet A, Gozlan J, et al. Induction and maintenance therapy of CMV central nervous system infection in HIV infected patients. AIDS 2000;**14**:517–24.
5. Janowicz D, Johnson R, Gupta S. Successful treatment of CMV ventriculitis immune reconstitution syndrome. J Neurol Neurosurg Pscyhiatry 2005;**76**:691–2.
6. Arribas J, Clifford D, Fichtenbaum C, et al. Level of cytomegalovirus (CMV) DNA in cerebrospinal fluid of subjects with AIDS and CMV infection of the central nervous system. J Infect Dis 1995;**172**:527–31.
7. Tunkel A, Glaser C, Bloch K, et al. The management of encephalitis: clinical practice guidelines by the Infectious Diseases Society of America. Clin Infect Dis 2008;**47**:303–27.

CASE 21

Same Family, Different Genus?

Michael Grosdenier and Rachel Kneen

History

An 8-day-old female neonate presented to a local hospital with two brief focal seizures involving the face and upper limbs. She had a 12-hour history of a change in her breathing pattern (noted to be rapid and shallow), a rash on her abdominal wall and trunk, intermittent irritability and reduced interest in feeding. The baby was born to a gravid 4 para 2 mother by elective caesarean section at 39 weeks gestation. The pregnancy had been uncomplicated and there were no risk factors for sepsis. There were no immediate neonatal problems and the mother and infant went home on day 4 with breast-feeding established. The infant's birth weight and growth parameters, including the occipitofrontal circumference, were on the 50th centile. All members of the family were well.

Examination

The infant had an axillary temperature of 38.8°C, a heart rate of 150 beats per minute, respiratory rate of 50 per minute, oxygen saturation of 97% in air and a capillary refill time of 3–4 seconds centrally. She looked pale, her skin was mottled and she had a faint, blanching macular rash over her abdomen and arms. She was irritable on handling and the anterior fontanelle was tense. There were signs of mild respiratory distress, with tachypnoea and some intercostal recession. The heart sounds and peripheral pulses were normal and lung fields were clear. Her abdomen was soft and she had normal female genitalia. Her nappy was filled with a normal yellow, seedy (breast milk) stool, but were described as being more loose than previously by the mother. She was generally hypotonic and drowsy, but there were no focal neurological signs present, and no abnormal movements were observed. Her blood glucose was 2.6 mmol/l.

Initial Differential Diagnosis

- Meningitis: viral, bacterial
- Meningoencephalitis: viral, bacterial, e.g. herpes simplex virus (HSV) type 2
- Sepsis, e.g. urinary tract infection or pneumonia with symptomatic (e.g. electrolyte-disturbance) related seizures.
- Inborn error of metabolism, e.g. organic acidaemia
- Early infantile epileptic encephalopathy, e.g. Ohtahara syndrome
- Cerebral haemorrhage or venous sinus thrombosis and secondary infarction

Results of Initial Investigations

Full blood count, renal function test, calcium and magnesium were normal. The C-reactive protein was 340 mg/l. Urine microscopy was normal. Cerebrospinal fluid (CSF) analysis after a lumbar puncture revealed the following: white cell count (WCC) 8/mm^3, red blood cells 2/mm^3, protein 0.85 g/l and glucose 4.1 mmol/l (paired blood glucose was 6 mmol/l). The CSF analysis was considered to be normal for a term neonate (i.e. WCC < 15 cells/mm^3). Gram stain was negative. A chest radiograph showed only a normal thymus shadow but no focal consolidation. A computer tomography scan of the brain was normal.

Progress and Further Investigations

Intravenous (IV) antibiotics and aciclovir were commenced. The infant had several further seizures that were treated with a dose of IV lorazepam and phenytoin loading. She remained febrile for 3 days with temperatures recorded up to 39.5°C. Blood and CSF cultures were negative. An electroencephalogram showed an immature cortical rhythm but no seizures were recorded during the investigation.

A magnetic resonance imaging (MRI) of the brain was performed (**Figure 21.1**).

She required nasogastric tube feeding for 24 hours. Antibiotics and aciclovir were stopped on day 5 when bacterial cultures and polymerase chain reaction (PCR) for HSV from the CSF were reported as negative and the child had made a good recovery. She was discharged the following day.

Definitive Investigation Results

Viral PCR testing was positive on the CSF and stool samples for human parechovirus type 3.

Diagnosis

Neonatal encephalitis caused by human parechovirus type 3.

Figure 21.1. Coronal FLAIR and T1-weighted MRI of an 8-day-old neonate with focal seizures and a faint macular rash.

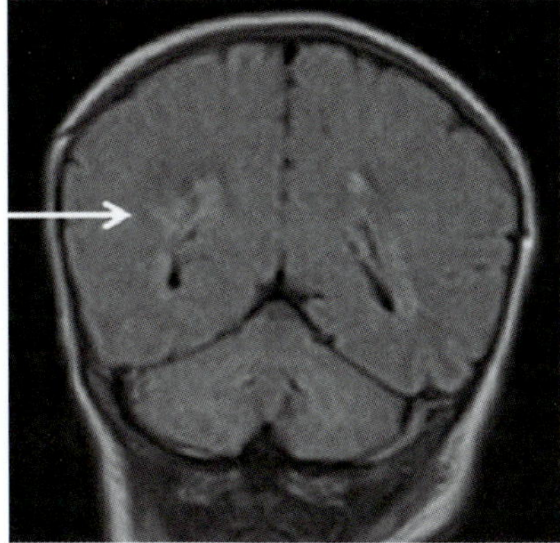
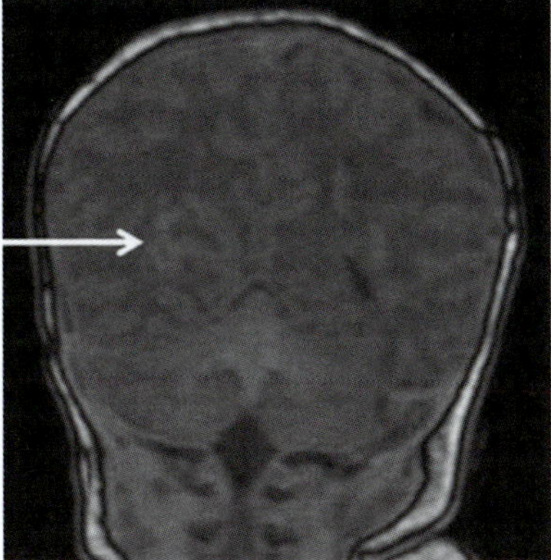

These demonstrate abnormal signal (arrow) in the periventricular regions of the right parietal lobe.

Management and Outcome

The child remained well at home and was reviewed aged 3 and 9 months. She had no further seizures and was making normal developmental progress.

Prevention

Epidemiological studies have shown that human parechovirus (HPeV) infection is common in children; the seroprevalence for HPeV type 1 (HPeV1) reaches 88% by the age of 2 years [1]. Placental passage of maternal antibodies during pregnancy offers passive prevention against neonatal infection to HPeV1 and HPeV2 until about 6 months of age. However, the recent emergence of HPeV3 and the lower seroprevalence in women of childbearing age has seen an emergence of infections in neonates, giving a lower median age of cases: 1.3 months for HPeV3 versus 6.6 months for other serotypes [1]. There is currently no immunisation available for parechovirus.

Discussion

Human parechoviruses are from the large Picornaviridae family. They are small, non-enveloped, single-stranded and positive-sense RNA viruses. They were initially placed within the *Enterovirus* genus, but new molecular-based techniques (specific reverse-transcriptase PCR [RT-PCR]) have shown they are sufficiently different to be placed in the separate *Parechovirus* genus. Most HPeV types have only recently been identified; hence, HPeV infection is probably underdiagnosed. At least 16 HPeV types have been discovered to date (www.picornastudygroup.com). The infection is usually mild, causing gastrointestinal and respiratory symptoms, but can also be severe with central nervous system (CNS) infection and hepatitis; the latter is reported for HPeV3 [2]. In a recent retrospective study assessing the characteristics of the CSF in young infants evaluated for sepsis, the incidence of HPeV infection was higher than enterovirus infection, and this has been confirmed in larger studies (**Figure 21.2**) [3]. In the majority of cases, there is no CSF pleocytosis and CSF glucose and protein levels are normal in HPeV3 [3]. This can be falsely reassuring or misleading when faced with such results in clinical practice. Patients with CNS infection due to HPeV3 can present with seizures, and imaging may show diffuse white matter changes on diffusion-weighted MRI [4,5]. More importantly, significant neuro-developmental complications including cerebral palsy, epilepsy and learning difficulties have been described following CNS infection with HPeV3 in cases with white matter changes [4]. Therefore, accurate diagnosis is necessary to allow appropriate neuro-developmental follow-up. Other peculiar characteristics of the HPeV3 infection are its peak incidence in the summer months and an as-yet unexplained biannual infection cycle in even years since 1988 in Europe [1].

Key Points

- HPeV infection is characterised by a seasonal occurrence (spring and autumn)
- Although parechovirus infections typically present with mild gastrointestinal or respiratory illness, HPeV type 3 can cause severe disease, sepsis and encephalitis.

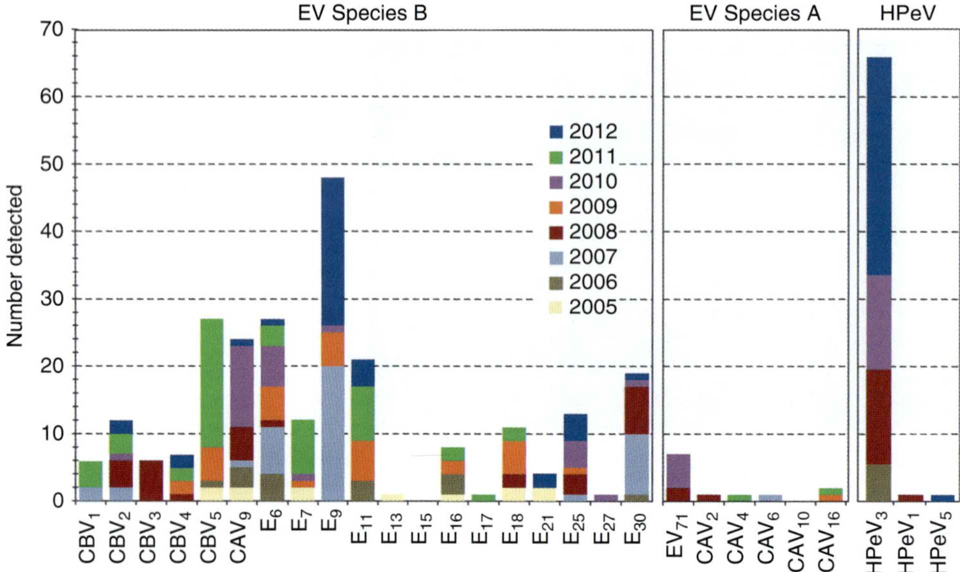

CAV: coxsackie A virus; EV: enterovirus; HPeV: human parechovirus.

Figure 21.2. Distribution of enterovirus and human parechovirus types in cerebrospinal fluid samples, Scotland, 2005–2012 ($n = 404$). (Reproduced from [6] under CC BY 4.0.)

- Think of HPeV in children less than 6 months old with meningeal irritation with or without encephalopathy, even if the routine CSF parameters are completely normal.
- Many hospitals now offer CSF PCR for parechovirus as part of a routine neonatal septic screen.

Looking Back

Human parechovirus types 1 and 2 were discovered in the 1950s. They were initially classified as echovirus 22 and 23, respectively, within the *Enterovirus* genus, before they were renamed and placed in the separate Parechovirus genus. Among the 16 parechoviruses type 3 causes the most severe manifestations.

Did You Know?

In the mid-1990s a new virus, Parechovirus B, was isolated from bank voles.

References

1. Harvala H, Simmonds P. Human parechoviruses: biology, epidemiology and clinical significance. J Clin Vir 2009;**45**:1–9.
2. Harvala H, Wolthers KC, Simmonds P. Parechoviruses in children: understanding a new infection. Curr Opin Infect Dis 2010;**23**:224–30.
3. Sharp J, Harrison CJ, Puckett J, et al. Characteristics of young infants in whom human parechovirus, enterovirus or neither were detected in cerebrospinal fluid during sepsis evaluations. Pediatr Infect Dis J 2013;**32**:213– 16.
4. Verboon-Maciolek MA, Groenendaal F, Hahn CD, et al. Human parechovirus causes encephalitis with white matter injury in neonates. Ann Neurol 2008;**64**:266–73.
5. Gupta S, Fernandez D, Siddiqui A, et al. Extensive white matter abnormalities associated with neonatal parechovirus (HPeV) infection. Eur J Paed Neurol 2010;**14**:531–4.
6. Harvala H, Calvert J, Van Nguyen D, et al. Comparison of diagnostic clinical samples and environmental sampling for Enterovirus and parechovirus surveillance in Scotland 2010–2012. Eurosurveillance 2014;**19**:pii–20772.

CASE 22

The Great Pretender

Richard J.B. Ellis

History

A 37-year-old gentleman was admitted to his local district general hospital with a history of sudden-onset speech disturbance and right-sided hemiplegia.

In the months prior to admission he had felt generally unwell. There had been an episode of transient facial weakness 6 months previously, which resolved spontaneously within 24 hours. There were also episodes of fleeting paroxysms of facial pain on the background of a progressive, bilateral headache. The family had noted some personality change and increasing forgetfulness over the preceding few years.

He had a past medical history of depression diagnosed 3 years previously, for which he took citalopram 20 mg once a day. He had been treated for *Chlamydia* in his late teens by his general practitioner without any complication. He had also had a painless ulcer on his lip, which was diagnosed as a cold sore and resolved spontaneously.

There was no family history of note. He was a non-smoker with no history of illicit drug use. He lived with his boyfriend and was currently unemployed. He had been fired from his job as a hairdresser due to several incidents where he had accidentally injured customers. He had been out of the country only once in the previous 10 years, a week-long holiday to Egypt. There was no report of illness while he had been abroad.

Examination

On admission he was drowsy with eyes opening spontaneously, localising to pain, and was noted to have a marked expressive aphasia. Pupils were equal with normal accommodation but were unresponsive to direct light stimuli. There was a normal range of eye movements with jerky saccades. Nystagmus was not noted. Funduscopy was unremarkable.

There was mild right-sided facial weakness with flattening of the nasolabial fold on the right with forehead sparing. Facial sensation was intact. Masseter and temporalis functions were normal. There were normal tongue, palatal and uvula movements.

There was a left-sided intention tremor and dysdiadochokinesis. Pronator drift was noted on the right. Tone was normal and he was noted to have a mild right-sided hemiparesis affecting both his upper and lower limb equally. He had extensor plantars, but with absent knee and ankle jerks, bilaterally.

Joint position sense, vibration, pin-prick and light touch were all intact on sensory examination.

He had a regular pulse at 70 beats per minute. Auscultation of the chest revealed normal heart sounds, with no murmurs or added heart sounds. Normal, vesicular breath sounds were heard with no superimposed wheeze, rhonchi or crackles. Abdominal examination did not reveal any masses or organomegaly.

No rashes or skin lesions were observed.

Initial Differential Diagnosis

The acute presentation was consistent with an acute stroke in the left cerebral hemisphere giving a mild right hemiparesis. However, the additional left-sided abnormalities on examination, and preceding history of transient facial weakness and clumsiness, suggest multiple events. The absent deep tendon reflexes in the lower limbs would not be explained by cerebral ischaemia, suggesting either multiple pathologies or a single disease which causes cerebral ischaemic events and peripheral nerve disease.

Causes of Multiple Cerebral Infarcts

- Cardioembolic
  - Bacterial endocarditis
  - Libmann Sachs endocarditis
  - Mural thrombus
  - Atrial myxoma
  - Carotid/vertebral artery dissection
  - Paradoxical embolus via patent foramen ovale/atrial septal defect
- Vasculitides
  - Polyarteritis nodosa
  - Takayasu's arteritis
  - Wegener's granulomatosis
  - Microscopic polyangiitis
  - Churg–Strauss
  - Primary angiitis of the central nervous system
  - Drug-induced, i.e. cocaine
  - Vasculopathies, i.e. intravascular lymphoma
  - Moya-Moya disease
  - Infective
    - HIV/AIDS

  - Lyme disease
  - Neurosyphilis
  - Bacterial meningitis
  - Tuberculosis meningitis
  - Neurocysticercosis
  - Fungal meningoencephalitis (by mycotic aneurysm and vessel invasion)
- Immune/inflammatory
  - Systemic lupus erythematous including cerebral lupus
  - Sarcoidosis
  - Bechet's
  - Susac's syndrome
- Thrombophilias
  - Hyperhomocystinaemia
  - Antithrombin deficiency (including nephrotic syndrome)
  - Hyperviscosity syndromes
  - Myeloproliferative disorders
  - Protein C and S deficiency
  - Sickle cell disease
- Inherited
  - Mitochondrial encephalomyopathy, lactic acidosis, and stroke-like episodes (MELAS)
  - Cerebral Autosomal Dominant Arteriopathy with Subcortical Infarcts and Leukoencephalopathy (CADASIL)
  - Connective tissue disorders, i.e. Ehlers–Danlos syndrome especially Type IV (Vascular) forms
  - Fabry's disease

Absent Ankle Jerks and Extensor Plantars

- Friedrich's ataxia
- Sub-acute combined degeneration of cord
- Conus medullaris lesion
- Tabes dorsalis
- Anterior horn cell disease
- Cervical myelopathy + peripheral neuropathy

Results of Initial Investigations

Bloods: full blood count, urea and electrolytes, liver function test, C-reactive protein, erythrocyte sedimentation rate, bone profile, B12, folate, thyroid function, iron studies were all normal.

Electrocardiogram showed normal sinus rhythm at 72 beats per minute, with no evidence of left ventricular hypertrophy, a normal axis, and no ST segment changes or T-wave inversion.

Figure 22.1. Axial CT scan of a 37-year-old gentleman with a sudden onset of speech disturbance and right-sided hemiplegia.

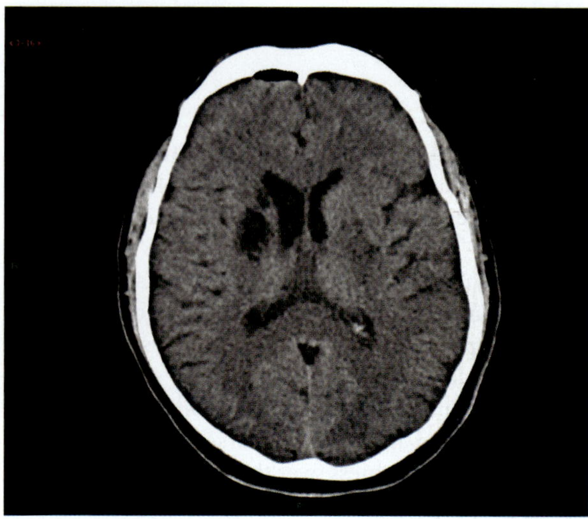

This shows ischaemic infarcts in both thalami.

A CT scan was performed in the emergency department (**Figure 22.1**).

A magnetic resonance image (MRI) of the head was performed (**Figure 22.2**).

A transthoracic echocardiogram showed no evidence of a patent foramen ovale, atrial or ventricular septal defect. There was also no valvular defect, vegetations or regurgitation. There was normal left ventricular size and function and normal aortic root dimensions.

Cerebrospinal fluid (CSF) had a normal opening pressure, with a lymphocytic pleocytosis, raised protein, and a normal glucose ratio. CSF cytological examination demonstrated non-specific chronic active inflammation.

Progress and Further Investigations

During the course of his admission the patient remained stable while further investigations were ordered. These included: HIV, Borrelia serology, antibodies associated with vasculitis, *NOTCH-3* mutation for cerebral autosomal dominant arteriopathy with subcortical infarcts and leukoencephalopathy (CADASIL), Pathergy test and computer tomography angiogram and venogram.

The Borrelia initially provided a positive IgM, but negative IgG result; further analysis at the national

Figure 22.2. Axial T2-weighted and diffusion-weighted MRI scans in the same patient.

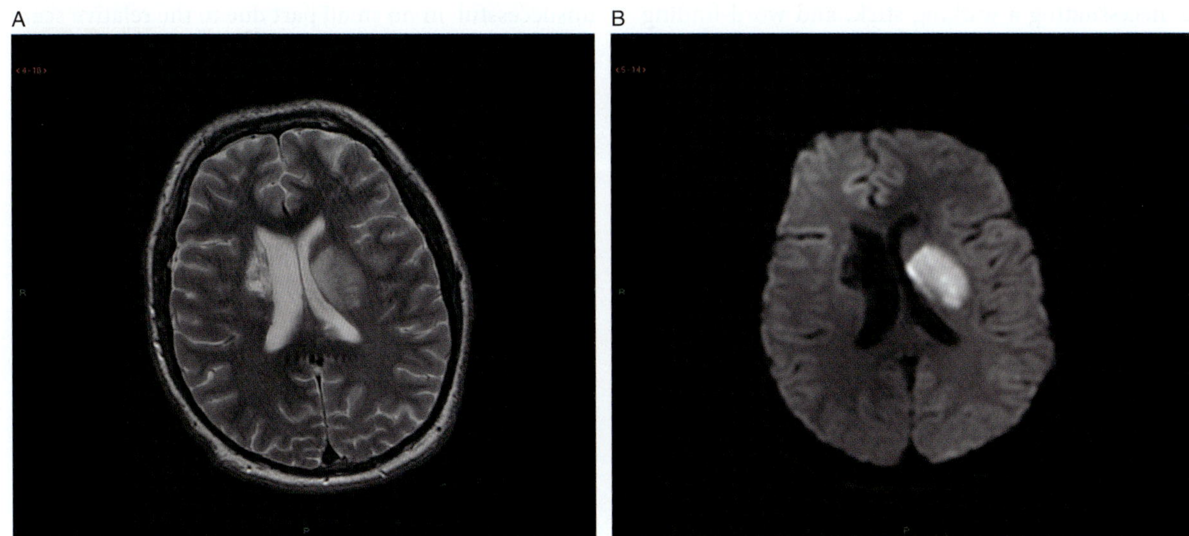

(A) The images shown here demonstrate two hyperintense lesions on the T2-weighted imaging. (B) However, diffusion-weighted imaging shows they are of different chronicity. There were also right inferior cerebellar infarcts and also old ischaemic change in the pons and the right basal ganglia, not shown here.

reference laboratory revealed this to be a false positive result.

Further episodes of paroxysmal retro-orbital and ophthalmic neuralgia occurred during his admission. Although they were not associated with autonomic features, attempts were made to treat these as one of the trigeminal autonomic cephalgias. These episodes were unfortunately refractory to treatments such as carbamazepine and lamotrigine. They eventually subsided once the underlying cause was diagnosed and treated.

Finally the definitive investigations returned from the laboratory.

Results of Definitive Investigations

The serum venereal disease reference laboratory (VDRL) test for syphilis was positive and further testing with *T. pallidum* haemagglutination (TPHA), treponemal enzyme immunoassay (EIA) and rapid plasma reagin (RPR) were requested on the CSF and serum samples, with the following results:

Serum

VDRL: reactive

Treponemal EIA: positive

TPHA: positive (> 1:40,960)

RPR: reactive (> 1:32)

CSF

VRDL: reactive

Diagnosis

Meningovascular neurosyphilis and tabes dorsalis.

Management and Outcome

Once the diagnosis was confirmed, procaine penicillin was started immediately.

Within hours of the administration of procaine penicillin the patient developed high fevers, rigors, hypotension and tachycardia. There was no evidence of sepsis; a Jarisch–Herxheimer reaction was diagnosed and supportive therapy was aggressively pursued.

The patient stabilised over the next 48 hours and subsequently underwent a period of neurorehabilitation with input from physiotherapists, speech and language therapists and occupational therapists to improve the patient's functional outcome.

The paroxysmal neuralgias were recognised as Pel's crises, also known as tabetic ocular crises, a known complication of neurosyphilis. They resolved with treatment of neurosyphilis. The pupillary defect described is the Argyll–Robertson pupil, colloquially known as the Prostitute's pupil as it 'accommodates but does not react'.

He was later discharged from hospital with weakness necessitating a walking stick, and word-finding difficulties requiring ongoing speech and language input in the community. Six-monthly lumbar punctures were performed until the CSF white cell count was normal.

Prevention

Syphilis is a sexually transmitted disease and the only guaranteed method of preventing transmission is through the practice of safe sex with condom use as barrier protection. *Treponema pallidum*, the causative organism, is transmitted by direct contact with syphilitic chancres. Only a few organisms are required to infect a person through abraded skin.

Active surveillance programmes exist within HIV-related care and current recommendations suggest regular testing may reduce complications as well as transmission of disease. Health education programmes are also essential for disseminating knowledge of this disease as well as other sexually transmitted infections (**Figure 22.3**) [1].

Attempts to develop a vaccine so far have been unsuccessful, in no small part due to the relative scarcity of surface proteins on *T. pallidum* for an antibody to be effective.

Discussion

Syphilis is the result of infection from the spirochete bacterium *Treponema pallidum*, transmitted by direct contact with an infectious lesion during sexual activity, vertically in pregnancy or through infected blood products (**Figure 22.4**) [2].

Syphilis can be classified as congenital or acquired, and acquired can be further classified into primary, secondary, early and late latent (tertiary) syphilis. Neurosyphilis can occur during any stage of infection. As a result, it is essential that clinicians are familiar with the disease, and its variety of clinical manifestations [3]. Most of our knowledge of neurosyphilis manifestations come from observations predating the advent of penicillin. Nowadays, in the era of effective antibiotic therapies, late latent neurosyphilis is rare. The case presented here highlights just one of the many 'masks' that central nervous

A

TWO MEN WHO HAD
SYPHILIS
He took treatments regularly.
He didn't.

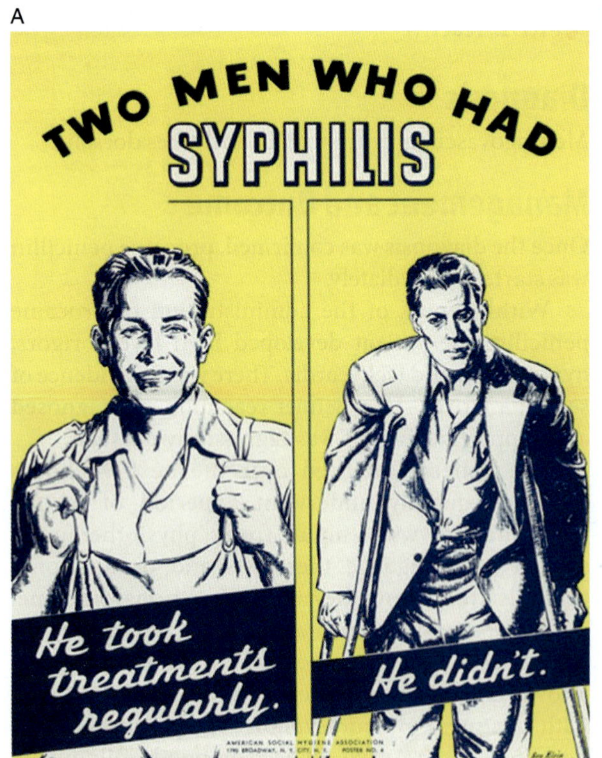

B

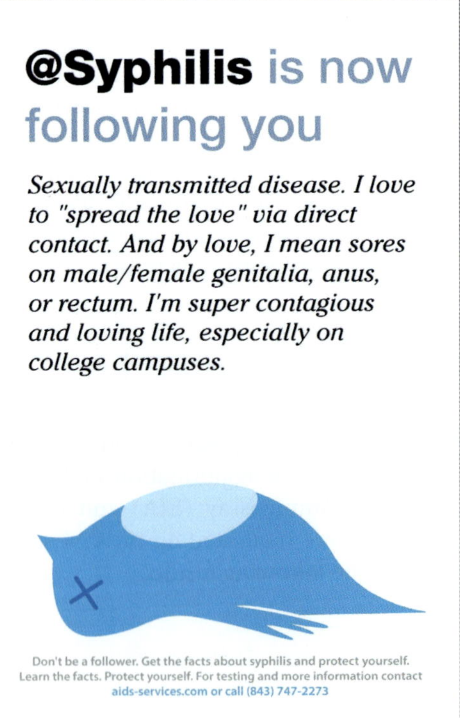

Figure 22.3. (A) American public service poster promoting early detection and treatment of syphilis in 1940. (With permission of the American Sexual Health Association and Social Welfare History Archives, University of Minnesota Libraries. All rights reserved.) (B) Modern syphilis awareness campaign poster from Lowcountry AIDS Services, Charleston, SC. (Created by Gil Shuler Graphic Design and reproduced with permission.)

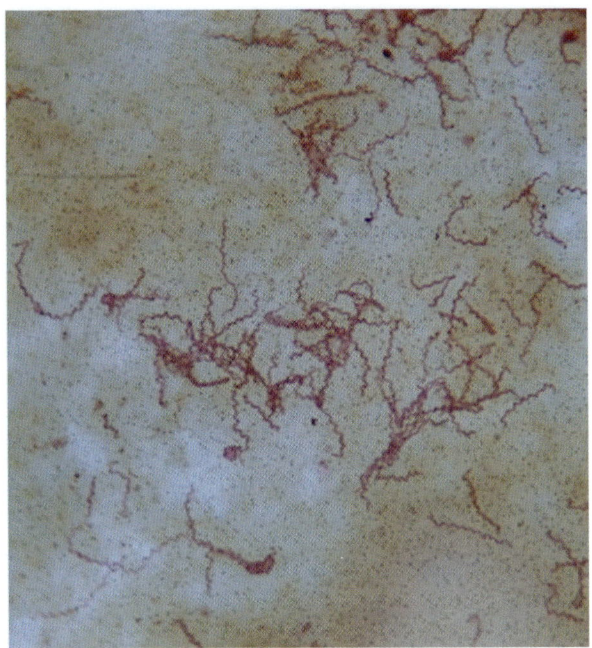

Figure 22.4. *Treponema pallidum* as seen on microscopy.

system infection with *T. pallidum* can wear. **Table 22.1** illustrates the forms late latent syphilis can take.

The case illustrates other salient points. His clinical features were caused by a combination of meningovascular syphilis and tabes dorsalis. The paroxysmal neuralgias were Pel's crises, also called tabetic ocular crises, a known complication of neurosyphilis. They resolved with treatment of neurosyphilis.

While antibiotic therapy will remove the causative organism from the system, the infarcts, resulting from small and medium vessel disease, are irreversible. The same is true of neurological deficit in tabes dorsalis, as demyelination in the posterior columns tends to leave irreversible damage and treatment merely prevents worsening.

Following the initiation of treatment, the patient suffered a Jarisch–Herxheimer reaction. This is the result of rapid cytokine and endotoxin release from the death of spirochetes following antibiotic initiation and can be fatal. There have been no randomised controlled trials of the prophylactic use of corticosteroids and experience is largely anecdotal. One small open-label trial found that primary prophylaxis with steroids was beneficial in some with early syphilis, and some physicians choose to cover the first few days of treatment of late syphilis with steroids [5]. In one small study, anti-tumour necrosis factor alpha was found to be efficacious as primary prophylaxis [5,6].

After discharge the patient described here had six-monthly lumbar punctures because CSF protein and VDRL can take over a year to normalise and VDRL is the only test that may return to normal after treatment. If the patient deteriorates then investigation should be undertaken and treatment may need to be re-started. Since the start of the antibiotic era, with the reduction in cases, syphilis has fallen away from public and physician consciousness. However, clinicians should be vigilant because the disease is back on the rise after decades of decline [7]. From 2003 to 2012, diagnoses of syphilis, in genitourinary clinics in England, increased by 61% in men, compared with a 16% decrease in women. This increased incidence has been focused on urban centres where higher proportions of the population are men who have sex with men [8]. There is a clear association

Table 22.1 Clinical features of symptomatic late syphilis.

Form	Timing after infection	Signs and symptoms
Asymptomatic	Early/late	Abnormal CSF with no signs or symptoms; this is of uncertain clinical significance given that CSF abnormalities have been found in 30% of primary and secondary syphilis, yet this becomes clinically significant in the majority of patients
Meningovascular	2–7 years	Focal arteritis inducing infarction and meningeal inflammation; signs dependent on location of vascular insult. Occasional prodrome; headache, emotional lability, insomnia
General paresis	10–20 years	Cortical neuronal loss; gradual decline in memory and cognitive functions, emotional lability, personality change, psychosis and dementia. Seizures and hemiparesis are late complications
Tabes dorsalis	15–25 years	Inflammation of spinal dorsal column/nerve roots; lightning pains, areflexia, paraesthesia, sensory ataxia, Charcot's joints, mal perforans, optic atrophy, Argyll Robertson pupil
Cardiovascular	10–30 years	Aortitis (usually ascending); asymptomatic, substernal pain, aortic regurgitation, heart failure, coronary ostial stenosis, angina, aneurysm formation
Gummatous	1–46 years (mean 15)	Inflammatory granulomatous destructive lesions can occur in any organ but most commonly affect bone and skin.

Adapted from [4].

with co-infection with HIV; strategies to screen for other sexually transmitted diseases in HIV-positive patients have resulted in more cases being treated in the early stages, reducing the risk of the devastating consequences of late latent infection [9].

Patients today rarely present with a known syphilis history. Stokes wrote in 1944 that 'the frequency of neurosyphilis in general medical practice depends to a large extent on the thoroughness of the search for signs of neuraxis involvement and the frequency with which the spinal fluid examination is employed'. This maxim remains unchanged after many decades [10,11].

Treatment regimes are more consistently agreed upon, and are largely based on Class III evidence. UK guidelines for the management of syphilis have been produced by the British Association for Sexual Health and HIV [4].

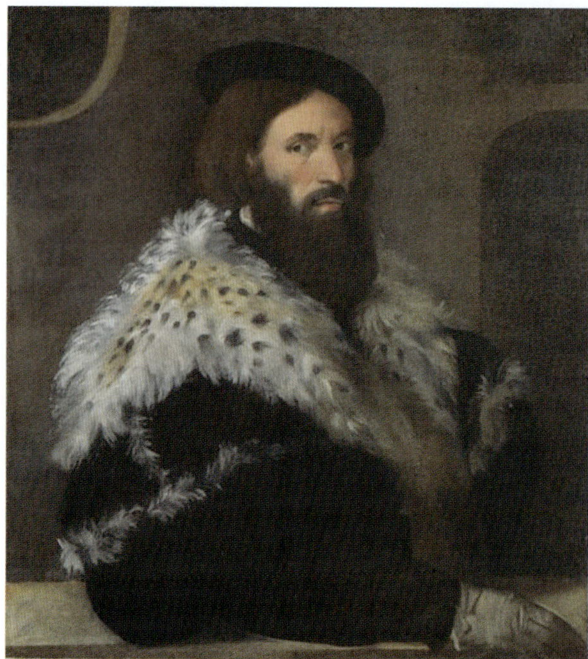

Figure 22.5. Girolamo Fracastoro c. 1528: credited with the name for syphilis, which is derived from his 1530 epic poem, *Syphilis sive morbus gallicus*, about a shepherd boy named Syphilus who insulted the Greek god Apollo and was punished with the disease to which his name is now given.

Key Points

- Syphilis is a treatable chronic infection, caused by *Treponema pallidum*, with a broad variety of clinical manifestations from primary through to tertiary disease.
- Knowledge of at-risk groups and its presentations is essential to establish a low index of suspicion in these cases.
- Early recognition and treatment reduces the risk of developing significant complications involving not only the central nervous system, but also cardiovascular structures (i.e. syphilitic aortitis) and granulomatous skin and bone disease (i.e. gummatous syphilis).

Looking Back

Syphilis was originally coined by the Italian physician and poet Fracastorius as the name of his poet's protagobist afflicted with the dreaded disease (**Figure 22.5**). It derives from the Greek word *syphlos*, meaning crippled or maimed, and has historically been used as a term of derision for political ends. During times of conflict in Italy it was known as 'Morbus Gallicus' or the 'French Disease', conversely in French it became the 'Italian Disease'.

Owing to the variety of symptoms and presentation associated with syphilis it is commonly referred to as 'the Great Imitator', a term attributed to Sir William Osler.

Did You Know?

`He who knows syphilis knows medicine' – Sir William Osler.

The long list of illustrious people who had syphilis is headed by Oscar Wilde.

Sir Arthur Conan Doyle, author of the Sherlock Holmes novels, completed his doctorate on tabes dorsalis in 1885.

'It is unthinkable for a Frenchman to arrive at middle age without having syphilis and the Cross of the Legion of Honor.' – *Andre Gide* (1869–1951)

References

1. Cohen CE, Winston A, Asboe D, et al. Increasing detection of asymptomatic syphilis in HIV patients. Sex Transm Infect 2005;**81**:217–19.
2. Hooshmand H, Escobar MR, Kopf SW. Neurosyphilis. A study of 241 patients. JAMA 1972;**219**(6):726–9.
3. Scheck DN, Hook EW. Neurosyphilis. Infect Dis Clin North Am 1994;**8**:769–95.
4. Kingston M, French P, Goh B, et al. UK National Guidelines on the Management of Syphilis 2008. Int J STD AIDS 2008;**19**:729–40.
5. Houston A, French P. Secondary syphilis. In Arnold AM, Griffin G, editors. *From Challenging Concepts in Infectious Diseases and Clinical Microbiology: Cases with Expert Commentary*. Oxford: Oxford University Press; 2014: 37.
6. Fekade D, Knox K, Hussein K, et al. Prevention of Jarisch–Herxheimer reactions by treatment with antibodies against tumor necrosis factor alpha. N Engl J Med 1996;**335**:311–15.
7. Nicoll A, Hamers FF. Are trends in HIV, gonorrhoea and syphilis worsening in Western Europe? BMJ 2002;**324**:1324–7.
8. Public Health England. Recent epidemiology of infectious syphilis and congenital syphilis. Infection Rep 2013;7(44). www.gov.uk/government/publications/infectious-syphilis-and-congenital-syphilis-recent-epidemiology (accessed May 14, 2018).
9. Parkes R, Renton A, Meheus A, et al. Review of current evidence and comparison of guidelines for effective syphilis treatment in Europe. Int J STD AIDS 2004;**15**:73.
10. Stokes JH, Beerman H, Ingraham NR. Modern Clinical Syphilology. 3rd ed. Philadelphia, PA: WB Saunders; 1944.
11. Marra CM, Maxwell CL, Smith SL, et al. Cerebrospinal fluid abnormalities in patients with syphilis: association with clinical and laboratory features. J Infect Dis 2004;**189**:369.

CASE 23

Word Salad

Sylviane Defres

History

A 41-year-old, right-handed, English Literature teacher with a past medical history of controlled hypothyroidism and asthma presented with a 3-day history of feeling generally unwell. Initially this began with a loss of appetite and vomiting for 1 day, followed by language disturbance, lack of concentration and strange sensations in her right hand, which felt cold and uncomfortable intermittently. The language difficulties worsened and she was admitted to her local hospital.

She had no history of headache or weakness, neck stiffness or pain, photophobia or any visual disturbances. There was no recent foreign travel. A vaccination history was not known, but she was thought to have had the routine UK immunisations during childhood.

Examination

On admission, general examination was normal with a temperature of 37.6°C, pulse 69 beats per minute, blood pressure 132/62 mmHg and pulse oximetry was normal. Her score on the Glasgow coma score was recorded as 14–15/15 (eyes 4/4, verbal 4–5/5, motor 6/6).

She appeared to have rambling speech and a reduced ability to focus on and answer the questions asked. There was also some degree of short-term memory impairment. Her mini-mental state examination was 23/30. Romberg's test was negative, power and coordination were normal. Tone was increased on the right lower limb and reflexes appeared brisk throughout; however, plantar responses were normal. Funduscopy was limited due to poor cooperation.

Initial Differential Diagnosis

- Sub-acute, progressive language and short-term memory impairment, potentially localising to the peri-sylviane structures of the left hemisphere and predominantly the temporal lobe
  - Encephalitis (viral, antibody-mediated, other inflammatory cause, or unknown)
  - Vascular event (ischaemia, haemorrhage, dissection or venous sinus thrombosis), although the history was not hyperacute
  - Space-occupying neoplasia, although the history was quite short for this

Results of Initial Investigations

Blood results were unremarkable, with a normal full blood count, urea and creatinine and liver function tests. Sodium was 133 mmol/l and C-reactive protein was < 0.1 g/l.

A computer tomography (CT) brain scan was performed (**Figure 23.1**), and after review by a neuroradiologist an urgent magnetic resonance imaging (MRI) scan, was also performed (**Figure 23.2**).

A lumbar puncture (LP) had an opening pressure of 19.5 cm H_2O, the cerebrospinal fluid (CSF) was clear and colourless, protein was 0.31 g/l, the glucose was 4.5 mmol/l and simultaneous serum glucose was 6.5 mmol/l. CSF red cell count was 2 cells/mm^3, the white cell count was 10 cells/mm^3, 80% lymphocytes, 20% polymorphs, no organisms were seen and there was no growth after 48 hours.

Results of Definitive Investigations

Viral polymerase chain reaction (PCR) of the CSF was performed for herpes simplex virus (HSV), varicella zoster virus (VZV), parechovirus and enteroviruses. CSF PCR was negative for HSV type 2, VZV, parechovirus and enterovirus, but was positive for HSV type 1.

Diagnosis

Herpes simplex type 1 encephalitis.

Management and Outcome

Intravenous (IV) aciclovir was commenced immediately after the LP, prior to the HSV PCR result being available.

In the first 2 days of her admission, she developed involuntary movements of her right limbs and

Figure 23.1. CT brain scan of a 41-year-old right-handed lady who presented with sub-acute language dysfunction and short-term memory loss.

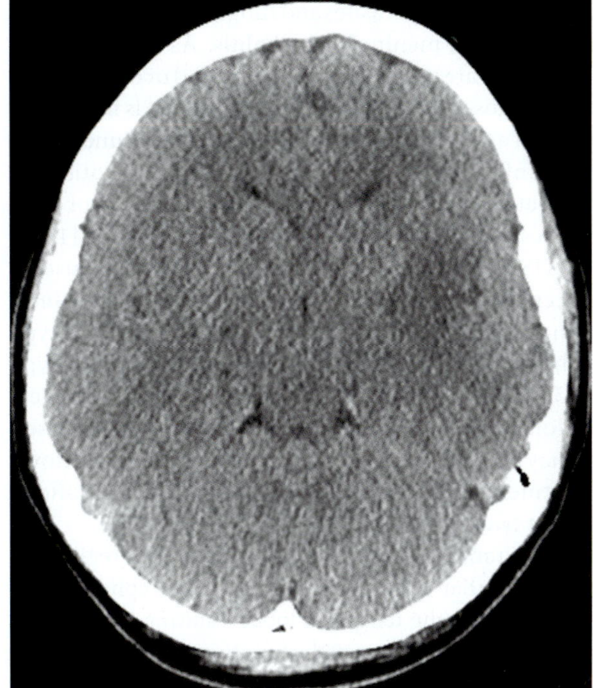

This was initially verbally reported as demonstrating a focal lesion, without evidence of ring enhancement, within middle cerebral artery territory, which may be ischaemic or an abscess.

a right-sided weakness. Her temperature rose to a maximum of 38.9°C. Subsequently, on day 5 her clinical condition deteriorated with both a receptive and expressive dysphasia, she developed pronator drift of the right arm and the frequency of the attacks of involuntary movements of her right arm and leg increased. She went on to have secondary generalised tonic–clonic seizures and her Glasgow coma score did not recover following these, despite IV phenytoin.

A repeat MRI brain scan was performed (**Figure 23.3**). An electroencephalogram was markedly abnormal, showing diffuse slowing background rhythm representing encephalopathy. However, there was no clear evidence of ongoing seizure activity. On account of the changes in the MRI, and deterioration despite aciclovir, adjunctive corticosteroids were commenced, and IV aciclovir was continued.

Towards the end of the subsequent week she started to improve, with some insight into her illness. She was able to appreciate that she had memory difficulties and was partially aware of her expressive dysphasia.

A repeat LP prior to stopping aciclovir on day 13 showed that she was now negative for HSV by PCR. Prior to discharge her Mini Mental State Examination was 28/30 and Addenbrookes Cognitive Examination

Figure 23.2. Axial T2-weighted (A, B) and coronal FLAIR (C) MRI scans from the same patient.

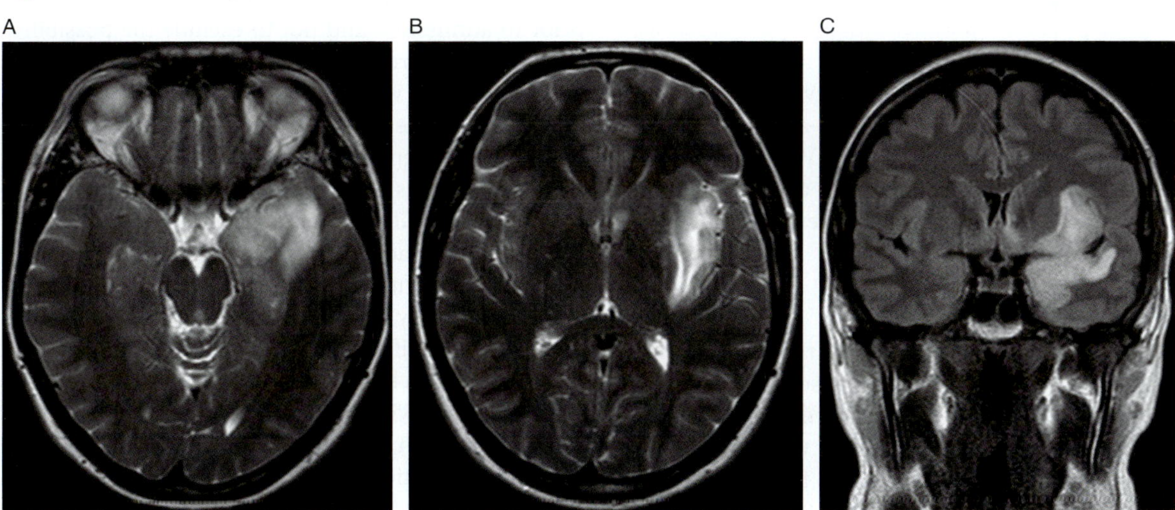

These demonstrate hyperintensity predominantly in the left mesial temporal lobe but also involving surrounding structures.

Figure 23.3. A coronal FLAIR MR image from the same patient after deterioration with increasing frequency and severity of seizures.

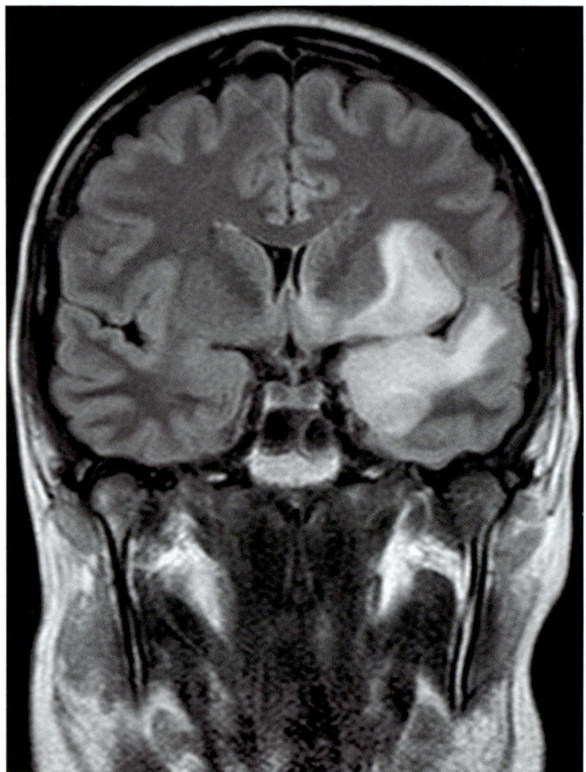

This demonstrates an increase in the volume of the lesion with surrounding oedema.

was 72/100. She was discharged with outpatient neurorehabilitation.

Prevention

At present there are no means to prevent HSV infection. There are no immunisations and no way of predicting who may go on to get HSV type 1 encephalitis, although there is a bimodal age distribution and individuals with immunosuppression may be at greater risk.

Discussion

Although encephalitis is relatively rare, its importance lies in the fact that for some causes there is effective treatment, provided it is started early, and delays in treatment can be devastating. In western settings the incidence of encephalitis ranges from 0.7 to 13.8 per 100,000 for adults and 10.5–13.8 per 100,000 in children [1,2].

Strictly speaking, encephalitis is a pathological diagnosis of inflammation of the brain, but in clinical practice surrogate markers of inflammation are used. Encephalitis has many infectious and non-infectious aetiologies, including numerous viruses and, to a lesser extent, bacteria, parasites and fungi, which may be associated with a meningoencephalitis. As some of these pathogens are geographically restricted or of particular risk to those with immune compromise, it is important to elicit a travel history and to establish immune status. Non-infective causes include those that are antibody-mediated, such as *N*-methyl D-aspartate receptor antibodies, which may be *de novo* or paraneoplastic [1,2].

HSV is the most commonly identified cause of encephalitis in the western setting with an annual incidence of 0.2–0.4 per 100,000. Most is due to HSV type 1, but approximately 10% may be caused by HSV type 2 [3,4]. It is diagnosed by a positive CSF PCR. If the test is done very early, within a few days of symptom onset, it may be falsely negative, and so presumptive aciclovir treatment should continue and the LP repeated after a day or two.

The range of presentations reflects the regions of the brain that are inflamed. In HSV encephalitis this is commonly the temporal lobe, resulting in language and short-term memory dysfunction, and seizures in a proportion. However, frontal lobe and more global dysfunction leads to most patients presenting with general, non-specific features including altered consciousness, behaviour or personality, and headache [5]. In addition, many patients will have a history of fever even if they are not febrile on admission. Therefore, it is important to specifically assess for a febrile or coryzal illness prior to admission, and not to exclude the possibility of encephalitis from the differential diagnosis simply because a fever was not documented on admission. Furthermore, the clinician should obtain a collateral history for evidence of altered behaviour, personality and cognition, as many mildly confused patients can have a normal Glasgow coma score on admission. In addition, it is unadvisable to attribute the combination of fever and confusion to infection outside of the brain (e.g. a respiratory or urinary infection), unless there is strong evidence; if there is any doubt, patients should be investigated for a brain infection.

All patients with suspected central nervous system infection need an immediate LP, unless there is a clinical contraindication, to establish or refute the diagnosis and to direct treatment [1,2].

Intravenous aciclovir for a minimum of 14 days is currently recommended in immunocompetent adults (**Figure 23.4**) [1,2]. Adjunctive corticosteroids

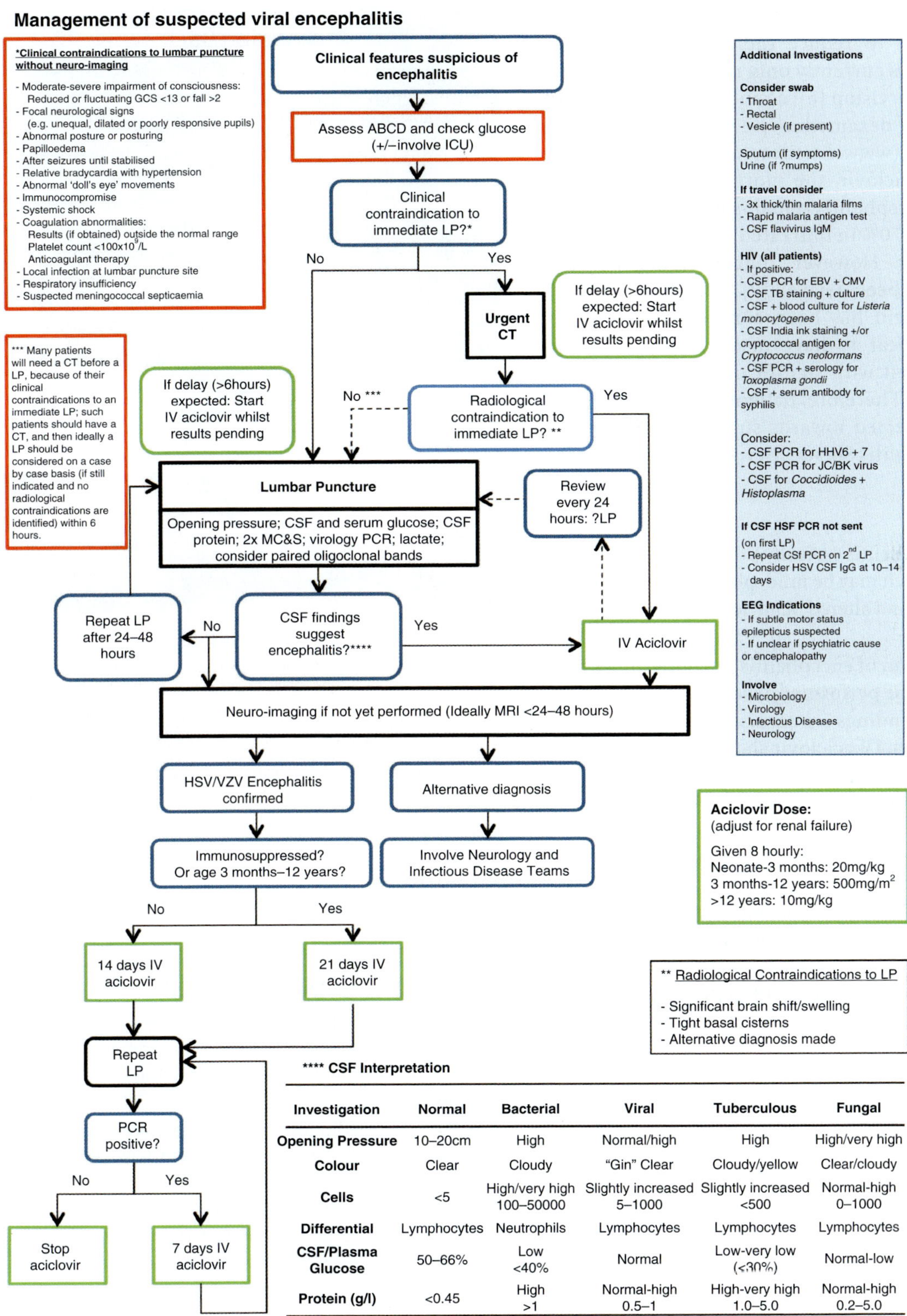

**** CSF Interpretation

Investigation	Normal	Bacterial	Viral	Tuberculous	Fungal
Opening Pressure	10–20cm	High	Normal/high	High	High/very high
Colour	Clear	Cloudy	"Gin" Clear	Cloudy/yellow	Clear/cloudy
Cells	<5	High/very high 100–50000	Slightly increased 5–1000	Slightly increased <500	Normal-high 0–1000
Differential	Lymphocytes	Neutrophils	Lymphocytes	Lymphocytes	Lymphocytes
CSF/Plasma Glucose	50–66%	Low <40%	Normal	Low-very low (<30%)	Normal-low
Protein (g/l)	<0.45	High >1	Normal-high 0.5–1	High-very high 1.0–5.0	Normal-high 0.2–5.0

Figure 23.4. Algorithm for the management of suspected viral encephalitis in adults from UK guidelines [1].

are sometimes used, as in the case described here, in an attempt to reduce the associated oedema, although this is currently only recommended under specialist supervision [6]; a randomised trial assessing the role of dexamethasone in HSV encephalitis began in 2016 (www.dexenceph.org.uk).

Despite aciclovir, the mortality and morbidity from HSV encephalitis remains high. Mortality has reduced from 70% in untreated to 20–30% if treated with aciclovir. However, outcomes are worse if treatment has been delayed [7]. Even those patients where treatment has been commenced early and who may appear to have made a good recovery may still be left with significant neuropsychological problems. Therefore, patients and their families should be directed towards support services, such as the Encephalitis Society (www.encephalitis.info).

Key Points

- HSV encephalitis typically presents with a febrile illness, which may be mild, plus headache, confusion and altered behaviour, which may be subtle.
- On suspicion of encephalitis, imaging and a LP should be performed as soon as possible, and if the findings are consistent with HSV encephalitis, IV aciclovir should be started as presumptively.
- The CSF may not be positive for HSV if done early in the course of the illness and so treatment should be continued and the LP repeated.
- Treatment of HSV encephalitis with IV aciclovir should continue for a minimum of 14 days in immunocompetent adults, and UK guidelines recommend repeating the LP at this stage to establish clearance of the virus before stopping treatment.

Looking Back

The term 'herpes' comes from the Greek word meaning to 'creep' or 'crawl', in reference to the creeping nature of the herpetic skin lesions (**Figure 23.5**).

For a long time, oral transmission was suspected. For example, the Roman Emperor Tiberius tried to cure a public outbreak of herpes by forbidding kissing during public ceremonies. However, it was not until 1893 when Jean Baptiste Emile Vidal, a French dermatologist, reported human-to-human transmission of herpes infections, identifying the necessity of intimate human contact for human spread.

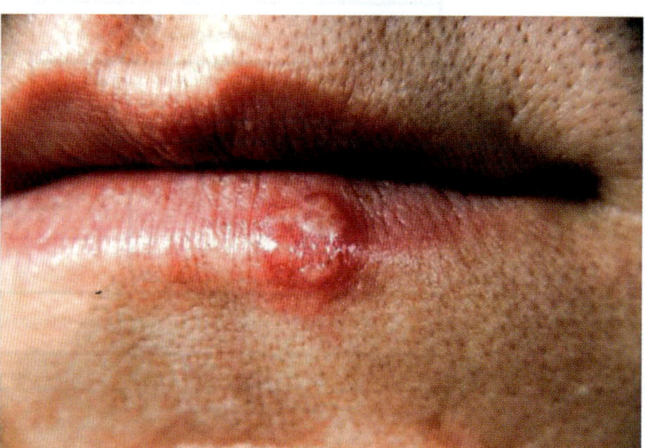

Figure 23.5. HSV causes 'creeping' cold sore lesions on the lips, although cold sores are not particularly associated with HSV encephalitis. (Reproduced with permission from Rassner G. *Atlas of Dermatology*, 3rd ed. Philadelphia, PA: Lea & Febiger; 1994: 42.)

Did You Know?

'Word salad' is a term used to describe a confused or unintelligible mixture of seemingly random words and phrases (**Figure 23.6**). The term is most often used in psychiatry.

Shakespeare is thought to have been referring to the transmission of herpes in Romeo and Juliet, when he wrote in Mercutio's speech about Queen Mab: *'O'er ladies lips, who straight on kisses dream, which oft the angry Mab with blisters plagues, because their breaths with sweetmeats tainted me'.*

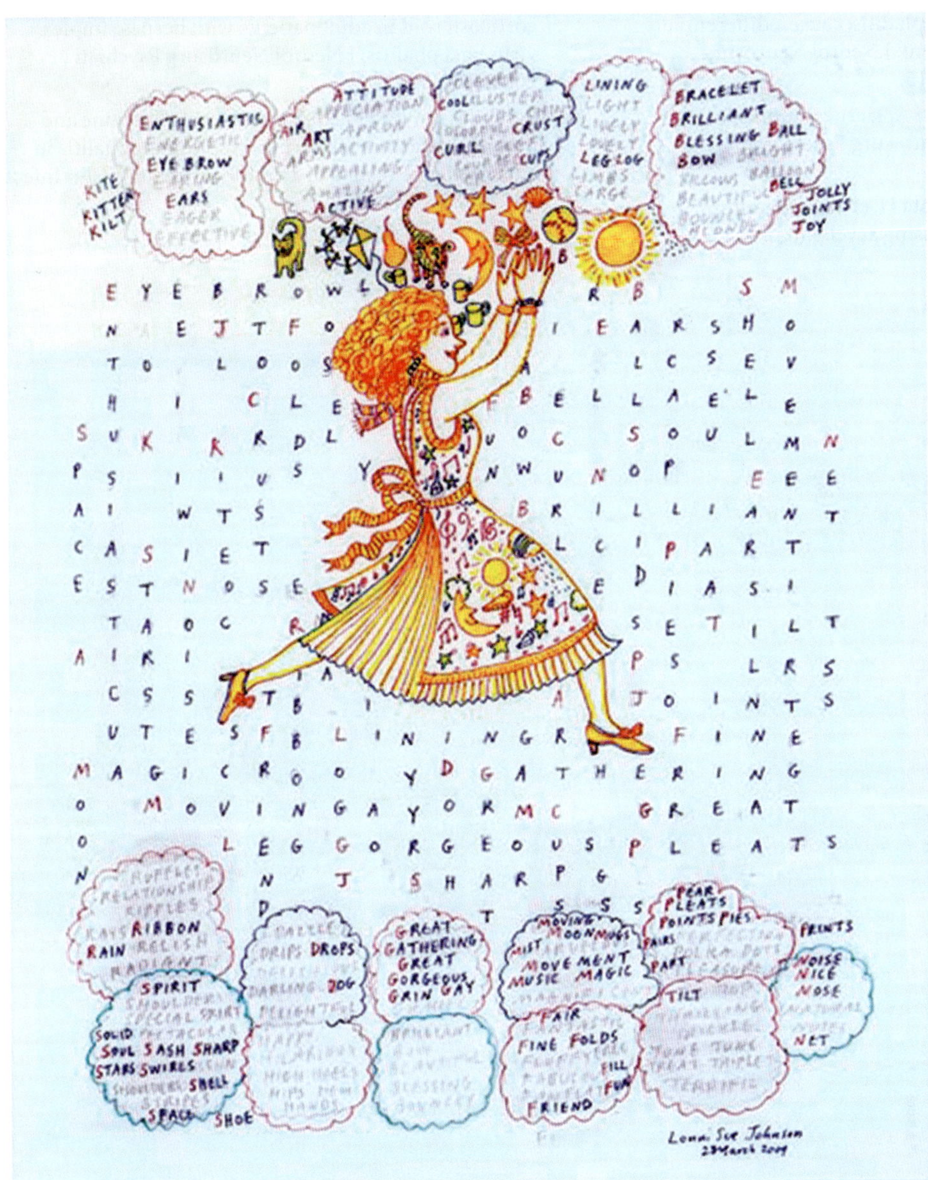

Figure 23.6. Difficulties in capturing words, expressed in this picture "'Enthusiastic' woman with pleated skirt" by artist Lonni Sue Johnson, who had HSV encephalitis a few years earlier. (© 2009 by Lonni Sue Johnson, used by permission from Aline M. Johnson. All rights reserved.)

References

1. Solomon T, Michael BD, Smith PE, et al. Management of suspected viral encephalitis in adults – Association of British Neurologists and British Infection Association National Guidelines. J Infect 2012;**64**: 347–73.

2. Kneen R, Michael BD, Menson E, et al. Management of suspected viral encephalitis in children – Association of British Neurologists and British Infection Association National Guidelines. J Infect 2012;**64**: 449–77.

3. Granerod J, Ambrose HE, Davies NWS, et al. Causes of encephalitis and difference in their clinical presentations in England: a multicentre, population-based prospective study. Lancet Infect Dis 2010;**10**:835–44.

4. Kennedy PGE. Viral encephalitis: causes, differential diagnosis and management. J Neurol Neurosurg Psychiatry 2004;**75**:i10–i15.
5. Kennedy PGE, Chaudhuri A. Herpes simplex encephalitis. J Neurol Neurosurg Psychiatry 2002;**72**:237–8.
6. Kamei S, Sekizawa T, Shiota H, et al. Evaluation of combination therapy using acyclovir and corticosteroid in adult patients with herpes simplex virus encephalitis. J Neurol Neurosurg Psychiatry 2005;**76**:1544–9.
7. Raschilas F, Wolff M, Delatour F, et al. Outcome and prognostic factors for herpes simplex encephalitis in adult patients: results of a multicentre study. Clin Infect Dis 2002;**35**:254–60.

CASE 24 A Mother and Baby

Anu Goenka and Rachel Kneen

History

A 2-day-old boy developed temperature instability and vomiting accompanied by two generalised seizures. He had been born at 34 weeks gestation with a birth weight of 1.9 kg (25th centile). The mother was a 30-year-old primagravida with no relevant past medical history. She had developed unplanned spontaneous preterm labour 1 week after a self-limiting febrile illness associated with coryzal symptoms and myalgia. There was no foetal distress noted before delivery, but the liquor was said to be meconium-stained. Following an uncomplicated vaginal delivery, the infant required five inflation breaths at delivery to establish good respiratory effort but then cried spontaneously. His arterial cord blood gas pH was 7.3 and venous pH was 7.35. There had been no antibiotic exposure *in utero*, and the baby had not been commenced on antibiotics at delivery.

Examination

On initial examination he handled poorly and was drowsy. His respiratory rate was 40 breaths per minute and there was mild respiratory distress. Oxygen saturations were 97% in room air. His heart rate was 160 beats per minute, blood pressure was 52/35 mmHg and central capillary refill time was 2 seconds. Cardiac and chest auscultation were normal, as was abdominal palpation. His anterior fontanelle was normotensive. A few hours after delivery, he was noted to be having subtle seizures with lip smacking and cycling movements of the lower limbs.

Initial Differential Diagnosis

- Early onset neonatal sepsis, e.g. Group B streptococcus
- Meningitis
- Meningoencephalitis, e.g. herpes simplex virus type 2
- Cerebral haemorrhage or venous sinus thrombosis and infarction
- Inborn error of metabolism

Results of Initial Investigations

He was neutropaenic, with a normal platelet count. C-reactive protein was 35 mg/l. Renal and liver function were normal. Serum glucose, calcium, lactate and ammonia were all normal. Blood gas showed a mild metabolic acidosis. Cerebrospinal fluid (CSF) examination revealed a white cell count of 324 cells/mm^3 with a neutrophil predominance, the glucose ratio was very low at 0.3 and the protein was elevated at 2.1g/l. Gram-positive bacilli was reported from both CSF and blood cultures, but was considered to be a diptheroid contaminant. Urine microscopy was normal. Chest X-ray and bedside cranial ultrasound on day 2 were normal. Cerebral function monitoring confirmed the presence of seizure activity.

Progress and Further Investigations

The seizures responded to intravenous midazolam and phenobarbitone. Initial antimicrobial treatment included intravenous benzylpenicillin and gentamicin, as well as aciclovir.

Results of Definitive Investigations

Listeria monocytogenes was cultured from the blood and CSF.

Diagnosis

Early onset neonatal sepsis and meningitis caused by *Listeria monocytogenes.*

Management, Progress and Outcome

In response to the culture results, benzylpenicillin and aciclovir were stopped and intravenous amoxicillin was commenced. He ultimately received 21 days of amoxicillin and gentamicin, making a gradual clinical recovery and establishing feeding. However, a repeat cranial ultrasound on day 7 of life showed worsening disease (**Figure 24.1**). Following this, serial cranial ultrasound demonstrated further progressive worsening (**Figure 24.2**). Therefore, a magnetic resonance imaging (MRI) brain scan was performed on day 19 of life (**Figure 24.3**).

Figure 24.1. Cranial ultrasound (coronal view) in a 7-day-old boy with temperature instability, vomiting and seizures.

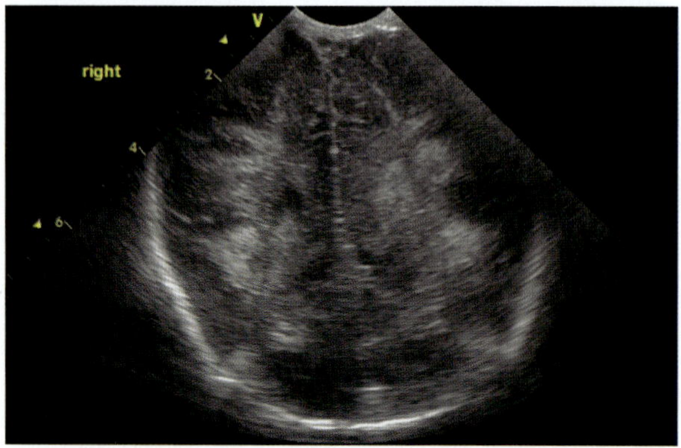

The image demonstrates bilateral intraventricular haemorrhage with a degree of ventricular dilatation, extensive increased echogenicity throughout the white matter indicative of oedema and possibly haemorrhage.

Figure 24.2. Cranial ultrasound on day 10 of life (coronal view) in the same infant.

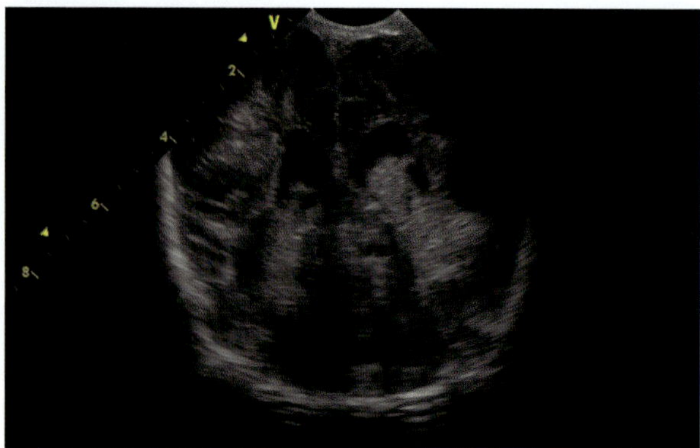

This demonstrates progression of ventricular dilatation, frank extension of intraventricular haemorrhage involving brain parenchyma on the left side and persistent white matter changes.

A

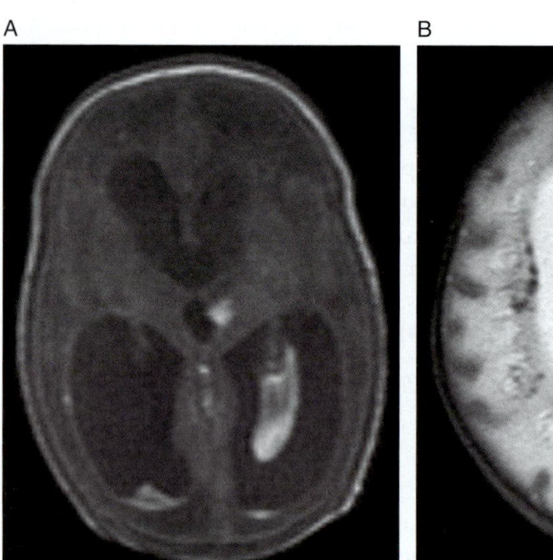

B

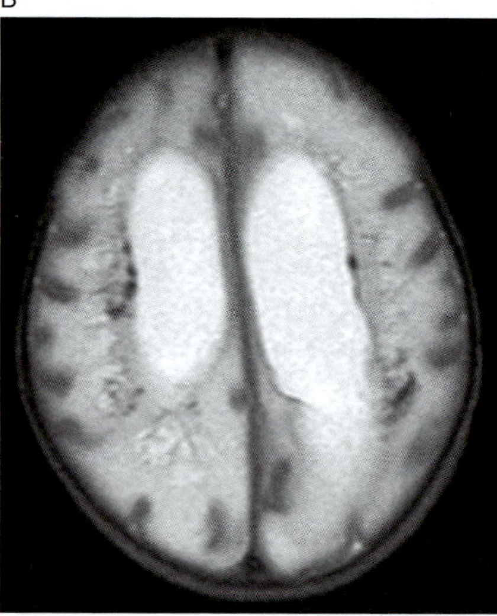

Figure 24.3. (A) A T1-weighted axial and (B) T2-weighted axial MRI brain scan image on day 19 of life in the same infant. This demonstrates ventriculomegaly and dependent haemorrhage in the occipital horns; the T2-weighted image shows additional diffuse haemorrhagic cystic changes, with widespread loss of grey–white differentiation in keeping with developing cystic encephalomalacia.

A ventricular tap was performed, removing 15 ml of CSF. Over the next 4 weeks clinical and ultrasound measurements were monitored (**Figures 24.4–24.5**). This prompted ventriculoperitoneal shunt insertion on day 50 of life.

At the last follow-up age 7 months there were some signs of delay in his gross and fine motor development: he was able to sit supported, but there was head lag when pulled to sit. He was visually attentive but had a hand preference, suggesting early signs of cerebral palsy. He was unable to transfer objects from hand to hand. He was able to participate in reciprocal babble, and audiology follow-up did not demonstrate any hearing loss.

Prevention

Prevention of *Listeria monocytogenes* infection rests largely on measures to reduce sporadic food-borne transmission. General food hygiene measures such as washing raw vegetables and storing raw meat away from other foods may reduce infection. Individuals at increased risk of infection, such as those who are pregnant, elderly or immunosuppressed, should avoid eating high-risk foods. High-risk foods include undercooked poultry, non-reheated hot dogs, soft cheeses and delicatessen counter foods. Consumption of hummus or melon at commercial establishments should also be avoided [1]. *L. monocytogenes* can be isolated

Figure 24.4. (A) Cranial ultrasounds (coronal views)on (A) day 25 and (B) day 29 in the same child.

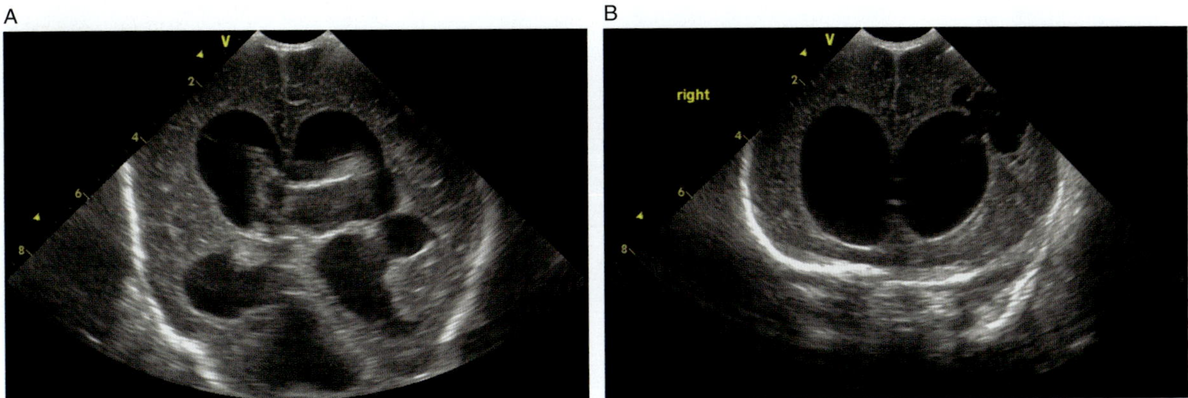

(A) demonstrates global ventricular dilatation and cystic changes in the white matter. (B) demonstrates progression of ventriculomegaly and left sided porencephalic cyst.

from foods stored as low as 4°C. Although the majority of infections are sporadic and not epidemic, *L. monocytogenes* remains notifiable in some countries. There can be a variable incubation period, making it difficult to establish the source of an infection, although most people develop symptoms within 1 month of infection and within 1–2 weeks for central nervous system (CNS) manifestations.

Discussion

Listeria monocytogenes is a Gram-positive bacillus that has a predilection for placental tissue and the CNS (**Figure 24.6**). It causes invasive bacterial infection including meningitis and septicaemia. Sporadic food-borne transmission is responsible for the majority of cases. Human-to-human transmission is rare, apart from vertical transmission, as in our case. Transient cellular immunodeficiency associated with pregnancy is associated with a 17-fold increased risk of acquiring infection [2,3]. Diagnosis in pregnancy is challenging due to the non-specific clinical presentation of febrile illness with coryza, myalgia, headache and backache, as in our case. Early diagnosis and antibiotic treatment of the pregnant woman can avoid the foetal and neonatal complications of chorioamnionitis, such as meningitis, sepsis, premature labour and intrauterine death [4]. Isolation of the organism is usually from blood or CSF culture, although culture from stool, as well as placental or high vaginal swab, is also possible.

This case highlights the non-specific clinical presentation of early onset neonatal sepsis. *L. monocytogenes* is the third most common cause of both early onset neonatal sepsis and meningitis, after Group B streptococcus and *Escherichia coli* [5]. In early onset neonatal sepsis, the clinical presentation of these organisms is largely indistinguishable. However, there are a few features that may alert the clinician to the specific possibility of *L. monocytogenes* infection. These include unplanned spontaneous preterm labour and foul-smelling meconium-stained amniotic fluid [6]. Some infants may also have a rash (**Figure 24.7**). Obtaining an accurate maternal history with regards to the potential food-borne source of infection is often challenging given the variable incubation time. A full septic screen including blood, urine and CSF culture should always be performed in suspected early onset neonatal sepsis. CSF findings in *L. monocytogenes* meningitis usually reflect a pyogenic bacterial picture, as in this case. Blood and CSF Gram staining may demonstrate the presence of Gram-positive bacilli, which can be easily mistaken for diptheroid skin contaminants, as they were initially in this case.

There are no controlled trials to inform choice and duration of antibiotic therapy for neonatal meningitis caused by *L. monocytogenes*. Intravenous amoxicillin was used in this case, although a potential synergistic effect of gentamicin has been noted in some studies [7].

Babies surviving neonatal meningitis caused by *L. monocytogenes* often suffer long-term neurological deficits. Factors which may influence the degree of neurological disability include how promptly antibiotic treatment was initiated and the degree of prematurity. This case developed intraventricular haemorrhage and obstructive hydrocephalus, both of which are

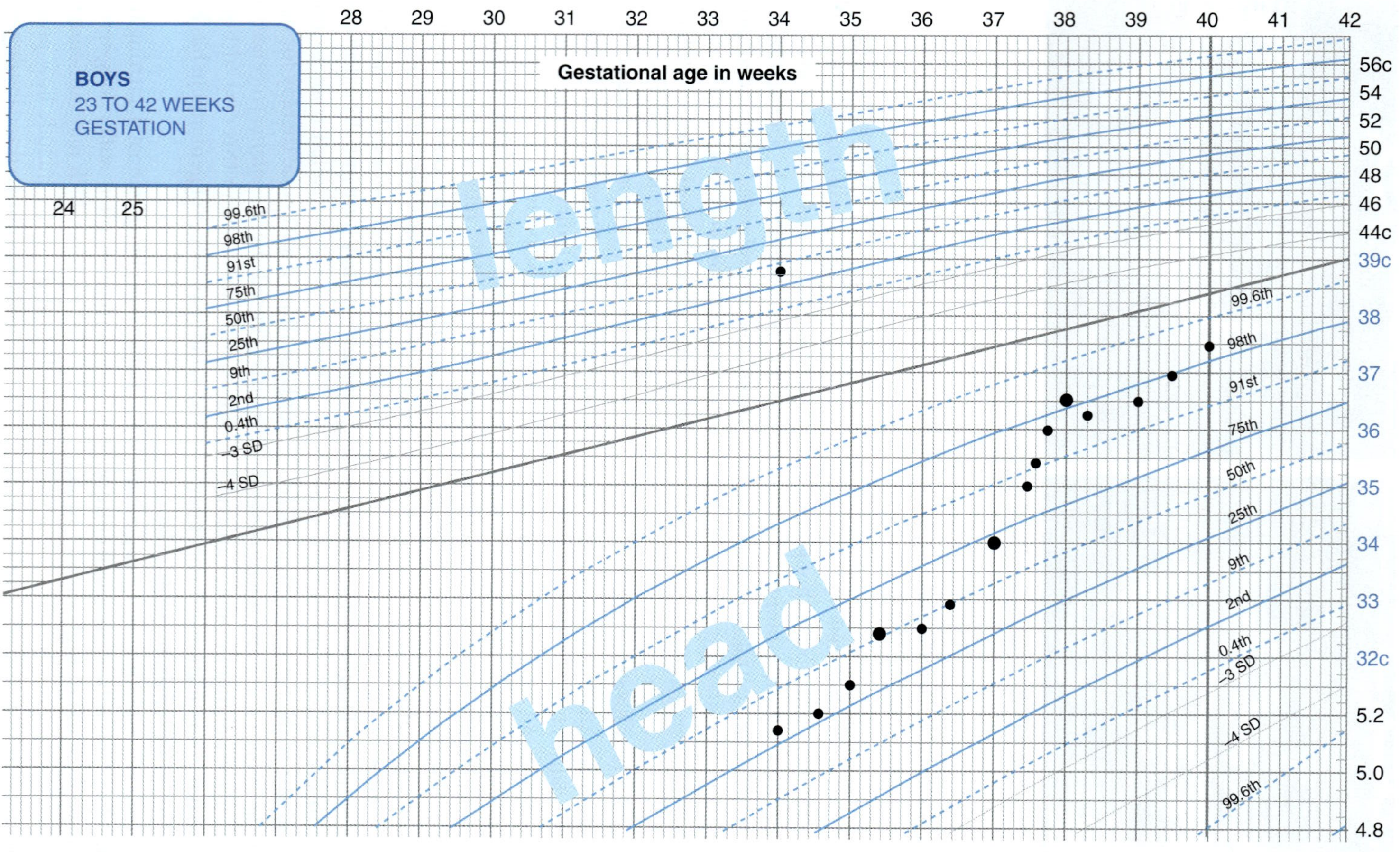

Figure 24.5. Serial head circumference measurement in the same child over this period. This illustrates progressive hydrocephalus despite the ventricular tap.

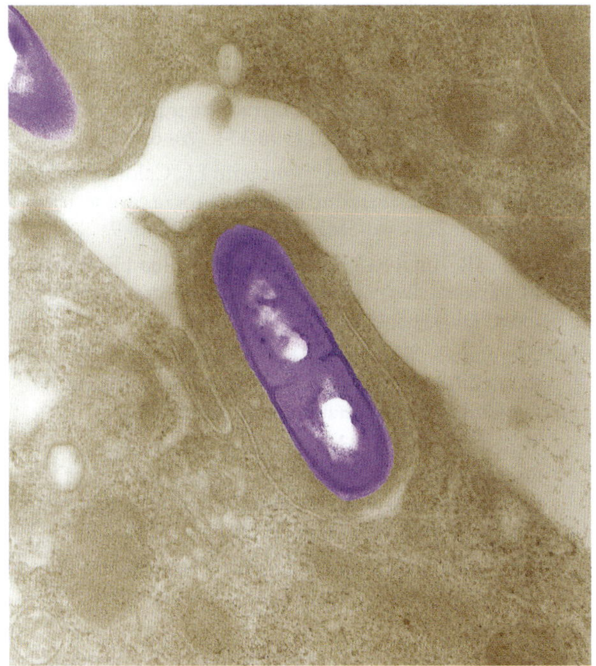

Figure 24.6. Electron micrograph of a *Listeria monocytogenes* bacterium in tissue. (Courtesy of Centers for Disease Control and Prevention, USA.)

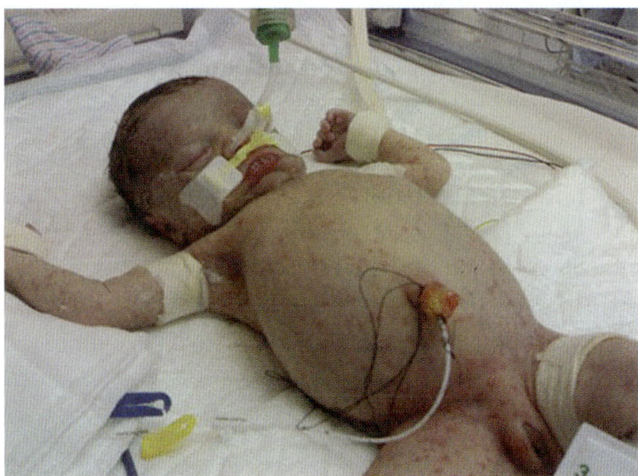

Figure 24.7. Generalised maculopapular rash present at birth that disappeared within a few hours of life in an infant with *Listeria monocytogenes* infection. (Reproduced with permission from [8].)

recognised complications of neonatal meningitis. Daily head circumference monitoring was vital in the early identification of the development of hydrocephalus, and for this baby allowed prompt further evaluation and treatment.

Key Points

- Presentation of *L. monocytogenes* is clinically non-specific in pregnant women and neonates alike. Early diagnosis and treatment in pregnant women protects neonates from severe disease.
- Unplanned spontaneous preterm labour and foul-smelling meconium-stained amniotic fluid may indicate that a neonate has Listeria infection.
- Be wary of accepting that Gram-positive bacilli found on CSF or blood microscopy are diptheroid contaminant; they could be could be *L. monocytogenes.*
- Daily head circumference monitoring is vital to identify hydrocephalus early.

Looking Back

In 1936, Burn described the first case series of three newborns with early onset sepsis caused by a Gram-positive bacillus. The post-mortem description of 'granulomatosis infantiseptica' associated with *L. monocytogenes*, characterised by multiple granulomas and microabscesses, was described later in 1951 [9]. The first association with food-borne transmission causing an epidemic was in 1983 and involved coleslaw [10].

Did You Know?

In 1989 a nosocomial outbreak of neonatal listeriosis was linked with mineral oil, which had been used to bathe babies, originating from a multi-dose container, from which *L. monocytogenes* was isolated [11].The genus *Listeria* was named in honour of the British pioneer of sterile surgery Joseph Lister, even though he had no role in its discovery (**Figure 24.8**) [12].

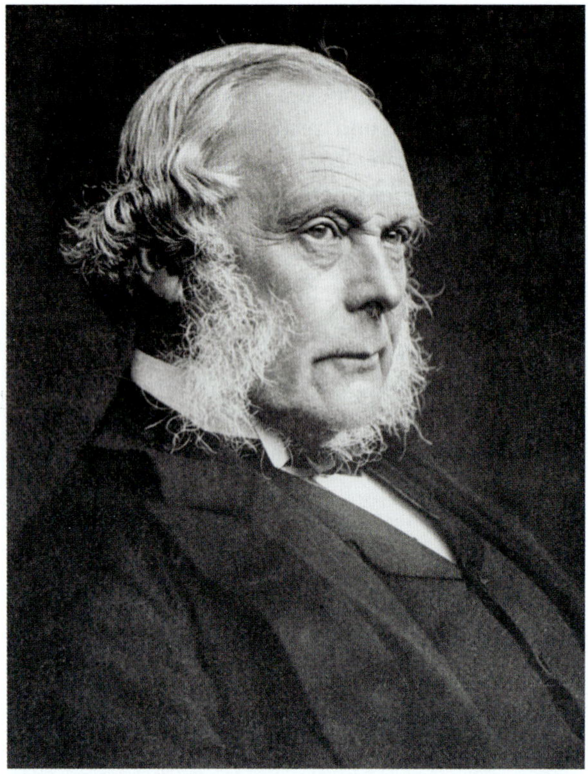

Figure 24.8. Joseph Lister, the British pioneer of sterile surgery, in whose honour Listeria is named, although he had no role in its discovery. Lister was famous for promoting antiseptic techniques, spraying carbolic acid (phenol) over surgical equipment, and the surgical incision site to prevent infection. (Photo courtesy of Photos.com.)

References

1. Varma JK, Samuel MC, Marcus R, et al. *Listeria monocytogenes* infection from foods prepared in a commercial establishment: a case-control study of potential sources of sporadic illness in the United States. Clin Infect Dis 2007;**44**:521–8.
2. Southwick FS, Purich DL. Intracellular pathogenesis of listeriosis. N Engl J Med 1996;**334**:770–6.
3. Mylonakis E, Paliou M, Hohmann EL, Calderwood SB, Wing EJ. Listeriosis during pregnancy: a case series and review of 222 cases. Medicine 2002;**81**:260–9.
4. Evans JR, Allen AC, Stinson DA, Bortolussi R, Peddle LJ. Perinatal listeriosis: report of an outbreak. Pediatr Infect Dis 1985;**4**:237–41.
5. Vergnano S, Menson E, Kennea N, Neonatal infections in England: the NeonIN surveillance network. Arch Dis Child Fetal Neonatal Ed 2010;**96**:F9–14.
6. Mazor M, Froimovich M, Lazer S, Maymon E, Glezerman M. *Listeria monocytogenes*. The role of transabdominal amniocentesis in febrile patients with preterm labor. Arch Gynecol Obstet 1992;**252**:109–12.
7. Hof H. An update on the medical management of listeriosis. Expert Opin Pharmacother 2004;**5**:1727–35.
8. Benitez-Segura I, Fiol-Jaume M, Balliu PR, Tejedor M. *Listeria monocytogenes*: generalised maculopapular rash may be the clue. Arch Dis Child Fetal *Neonatal Ed* 2013;**98**:F64.
9. Hof H. History and epidemiology of listeriosis. FEMS Immunol Med Microbiol 2003;**35**(3):199–202.
10. Schlech WF, Lavigne PM, Bortolussi RA, et al. Epidemic listeriosis – evidence for transmission by food. N Engl J Med 1983;**308**:203–6.
11. Schuchat A, Lizano C, Broome CV, et al. Outbreak of neonatal listeriosis associated with mineral oil. Pediatr Infect Dis J 1991;**10**:183–9.
12. Burn CG. Clinical and pathological features of a new pathogen of the genus *Listerella*. Am J Pathol 1936;**12**:341–8.

CASE 25

A Creeping Weakness

Liene Elsone and Mona Ghadiri-Sani

History

A 76-year-old right-handed retired female ward clerk presented to the local emergency department with excruciating, intermittent shooting and burning pain involving the left neck, shoulder and arm. The pain gradually spread over a week, to involve the tips of her fingers of her left hand. The shooting pain was exacerbated by movement or coughing and was accompanied by a constant background dull pain and paraesthesia in her left hand which disturbed her sleep. She also felt that her left grip was becoming weaker.

There was a past history of osteoporosis, hysterectomy and gastrectomy for peptic ulcers. She was an ex-smoker accumulating more than 30 pack-years. She had not had any significant recent travel history. There was a family history of breast and lung cancer

Examination

She had skin lesions over the left shoulder and down the outer arm (**Figure 25.1**). There was restricted movement of her left arm, in part due to pain. Power was preserved in all groups of muscles except for mild weakness (Medical Research Council power score 4/5) of left shoulder abduction and elbow flexion. Reflexes were intact with reduced sensation to pin-prick and light touch at the C5 and C6 dermatomes on the left. Proprioception and vibration sense were intact. Cranial nerve examination revealed a right-sided Horner's syndrome, but the rest of the cranial nerve examination was normal. There was no lymphadenopathy and breast examination was normal. She was not admitted initially, but re-presented 4 weeks later, complaining of further weakness (**Figure 25.2**).

She also had marked weakness (Medical Research Council power score 3/5) of the left supraspinatus, infraspinatus, serratus anterior, latissimus dorsi and deltoid muscles. She had grade 4/5 power in the left biceps, brachioradialis, triceps and finger flexors, abductors and extensors. The rest of the neurological examination remained unchanged, although a recurrence of the erythematous rash over the left shoulder was noted (**Figure 25.3**).

Initial Differential Diagnosis

The combination of wasting and progressive weakness with dermatomally distributed sensory loss suggested a disorder affecting the peripheral nerves. This could be mechanical, such as a compressive pathology (e.g. spondylosis, herniated cervical disc, tumour or

Figure 25.1. Skin lesions of a 76-year-old woman with a pain in the left neck, shoulder and arm, and a rash similar to this.

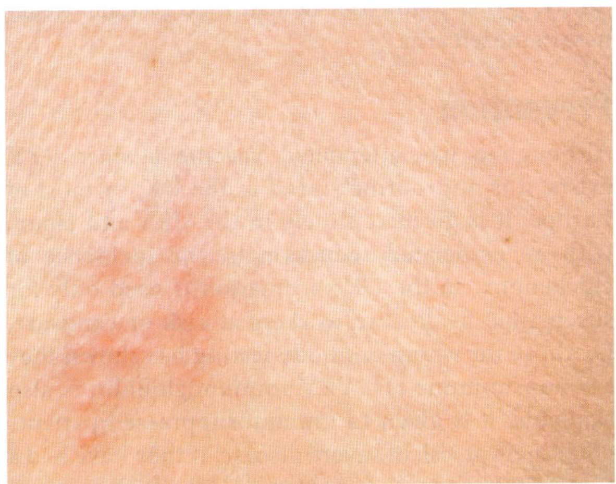

This shows a patchy erythematous rash with a few vesicles, which were present along the left C5 and C6 dermatomes. (Photo from: http://insidetheclinic.com/shingles-rash/)

Figure 25.2. The patient is pressing both arms against the wall.

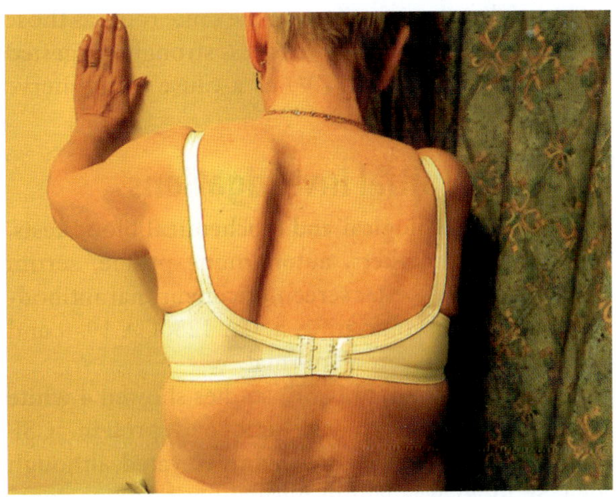

This shows winging of the left scapula, associated with wasting of the left infraspinatus muscle. (Photo: Tom Solomon.)

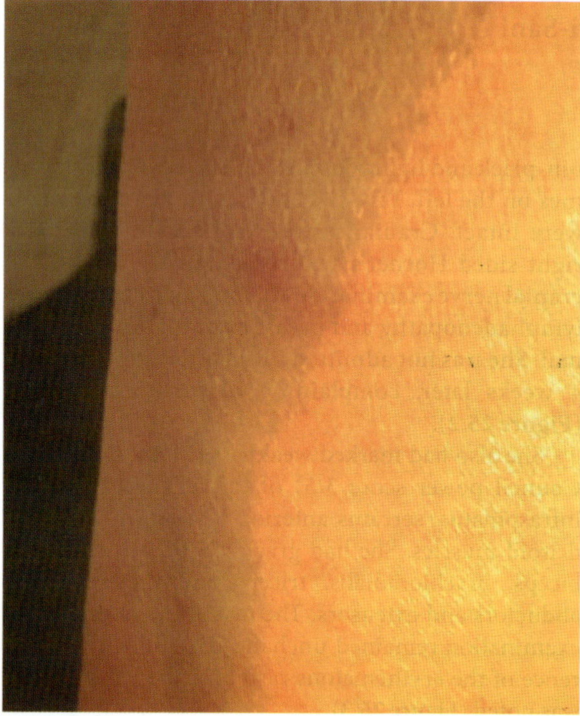

Figure 25.3. Recurrence of the patient's erythematous rash. (Photo: Tom Solomon.)

transection), or due to an inflammatory cause, which may be autoimmune (e.g. Sjogren's syndrome, vasculitis), idiopathic (i.e. neuralgic amyotrophy) or infective, including neurotropic herpes viruses, Lyme disease and HIV. Other possibilities included paraneoplastic disease, toxic or metabolic disturbances. Of all these possibilities, the erythematous vesicular rash in a dermatomal distribution affecting the same roots as those with lower motor neuron weakness strongly suggested varicella zoster virus (VZV) as a cause of the nerve damage.

Results of Initial Investigations

Routine haematological and biochemical blood tests, inflammatory markers, autoimmune profile, serum electrophoresis, coeliac screen, onconeuronal antibodies, carcinoembryonic antigen, CA 125, CA 19–9 and chest radiograph were all normal.

Cerebrospinal fluid (CSF) studies showed 4 white cells/mm^3, normal glucose ratio and protein. CSF immunoglobulin (Ig) G was slightly elevated, although the CSF index was within normal limits. Oligoclonal bands showed a type 3 pattern (i.e. oligoclonal IgG bands in the CSF not matched by bands in the serum), consistent with multiple sclerosis or nervous system inflammation.

Magnetic resonance imaging of her cervical spine and left brachial plexus, performed with contrast, showed no specific abnormality. Nerve conduction studies and electromyelogram were consistent with severe C6 and partial C7 root damage, dorsal root ganglion and anterior horn cell involvement at the left C6 level.

Results of Definitive Investigations

Blood serology showed VZV IgG suggestive of past VZV infection. Polymerase chain reaction (PCR) of the CSF was negative for both herpes simplex virus and VZV. HIV serology and antigen studies were negative.

Diagnosis

Varicella zoster virus causing shingles and radiculopathy.

Management and Outcome

When she first presented to the emergency department, based on the initial observations (the rash), the patient was diagnosed with shingles and she was given oral aciclovir 800 mg 5 times a day for 7 days and discharged home. However, 4 weeks later when she re-presented with progressive weakness of the left-hand grip and recurrence of the rash over the left shoulder (**Figure 25.3**), she was investigated thoroughly and treated with intravenous aciclovir. She had significant improvement of her symptoms over the coming year. On examination at 1-year follow-up she had mild residual weakness in the left arm.

Prevention

Although a live attenuated vaccine against VZV exists, it is not routinely used in the UK, or most of Europe. It is given routinely in the USA and Japan, with an associated reduction in the incidence of chickenpox. In the UK vaccination is used only for susceptible healthcare workers at risk of exposure, i.e. those for whom antibody testing has shown they are non-immune [1]. VZV immunoglobulin is also available; it is given to immunosuppressed patients and others at risk of severe disease, if they have had a significant exposure to someone with chickenpox or herpes zoster.

Discussion

VZV belongs to the alpha herpes virus sub-family of the herpes virus family. Primary infection results in chickenpox, which is a relatively mild and common childhood infection, only rarely causing complications. The virus can then become latent for decades, remaining in the nervous system particularly in neural ganglions and rarely nerve roots [2]. In up to 20% of people, especially in immunocompromised patients, the virus can reactivate, causing the cutaneous condition herpes zoster or shingles, which can cause recurrent attacks.

Herpes zoster usually presents initially with flu-like symptoms, dermatomal pain and paraesthesia associated with a vesicular erythematous rash. This may precede the onset of the other symptoms or follow them, typically by 24–72 hours. The thoracic dermatomes are most commonly affected; however, VZV can affect any dermatome or the trigeminal nerve, supplying the skin of the face. The reactivation of the rash can involve multiple dermatomes both contiguous and non-contiguous (known as '*Zoster Multiplex*'). In *Zoster sine herpete*, reactivation of the virus occurs, causing pain in the absence of a rash or vesicles [3].

Neurological complications of VZV can occur at the same time as the acute skin eruption, as in this case, or up to several months after resolution of the rash (**Table 25.1**). The most common complication is post-herpetic neuralgia, severe pain, which can be persistent. Rarer complications include neuropathy (such as Guillain–Barré syndrome and radiculopathy), meningitis, myelitis, encephalitis, herpes zoster ophthalmicus and herpes zoster oticus (Ramsay Hunt Syndrome) [4]; stroke can occur as a complication of shingles due to an associated vasculitis. Non-neurological complications include bacterial skin infections, uveitis, keratitis and acute retinal necrosis.

Shingles is usually diagnosed clinically and is not a hard diagnosis to make when there is the typical dermatomal vesicular rash with the prodromal symptoms. Supportive tests include serological testing with detection of IgM and IgG antibodies to VZV, PCR for VZV, culture of the skin lesion or CSF; direct florescent antibody testing on skin scrapings can also be used for diagnosis [5].

Diagnosing the neurological complications of shingles may be harder because the rash may no longer be present or obvious when the neurological features begin: asking carefully about a rash is thus important.

Table 25.1 Neurological complications of varicella zoster virus, modified from [6].

Complications of acute infection (varicella)	
Cerebellitis	
Acute encephalitis	
Complications of viral reactivation (zoster)	
Post-herpetic neuralgia	
Cranial neuropathies	
	Ramsay Hunt syndrome
	Herpes zoster ophthalmicus
	Trigeminal neuronitis
	Optic and oculomotor neuropathies/retinitis
	Mononeuritis of other cranial nerves
	Polyneuritis cranialis
Stroke syndromes	
	Herpes zoster ophthalmicus with delayed contralateral hemiparesis
	Cervical zoster with posterior circulation infarcts
	Granulomatous angiitis of the basilar artery
Encephalitis syndromes	
	Encephalitis
	Diffuse small/medium vessel arteritis
Myelitis	

In the patient described above the presence of VZV IgG in the serum was supportive of the diagnosis; in other patients VZV may be detectable in the CSF by PCR because the virus has been reactivated.

Management of shingles is usually dependent on the patient's age, severity of disease, immune status and presence of complications. Antiviral therapy, typically with the virostatic agent aciclovir, is the main therapy. Other antiviral medications which can be effective are valaciclovir, famciclovir and penciclovir [7]. Symptomatic treatments include pain management and antihistamines. Prompt initiation of antiviral drugs is crucial to reduce morbidity and mortality, especially in immunocompromised patients and those with neurological and ophthalmological complications. Oral steroids are also often used.

Key Points

- Shingles usually presents with a prodromal illness followed by a vesicular rash which can be contagious, and is usually diagnosed on clinical features alone.

- A wide range of neurological complications are associated with VZV reactivation, that can occasionally occur without the rash
- Neurological complications of shingles are treated with intravenous aciclovir or related antiviral drugs.

Looking Back

The words herpes, meaning 'to creep', and zoster, meaning 'zone or girdle', are derived from the Greek *herpein* and *zoster*, respectively.

Vesicular rashes have been described since the ancient civilisations, but by the end of the nineteenth century a link between herpes zoster and chickenpox was made. The link was finally proven a century later in the 1950s.

Did You Know?

Zoster is the name of a rock music band from Bosnia and Herzegovina. It was named after one of the band recovered from herpes zoster, diagnosed by a physician who was a fan of the band.

References

1. Public Health England. Varicella. In: The Green Book (chapter 34). London: Department of Health. Retrieved from www.gov.uk/government/publications/varicella-the-green-book-chapter-34; 2013 (accessed June 4, 2014).
2. Gilden D, Mahalingam R, Nagel MA, et al. The neurobiology of varicella zoster virus infection. Neuropathol Appl Neurobiol 2011;**37**:441–63.
3. Lewis GW. Zoster sine herpete. Br Med J 1958;**2**: 418–21.
4. Galil K, Choo PW, Donahue JG, et al. The sequelae of herpes zoster. Arch Intern Med 1997;**157**:1209.
5. Leung J, Harpaz R, Baughman AL, et al. Evaluation of laboratory methods for diagnosis of varicella. Clin Infect Dis 2010;**51**:23–32.
6. Solomon T. Encephalitis, and infectious encephalopathies. In: Donaghy M, editor. *Brain's Diseases of the Nervous System*. 12th ed. Oxford: Oxford University Press; 2009: 1355–428.
7. Tyring SK. Management of herpes zoster and postherpetic neuralgia. J Am Acad Dermatol 2007;**57**:136–42.

CASE 26

Preventable Neuropathy

Anand Iyer and Rachel Kneen

History

A 13-year-old girl was admitted to hospital in Vietnam with difficulty swallowing, nasal regurgitation of fluids, altered voice, blurring of near vision and aspiration pneumonia. She had a history of a febrile illness 5 weeks earlier, with severe sore throat, facial and neck swelling, hoarse voice and difficulty breathing. She had been treated with antibiotics at this time and her symptoms resolved after 10 days. She had no significant medical history. Her parents reported one dose of primary immunisations at the age of 2 years, but were unsure of the details.

Examination

On examination, she was afebrile and did not have a 'toxic' appearance suggestive of acute bacterial infection. Her pulse was regular at 60 per minute and her blood pressure was 100/50 mmHg. She had occasional palpable ventricular ectopic beats. Cranial nerve examination was abnormal (**Figure 26.1**). She also had a nasal quality to her speech with an absent gag reflex and absent palate movement, and failure of pupillary restriction on accommodation. She walked with a wide-based gait and examination showed 4/5 on the Medical Research Council power scale symmetrically in both proximal and distal, flexor and extensor muscle groups. She had generalised areflexia and her Babinski response was negative. She had distal sensory loss in the lower limbs to all modalities in a glove and stocking distribution up to mid-calf.

Figure 26.1. Facial appearance of a 13-year-old Vietnamese girl who presented with a sore throat, following a febrile illness. In (A) she is being asked to keep her eyes tightly closed. In (B) she is being asked to smile.

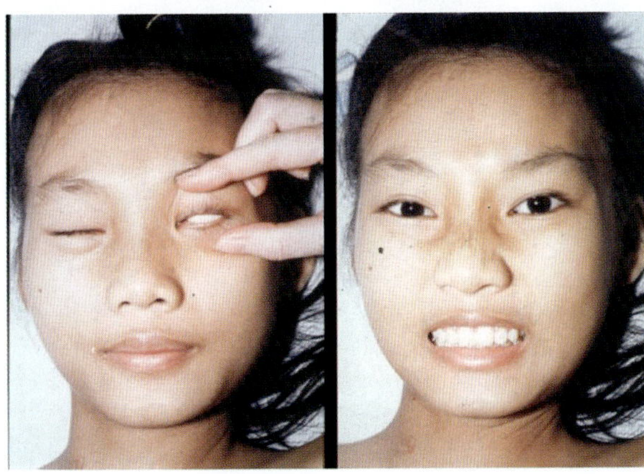

The images show bilateral facial weakness of a lower motor neuron type with symmetrical involvement of the frontalis, orbicularis oculi (including Bell's phenomenon) and orbicularis ori. (Photo: Tom Solomon.)

Initial Differential Diagnosis

The symptoms and signs were suggestive of an acute, evolving motor and sensory polyneuropathy. Potential causes include:

- acute infection (e.g. central nervous system Lyme disease, tick paralysis, diphtheritic polyneuropathy, botulism)
- post-/para-infectious process (i.e. Guillain–Barré syndrome)
- vasculitis polyneuropathy.

Investigations

Basic blood tests were normal and culture of a throat swab was negative. An electrocardiogram (ECG) revealed a prolonged PR interval and frequent ventricular ectopic beats. Nerve conduction studies were initially normal; the conduction velocity was 44.4 m/s in the posterior tibial nerve (normal values > 42.5 m/s) with distal motor latency of 5.02 ms (normal values < 5.2 ms). However, when repeated three weeks later, abnormalities were detected including a delayed conduction velocity of 35.3 m/s and distal motor latency of 7.02 ms. This is in keeping with a demyelinating peripheral neuropathy.

Progress and Outcome

The girl's bulbar symptoms and accommodation difficulties improved over the next 2 weeks. She developed persistent sinus tachycardia for the following 4 weeks, which gradually improved and did not need any specific intervention. Her peripheral weakness continued to deteriorate and reached its peak at 7 weeks, followed by a slow improvement. She did not require any respiratory support. She was able to walk again 5 months after presentation with supportive treatment and rehabilitation.

Diagnosis

Diphtheritic demyelinating motor and sensory polyneuropathy. with a bi-phasic presentation: initial cranial neuropathies with bulbar symptoms followed by a generalised weakness. This presentation with a sore throat followed by progressive neuropathy is characteristic of diphtheria, especially if it begins with the cranial nerves and then progresses. The prolonged PR interval and frequent ventricular ectopics on ECG are suggestive of myocarditis, also caused by diphtheria, and confirming the diagnosis.

Prevention

Immunisation with diphtheria toxoid is the only effective control. The minimum protective level of serum antitoxin is 0.01 IU/ml. A vaccine containing diphtheria and tetanus toxoid with acellular pertussis and Haemophilus Influenza B is currently given to children in the UK. Vaccination programmes in Vietnam when this patient presented, and in the preceding years, were patchy. Antitoxin levels wane over time and a tetanus and diphtheria toxoid may be given every 10 years. Acquiring diphtheria does not confer immunity and individuals recovering from the disease are given active immunisation during convalescence.

Discussion

Diphtheritic polyneuropathy is a toxin-mediated acute demyelinating polyneuropathy, which occurs as a complication of severe infection with the Gram-positive aerobic bacillus *Corynebacterium diphtheriae* (**Figure 26.2**). *C. diphtheriae* predominantly resides in the mucous membranes and is spread by airborne respiratory droplets. It initially causes a severe pharyngitis with development of a typical whitish grey membranous exudate over the pharyngeo-tonsillar area that bleeds when scraped (**Figure 26.3**). There is profound lymphadenopathy with surrounding oedema causing facial and neck swelling, which is recognised as a 'bull-neck' appearance.

Local toxic effects occur by direct spread of the toxin and results in early bulbar symptoms while the generalised neuropathy arises from haematogenous dissemination of the toxin. The polyneuropathy occurs in approximately 10% of moderate infections and up to 75% of severe infections and follows a biphasic course, as seen in this case [1]. Initially there may be oculomotor palsy and phrenic nerve involvement causing respiratory paralysis; other symptoms suggestive of cranial neuropathies are numbness in

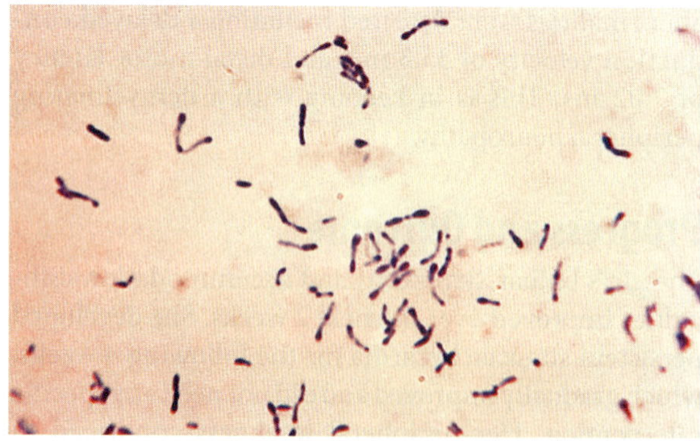

Figure 26.2. Photomicrograph showing Gram-positive *Corynebacterium diphtheriae* stained with methylene blue. (From: www.cdc.gov/diphtheria/about/photos.html)

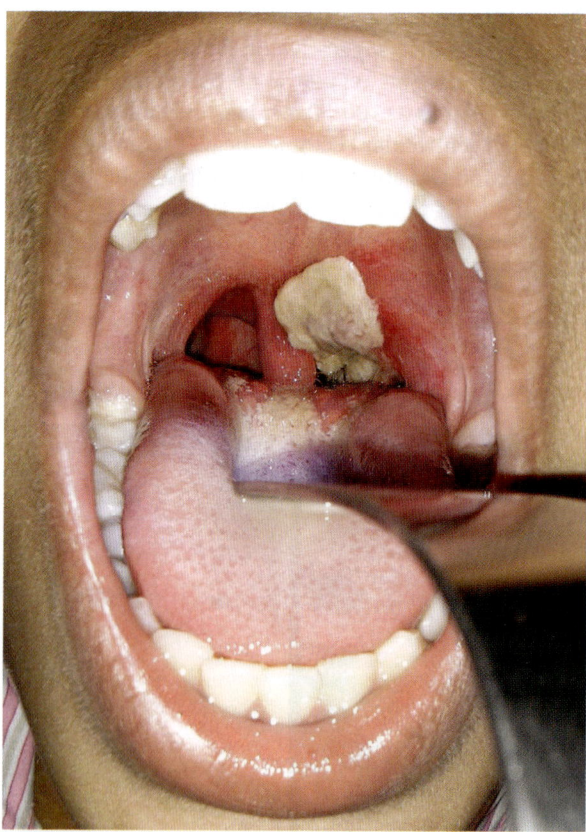

Figure 26.3. The grey-white pseudomembrane covering the tonsils in diphtheria. (Photo courtesy of Dileepunnikri, reproduced under CC BY-SA 3.0.)

gingivae, tongue and face, nasal speech and regurgitation, dysphonia and dysphagia. This may then be followed by neuropathy affecting the longer nerves in the limbs. The parasympathetic autonomic nervous system is also affected leading to blurred vision, abnormal pupil reactions and cardiac conduction defects, as seen in this case. Vagal denervation leads to persistent tachycardia.

Logina and Donaghy [2] studied 51 patients with diphtheritic polyneuropathy during an outbreak in Latvia in 1994: 30 (60%) had survived severe diphtheria (neck swelling, toxic shock, acute renal failure or myocarditis). Bulbar symptoms were present in 49 with a median (range) time of onset of 10 (2–50) days after the primary infection. This improved over the next 30 days, followed by a further bulbar deterioration at 40 (17–54) days in 19 patients. Limb weakness followed the bulbar symptoms in 45, with median onset at 37 (12–6) days and reached its peak severity at 49 days. Improvement began at 73 (20–115) days. This cohort was compared with 20 patients with Guillain–Barré syndrome, and those affected with Guillain–Barré syndrome showed peak deterioration at 10 (2–28) days and improvement at 21 (4–49) days, and usually followed a monophasic course. At 1-year follow-up, 6% of patients with diphtheritic polyneuropathy and 13% of patients with Guillain–Barré syndrome were unable to walk independently. **Table 26.1** summarises the key differentiating features between diphtheritic polyneuropathy and Guillain–Barré syndrome.

The pathogenesis of diphtheritic polyneuropathy is characterised by paranodal and segmental demyelination with preservation of the axonal continuity in most cases. *C. diphtheriae* produces a 62-kDa polypeptide exotoxin that inhibits protein synthesis and causes local tissue necrosis. The toxin inhibits synthesis of myelin protetolipid leading to demyelination.

Investigations to confirm diphtheria during the acute infection is by isolation of *C. diphtheriae* on culture from a throat swab which is inoculated in an aerobic tellurite medium. Cerebrospinal fluid (CSF) studies are variable and can show lymphocytosis or dissociated increase in protein. There is no correlation between CSF changes and severity of clinical presentation [3]. Nerve conduction studies demonstrate prolongation of distal motor latency, delayed F-wave latency, slowing of conduction velocity and conduction block [4].

Table 26.1 Differentiating features between diptheretic polyneuropathy and Guillain–Barré syndrome.

	Diphtheritic neuropathy	Guillain–Barré syndrome
Phases	Biphasic	Monophasic
Time course	Onset time equals recovery time	Rapid onset, slower recovery
Facial muscle involvement	Rare	Common
Autonomic symptoms	Vagal dysfunction, tachycardia	Sympathetic and parasympathetic
Other features	Blurred near vision, palatal weakness	Not typically seen

The overall case fatality rate of diphtheria was 2–3% during an outbreak in Russia [5]. The most common cause of death was severe myocarditis or respiratory failure. The risk of death from cardiomyopathy increases with the amount of membrane that is visible in the oropharynx at presentation [6]. Antibiotic therapy with antitoxin administration within 48 hours of presentation has been reported to decrease the subsequent development of diphtheritic polyneuropathy by 50% [7]. There is no specific treatment for diphtheritic polyneuropathy and the management is mainly supportive. Monitoring of lung vital capacity with physical rehabilitation is the mainstay of treatment. The only measure for effective control against diphtheria infection is universal immunisation with diphtheria toxoid throughout life. In the UK, the classical disease is very rare and milder infections (without the effects of toxin) resemble streptococcal pharyngitis. Based on serosurveillance studies, approximately 50% of adults over 30 years are susceptible to diphtheria and this increases to over 70% in older age groups [8].

Key Points

1. Diphtheritic polyneuropathy occurs in 75% of survivors of severe diphtheria pharyngitis.
2. Diphtheritic polyneuropathy follows a bi-phasic course and is a form of demyelinating polyneuropathy, with similarities to Guillain–Barré syndrome, but typically affecting cranial and then peripheral nerves.
3. It naturally slowly recovers over weeks, and so survival rates are good for patients supported through intensive care.

Looking Back

In Spain, the year 1613 is known as *El Año de los Garrotillos* (The Year of Strangulations) because of the large diphtheria epidemic during that year.

The discovery of the toxin in 1888 by Roux and Yersin led to the formation of the toxoid and mass immunisation.

Prior to the 1940s, diphtheria was common in the UK.

Did You Know?

The name diphtheria comes from the Greek for leather '*diphtheria*', 'leather' because of the leathery appearance of the pseudomembrane in the throat.

Large outbreaks occurred in the former Soviet Union, in the 1990s, and among Rohingya refugees in Bangladesh; in both cases the outbreaks were linked to low immunisation coverage in young children, waning immunity in adults and large-scale population movements.

References

1. Krumina A. Diphtheria with polyneuropathy in a closed community despite receiving recent booster vaccination. J Neurol Neurosurg Psychiatr 2005;**76**:1555–7.
2. Logina I, Donaghy M. Diphtheritic polyneuropathy: a clinical study and comparison with Guillain–Barré syndrome. J Neurol Neurosurg Psychiatr 1999;**67**:433–8.
3. Piradov MA, Pirogov VN, Popova LM, Avdunina IA. Diphtheritic polyneuropathy: clinical analysis of severe forms. Arch Neurol 2001;**58**:1438–42.
4. Créange A, Meyrignac C, Roualdes B, Degos JD, Gherardi RK. Diphtheritic neuropathy. Muscle Nerve 1995;**18**:1460–3.
5. Rakhmanova AG, Lumio J, Groundstroem K, et al. Diphtheria outbreak in St. Petersburg: clinical characteristics of 1,860 adult patients. Scand J Infect Dis 1996;**28**: 37–40.
6. Kneen R, Dung MN, Solomon T, et al. Clinical features and predictors of diphtheritic cardiomyopathy in Vietnamese children. Clin Infect Dis 2004;**39**:1591–8.
7. Roche S, Stone S, Allen CM, Lange LS. Diphtheritic polyneuritis in an elderly woman: clinical and neurophysiological follow-up. Br J Clin Pract 1990;**44**:285–7.
8. Maple PA, Jones CS, Wall EC, et al. Immunity to diphtheria and tetanus in England and Wales. Vaccine 2000;**19**:167–73.

CASE 27

It's In the Genes

Mona Ghadiri-Sani and Sylviane Defres

With thanks to Dr Ian Hart and Dr Katherine Ward

History

A 52-year-old man with a long history of hypertension and rheumatoid arthritis, which had been stable for several years on methotrexate, presented with a 5-month history of early morning headaches, which improved during the day. Initially the headaches were diagnosed as migraines, but he subsequently had a 1-week history of confusion, auditory hallucinations, disorientation and short-term memory impairment. He was also complaining of restriction of his visual fields, particularly on the left.

He was self-employed, working on a farm, and lived with his mother. There was no recent history of vaccination, foreign travel or contacts.

Examination

On examination his abbreviated mental test score was 6/10. He had bilateral partial ptosis, left homonymous hemianopia with normal visual acuity. The remainder of the cranial nerve examination, including funduscopy, was normal.

He had an unsteady gait but examination of the upper and lower limbs demonstrated normal tone, power and sensation with symmetrical reflexes and flexor plantars.

Initial Differential Diagnosis

- Encephalitis
  - Inflammatory, including vasculitis
  - Infective, typically viral
  - Paraneoplastic

Other differentials include neoplasia, demyelination.

Results of Initial Investigations

His routine bloods including full blood count, electrolytes, urea and creatinine, liver and bone profile, glucose, lactate dehydrogenase and inflammatory markers were all normal. Following a computed tomography head scan a magnetic resonance imaging (MRI) brain scan was performed (**Figure 27.1**).

A subsequent magnetic resonance angiogram was normal. He had a lumbar puncture (LP) which showed a white cell count of 40 cells/mm^3 (100% lymphocytes), protein of 4.6 g/l and glucose of 4.8 mmol/l (8.1 mmol/l in the serum).

Cerebrospinal fluid (CSF) polymerase chain reaction (PCR) was negative for herpes simplex virus 1+2, parechovirus, enterovirus, varicella zoster virus and subsequently for Epstein–Barr virus (EBV), JC virus, toxoplasma, tuberculosis, Lyme and paraneoplastic screen.

Progress and Further Investigations

Over the next few days his visual acuity reduced and eventually he developed cortical blindness. He became densely amnesic and continued to confabulate. He had several events during which he became unresponsive with associated hypotension and hyponatraemia (sodium 117), which investigations showed was consistent with the syndrome of inappropriate diuretic hormone secretion (SIADH). One of these events precipitated an intensive therapy unit admission. He was also spiking temperatures; however, despite being investigated several times with septic screens and repeat lumber punctures, no cause was found. The pyrexia was eventually thought to be secondary to thalamic involvement.

His vasculitic screen, Venereal Disease Research Laboratory and HIV serology and Whipple's screen, aquaporin 4 antibodies and paraneoplastic screen were all negative.

A repeat MRI scan was performed (**Figure 27.2**).

Refined Differential Diagnosis

- Encephalitis
  - Neoplastic – lymphoma, glioma or metastatic
  - Infective – viral, atypical
  - Paraneoplastic

Results of Further Investigations

PCR of the CSF was positive for human herpes virus (HHV) 6. The initial viral load was 1000 copies/ml and on a subsequent LP was 6600 copies/ml. However, subsequently blood samples were also found to be positive at 44,000 copies/ml in serum and 2.7 million copies/ml in whole blood. This is consistent with chromosomal integration of HHV6, potentially giving a false positive

Figure 27.1. Axial MRI scans in a 52-year-old gentleman with a history of rheumatoid arthritis receiving methotrexate, who presented with sub-acute headache and progressive confusion. He was found to have mild bilateral ptosis and a left homonymous hemianopia.

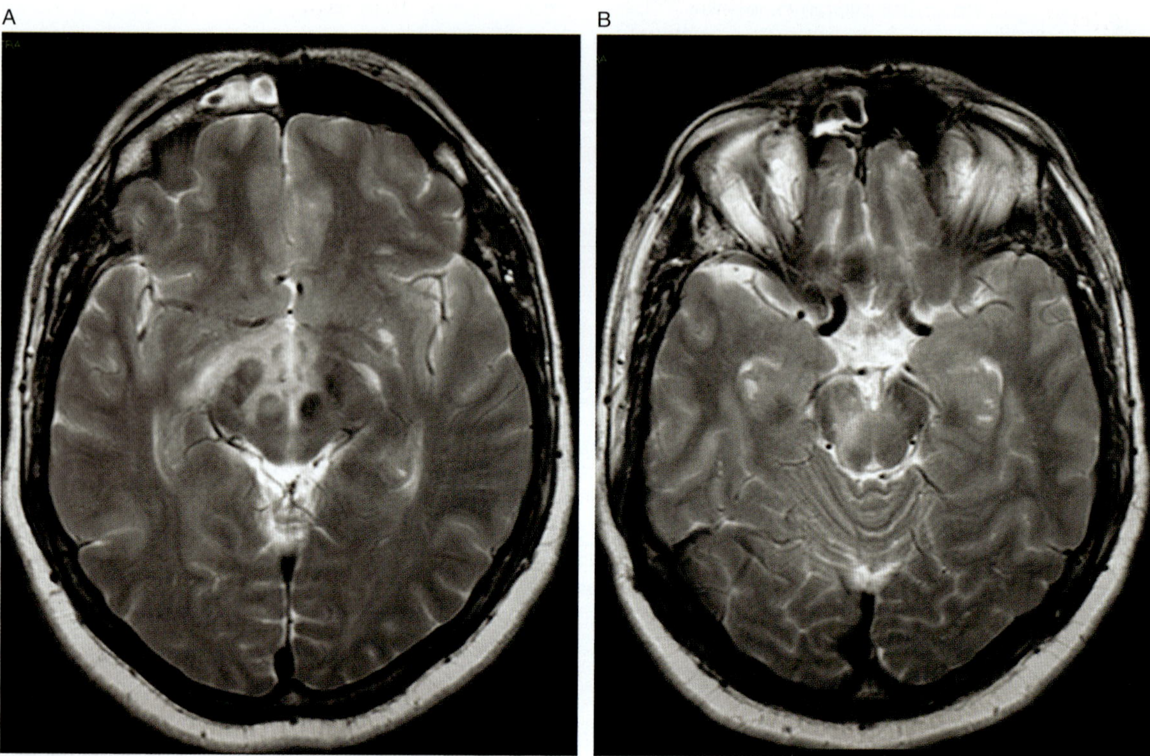

This shows high signal changes in the right thalamus, hypothalamus, basal ganglia, midbrain and cerebral peduncles.

in the CSF, rather than acute central nervous system (CNS) infection. No other infectious or autoimmune cause of the encephalitis could be found.

Diagnosis

The patient was diagnosed with rhombencephalitis (brainstem encephalitis) of uncertain aetiology, and incidental chromosomal integration of HHV6.

Management and Outcome

To reduce the risk of ongoing infection with any pathogen, his methotrexate was stopped. He was treated initially with intravenous immunoglobulin, steroids and, subsequently, plasma exchange to cover a potential autoimmune encephalitis. When the initial CSF HHV6 result was available, he was started on intravenous ganciclovir for 3 weeks followed by oral valganciclovir for a further 3 weeks. This treatment plan was pursued even when the results suggesting chromosomal integration became available.

He showed significant improvement clinically and radiologically (**Figure 27.3**). He had no further episodes of unresponsiveness or pyrexia, he became alert to the extent that he was able to recognise family members and started to recall memories from the past. However, he continued to have dense anterograde amnesia and remained cortically blind. He was eventually discharged to a local rehabilitation centre prior to going home.

Prevention

There is no vaccination for HHV6. A prospective multi-centre study was conducted to assess the safety and efficacy of pre-emptive therapy with foscarnet sodium for the prevention of HHV6 encephalitis in haematopoietic stem cell transplant patients, who are especially vulnerable. The treatment proved safe, and only one patient developed mild limbic encephalitis just after pre-emptive therapy started [1].

Figure 27.2. Repeat axial MRI scan in the same patient who had developed worsening confusion, cortical blindness, pyrexia and SIADH.

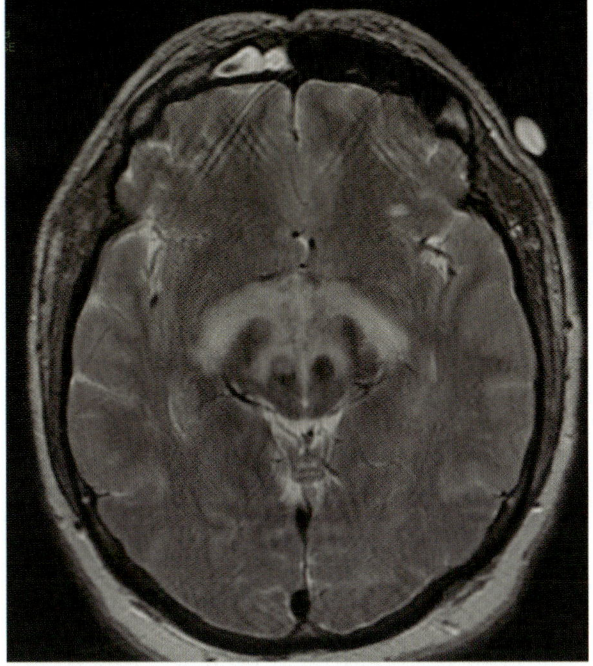

This shows high signal involving the left thalamus, hypothalamus and midbrain.

Discussion

Human herpes virus 6 is a member of the *Roseolovirus* genus, in the Betaherpesviridae subfamily of the Herpesvirus family [2]. It is characteristically T-lymphotrophic, but can infect other cell types, including neurons and hair follicles [3]. More recently, two variants have been distinguished: HHV6A and HHV6B. As with all herpesviruses, after primary infection, HHV6 remains latent in the CNS, monocytes and bone marrow progenitor cells. It is subsequently shed chronically in the saliva [4]. Transmission thus occurs through kissing, particularly mother to infant, and also through blood products.

Almost all children are seropositive by the age of 2, making late-onset primary infections rare [5]. Primary infection with HHV6, although usually asymptomatic, can cause exanthema subitum, also known as roseola or 6th disease. This is a febrile illness typically associated with a rash and leucopaenia, and sometimes also thrombocytopaenia and hepatitis (**Figure 27.4**). There is also a relatively high incidence of febrile seizures, particularly prolonged seizures in HHV6 infection. Primary infection can also cause a mononucleosis-like illness, or when the CNS is infected, HHV6 type B can cause encephalitis or intractable seizures.

A

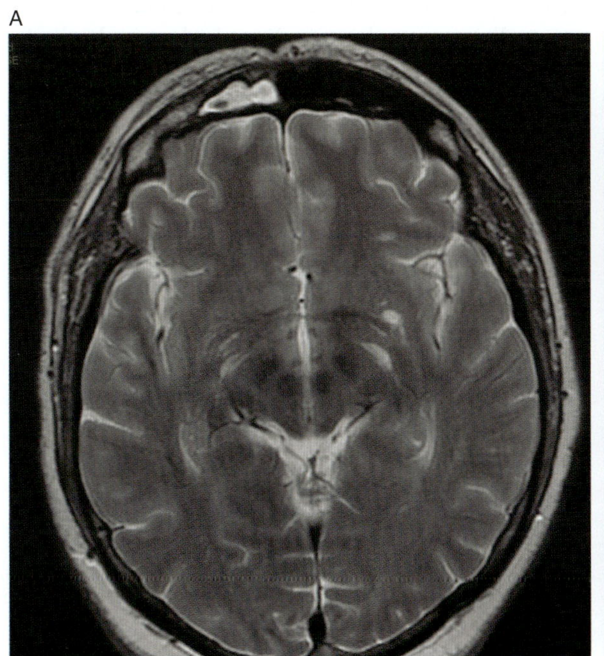

B

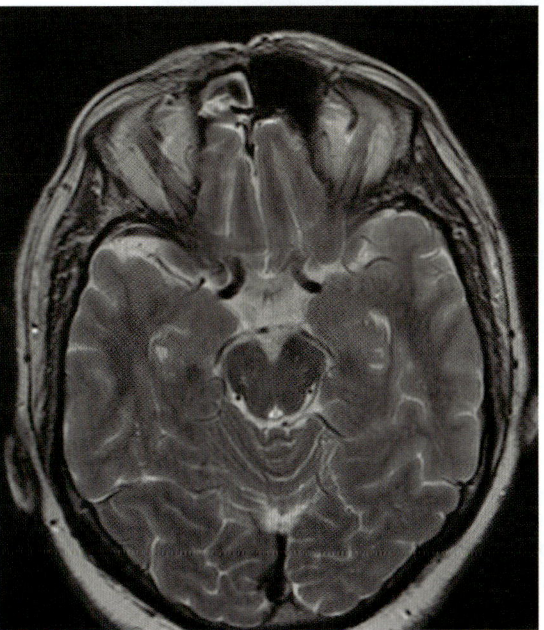

Figure 27.3. Improvements in MRI after initiation of treatment.

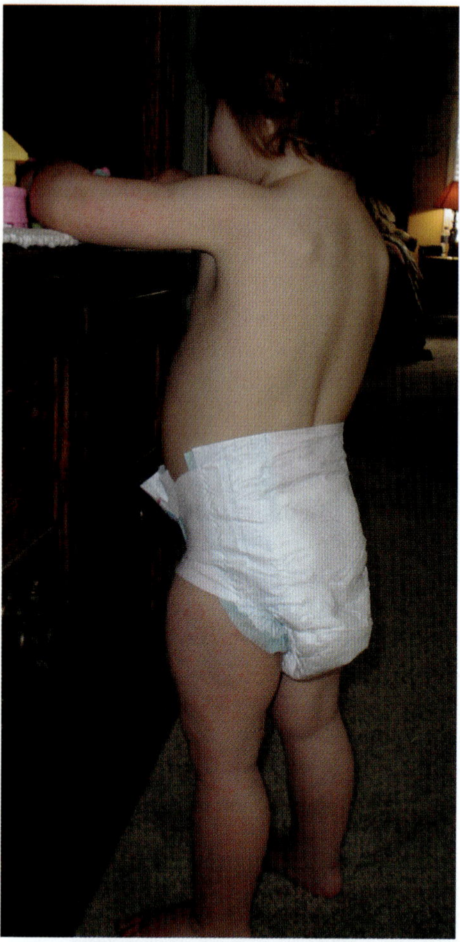

Figure 27.4. Roseola rash. This is the most common presentation of HHV6 infection. After a few days of fever, as the temperature reduces the rash begins on the trunk then spreads to the arms, legs and neck. (From: https://en.wikipedia.org/wiki/File:Roseola_on_a_21-month-old_girl.jpg)

Like the other herpes viruses, reactivation can occur in later life; clinical manifestations include encephalitis, both in the immunocompetent and immunocompromised, although predominantly in the latter.

There is antibody cross-reactivity between HHV6 and the related virus HHV7; in addition, HHV6 antibody titres may rise following primary Cytomegalovirus and EBV infections [6].

HHV6 is the only herpesvirus that is known to be associated with chromosomal integration and this may be found in approximately 1(0.8–1.5)% of the healthy population in the UK and the USA [7,8]. In those with chromosomal integration, viral replication has also been identified in some [9,10]. Therefore, establishing that HHV6 is the cause of encephalitis can be complicated. Definitive proof of active infection would require isolation of virus in tissue culture or identification by fluorescent in-situ hybridisation, but this is not routinely available. Definitive proof of viral chromosomal integration has been demonstrated on sequencing from hair follicles, although again, this is not routinely available. However, some other results can be informative although they require cautious interpretation. Viral species may be useful as HHV6A is an orphan virus and has not been proven to cause human disease; therefore, only HHV6B is thought to be of significance. Viral load may be useful because integrated virus typically results in very high levels detectable by PCR of serum or whole blood, as in this case. Furthermore, in viral integration the viral load will be approximately 50-fold lower in serum than whole blood, also as in this case. Sequential testing for HHV6 by PCR is required to detect acute infection, as peak viral loads are very brief in primary infection. In contrast, in chromosomal integration the PCR titre remains persistently high. Nevertheless, these high levels can mask any HHV6 DNA due to active infection. If active infection is established, ganciclovir is recommended. Some case reports describe reduction in the CSF viral load in active infection, and this is typically > 10-fold after about 2 weeks of therapy.

In the patient described here, treatment had been started by the time the results of the blood PCR, indicating chromosomal integration, had come back. As this may have masked encephalitis caused by HHV6, the treatment course was completed.

Key Points

- HHV6 commonly causes a febrile illness with rash in children known as exanthema subitum, roseola or 6th disease; it is also responsible for many cases of febrile seizures.
- HHV6 encephalitis can occur in both the immunocompromised and the immunocompetent, although predominantly in the former, either during primary infection or as a result of reactivation or reinfection.
- Asymptomatic chromosomal integration of HHV6 occurs, and can thus give misleading positive viral detection by PCR.
- It is important to differentiate between active HHV6 infection and chromosomal integration in order to prevent unnecessary exposure to potentially toxic antiviral drugs.

Table 27.1 The six exanthemas as historically recognised and the associated pathogen now thought responsible.

Name	Number	Virus
Rubeola (measles)	First disease	Measles virus
Scarlet fever	Second disease	*Streptococcus pyogenes*
Rubella (German measles)	Third disease	Rubella virus
*	Fourth disease	*Staphylococcus aureus*
Erythema infectiosum	Fifth disease	Parvovirus B19
Roseola infantum	Sixth disease	HHV6 and HHV7

* There is controversy around whether a separate 'fourth disease' really existed; experts now think it was staphylococcal skin infection, also known as scalded skin syndrome.

Looking Back

HHV6 was discovered in 1986 when Dharam Ablashi, Syed Zaki Salahuddin and Robert Gallo cultivated peripheral blood mononuclear cells from patients with advanced HIV infection and lymphoproliferative disorders. It was formerly called human B-lymphotrophic virus (HBLV).

Did You Know?

Historically, six exanthemas (or cutaneous eruptions) caused by infections have been recognised, some for centuries [11]. Initially they had rather evocative names, numbers were allocated in the early twentieth century, and associated pathogens identified subsequently (**Table 27.1**).

References

1. Ishiyama K, Katagiri T, Hoshino T, et al. Pre-emptive therapy of human herpesvirus-6 encephalitis with foscarnet sodium for high-risk patients after haematopoietic SCT. Bone Marrow Transplant 2011;**46**:863–9.
2. Ward KN. Human herpesviruses-6 and -7 infections. Curr Opin Infect Dis 2005;**18**:247–52.
3. Kleinschmidt-DeMasters BK, Gilden DH. The expanding spectrum of herpes virus infections of the nervous system. Brain Pathol 2001;**11**:440–51.
4. Luppi M, Barozzi P, Morris C, et al. Human Herpesvirus 6 latently infects early bone marrow progenitors in vivo. J Virol 1999;**73**:754–9.
5. Ward KN. The natural history and laboratory diagnosis of human herpesviruses-6 and -7 infections in the immunocompetent. J Clin Virol 2005;**32**:183–93.
6. Ward KN, Gray JJ, Fotheringham M, Sheldon MJ. IgG antibodies to human herpesvirus-6 in young children: changes in avidity of antibody correlate with time after infection. J Med Virol 1993;**39**: 131–8.
7. Hall CB, Caserta MT, Schnabel KC, et al. Congenital infections with human herpes virus 6 (HHV6) and human herpesvirus 7 (HHV7). J Pediatr 2004;**145**: 472–7.
8. Clark DA, Nacheva EP, Leong HN, et al. Transmission of integrated human herpesvirus 6 through stem cell transplantation: implications for laboratory diagnosis. J Infect Dis 2006;**193**:912–16.
9. Arbuckle JH, Medveczky MM, Luka J, et al. The latent human herpesvirus-6A genome specifically integrates in telomeres of human chromosomes in vivo and in vitro. Proc Natl Acad Sci USA 2010;**107**:5563–8.
10. Ward KN, Leong HN, Nacheva EP, et al. Human herpesvirus 6 chromosomal integration in immunocompetent patients results in high levels of viral DNA in blood, sera and hair follicles. J Clin Microbiol 2006;**44**:1571–4.
11. Bialecki C, Feder HM Jr, Grant-Kels JM. The six classic childhood exanthems: a review and update. J Am Acad Derm 1989;**21**:891–903.

CASE 28

Sutton's Law

Sylviane Defres

History

A 72-year-old right-handed woman was transferred by emergency back to the UK from her holiday in Italy. In Italy, while enjoying a coffee and reading the newspaper, she was described as becoming angry and annoyed, she quickly then became vacant and unresponsive and proceeded to develop tonic then clonic movements of her limbs with blood visible in her mouth. At this time she was admitted to the local hospital in Italy.

She had been suffering with headaches, particularly early in the morning, for about 3 months prior to admission. She also had a vague history of tiredness during this period and had noticed unintentional weight loss over this time. There was no history of fever or sweats.

Her only significant past medical history included an episode of transient lymphadenopathy and parotid swelling about 6 years prior for which a fine-needle aspirate was non-diagnostic and a biopsy was not performed.

Examination

General examination including cardiovascular, respiratory, gastrointestinal systems was normal and she was apyrexial, although she looked underweight.

Neurological examination revealed she was unsteady on her feet, although Romberg's test was negative and she had no cerebellar signs. She had a degree of dysphasia, which was predominantly receptive.

Initial Differential Diagnosis

This was an acute presentation of a seizure (complex partial progressing to a secondary generalized), on top of a 3-month history of headaches, tiredness and weight loss, in an elderly lady. A neoplasm was at the top of the differential, although other space-occupying causes of seizure should be considered. There is no history of fever, but fever may not be apparent in some chronic infections, such as tuberculosis or cerebral abscesses; the lymphadenopathy 6 years earlier could have suggested some chronic indolent process, such as lymphoma. Cerebrovascular disease is another common cause of a first seizure in the elderly, although this would not explain the weight loss.

Results of Initial Investigations

Routine blood tests were normal.

A computer tomography (CT) head scan was performed on admission to the UK hospital (**Figure 28.1**).

Four days later a magnetic resonance imaging (MRI) head scan was performed (**Figure 28.2**).

Refined Differential Diagnosis

With the multiple lesions seen on imaging, cerebral metastases were felt to be most likely. However, the differential included:

- tuberculomas
- lymphoma
- cerebral toxoplasma
- abscesses
- cryptococcomas

Results of Definitive Investigations

A biopsy was performed for both diagnosis and to reduce the mass-effect of the largest lesion (**Figure 28.3**).

On account of these findings, serological tests were requested for *Toxoplasma gondii*, and HIV, both of which were positive.

Diagnosis

Cerebral toxoplasmosis secondary to HIV infection.

Management and Outcome

The toxoplasma serology was negative for IgM and positive for IgG antibody, indicating this was not an acute toxoplasma infection, but that she had been infected previously. To further assess her HIV disease, she had an HIV viral load test which was 25,000 copies/ml and a CD4 count which was 10 cells/μl, indicating profound immunocompromise. She also had investigations for any other possible opportunistic infections or risks thereof; these included: hepatitis screen, Epstein–Barr virus (EBV), cytomegalovirus (CMV) and cryptococcal antigen testing.

Treatment was started for cerebral toxoplasmosis with sulphadiazine, pyrimethamine and folinic acid. In addition she was given corticosteroids to reduce the cerebral oedema, and an anticonvulsant drug.

Figure 28.1. CT head scan of a 72-year-old lady presenting with a complex–partial seizure.

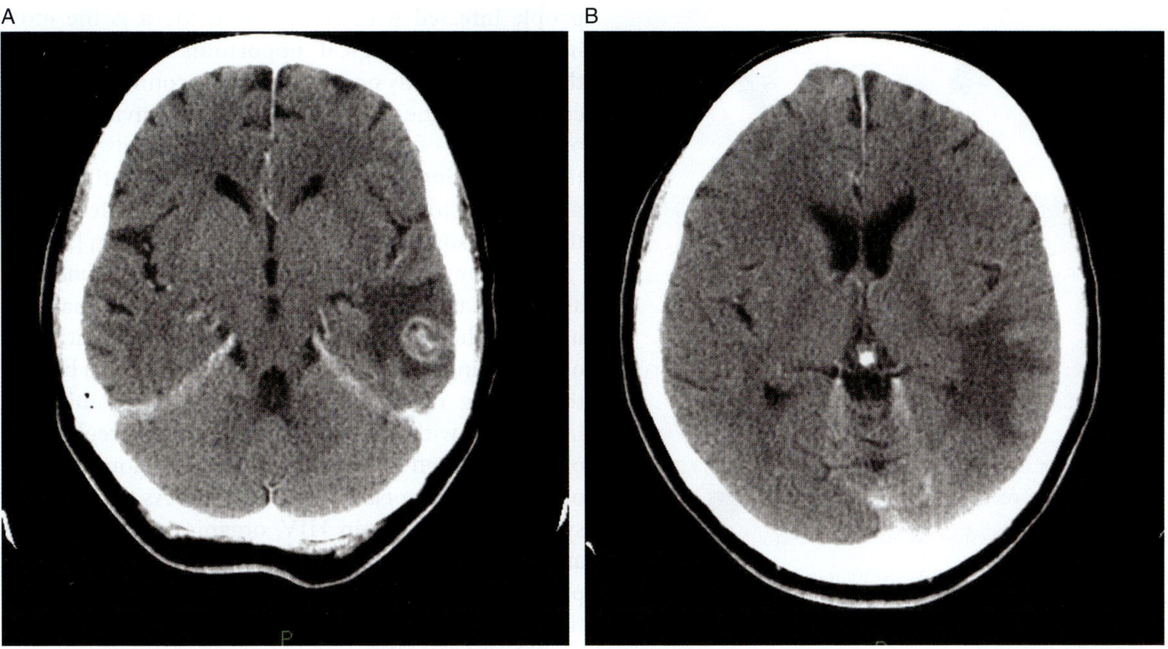

This shows a left temporal space-occupying lesion with surrounding oedema and a small left superficial lesion.

Figure 28.2. MRI head scan (coronal and axial images) in the same patient.

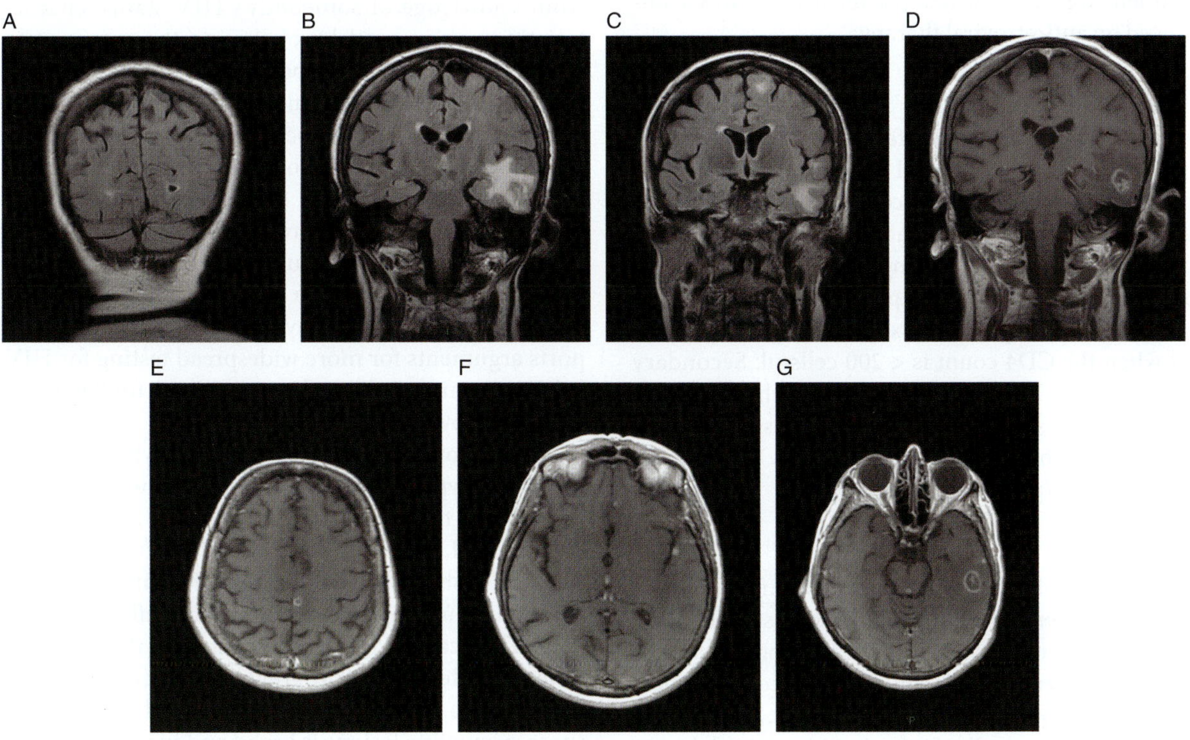

This shows a number of discrete lesions throughout both hemispheres, which were initially missed on CT.

Figure 28.3. Neurohistopathology from the largest of these lesions from a biopsy and stained with haematoxylin and eosin.

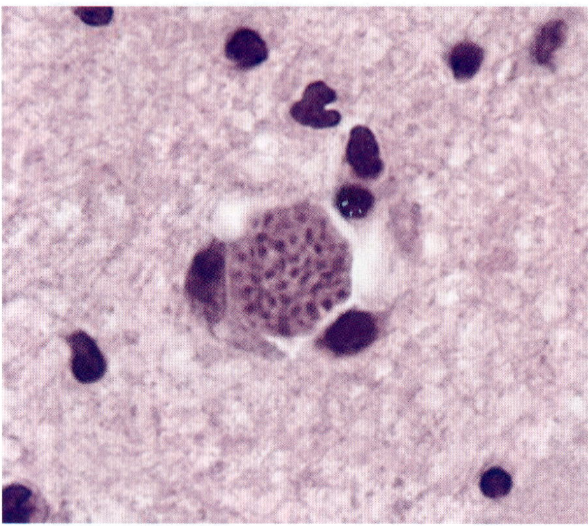

This shows necrotising abscesses, with multiple Toxoplasma cysts containing bradyzoites and tachyzoites, and free organisms.

Clinically, she improved gradually, and a repeat MRI scan 3 weeks later showed an improvement in the oedema of the left temporal lobe. About 4 weeks into treatment for cerebral toxoplasmosis, she was commenced on antiretroviral therapy.

Prevention

Prevention of toxoplasma infection for those who are IgG-negative (when screened for in immunocompromised individuals) includes counselling about avoiding eating undercooked meat and about the risks of infection from cats, e.g. using gloves when cleaning out cat litter. In HIV, primary prophylaxis against toxoplasma should be given if toxoplasma IgG is positive and when the CD4 count is < 200 cells/μl. Secondary prophylaxis in HIV is given to those who have had central nervous system (CNS) toxoplasma disease. Maintenance should continue until the CD4 count is above 200 cells/μl for 6 months [1].

Discussion

Cerebral toxoplasmosis is caused by infection with *Toxoplasma gondii*, an intracellular parasite acquired from ingestion of oocysts from the environment (contaminated water or food, soil or cat faeces) or ingestion of tissue cysts in undercooked meat. Acquisition can also occur vertically if infection is acquired during pregnancy (**Figure 28.4**).

Cerebral toxoplasmosis is most often found in people infected with HIV; worldwide it is the most important neurological opportunistic infection in this group, usually occurring at CD4 counts below 200 cells/μl, with the greatest risk at <50. Individuals with other causes of immunosuppression are also susceptible, including those receiving steroids, anti-tumour necrosis factor therapies, transplant recipients and those with some haematological malignancies [2,3].

Primary infection with *Toxoplasma gondii* is asymptomatic in about 80% of cases, the remainder having a flu-like illness. Very rarely encephalitis can occur during the primary infection, which can be life-threatening in those with immunocompromise. In individuals with an intact immune system, replication of the pathogen is controlled and no serious damage occurs from *Toxoplasma gondii* cysts. As the immune system deteriorates in HIV, organisms can replicate and invade the surrounding tissue. Thus, CNS toxoplasmosis is usually due to reactivation of latent infection resulting in cerebral abscesses, although diffuse encephalitis can also occur [4,5].

Definitive diagnosis of cerebral toxoplasmosis can only be achieved by brain biopsy; however, this can usually be avoided because the diagnosis is likely from knowledge of somebody's HIV status, characteristic imaging, and by observing the response to presumptive treatment; positive toxoplasma serology status may be helpful, though it is positive in many individuals, and occasionally is negative in someone with HIV and toxoplasma through severe immunosuppression.

The case described here was unusual in that the patient's positive HIV status was unexpected because of her age. However, it is a reminder that a diagnosis of HIV can be made in any one, of any age, and supports arguments for more widespread testing for HIV [6]. It is certainly indicated in people with undiagnosed space-occupying lesions [7].

Brain biopsy should be considered where the history is not typical, for solitary lesions or when there is no response to presumptive therapy after 2 weeks.

On MRI, toxoplasmosis usually causes multiple solid or cystic spherical lesions with ring enhancement, surrounding oedema and mass effect, as seen here. They can be located anywhere in the CNS but have a predilection for the grey/white interface and the basal ganglia. In patients with AIDS, the differential for space-occupying lesions is broad and includes cryptococcosis, histoplasmosis, aspergillosis, tuberculosis

Table 28.1 Intracranial space occupying infections and neurological HIV disease.

		Toxoplasmosis	Lymphoma	Progressive multifocal leukoencephalopathy	Tuberculoma	HIV-associated dementia
Clinical features		Subacute onset 2-8 weeks, with confusion, focal neurology, seizures in 15%	Gradual onset (weeks-months) cognitive decline, hemiparesis, hemianopia, dysphasia, ataxia; seizures rare, systemically well	Subacute presentation +/- meningitis, or cognitive impairment with or without focal signs, and seizures	Chronic onset of dementia, often with sphincter disturbance, may have associated and movement disorders	
Imaging	SOL location	SOLs occur at cortical interface of grey and white matter, and basal ganglia	Anywhere, but esp periventricular	White matter lesions, extending up to edge, esp parieto-occipital, and frontal lobes. If contrast enhancement - good prognostic signs	Small multiple, associated with meningeal enhancement (tuberculomas); or larger (Tb abscess)	No SOL, but may have diffuse high signal white matter change, with no enhancement. Usually just atrophy
	Number	Multiple - usually	Single or few	Diffuse changes	Single or several	None
	Oedema	Marked oedema	Moderate oedema	Usually not	Marked	None
	Enhancement?	Ring enhancing lesions	Homogeneous enhancement	Usually not	Ring enhancing	None
Ancillary Investigations		CSF EBV PCR pos; PET scan pos	CSF JC PCR positive	CSF acid fast bacillus and culture; CXR; Tuberculin; Gamma interferon test*	HIV viral load in CSF? Diagnosis of exclusion of other causes	
Treatment		Toxoplasma treatment	Radiotherapy / Palliation	Antiretroviral therapy	Quadruple therapy plus steroids	Antiretroviral therapy

CXR: Chest X-ray, EBV: Epstein–Barr Virus, PCR: Polymerase Chain Reaction, SOL: Space Occupying Lesions

(Modified from Solomon T. Intracranial space occupying infections and neurological HIV disease In: Donaghy M, ed. Brain's Diseases of the Nervous System. 12th ed. Oxford: Oxford University Press; 2009: 1429-57. By permission of Oxford University Press.)

and CNS lymphoma. The presence of a single lesion favours lymphoma [8]. The presence of multiple lesions, particularly in the locations described, in addition to unrestricted diffusion on diffusion-weighted imaging, and an apparent diffusion coefficient of the core that exceeds that of the white matter favours toxoplasmosis over lymphoma.

Clinicians should liaise with infectious disease physicians regarding management of toxoplasmosis as there are a number of regimens; there can also be difficult decisions around the choice and timing of the introduction of antiretroviral drugs. Moreover, clinicians need to be vigilant for the possibility of the patient having other opportunistic infections or developing an immune reconstitution syndrome once antiretroviral treatment is started [8]. Typically, first-line therapy for toxoplasmosis includes sulphadiazine and pyrmethamine (with folinic acid) [9]. Steroids may be necessary to reduce swelling and in severe cases surgical decompression may be necessary. Anticonvulsants should only be given to those with a history of seizures, not routinely to all patients with cerebral toxoplasmosis.

Prognosis depends on whether immune restoration can be achieved. Residual neurological impairment occurs in around 40% of patients and seizures are common.

Key Points

- An HIV test should be performed in anyone with a space-occupying lesion where the cause is uncertain, whatever their age.
- Toxoplasmosis is the most common cause of multiple mass lesions in advanced HIV, although it can also present with diffuse encephalitis.
- Primary infection with *Toxoplasma gondii* is usually asymptomatic and 30–65% of the world's population has been exposed through contaminated water or undercooked meat.
- The differential diagnosis of cerebral toxoplasmosis on neuroimaging includes primary CNS lymphoma and tuberculosis. In most situations presumptive treatment for toxoplasmosis should be given and response to treatment observed.
- Following successful treatment, prophylactic anti-toxoplasma therapy should be continued until immune function has been restored.

Looking Back

In 1908, Nicolle and Manceaux, working at the Pasteur Institute in Tunis, discovered the *Toxoplasma gondii* protozoan in the hamster-like rodent, *Ctendactylus gundi*, which was being used for Leishmania research [10]. They named the organism based on its morphology ('toxo': arc or bow, 'plasma': life) and the name of the host.

Did You Know?

For the parasite's normal reproductive cycle, infected rodents need to be eaten by cats (**Figure 28.4**). Infection with *Toxoplasma gondii* has been shown to alter rodents' behaviour in a way which is favourable to their chance of being eaten. The rodents' natural aversion to cat odours, which is thought to be a protective instinct, is reversed; infected rodents actually show a preference for cat odours (**Figure 28.5**).

Sutton's Law is that one should first consider the most obvious diagnosis; though in this case the most obvious was cerebral metastases! It is named after the American William Sutton, a bank robber for forty years, who is reputed to have responded to the question as to why he robbed banks with the answer 'because that's where the money is.'

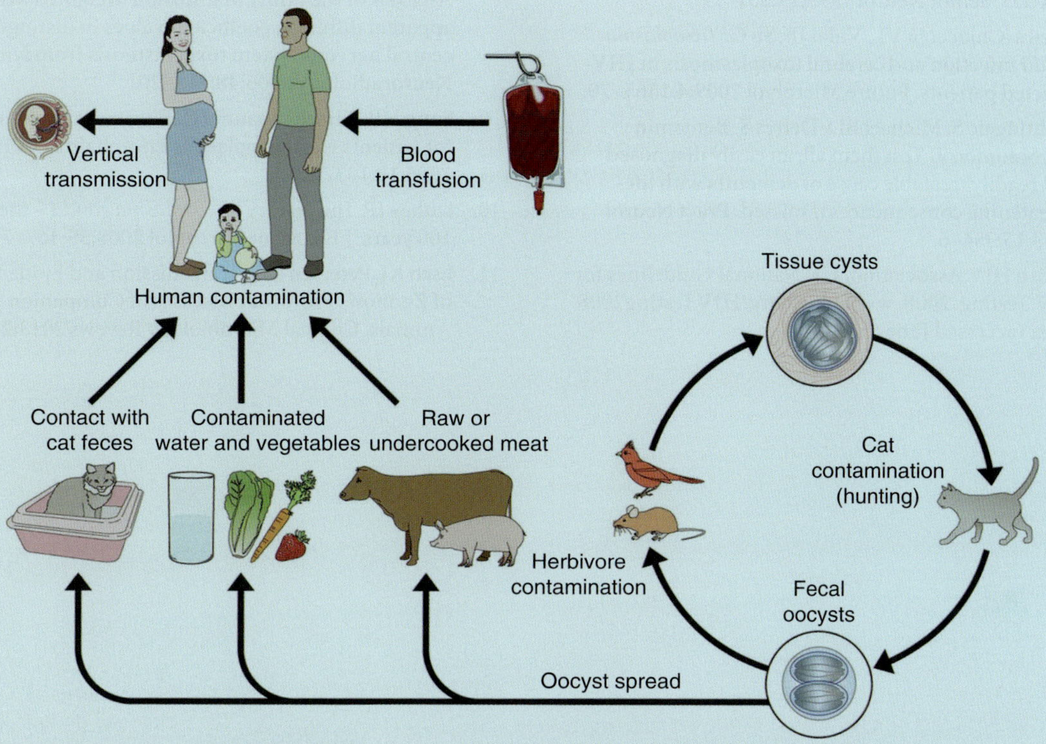

Figure 28.4. *Toxoplasma gondii* life cycle. Domesticated and wild cats are the definitive hosts of *T. gondii* and become infected after the consumption of animals containing infective tissue cysts. Faecal oocysts are shed in large numbers by acutely infected cats for approximately 2 weeks. After shedding, parasite sporulation into infective oocysts takes place in 1–5 days. The ingestion of oocysts by other species leads to the formation of tissue. *T. gondii* rapidly excysts within the intestine, developing into the highly invasive tachyzoite form. Cellular infection results in bradyzoite-containing tissue cysts. (Reproduced from [11] with permission.)

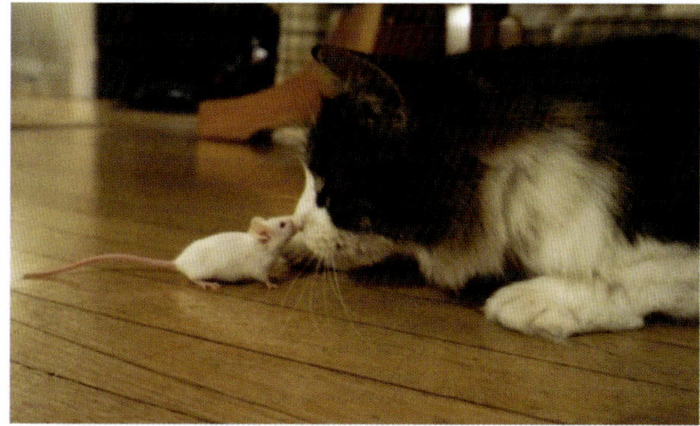

Figure 28.5. Altered behaviour of an infected rodent. (From www.nature.com/news/parasite-makes-mice-lose-fear-of-cats-permanently-1.13777)

References

1. Centers for Disease Control and Prevention, National Institutes of Health, Infectious Diseases Society of America/HIV Medicine Association. Guidelines for Prevention and Treatment of Opportunistic Infections in HIV-infected Adults and Adolescents. MMWR Recomm Rep 2009;**58**:1–207.
2. Mandell JE, Bennett JE, Dolin R, editors. *Toxoplasma gondii*. In: *Mandell, Douglas, and Bennett's Principles and Practice of Infectious Diseases*. 7th ed. Philadelphia, PA: Saunders.
3. Cibickova L, Horacek J, Prasil P, et al. Cerebral toxoplasmosis in an allogeneic peripheral stem cell transplant recipient: case report and review of literature. Transpl Infect Dis 2007;**9**:332–5.

4. Cohen BA. Neurologic manifestations of toxoplasmosis in AIDS. Semin Neurol 1999;**19**:201–11.
5. Pereira-Chioccola VL, Vidal JE, Su C. *Toxoplasma gondii* infection and cerebral toxoplasmosis in HIV-infected patients. Future Microbiol 2009;**4**:1363–79.
6. Nightingale S, Michael BD, Defres S, Benjamin LA, Solomon T. Test them all; an easily diagnosed and readily treatable cause of dementia with life-threatening consequences if missed. Pract Neurol 2013;**13**:354–6.
7. British HIV Association. UK National Guidelines for HIV Testing. 2008. www.bhiva.org/HIVTesting2008.aspx (accessed June 6, 2008).
8. Schroeder PC, Donovan Post MJ, Oschatz E, et al. Analysis of the utility of diffusion-weighted MRI and apparent diffusion coefficient values in distinguishing central nervous system toxoplasmosis from lymphoma. Neuroradiology 2006;**48**:715–20.
9. Fung HB, Kirschenbaum HL. Treatment regimens for patients with toxoplasmic encephalitis. Clin Ther 1996;**18**:1037–56.
10. Dubey JP. The history of *Toxplasma gondii* – the first 100 years. J Eukaryot Microbiol 2008;**55**:467–75.
11. Esch KJ, Petersen CA. Transmission and Epidemiology of Zoonotic Protozoal Diseases of Companion Animals. Clinical Microbiology Revews 2013;**26**:58–85.

CASE **29**

'No Milk For Me, Please'

Michael Grosdenier

History

A 12-day-old girl was brought to her local hospital with pyrexia, laboured breathing, lethargy, irritability, pallor and poor feeding which had developed over a 24-hour period. In the emergency department she had two brief focal seizures. She was born at term via a normal vaginal delivery with growth parameters on the 25th centile. Her mother's pregnancy was uneventful except for a urinary tract infection at 32 weeks which was treated with nitrofurantoin.

On examination, a temperature of 38.9°C was recorded. The baby was pale and slightly mottled. The respiratory rate was 50 breaths per minute and heart rate was 180 per minute. The capillary refill time was 2–3 seconds. The anterior fontanelle was full. Systems examination was otherwise normal. There were no signs of local skin infection. Her umbilical stump and surrounding skin looked healthy.

Initial Differential Diagnosis

- Bacterial meningitis or meningoencephalitis, e.g. herpes simplex virus (HSV) type 2 encephalitis
- Necrotising enterocolitis following bacterial translocation leading to septicaemia
- Septicaemia from another source, e.g. urinary tract infection or pneumonia
- Neonatal disseminated HSV-2 infection
- Other cause of neonatal shock, e.g. cardiac failure

Results of Initial Investigations

Baseline bloods showed a C-reactive protein (CRP) of 21.7 mg/l, a white cell count (WCC) of 11.6 × 10^9/l with neutrophils of 8.1 × 10^9/l. A capillary blood gas showed a very mild respiratory acidosis and a lactate of 2 mmol/l. A computer tomography (CT) brain scan was performed (**Figure 29.1**). A chest X-ray and urine microscopy and culture were normal.

Progress/Further Investigations

The patient was intubated and ventilated for ongoing seizure activity, and leveritacetam given to control seizures. She was given a fluid bolus and was started on cefotaxime and amoxicillin as per the hospital neonatal antibiotic policy, after obtaining the blood cultures. A lumbar puncture (LP) taken 6 hours after admission showed a WCC of 392/mm^3 (73% polymorphs, 12% lymphocytes), red cells of 96/mm^3, cerebrospinal fluid (CSF) glucose of < 0.5 mmol/l (blood glucose at time of the LP was 5.9 mmol/l), CSF protein was 11 g/l. Gram stain examination was negative but antibiotics had been given prior to the LP. Repeat blood tests showed a rise in CRP to 131 within 24 hours and a high WCC of 31.1 × 10^9/l with neutrophilia of 19.9 × 10^9/l.

Results of Definitive Investigations

The results of blood cultures were available within the first 24 hours; group B streptococcus (GBS) was isolated. CSF culture was negative but GBS antigen testing was positive.

Diagnosis

Late-onset group B *streptococcus* (GBS) meningitis and septicaemia.

Figure 29.1. Contrast CT scan of a 12-day-old girl with fever, lethargy and seziures.

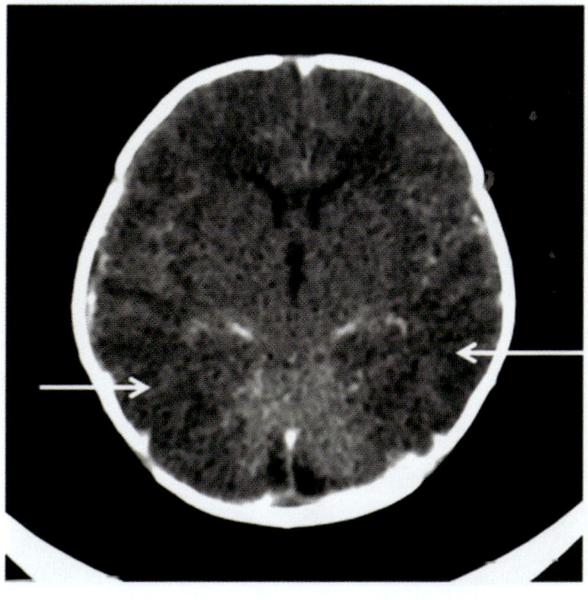

The scan shows low attentuation in the parietal and occipital lobes (arrows). No enhancing lesions are seen.

Management and Outcome

She was extubated after 2 days with no further seizures. A magnetic resonance imaging (MRI) scan 3 days after admission confirmed the CT findings (**Figure 29.2**).

She was an inpatient for 3 weeks to complete a 14-day course of intravenous cefotaxime; amoxicillin was discontinued when the blood and CSF culture results were available. She was discharged on anti-epileptic drugs, and was referred to the physiotherapists for developmental follow-up. When reviewed at 20 weeks of age, she had an enlarging occipitofrontal head circumference, and an outpatient CT scan revealed an obstructive hydrocephalus. She was admitted for ventriculoperitoneal shunt insertion. At this point she had global developmental delay including a delay in visual maturation and an evolving picture of a four-limb cerebral palsy (quadriplegia).

Prevention

Up to 30% of women carry group B streptococcus. Infants acquire the bacteria from their mother's through the birth canal during delivery or in labour because of ascending infection through chorioamnionitis or during premature rupture of the membranes. The best approach to prevention of group B streptococcus disease is debated. In the USA, all pregnant women are screened for carriage and treated if positive, but this approach has not been adopted in other western countries due to the lack of strong evidence [1]. Current UK guidance is available through the Royal College of Obstetricians and Gynaecologists [2]. Intrapartum antibiotic prophylaxis is offered to women with a previous infant with invasive group B streptococcus infection, if the mother is found to have group B streptococcus bacteriuria or a positive vaginal swab in the current pregnancy, or if she is in preterm labour or develops pyrexia (> 38°C) in labour. The recommended antibiotic prophylaxis is intravenous benzylpenicillin (3 g as soon as possible then 1.5 g every 4 hours until delivery). If there is an allergy to penicillin, either a cephalosporin or vancomycin should be used, depending on the severity of the allergy. Since a raised temperature can indicate chorioamnionitis, a broad–spectrum antibiotic, not penicillin G, is recommended in this situation. The antibiotic regimen of choice will depend on local microbiology guidance. Although intrapartum antibiotic prophylaxis shows benefit in reducing the risks of early onset group B streptococcus disease, this is not supported by strong evidence. There is no evidence it reduces late-onset disease [3]. There are no available vaccines against group B streptococcus, although they are in development. Although this is felt to be technically achievable, an obstacle to such a vaccine has been a shifting pattern of the prevalent group B streptococcus serotype as well as legal and regulatory issues [4].

Figure 29.2. T2-weighted MRI axial scan on the same child.

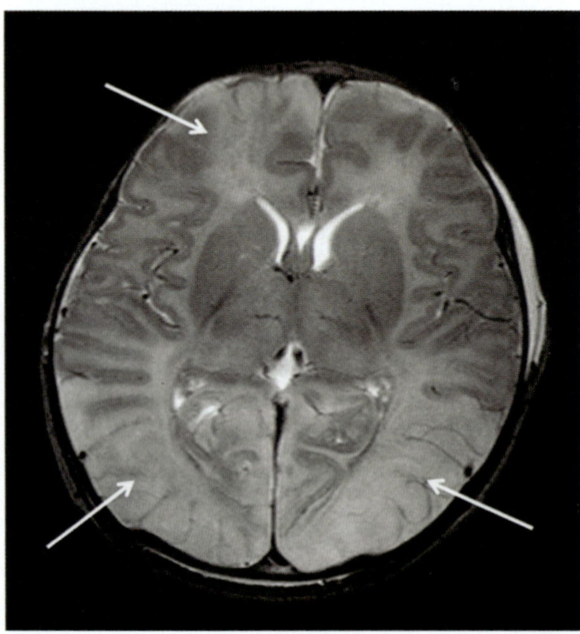

This demonstrates diffuse high signal abnormalities extending into the cortical grey matter of the right frontal, and both parietal and occipital lobes (arrows).

Discussion

Streptococcus agalactiae, more commonly known as group B streptococcus, is a Gram-positive coccus. It is one of the most common culprits for late infection in the neonatal population, along with other coagulase-negative staphylococci, enterobacteriaceae, *Staphylococcus aureus* and fungi [5]. Group B streptococcus is characterised by the presence of Group B Lancefield antigen and its capacity to hydrolyse sodium hippurate, which is the basis for its identification (**Figure 29.3**). Group B streptococcus is the commonest cause of neonatal meningitis in the UK and Ireland. An estimated 20–30% of pregnant women carry the bacteria [4]. The bacteria live in the bowel or vagina and sometimes in the nose and throat. The risk is due to the potential transmission to the newborn infant through the birth canal during delivery, or during labour by ascending infection through chorioamnionitis or premature rupture of the membranes. In neonatal sepsis it is therefore important to consider previous maternal history, the results of high vaginal swabs, any baby's skin swab results, as well as finding out from the hospital infection control team whether there has been any

Purple colour is positive for hippurate hydrolysis

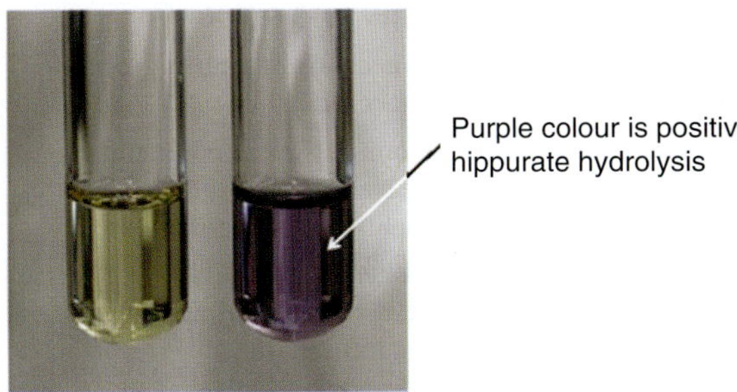

Figure 29.3. The hippurate test detects the amino acid serine cleaved from hippuric acid by hippuricase. A reagent (ninhydrin) is added and a purple discolouration signifies a positive test: presence of hippuricase is presumptive of GBS. (From: www.cdc.gov/groupbstrep/lab/lab-photos.html)

bacterial colonisation of the neonatal unit. The incidence of group B streptococcus infection in the newborns is estimated at around 0.7 per 1000 live births in the UK and Ireland [6], with a worldwide estimate of 0.59 per 1000 live births [7]. Two distinct patterns of infection have been described: early (within the first 6 days of life) and late (7–90 days after birth). The early form accounts for two-thirds of group B streptococcus infections and tends to cause septicaemia, sometimes with pneumonia. Late-onset disease presents principally as meningoencephalitis [6]. Group B streptococcus is a major cause of mortality and morbidity with an overall mortality rate of almost 10% reported in the UK [6]. Comparable case fatality rates have been described in other European countries [8]. Group B streptococcus meningoencephalitis is associated with sequalae in up to 50% of cases, with hearing impairment, developmental delay and cerebral palsy being common [9,10]. Finally, although a reduction of the incidence of early onset group B streptococcus disease has been demonstrated in the USA following the introduction of universal screening and intrapartum intravenous antibiotics prophylaxis, the strategy has not demonstrated a reduction in group B streptococcus-related mortality overall [3].

Key Points

- Up to 30% of women carry group B streptococcus, and their infants are at risk of acquiring the infection from the birth canal during delivery, or shortly before.
- Neonates with group B streptococcus present with septicaemia and sometimes pneumonia within the first week, or with meningoencephalitis between 1 week and 3 months.
- The role of screening for group B streptococcus is controversial. In the USA there is universal screening of pregnant women, and intrapartum intravenous antibiotic prophylaxis for those who are positive, but the evidence in support of this is not conclusive.

Join the national campaign
WHY GUESS?
when you can test
www.gbss.org.uk tel: 01444 416176
Group B Strep Support
www.gbss.org.uk
WORKING TO STOP GBS INFECTION IN BABIES.
Registered Charity number: 1112065

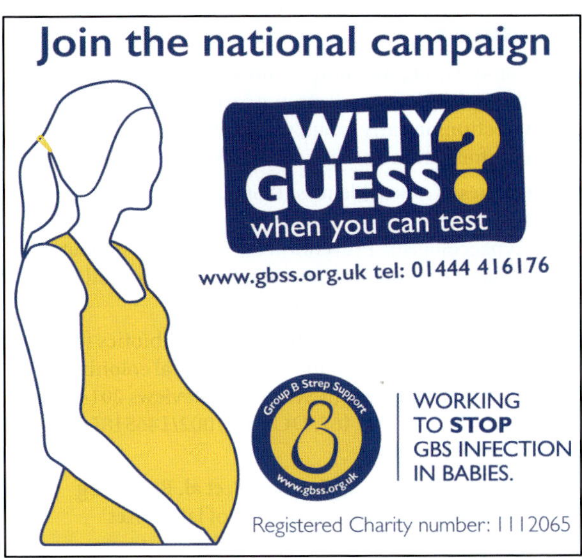

Figure 29.4. A poster for the campaign for all UK women to be offered a test for group B streptococcus carriage in late pregnancy. (Reproduced with kind permission of GBSS.)

Looking Back

Group B streptococcus has been a recognised cause of mastitis in cattle in the post Second World War era. The infection of the cow's udder led to diminished milk production. Hence the name *Streptococcus agalactiae*, as agalactiae means 'no milk'.

Did You Know?

In the UK there is a strong lobby pushing for universal screening for group B streptococcus, although an independent committee in the UK did not recommend it, because it would result in many women receiving unnecessary antibiotics (**Figure 29.4**).

References

1. Colbourn TE, Asseburg C, Bojke L, et al. Preventive strategies for group B streptococcal and other bacterial infections in early infancy: cost effectiveness and value of information analyses. BMJ Res 2007;**335**:655.
2. Hughes RG, Brocklehurst P, Steer PJ, Heath P, Stenson BM on behalf of the Royal College of Obstetricians and Gynaecologists. Prevention of early-onset neonatal group B streptococcal disease. Green-top Guideline No. 36. BJOG 2017; 124:e280–e305.
3. Ohlsson A, Shah VS. Intrapartum antibiotics for known maternal Group B streptococcal colonization. Cochrane Database of Systematic Reviews 2014, Issue 6. Art. No.: CD007467. DOI: 10.1002/14651858. CD007467.pub4.
4. Jordan HT, Farley MM, Craig A, et al. Revisiting the need for vaccine prevention of late-onset neonatal group B streptococcal disease: a multistate, population-based analysis. Pediatr Infect Dis J. 2008 Dec;27(12):1057-64. doi: 10.1097/ INF.0b013e318180b3b9.
5. Ohlsson A, Shah VS. Intrapartum antibiotics for known maternal Group B streptococcal colonization. Cochrane Database Syst Rev 2013;**6**:CD07467.
6. Heath PT, Feldman RG. Vaccination against group B Streptococcus. Exp Rev Vaccines 2005;**4**:207–18.
7. Vergnano S, Menson E, Kennea N, et al. Neonatal infections in England: the NeonIN surveillance network. Arch Dis Child Fetal Neonatal Ed 2011;**96**:F9–14.
8. Heath PT, Balfour G, Weisner AM, et al. Group B streptococcal disease in UK and Irish infants younger than 90 days. Lancet 2004;**363**:292–4.
9. Edmond KM, Kortsalioudaki C, Scott S, et al. Group B streptococcal disease in infants aged younger than 3 months: systematic review and meta-analysis. Lancet 2012;**379**:547–56.
10. Trijbels-Smeulders M, de Jong GA, Pasker-de Jong PCM, et al. Epidemiology of neonatal group B streptococcal disease in the Netherlands before and after introduction of guidelines for prevention. Arch Dis Child Fetal Neonatal Ed 2007;**92**:F271–6.
11. Heath PT. Neonatal meningitis. Arch Dis Child Fetal Neonatal Ed 2003;**88**:F173–8.
12. Doctor BA, Newman N, Minich NM, et al. Clinical outcomes of neonatal meningitis in very low birth weight infants. Clin Pediatr (Phila) 2001;**40**:473–80.

CASE 30

More than Mononucleosis

Karolina Griffiths, Lynsey C. Goodwin and Alastair Miller

History

A 21-year-old university student presented to her local student health centre with left-sided face weakness, blurred vision and diplopia. She was previously fit and well, a non-smoker, with no history of excessive alcohol or illicit drug use, and lived in student halls. She was on no regular medication and had no known allergies. Preceding this she complained of a 3-week history of sore throat, enlarged cervical lymph nodes and a high fever, associated with diarrhoea, vomiting and general malaise. Her general practitioner had treated her presumed tonsillitis with a 3-week course of erythromycin, but no improvement had been seen.

Examination

On examination in the Accident and Emergency department she was afebrile with normal vital signs. She was alert and coherent. No enlarged tonsils were noted and there were no features of meningism. Respiratory, cardiovascular and gastrointestinal examinations were normal and there was no axillary or inguinal lymphadenopathy. In addition there was no evidence of vesicles at the external auditory meatus. On neurological examination she had an obvious lower motor neuron facial weakness on the left. The rest of the cranial nerve examination was unremarkable. There was normal limb power and tone; however, she had upgoing plantars and brisk knee jerk bilaterally; in addition, biceps, supinator and triceps reflexes were brisk in the right arm.

Initial Differential Diagnosis

The differential diagnosis on this admission was that for a new lower motor neuron facial weakness with upper motor neuron signs in the limbs, indicating either a single lesion involving the midbrain or pons or two separate lesions, which could include both peripheral and central nerve involvement. The differential included infections causing a brainstem encephalitis (rhombencephalitis), such as Lyme disease or HIV seroconversion, a post-infectious, or other inflammatory disease, including demyelination or sarcoid.

Results of Initial Investigations

HIV antibody was negative. She underwent a lumbar puncture (LP), which demonstrated an opening pressure of 24 cm H_2O, white cell count (WCC) 9 cells/mm^3 (100% lymphocytes), red cell count (RCC) 20 cells/mm^3, CSF/serum glucose ratio 3, protein 5.8 g/l; polymerase chain reaction (PCR) was negative for varicella zoster virus (VZV), enterovirus and parechovirus, but was positive for herpes simplex virus (HSV).

Epstein–Barr virus (EBV) IgM and IgG were positive, and EBV nuclear antigen (EBNA) testing was negative consistent with an acute primary EBV infection. She also had a positive lupus anticoagulant and anticardiolipin antibody.

Progress and Second Presentation

She was treated with aciclovir and steroids, made a good recovery and was discharged after 6 days.

However, 4 weeks later she was readmitted with ongoing fevers and a fine tremor. The facial weakness had resolved. Initial investigations at that time showed she had a neutropaenia, lymphopaenia, with normal haemoglobin and platelet count, and a raised erythrocyte sedimentation rate (> 120 mm/hour).

While on the ward, she developed episodes of myoclonic jerks in all four limbs with lip smacking. These jerks were more prominent on the right and were not associated with alterations in consciousness. Phenytoin was started, but then quickly discontinued as it caused a maculopapular rash. Therefore, lamotrigine was commenced and the jerking episodes were controlled and did not reoccur.

A repeat LP demonstrated an opening pressure of 27.5 cm H_2O cerebrospinal fluid (CSF), WCC 4 cells/mm^3 (100% lymphocytes), RCC 2 cells/mm^3, glucose 33 mg/l, protein 2.7 g/l; PCR for HSV, VZV and cytomegalovirus (CMV) were negative and acid-fast bacillus stain for tuberculosis was also negative. pANCA, cANCA, anti-GBM, RF, ANA, dsDNA, ENA and anti-CCP were negative. Her ferritin was elevated at 246 ng/ml.

Serology for EBV was consistently positive (positive IgM, IgG, negative EBNA); however, EBV PCR was negative (< 500 copies/ml). A diagnosis of encephalitic illness secondary to EBV infection was made.

Because of the leukopaenia a bone marrow trephine was performed, which showed no evidence of myelo- or lympho-proliferative disorder and no evidence of myelodysplastic syndrome, infection or infiltrative process. However, a marked CD4 immunodeficiency was noted, at 0.085×10^9/l. There was also reduced CD3, CD8, CD19 and natural killer cells.

Further discussion with the family revealed that her mother had been noted since her thirties to have a cellular immunodeficiency, with neutropaenia, low platelets and normal haemoglobin, but this had never been symptomatic and all attempts to find an underlying cause had been unsuccessful.

The patient was commenced on intravenous (IV) aciclovir for 10 days, followed by valaciclovir for 2 weeks. She spent a month in hospital undergoing the above investigations and ensuring the seizures were controlled. She was discharged home.

Further Progress and Third Presentation to Hospital

Seven days later she was admitted for the third time with a severe right lower lobe pneumonia and sepsis. Hepatomegaly was noted on examination. She was pyrexial at 39.3°C, with a heart rate of 112 beats per minute, and a blood pressure of 100/54 mmHg. She had respiratory difficulties and her oxygen saturation was 98% on 35% oxygen. Despite aggressive treatment, she remained hypotensive and her blood pressure dropped further to 60 mmHg systolic. She was therefore transferred to the intensive care unit for inotropic support, intubation and ventilation. EBV PCR was consistently positive, both in blood (log 4.4 copies/ml) and bronchoalveolar lavage fluid (log 3.9 copies/ml). Although she appeared to have chronic EBV infection, the exact disease process was unclear at this time; therefore, empirical treatment was started with aciclovir and broad-spectrum antibiotics. Co-trimoxazole was also given as *Pneumocystis jiroveci* prophylaxis in view of the patient's low CD4 count. Imaging of the patient's brain with computer tomography and magnetic resonance imaging scanning was unremarkable.

The patient developed a reticular rash, raising concern about autoimmune vasculitis. Therefore, a weekly dose of 15 mg/kg cyclophosphamide was started and along with IV methylprednisolone 500 mg daily. She spent 2 days in the intensive care unit, slowly recovered and was transferred back to the infectious diseases ward. Here she continued to receive high doses of steroids and further investigations were performed.

Results of Definitive Investigations

With the diagnosis remaining unclear, a repeat bone marrow examination was performed on her third admission; this demonstrated haemophagocytes, indicating a diagnosis of haemophagocytic lymphohistiocytosis syndrome.

Diagnosis

Chronic active Epstein–Barr Virus (EBV) infection causing haemophagocytic lymphohistiocytosis syndrome and presenting with EBV encephalitis.

Management and Outcome

Her care was taken over by the haematology team, and treatment followed the haemophagocytic lymphohistiocytosis (HLH) protocol, with the patient receiving cyclophosphamide and dexamethasone (but no etoposide). After just one month her EBV PCR was negative. She has continued on this protocol as an outpatient, receiving aciclovir (initially 800 mg twice daily, reduced to 400 mg twice daily) and cyclosporin 75 mg twice daily. In view of the mother's immune abnormality, a geneticist was involved but no genetic abnormality was identified.

Prevention

There is no vaccine available currently for EBV and many people will become infected during their lifetime. While infection often results in minor symptoms or a typically self-limiting syndrome of pharyngitis, adenitis and fever termed 'infectious mononucleosis' or 'glandular fever', EBV can cause serious disease in those with immune compromise. Early establishment of familial risk factors, such as in this case, or risk of HIV are important in the prompt identification of EBV as the cause of an acute neurological syndrome.

Discussion

Haemophagocytic lymphohistiocytosis syndrome is so named because the immune system produces too many lymphocytes and macrophages (histiocytes), and there is phagocytosis of the blood-producing cells in the marrow. Also known as haemophagocytic syndrome, it is a spectrum of both inherited and acquired conditions (**Figure 30.1**) [1,2]. Acquired or 'reactive'

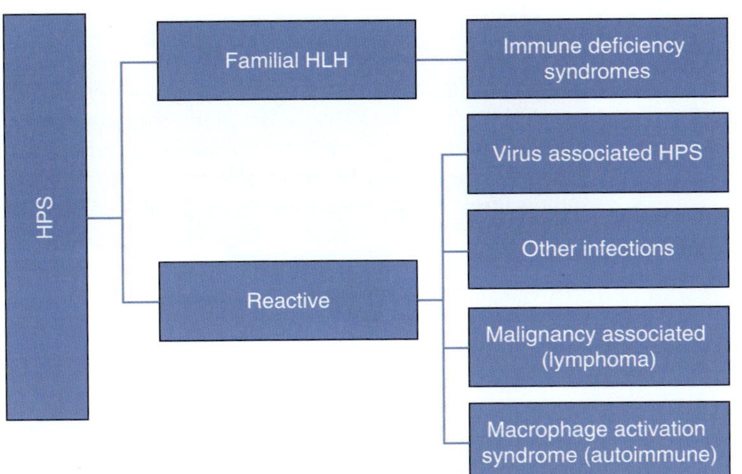

Figure 30.1. Classification of haemophagocytic syndrome. (Modified from [3] with permission of Elsevier.)

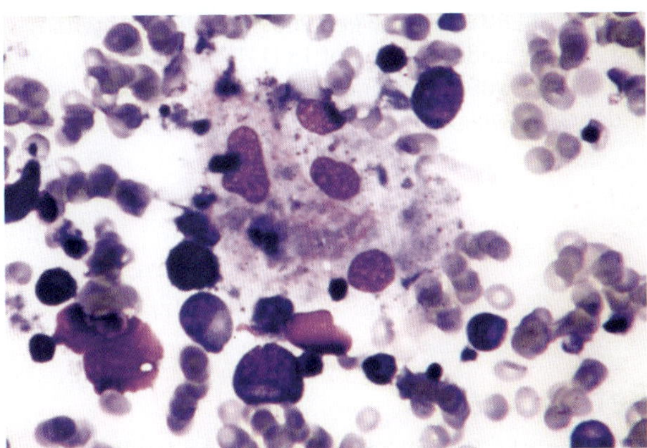

Figure 30.2. Bone marrow aspirate showing phagocytosis of neutrophils, nucleated erythrocyte, and platelets by benign histiocytes (Wright stain, ×400). (Reproduced from [4].)

HLH is associated with infections. The most common virus associated with HLH is EBV, but other causative agents include CMV, HSV, VZV and influenza virus. EBV predominantly affects B cells, but severe disease is associated with other targets in the immune system [1]. During EBV HLH, the virus infects primary CD8+ T cells with a failure to produce sufficient EBV-specific cytotoxic T cells, suggesting a natural killer T-cell dysfunction (**Figure 30.2**). This provokes a macrophage response and a large cytokine storm, proceeding to organ dysfunction, coagulopathy and cytopaenia. It is thought the infected CD8+ cells have a prolonged cytotoxic activity as an EBV protein (BHRF1) can reduce the susceptibility of the cells to apoptosis [1]. Other related conditions include leishmania or malignancy-associated haemophagocytic syndrome. [3]

Most cases occur in immune-competent children and adults; however, EBV HLH cases have been seen in immune deficiencies, both from familial and non-familial cases [3]. Published reports have identified an association between chronic active EBV infection with HLH and two missense mutations in *PRF1* [5]. In this case, the patient's mother reported a cellular immunodeficiency; therefore, potentially EBV had triggered a familial form. However, no genetic abnormalities were identified. The distinctions between familial and reactive forms are increasingly blurred as new genetic defects come to light, and infections can trigger the onset of familial HLH. Diagnosis of HLH is often late, with criteria established by the Histiocyte Society (**Table 30.1**) [6]. An initial bone marrow biopsy may not always demonstrate haemophagocytosis; therefore, this needs to be repeated [3].

EBV viral load provides information on diagnosis, prognosis and efficacy of treatment. EBV HLH has the worst prognosis of all virus-associated HLH [7].

Case reports have based treatment on Histiocyte Society 2004 guidelines, an evidence-base from children with familial HLH [6,8,9]. Concerns have been raised that this regimen is too toxic. Etoposide, a pro-apoptopic agent that acts on lymphocytes, has severe immunosuppressant effects and has been linked to acute myeloid leukaemia. Methylprednisolone has been used instead, with or without immunoglobulins, with mixed results. However, there are indications that etoposide has a crucial role in EBV HLH by inhibiting EBV nuclear antigen in infected cells [10] with small studies demonstrating a survival benefit [7,11]. Reports demonstrate that elevated cytokines differ

Table 30.1 Revised diagnostic guidelines for haemophagocytic lymphohistiocytosis (HLH). (Reproduced from [6] with permission from John Wiley & Sons, Inc.)

The diagnosis of HLH can be established if one of either 1 or 2 below is fulfilled
(1) A molecular diagnosis consistent with HLH
(2) Diagnostic criteria for HLH fulfilled (five out of the eight criteria below)
(A) Initial diagnostic criteria *(to be evaluated in all patients with HLH)*
Fever
Splenomegaly
Cytopaenias (affecting > 2 of 3 lineages in the peripheral blood):
Haemoglobin < 90 g/l (in infants < 4 weeks: haemoglobin < 100 g/l)
Platelets < 100 × 10⁹/l
Neutrophils <1.0 × 10⁹/l
Hypertriglyceridaemia and/or hypofibrinogenaemia:
Fasting triglycerides > 3.0 mmol/l (i.e. > 265 mg/dl)
Fibrinogen < 1.5 g/l
Haemophagocytosis in bone marrow or spleen or lymph nodes
No evidence of malignancy
(B) New diagnostic criteria
Low or absent NK-cell activity (according to local laboratory reference)
Ferritin > 500 pg/l
Soluble CD25 (i.e. soluble IL-2 receptor) > 2400 U/ml

between the different HLH subtypes [12]; further HLH protocol developments should allow for variations in pathogenesis. Potential specific treatment strategies include the use of interleukin-1β blockade, allogeneic stem cell transplant for familial HLH and rituximab as a treatment adjunct for EBV HLH (by quickly clearing infected B cells) [13,14].

Key Points

- EBV can cause a range of neurological and other disorders, particularly in those with immunocompromised.
- If initial investigations fail to identify a cause of immunocompromised it is worth repeating investigations.
- EBV is the most common cause of acquired haemophagocytic lymphohistiocytosis (HLH) syndrome.

Looking Back

Scott and Robb-Smith first reported four patients with a HLH-like picture in 1939, naming the condition 'histiocytic medullary reticulosis' [8]. One of this book's editors (TS) was taught by Robb-Smith in Oxford, who himself was taught there by the great Sir William Osler!

Did You Know?

There is a particularly high incidence of EBV HLH in Asia [15], but it has also been described elsewhere [16]. A national survey in Japan demonstrated 163 cases of EBV HLH between 2001 and 2005, of whom 126 were under the age of 15 [11]. There is a slightly higher frequency in girls than boys with a peak incidence between 1 and 2 years [3].

References

1. Dexter LJ. The pathogenesis of primary, latent and reactivated Epstein–Barr virus infections: an update on clinically relevant interactions between Epstein–Barr virus and the human immune response. Rev Med Microbiol 2011;**22**:48–54.
2. Okano. Acute or chronic life-threatening diseases associated with Epstein–Barr virus infection. Am J Med Sci 2012;**343**:483–9.
3. Rouphael NG, Talati NJ Vaughan C, et al. Infections associated with haemophagocytic syndrome. Lancet Infect Dis 2007;7:814–22.
4. Lee J, Chung I, Shin D, et al. Hemorrhagic fever with renal syndrome presenting with hemophagocytic lymphohistiocytosis. Emerg Infect Dis. 2002;**8**: 209–10.
5. Zhang K, Filipovich AH, Johnson J, Marsh RA, Villanueva J, editors. Hemophagocytic Lymphohistiocytosis, Familial. Seattle, WA: University of Washington; 2006.

6. Henter J, Horne A, Aricó M, et al. HLH-2004: diagnostic and therapeutic guidelines for hemophagocytic lymphohistiocytosis. Pediatr Blood Cancer 2007;**48**:124–31.
7. Imashuku S, Teramura T, Tauchi H, et al. Longitudinal follow-up of patients with Epstein–Barr virus-associated hemophagocytic lymphohistiocytosis. Haematologica 2004;**89**:183–8.
8. Berry PA, Bernal W, Pagliuca A, et al. Multiple organ failure and severe bone marrow dysfunction in two 18 year-old Caucasian patients: Epstein–Barr virus and the haemophagocytic syndrome. Anaesthesia 2008;**63**:1249–54.
9. Torti L, Larocca LM, Massini G, et al. Epstein–Barr Virus (EBV)-associated haemophagocytic syndrome. Mediterr J Hematol Infect Dis 2012;**4**:e201.
10. Imashuku S, Kuriyama K, Teramura T, et al. Requirement for etoposide in the treatment of Epstein–Barr virus-associated hemophagocytic lymphohistiocytosis. J Clin Oncol 2001;**19**:2665–73.
11. Ishii E, Ohga S, Imashuku S, et al. Nationwide survey of hemophagocytic lymphohistiocytosis in Japan. Int J Hematol 2007;**86**:58–65.
12. Canna SW, Behrens EM. Not all hemophagocytes are created equally: appreciating the heterogeneity of the hemophagocytic syndromes. Curr Opin Rheumatol 2012;**24**:113–18.
13. Balamuth NJ, Nichols KE, Paessler M, Teachey DT. Use of rituximab in conjunction with immunosuppressive chemotherapy as a novel therapy for Epstein Barr virus-associated hemophagocytic lymphohistiocytosis. J Pediatr Haem Oncol 2007;**29**:569–73.
14. Darteyre S, Ludwig C, Jeziorski E, Schved J-F, Rodière M. Syndrome d'activation macrophagique et infection à virus d'Epstein–Barr chez l'enfant. Méd Malad Infect 2010; **40**:18–26.
15. Janka G, Imashuku S, Elinder G, Schneider M, Henter JI. Infection- and malignancy-associated hemophagocytic syndromes. Secondary hemophagocytic lymphohistiocytosis. Hematol Oncol Clin North Am 1998;**12**:435–44.
16. Beutel K, Gross-Wieltsch U, Wiesel T, et al. Infection of T lymphocytes in Epstein–Barr virus-associated hemophagocytic lymphohistiocytosis in children of non-Asian origin. Pediatr Blood Cancer 2009;**53**: 184–90.

CASE 31

Return of an Old Foe

Syed Hyder

History

A 49-year-old right-handed man presented with a 5-year history of a progressive weakness and difficulty using his left arm and leg. He noticed his left foot was dragging, and he had fallen twice. He also complained of generalised fatigue but there was no diurnal variation in his weakness, or ptosis. There was dull persistent joint pain in his knees and back. Although there were no sensory symptoms, the patient described his limbs as feeling cold at all times, even in hot weather. He did not complain of any bowel or bladder symptoms. There were no vision, speech, swallowing or breathing problems.

When he was 12 years old he had become severely weak and unwell and had spent 2 weeks in the intensive therapy unit with respiratory support. However, he went on to make a good recovery and after 6 months of intensive physiotherapy and exercise he could walk completely normally.

Examination

On observation he had a scoliosis. There was wasting of the intrinsic hand muscles, and although there was no wasting in the lower limbs, there were occasional fasciculations in the thighs and calves. Power was reduced in the upper and lower limbs to 4– to 4+/5, on the Medical Research Council power grading, in most groups. In addition, dorsiflexion of the left ankle was 3/5, consistent with a left foot drop. Deep tendon reflexes were reduced in both arms and absent in both lower limbs; both planters were down-going. The sensory examination for temperature, pin-prick, vibration and proprioception was normal. Cranial nerves examination, including funduscopy, was normal. There were no dermatological lesions or lymphadenopathy. General cardiovascular, respiratory and abdominal examinations were normal.

Initial Differential Diagnosis

The 5-year history and examination findings were suggestive of a progressive lower motor neuron syndrome, with no apparent upper motor neuron or sensory involvement; this might be seen in:

- Motor neuron disease
- Chronic inflammatory demyelinating polyneuropathy
- Multifocal motor neuropathy
- Inclusion body myositis

The history of severe weakness when aged 12 requiring ventilator support on the intensive therapy unit, followed by months of physiotherapy was suggestive of acute poliomyelitis, which raised the possibility that this current presentation is:

- Post-polio syndrome

Results of Initial Investigations

Initial blood tests showed a normal CK, renal and thyroid function. The patient underwent a lumbar puncture. Routine cerebrospinal fluid (CSF) studies, including white cell count, red cell count, glucose ratio and protein, were normal. A magnetic resonance imaging scan of the whole spine showed degenerative changes at L4 and L5 regions, in the absence of any cord or nerve root compression. Nerve conduction studies were normal.

On further questioning it became apparent that at the time of the illness when he was 12 years old, his mother was told he had suffered with polio. An electromyogram showed no evidence of active denervation. However, there was significant evidence of chronic denervation and reinervation changes, producing giant units, consistent with previous poliomyelitis.

Diagnosis

Post-polio syndrome (post-poliomyelitis progressive muscular atrophy).

Management and Outcome

Over the next few years he was treated with supportive care through a multi-disciplinary team approach, which included physiotherapy, occupational therapy, social work and input from the orthotist, who made a foot splint and other devices. Under supervision of the physiotherapist he had a graded exercise programme. This was aimed at retaining muscle mass, strength and function and alleviating symptoms without causing excessive fatigue and damaging muscles and joints. He slowly became progressively weaker and needed more input. His home was adapted with ramps and rails, and ultimately he needed a wheelchair.

Prevention

Poliomyelitis is prevented by vaccination with the inactivated vaccine or the live attenuated vaccine. There are no known ways of preventing post-poliomyelitis syndrome in someone who has had poliomyelitis.

Discussion

A range of neurological problems can occur many years after poliomyelitis; these include increasing scoliosis and associated compression of the nerve roots, compression related to the use of orthotic devices, and symptoms related to joint instability and weight gain. However, a specific neurological syndrome of post-poliomyelitis progressive muscular atrophy was recognized from the 1970s onwards [1–3]. The diagnostic criteria for post-poliomyelitis progressive muscular atrophy, or post-polio syndrome, require a credible history of acute poliomyelitis; partial recovery of function afterwards with a minimum 15-year period of stabilisation, which is followed by new weakness or abnormal muscle fatigue, decreased endurance, muscle atrophy or generalised fatigue. The diagnosis requires exclusion of medical, orthopaedic and neurologic conditions that may be causing the symptoms.

Post-polio syndrome develops in approximately 20–30% of polio survivors; there are thought to be around 250,000 patients with post-polio syndrome in Europe and an estimated 20 million worldwide. The syndrome develops with a peak incidence 20–35 years after the initial attack; the interval is shorter if the initial attack was more severe.

Risk factors for developing post-polio syndrome include being more than 10 years old when struck by the initial attack of acute poliomyelitis; severe limb, bulbar or respiratory involvement during the acute illness; incomplete recovery after that illness, with residual disability and paralytic involvement in all four limbs; recent weight gain; and muscle pain associated with exercise.

The pathogenesis of post-polio syndrome is uncertain. In acute poliomyelitis, polio virus destroys lower motor neurons in the anterior horns of the spinal cord [4,5]. The surviving lower motor neurons send out sprouts to denervated muscle fibres, thus forming giant motor units. In some patients the persistence of viral RNA and presence of inflammatory cytokines in the CSF suggests chronic infection and inflammation may be important. Electromyographic findings show large motor units with ongoing chronic denervation and jitter on single fibre studies, as seen in this case. This has led to the suggestion that the deterioration is a result of the physiological attrition of the large unstable motor units [6,7].

Key Points

- Post-polio syndrome is not uncommon in survivors of acute poliomyelitis, occurring decades afterwards. There is no specific treatment for this progressive muscular atrophy.

Looking Back

The earliest record of a withered shortened leg with the characteristic appearance of poliomyelitis is an Egyptian stele of the eighteenth dynasty (approximately 1580–1350 BC) (**Figure 31.1**).

In 1908, Landsteiner and Popper demonstrated the transmissible nature of polio by injecting spinal cord homogenates from a patient who died of poliomyelitis into non-human primates.

Did You Know?

The name poliomyelitis is derived from the Greek 'polio' meaning grey and 'myelos' meaning marrow, thus referring to the grey matter in the anterior horn of the spinal cord, the suffix '–itis' meaning inflammation.

Culture of the virus (**Figure 31.2**) in 1949, for which Enders, Weller and Robbins received a Nobel Prize, led to the development of the inactivated vaccine by Salk and the live attenuated vaccine by Sabin. Their work, which saved millions of lives, was never recognised by the Nobel Committee.

Attempts to eradicate poliomyelitis by the year 2000 did not quite succeed, largely because of difficulties in areas of conflict. At the 2012 UN General Assembly world leaders renewed their commitment to eradicate the disease.

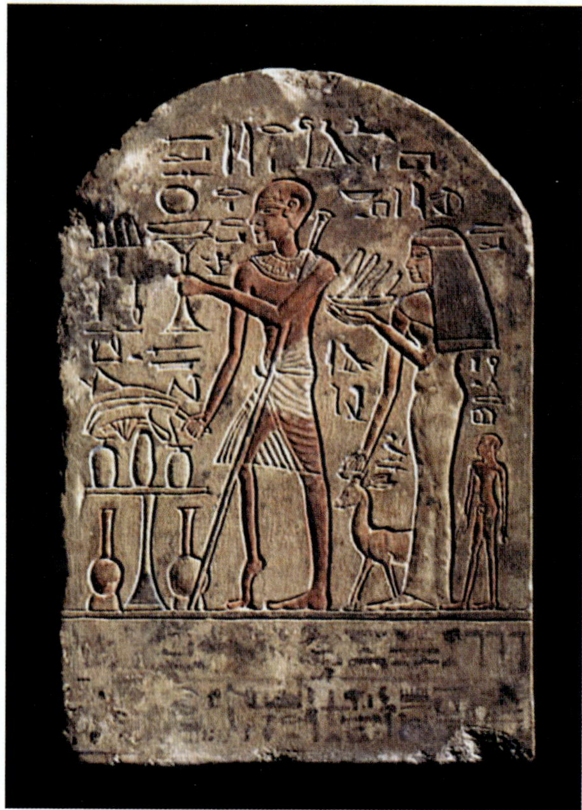

Figure 31.1. An Egyptian stele thought to represent a Polio victim. Eighteenth dynasty (approximately 1580–1350 BC). (From: http://en.wikipedia.org/wiki/File:Polio_Egyptian_Stele.jpg)

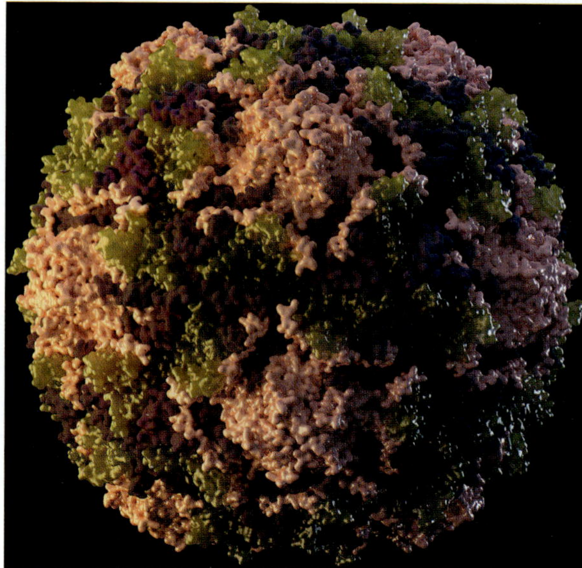

Figure 31.2. A 3D representation of a single poliovirus virion. It was reconstructed by Centers for Disease Control and Prevention, USA medical illustrators, and is based on electron micrographic data.

References

1. Howard RS. Clinical review poliomyelitis and post-polio syndrome BMJ 2005;**330**:1314–16.
2. Kidd D, Howard RS, Williams AJ, et al. Late functional deterioration following paralytic poliomyelitis. Q J Med 1997;**90**:189–96.
3. Howard RS. Late post-polio functional deterioration. Pract Neurol 2003;**3**:66–77.
4. Windeback AJ, Lichty WJ, Dube JR. Prospective cohort study of polio survivors in Olmstead county, Minnesota in the post-polio syndrome: advances in the pathogenesis and treatment Ann N Y Acad Sci 1995;**753**:81–6.
5. Mulder DM. Post-polio syndrome – past, present and future. In: Munsat TL, editor, *Post-polio Syndrome – Past, Present and future*. Boston, MA: Butterworth Heinemann; 1991: 1–8.
6. Carrington-Gowne A, Halstead LS. Post-polio syndrome pathophysiology and clinical management, clinical reviews in physical and rehabilitation medicine 1995;7:147–88
7. Dalakas MC, Sever JL, Madden DL, et al. Late postpoliomyelitis muscular atrophy: clinical, virologic, and immunologic studies. Rev Infect Dis 1984; Suppl 2:S562–7.

CASE 32

The Lethal Masquerader

Anand Iyer

History

A previously healthy, completely immunised, developmentally normal 12-month-old girl presented to the emergency department in the UK with features of severe rapidly progressive fever, purpuric rash and shock, consistent with meningococcal sepsis. She required extensive resuscitation, intravenous (IV) cefotaxime, and multi-organ support in the paediatric intensive care unit. She had no clinical evidence of meningism and did not have a lumbar puncture during the admission. *Neisseria meningitidis* group B was isolated from culture of her admission blood samples. She showed signs of improvement in the next 4 days and was extubated and transferred to the ward. Treatment with IV cefotaxime was continued for 10 days.

On day 11 after presentation her clinical condition deteriorated suddenly with high-grade intermittent fever, irritability, the development of a fine maculopapular rash all over her trunk and frequent focal seizures.

Examination

She was encephalopathic with a Glasgow coma score of 9/15. She had a generalised maculopapular rash and hepatosplenomegaly. She had a prolonged central capillary refill time of 4 seconds, tachycardia, hypotension and was febrile at 38.5°C. There were no signs of meningism or focal neurological impairment. No focus of infection was detected, but she was treated clinically as having sepsis and given antibiotics and fluid resuscitation. She required readmission to the intensive care unit for inotropic support.

Initial Differential Diagnosis of Acute Encephalopathy Following Recent Sepsis

- Cerebral venous sinus thrombosis, potentially with secondary venous infarction
- Acute ischaemic stroke secondary to cerebral vasculitis of the cerebral vasculature, secondary to possible meningitis
- Deranged electrolytes (hyponatremia)
- Infective space-occupying lesion
  - Subdural empyema
  - Brain abscess from infective emboli
- Metabolic disorder with decompensation precipitated by infection, e.g. mitochondrial encephalopathy
- Haemophagocytic lymphohistiocytosis (HLH)

Investigations

Initial investigations revealed normal renal function and electrolytes, low platelets 80 × 10^9/l, mildly elevated C-reactive protein 20 mg/l. Analysis of cerebrospinal fluid (CSF) revealed a white cell count of 120/mm^3 (predominantly lymphocytes), protein 0.56 g/l, glucose 3.2 mmol/l (serum glucose 5 mmol/l; ratio 0.64). CSF and blood culture were negative and a CSF polymerase chain reaction viral screen was negative. A computer tomography (CT) brain and venogram were normal.

Further biochemical investigations revealed a markedly elevated ferritin of 2010 μg/l, triglyceride of 6 mmol/l and fibrinogen of 1.2 g/l. A magnetic resonance imaging (MRI) brain scan was performed (**Figure 32.1**), as was bone marrow aspiration (**Figure 32.2**).

Diagnosis

Haemophagocytic lymphohistiocytosis secondary to primary meningococcal sepsis.

Progress and Further Management

HLH was treated with methylprednisolone, etoposide and cyclosporine. The child made a slow and steady improvement and required several weeks of neurological rehabilitation. She was scheduled for haematopoietic stem cell transplantation. She continued to remain developmentally delayed for age; however, she had made considerable progress. Investigations for a primary immunodeficiency disorder and molecular genetic testing for familial HLH have been negative.

Discussion

Haemophagocytic lymphohistiocytosis (HLH, also known as haemophagocytic syndrome) is one of the large number of reactive and neoplastic histiocytic

Figure 32.1. An axial T2-weighted MRI scan in a 12-month-old who presented with clinical features consistent with meningococcal septicaemia and then developed a rapidly deteriorating coma score despite antibiotic treatment (MRI performed 3 weeks after the initial presentation).

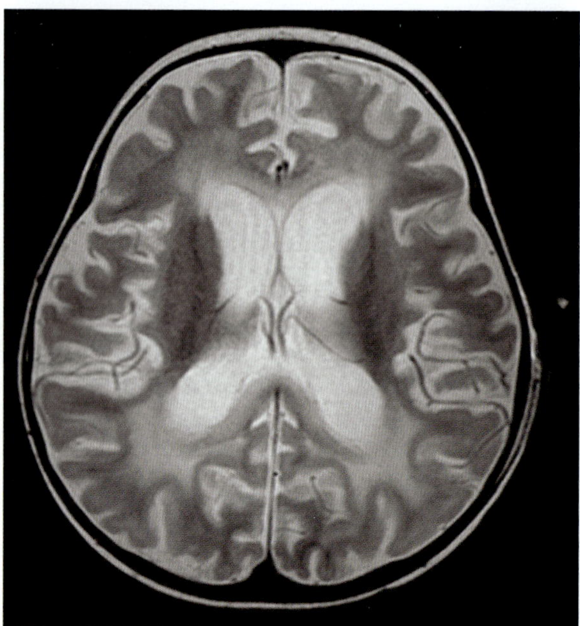

This shows generalised cerebral atrophy with symmetrical diffuse high signal in the periventricular white matter.

Figure 32.2. Bone marrow aspirate from the same child.

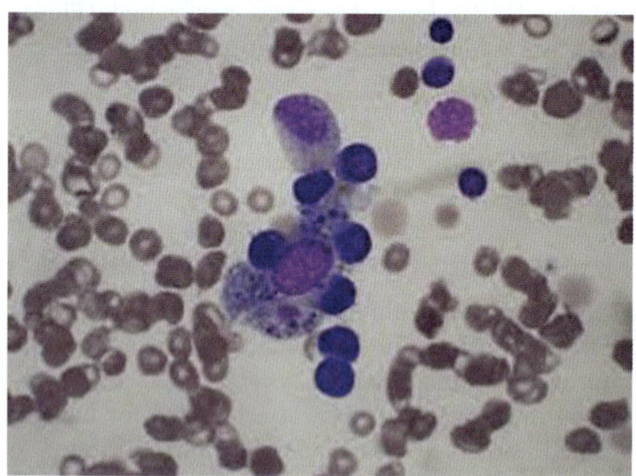

This shows evidence of haemophagocytosis, consistent with haemophagocytic lymphohistiocytosis.

disorders in which there is proliferation of 'histiocytes', i.e. cells from the monocyte/macrophage or Langerhans/dendritic cell lineages [1]. These include reactive macrophage storage diseases, like Gaucher's disease, malignant diseases like acute monocytic leukaemia, and reactive Langerhans cell diseases.

Table 32.1 Diagnostic criteria for haemophagocytic lymphohistiocytosis (2004, reproduced with permission of John Wiley & Sons, Inc. from [2]).

The diagnosis of HLH can be established if one of either 1 or 2 below is fulfilled:
1. A molecular diagnosis consistent with HLH is made.
2. Diagnostic criteria for HLH are fulfilled (5 of the 8 criteria below):*
Fever
Splenomegaly
Cytopaenias (affecting ≥ 2–3 lineages in the peripheral blood):
Haemoglobin < 90 g/l (haemoglobin < 100 g/l in infants < 4 weeks),
Platelets < 100×10^9/l,
Neutrophils < 1.0×10^9/l
Hypertriglyceridaemia and/or hypofibrinogenaemia
Fasting triglycerides ≥ 3.0 mmol/l, fibrinogen ≤ 1.5 g/l
Haemophagocytosis in bone marrow, spleen or lymph nodes
Low or absent natural killer cell activity
Ferritin ≥ 500 µg/l
Soluble CD25 ≥ 2400 U/ml

* Supportive criteria include neurologic symptoms, CSF pleocytosis, conjugated hyperbilirubinaemia and transaminitis, hypoalbuminaemia, hyponatraemia, elevated D-dimers and lactate dehydrogenase. The absence of haemophagocytosis in bone marrow does not exclude the diagnosis of HLH.

HLH is a clinical syndrome of hyper-inflammation resulting in an uncontrolled and ineffective immune response. It is characterised by persistent fever, pancytopaenia, hypofibrinogenaemia, hypertriglyceridaemia and hepatosplenomegaly (**Table 32.1**) [2]. Most cases reported in children less than 1 year of age are due to genetic defects predisposing to immune hyper-activation and are termed familial HLH. These are typically autosomal recessive conditions and the presentation is usually triggered by infection, with Epstein–Barr virus (EBV) being the most common pathogen identified (see also Case 31)[2–5]. In older children and adults, HLH typically occurs in the presence of another predisposing condition, such as severe infection, acquired immunodeficiency syndrome, malignancy or autoimmune disease, and these cases are termed secondary HLH (**Table 32.2**).

In 1991, diagnostic guidelines for HLH were presented by the Histiocyte Society and were based on five criteria: fever, splenomegaly, bicytopaenia, hypertriglyceridaemia and/or hypofibrinogenaemia, and haemophagocytosis. These were modified in 2004 with the inclusion of the molecular diagnosis of familial HLH.

Table 32.2 Causes of secondary (acquired) haemophagocytic lymphohistiocytosis.

Infection	Virus (e.g. EBV, CMV, Dengue, Parvovirus), bacteria (e.g. *E. coli*), parasite (e.g. malaria), protozoa, fungi
Autoimmune	JIA, SLE, Systemic sclerosis, Crohn's disease
Malignancies	T cell-derived – leukaemias and lymphomas
Acquired immune deficiency	Immunosuppression, BMT, renal transplant, AIDS
Poisoning	Ethylene glycol ingestion
Metabolic	Lysinuric protein intolerance, multiple sulphatase deficiency

JIA, juvenile idiopathic arthritis; SLE, systemic lupus erythematosus; BMT, bone marrow transplant; AIDS, acquired immunodeficiency syndrome; CMV, cytomegalovirus.

Certain genetic mutations leading to decreased apoptosis triggering have been identified in familial HLH [1,2]. These include autosomal recessive inheritance (*PRF1* [perforin], *MUNC13-4, STX11, STXBP2* and *RAB27A*) and X-linked recessive mutations (*SH2D1A, BIRC4*). Because differentiation between familial cases and secondary HLH is difficult on clinical grounds alone, it has been recommended that all children be tested for commonly identified genetic mutations causing familial HLH.

There is a huge variability in the presentation of HLH; however, early clinical suspicion and investigation may allow the clinician to diagnose this condition early. Particularly prolonged pyrexia of unknown origin, hepatitis and coagulopathy suggesting acute liver failure and cytopaenias are common features. Some patients also have a variety of dermatological manifestations including a generalised maculopapular erythematous rash, generalised erythroderma, oedema, panniculitis, morbilliform erythema, petechiae and purpura [4].

Horne et al. studied the neurological involvement in a large (n = 193) cohort of children with HLH and reported neurological symptoms in 37%, CSF abnormalities in 52% (pleocytosis and elevated protein) and both were present in 63% [2]. The most common clinical features were seizures, irritability and meningism. Children with abnormal CSF and neurological symptoms had a higher incidence of neurological sequelae and an increased risk of mortality. In another study of 46 children with primary HLH, 29 (63%) had neurological symptoms, 23 (50%) had abnormal CSF and 15 (33%) had an abnormal MRI brain scan, with the most common findings being symmetric periventricular white matter lesions with the absence of thalamic and brainstem involvement [3].

The main challenge in treating patients with HLH is making a timely diagnosis. Etoposide, dexamethasone and cyclosporine are often used in the initial treatment, as in the case described here. Stem cell transplant has been reported for familial HLH and in acquired cases in whom a relapse occurs. Intrathecal therapy with methotrexate and hydrocortisone has been reported for neurological involvement. Despite advances in recognition and treatment, the morbidity and mortality is high, with a 55% 3-year survival rate [3,4].

Key Points

- HLH should be considered if there is a clinical picture of sepsis, which is 'unusual' and/or not responsive to initial treatment.
- Serum ferritin, triglyceride and fibrinogen levels are useful tests.
- Early aggressive treatment improves survival; however, a significant number of children are left with long-term neurodevelopmental sequelae.

Looking Back

The earliest description of a histiocytic disorder is thought to be that of 25-year-old medical resident Alfred Hand, Jr, who presented a paper to the Philadelphia Pathological Society in 1893, describing the autopsy of a patient with several defects in cranial bone, although he entitled the paper Polyuria and Tuberculosis.

Later, Hand Schuller-Christian disease was named after him and two others who later described similar syndromes.

Did You Know?

Noting that Hand-Schuller–Christian disease, Letterer–Siwe disease and eosinophilic granuloma of bone have similar histological features, Lichenstein coined the term histiocytosis X to encompass them all, but more recently the term Langerhans cell histiocytoses has become the preferred term.

The nomenclature and categorisation of the histiocytic disorders is acknowledged to be one of the most confusing for any area of human disease [1]!

References

1. Cline MJ. Histiocytes and histiocytosis. Blood 1994;**84**:2840–53.
2. Henter J-I, Horne A, Aricó M, et al. HLH-2004: diagnostic and therapeutic guidelines for hemophagocytic lymphohistiocytosis. Pediatr Blood Cancer. 2007;**48**:124–31.
3. Horne A, Trottestam H, Aricó M, et al. Frequency and spectrum of central nervous system involvement in 193 children with haemophagocytic lymphohistiocytosis. Br J Haematol 2008;**140**:327–35.
4. Deiva K, Mahloaoui N, Beaudonner F, et al. CNS involvement at the onset of primary hemophagocytic lymphohistiocytosis. Neurology 2012;**78**:1150–6.
5. Jordan MB, Allen CE, Weitzman S, et al. How I treat hemophagocytic lymphohistiocytosis. Blood 2011;**118**:4041–52.

CASE 33 Bitten in the Hampshires

Heli Harvala and Tom Solomon

History

A previously healthy 35-year-old man presented with headache, nausea and vomiting to his general practitioner. At the practice, while being examined, he had a generalised tonic–clonic seizure and was thus admitted directly to a district general hospital.

One day prior to this presentation he had returned from a 6-week holiday in the USA, where he visited relatives in North Conway, New Hampshire and Rhode Island. Towards the end of his holiday, he had gone for a 5-day fishing trip in River Saco, in North Conway, and stayed in a log cabin.

Examination

On admission to hospital, he was noted to have several mosquito bites on his legs but the systemic examination was otherwise normal. He was fully conscious and the physical examination, including full neurological assessment, was unremarkable. However, the next day, he developed a pyrexia of 40.3°C and his neurological condition deteriorated rapidly. He became dysarthric and confused and soon after was admitted to intensive care because of a worsening coma score.

Initial Differential Diagnosis

The presentation of seizure and altered consciousness in the context of a febrile illness suggest a possible central nervous system infections, particularly:

- Viral encephalitis, e.g. herpes simplex virus, varicella zoster, enterovirus, West Nile virus
- Bacterial infection, e.g. *Listeria monocytogenes*
- Autoimmune encephalitis, e.g. paraneoplastic or primarily immune-mediated

Results of Initial Investigations

Baseline bloods showed a lymphopaenia (600 cells/μl), a thrombocytopaenia (46,000 cells/μl) and mild hyponatraemia.

A computer tomography (CT) scan of the brain was initially reported as normal. A lumbar puncture (LP) revealed 68 white blood cells/mm^3 (70% neutrophils, 30% lymphocytes) and an elevated total protein level (1.03 g/l).

Progress and Further Investigations

He was given intravenous (IV) antibiotics and aciclovir to cover possible listeria meningitis and herpes simplex virus encephalitis, respectively.

A magnetic resonance imaging (MRI) scan of the brain was performed (**Figure 33.1**).

The CT brain scan was reviewed and thought, on hindsight, to show low attenuation lesions in the external capsules with loss of definition of the caudate heads. A second LP demonstrated 26 white blood cells/mm^3 (100% lymphocytes) and an elevated total protein level (1.04 g/l).

Seven days later, when he had not improved, IV methylprednisolone was added to reduce cerebral inflammation.

Blood and cerebrospinal fluid (CSF) cultures for bacteria were negative, as was CSF polymerase chain reaction (PCR) for herpes viruses and enteroviruses. HIV testing was negative. Autoantibodies including anti-parietal cell, mitochondrial, smooth muscle, thyroid peroxidase and nuclear antibodies were also negative. Because of the travel history, mosquito bites and MRI findings, paired serum and CSF samples were tested for arthropod-borne viruses including West Nile virus, St Louis encephalitis virus and eastern, western and Venezuelan equine encephalitis viruses. These latter viruses were only considered because of a careful assessment of the detailed travel history, and a review of recent reports of disease activity on the Program for Monitoring Emerging Diseases (ProMed) Mail website.

Results of Definitive Investigations

There was a greater than 10-fold rise in antibody titre against eastern equine encephalitis virus in serum samples taken from day 7 (1:256) and day 13 (1:4004). The day 7 serum sample and CSF were also strongly positive for anti-eastern equine encephalitis virus IgM, and all serum samples had neutralising antibodies against eastern equine encephalitis virus as measured by a plaque-reduction neutralisation test. No sample was positive for eastern equine encephalitis virus RNA by PCR. Antibody testing was negative for the other arboviruses.

Figure 33.1. Axial (A,B) T2-weighted MRI in a 35-year-old man presenting with a generalised tonic–clonic seizure, encephalopathy and fever, having returned from North America.

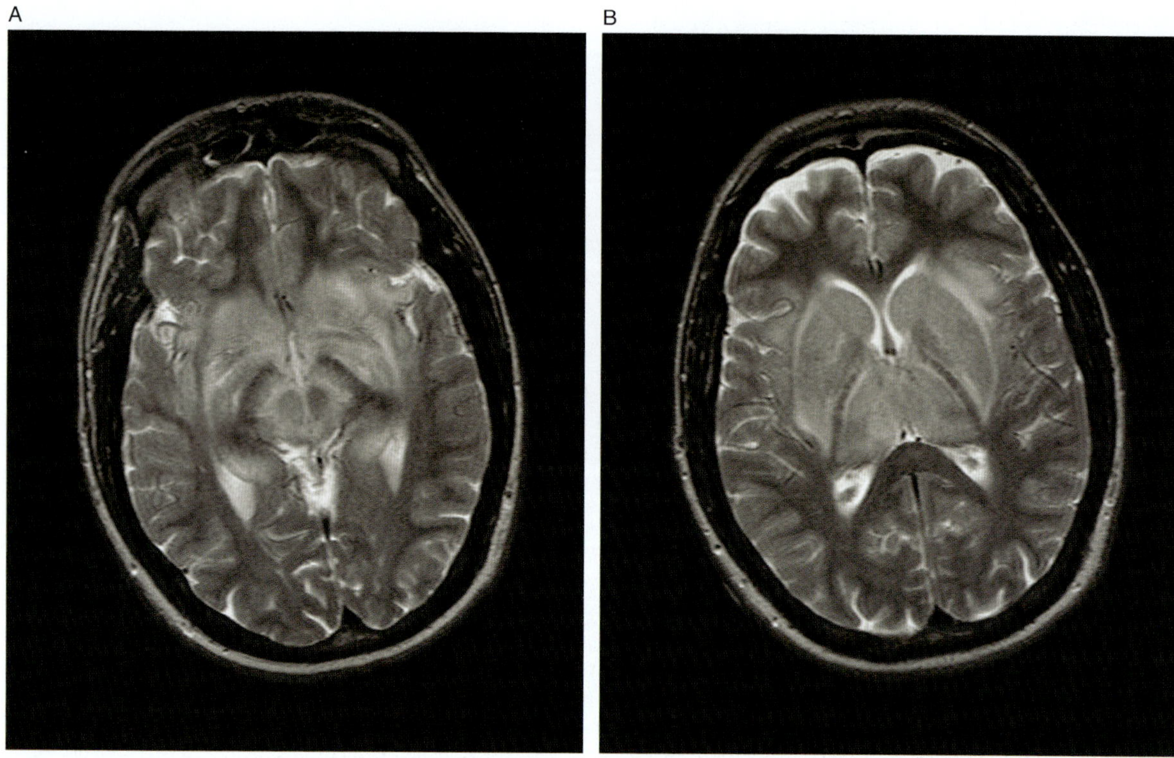

This demonstrates hyperintense T2-weighted signal in the brainstem (A) and the basal ganglia (B); reproduced with permission from [4].

Diagnosis

This was the first diagnosed case of encephalitis due to eastern equine encephalitis virus in Europe.

Management and Outcome

Treatment continued with amoxicillin, ceftriaxone and aciclovir until the diagnosis of eastern equine encephalitis was confirmed. He also received a 3-day course of methylprednisolone and antiepileptic medications. He remained comatose for 4 weeks, and 6 months later remained severely disabled with a spastic quadriparesis and tracheotomy in place.

There is no specific treatment of eastern equine encephalitis, although one individual was apparently treated successfully with immunotherapy [1].

Prevention

There is currently no vaccine to protect humans from against eastern equine encephalitis, although there are vaccines for horses.

The best way to avoid the disease is to minimise exposure to mosquitoes in affected areas by using personal protective measures and to reduce the population of infected mosquitoes through public health interventions.

Discussion

Eastern equine encephalitis virus is an arthropod-borne virus in the genus *Alphavirus* within the family Togaviridae. Western and Venezuelan equine encephalitis viruses are closely related alphaviruses known for causing neurological disease outbreaks in horses. Eastern equine encephalitis virus is transmitted between birds by *Culiseta melanura* and other mosquitoes; humans and horses become infected when they are bitten by mosquitoes (mainly *Aedes* species) which have fed on infected birds [2]. After birds, horses are the most frequent host of eastern equine encephalitis virus. Although human infections are rare, they are most commonly associated with recreational outdoor activities in and around freshwater hardwood swamps, where the mosquitos breed. Eastern equine encephalitis virus is endemic in a large geographical area extending from Ontario, Quebec and Nova Scotia provinces in Canada, down to the eastern USA and Gulf Coast and into South America as far as Argentina [2,3]. Approximately 270 human cases of eastern equine encephalitis have been confirmed since 1964 in the USA, most cases occurring between June and October (**Figure 33.2**). The case presented here is so far the only example of an imported case to Europe [4].

Most human infections are asymptomatic or mild, but approximately 4–5% of eastern equine encephalitis virus infections progress to encephalitis. Individuals younger than 15 years or over the age of 50 years are at higher risk for developing severe disease. The incubation period is throught to be between 2 and 10 days. Eastern equine encephalitis is characterised by a non-specific febrile prodrome followed by high fevers, severe headache, lethargy and seizures [5,6]. The evolution of neurological symptoms is often rapid, as it was in the case described here, leading to coma and, not infrequently, death. A short prodrome has been associated with an increased risk for death or severe disease in children [7]. MRI changes including non-enhancing high signal intensities in the basal ganglia, thalamus and brainstem as seen in this case, are described in eastern equine encephalitis virus infection, as in other arboviral encephalitides [1,4,6].

Eastern equine encephalitis is one of the most severe mosquito-borne encephalitides with a high case fatality rate of 30% [5]. Furthermore, at least half of the recovered patients have severe neurological deficits. There is no specific treatment for eastern equine encephalitis virus infection [1], but knowing the diagnosis helps to guide prognosis and has also public health implications.

Key Points

- Taking a detailed travel history, including exposure to mosquito bites, can be very important.
- High signal intensity changes on T2-weighted scans in the brainstem, thalamus and other basal ganglia may indicate an arboviral cause of encephalitis.
- The latest information on disease outbreaks can be readily obtained from ProMED-mail – the Program for Monitoring Emerging Diseases, an Internet-based reporting system dedicated to rapid global dissemination of information on outbreaks of infectious diseases and acute exposures to toxins (www.promedmail.org/).
- The case also serves as a timely reminder for travellers of the importance of avoiding mosquito bites wherever possible.

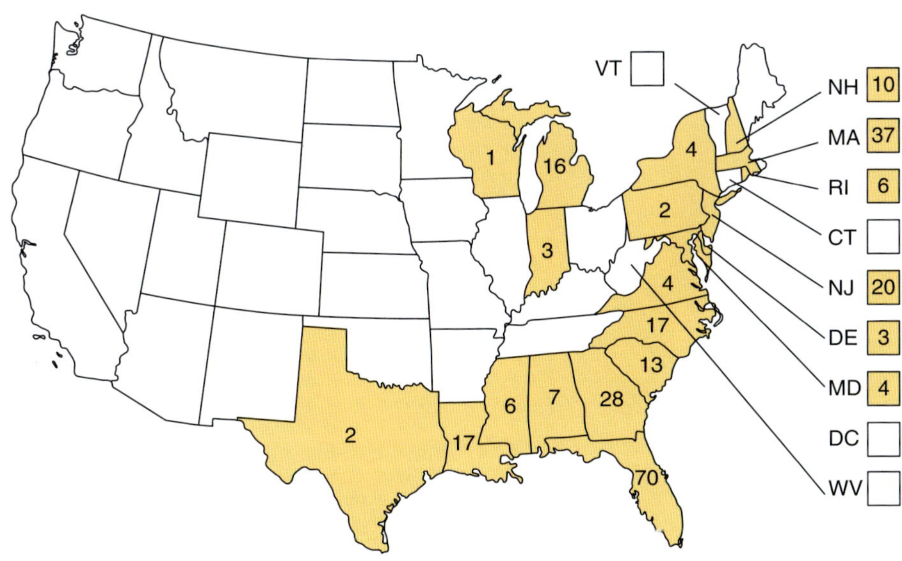

Figure 33.2. Eastern Equine Encephalitis Virus Neuroinvasive Disease Cases in the USA, Reported by State, 1964–2010, (Courtesy of Centers for Disease Control and Prevention, USA).

Looking Back

Eastern equine encephalitis was first recognized in Massachusetts, USA in 1831 when 75 horses died of encephalitic illness. The virus was first identified following its isolation from a horse brain in 1931 [8] and a human in 7 years later [9,10].

Did You Know?

Eastern equine encephalitis virus is also known as 'triple E virus' for its acronym. It is closely related to western equine encephalitis virus and Venezuelan equine encephalitis virus, which also occur in the Americas, in the approximate geographical locations described by their names.

References

1. Golomb MR, Durand ML, Schaefer PW, et al. A case of immunotherapy-responsive eastern equine encephalitis with diffusion-weighted imaging. Neurology 1991;**56**:420–1.
2. Davis LE, Beckham JD, Tyler KL. North American encephalitic arboviruses. Neurol Clin 2008;**26**:727–57.
3. Centers for Disease Control and Prevention, USA. Eastern equine encephalitis: epidemiology and geographic distribution (cited April 24, 2013). www.cdc.gov/easternequineencephalitis/tech/epi.html (accessed May 19, 2018).
4. Harvala H, Bremner J, Kealey S, et al. Case report: Eastern equine encephalitis virus imported to the UK. J Med Virol 2009;**81**:305–8.
5. Przelomski MM, O'Rourke E, Grady GF, Berardi VP, Markley HG. Eastern equine encephalitis in Massachusetts: a report of 16 cases, 1970–1984. Neurology 1988;**38**:736–9.
6. Deresiewicz RL, Thaler SJ, Hsu L, Zamani AA. Clinical and neuroradiographic manifestations of eastern equine encephalitis. N Engl J Med 1997;**26**:1867–74.
7. Silverman MA, Misasi J, Smole S, et al. Eastern equine encephalitis in children, Massachusetts and New Hampshire, USA, 1970–2010. Emerg Infect Dis 2013;**19**:194–201.
8. Meyer KF, Haring CM, Howitt B. The etiology of epizootic encephalomyelitis of horses in the San Joaquin Valley. Science 1931;**74**:227–8.
9. Webster LT, Wright FH. Recovery of eastern equine encephalomyelitis virus from the brain tissue of human cases of encephalitis in Massachusetts. Science 1938;**88**:305–6.
10. Feemster RF. Outbreak of encephalitis in man due to the eastern virus of equine encephalomyelitis. Am J Public Health Nations Health 1938;**28**:1403–10.

CASE 34 Racing Heart

Rachel Kneen

History

A 14-year-old boy presented to his local hospital with an episode of loss of consciousness and a generalised seizure. He had a 2-week history of non-specific and fluctuating lethargy, headaches and dizziness prior to his admission. During this time, he had also experienced several unusual stereotypical paroxysmal events lasting a few seconds only, where his heart 'would race', he would feel frightened and he felt his legs would not move properly. His mother had taken him to the general practitioner and he had an electrocardiogram that was normal. There was no eyewitness to these events, but in retrospect these were considered to be focal seizures. He had also suffered with some periods of rather paranoid behaviour. There was no significant past medical history. His mother suffered from transient post-natal hypothyroidism and his older brother had autoimmune hypothyroidism and temporal lobe epilepsy.

Examination

The patient was noted to be obese (weight 94 kg). He was afebrile, his pulse was 60 beats per minute and the other vital signs were normal. There was no rash, lymphadenopathy or signs of meningism. There were no other abnormal systemic findings. He was unconscious (Glasgow coma score 7/15). In so far as could be tested, there were no focal neurological signs.

Differential Diagnosis

- Acute encephalitis syndrome
    - Viral
    - Bacterial
    - Inflammatory: post- or para-infectious, e.g. acute disseminated encephalomyelitis, or autoimmune (e.g. limbic)
    - Other encephalopathy, e.g. toxic, or metabolic

Results of Initial Investigations

Baseline blood tests revealed a C-reactive protein of 14 mg/l and erythrocyte sedimentation rate 33 mm/hour. The full blood count, electrolytes and liver function tests, including ammonia, were normal. Thyroid function tests were slightly abnormal revealing an elevated thyroid-stimulating hormone (TSH) of 8.5 mu/l (range 0.3–3.8), but the thyroxine (T4) was 7.8 pmol/l (range 9–19). Cerebrospinal fluid (CSF) analysis revealed a pleocytosis with white cell count 15 cells/mm^3 (predominantly lymphocytes), red cell count 0 cells/mm^3; Gram stain and culture were negative. A computed tomography brain scan with contrast was normal. A routine electroencephalogram showed a diffusely slow pattern, indicating an encephalopathy, and no paroxysmal activity was seen.

Progress and Further Investigations

He was treated for suspected encephalitis with intravenous (IV) cefotaxime, and IV aciclovir and was moved to the intensive care unit where he was ventilated for 3 days. Following extubation he remained drowsy and confused for 1 day. Magnetic resonance imaging (MRI) of the brain was performed on day 2 of admission (**Figure 34.1**).

Figure 34.1. Coronal T2-weighted MRI brain scan in a 14-year-old male who presented with an episode of loss of consciousness and a generalised seizure.

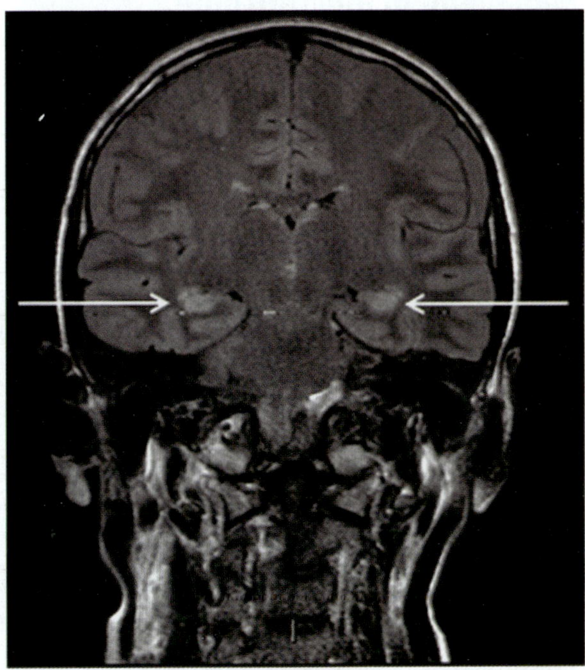

This shows symmetrical abnormal high signal within the medial temporal lobes/along the hippocampal formations bilaterally (arrows).

Extensive infective inflammatory and neurometabolic screens were normal. Ophthalmology review showed no signs of uveitis or vasculitis. Testing for anti-voltage-gated potassium channel (VGKC)-complex antibodies, anti-*N*-methyl-D-aspartate (NMDA) receptor antibodies, glutamic acid decarboxylase (GAD) antibodies and paraneoplastic antibodies was negative. Oligoclonal bands in the CSF were also negative.

Further Investigation Results

The raised TSH and low T4 were in keeping with hypothyroidism. Thyroid antibodies were raised with anti-thyroid peroxidase (TPO) microsomal antibodies measuring 178 IU/ml (range 0–50). Although he had hypothyroidism, antithyroid antibodies and a clinical presentation consistent with Hashimoto's encephalopathy, the imaging findings of high signal in the medial temporal lobe, with this clinical presentation, were felt to be more in keeping with a limbic encephalitis.

Diagnosis

He was diagnosed with limbic encephalitis and TPO antibodies, which were felt to be a marker of autoimmunity, rather than causal.

Management and Outcome

Initial treatment consisted of IV methylprednisolone (1 g once daily) for 3 days and intravenous immunoglobulin (IVIG) 2 g/kg over 2 days. He slowly improved, but was noted to have short-term memory impairment. He would also be quieter than usual and he had problems with sequencing and problem solving. He was discharged from hospital on a tapering course of oral prednisolone with a plan to complete a course of IV cyclophosphamide given monthly over 6 months in total. He continued to have ongoing short-term memory problems and had seizures with an intercurrent illness 3 months later. The fact that he had not responded dramatically to steroids further supported the idea that this was not Hashimoto's encephalopathy.

He had repeat MRI 6 months later (**Figure 34.2**). At this time, mycophenolete mofatil was commenced as a maintenance treatment with a plan to continue for 2 years and to monitor TPO antibodies. A detailed screen for an occult malignancy was negative.

Discussion

Limbic encephalitis is diagnosed in a patient with clinical and investigative features consistent with involvement of the limbic system, particularly the temporal lobes. The clinical features are typically sub-acute onset of short-term memory loss, behavioural change and seizures, and the investigatory findings are usually a combination of radiological, neurophysiological and histological features. Purely paraneoplastic antibodies associated with the condition include anti-Hu, Ma, and Ma2/Ta. Additional antibodies which can be paraneoplastic or *de novo* autoimmune conditions include anti-VGKC-complex, NMDA receptor and GAD antibodies. Limbic encephalitis was first described in adult patients and assumed initially to be a mainly paraneoplastic disorder; however, more recently limbic encephalitis in adults and children not associated with an underlying neoplasm has been recognised increasingly [1].

Encephalopathy associated with high titres of serum anti-thyroid antibodies was first described in 1966, and was given the term 'Hashimoto

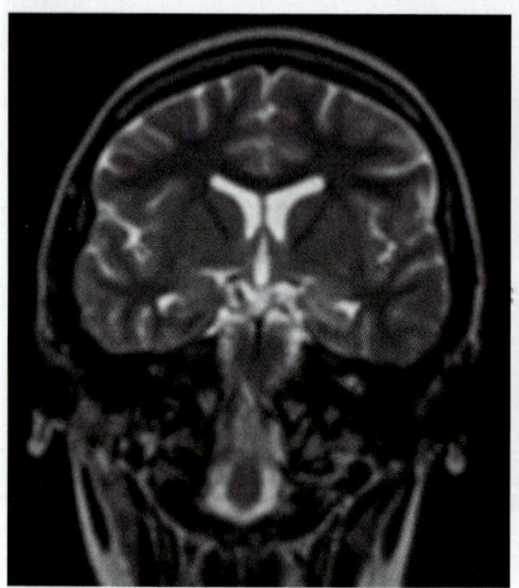

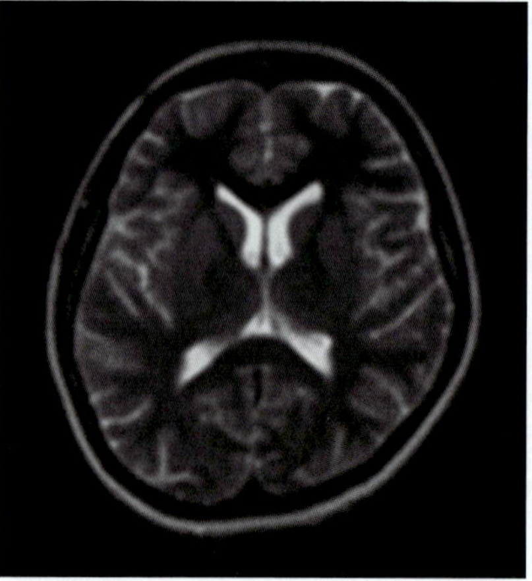

Figure 34.2. Coronal T2-weighted MRI brain scan in the same child 6 months after treatment with methylprednisolone, IVIG and cyclophosphamide.
This shows signal abnormality and volume loss in both hippocampi with enlargement of the temporal horns of the lateral ventricles.

encephalopathy' or steroid responsive encephalopathy. The laboratory and radiological findings are heterogeneous and the pathogenic role of the thyroid antibodies remains uncertain [2]. Hashimoto's encephalopathy is more common in young women and the presentation can include stroke-like episodes. The course may be relapsing and the outcome is generally considered to be good. MRI is usually normal; there are sometimes non-specific subcortical white matter abnormalities, but not the medial temporal lobe abnormalities as seen in this case are not considered part of the spectrum of Hashimoto's encephalitis. The combination of encephalopathy, elevated serum anti-thyroid antibody titres and clinical response to steroid therapy and association with other autoimmune diseases suggests that Hashimoto's encephalitis is an immune-mediated central nervous system (CNS) disorder [3]. However, the patient described here did not respond fully to the immunotherapy, and his clinical presentation, radiological findings and progress was felt to be more in keeping with limbic encephalitis.

Patients with limbic encephalitis are more likely to have a higher incidence of thyroid antibodies than the normal population (30% versus 15%) [4], but little has been published to convincingly demonstrate their pathogenic role [5,6]. It is more likely that thyroid antibodies in encephalopathic patients reflect epiphenomena of an immune-mediated process directed at an as-yet unidentified CNS antigen. Therefore, TPO antibodies represent a useful diagnostic biomarker even if direct pathogenicity is not established. Patients with thyroid antibody-associated limbic encephalitis may have a late response to immunotherapy; therefore, treatment should continue in the same way that is recommended for other types of limbic encephalitis [5,6].

Key Points

- Autoimmune limbic encephalitis is being recognised increasingly and many cases have specific associated antibodies in the serum and CSF directed at neuronal surface proteins.
- Immunomodulatory treatments can improve the outcome and prevent relapse, but currently the most effective treatments are unknown, including the length of treatment required.
- Hashimoto's encephalitis mainly affects young women, presents typically with stroke-like episodes and seizures, and is steroid responsive.

Looking Back

Hakaru Hashimoto graduated from Kyushu University, Japan in 1907. He described a condition that he named 'lymphomatous goitre' in 1912. Later this was renamed Hashimoto's thyroiditis.

Did You Know?

There is a street named after Hashimoto at the Maidashi Campus at Kyushu University in honour of his achievements. Hashimoto's encephalopathy was first described by the British neurologist, Brain in 1966.

References

1. Vincent A, Bien CG, Irani SR, Waters P. Autoantibodies associated with diseases of the CNS: new developments and future challenges. Lancet Neurol 2011;**10**:759–72.
2. Brain L, Jellinek EH, Ball K. Hashimoto's disease and encephalopathy. Lancet 1966;**2**:512–14.
3. Schiess N, Pardo CA. Hashimoto's encephalopathy. Ann N Y Acad Sci 2008;**1142**:254–65.
4. Castillo P, Woodruff B, Caselli R, et al. Steroid-responsive encephalopathy associated with autoimmune thyroiditis. Arch Neurol 2006;**63**: 197–202.
5. Hacohen Y, Joseph S, Kneen R, et al. Limbic encephalitis associated with elevated antithyroid antibodies. J Child Neurol 2014;**29**:769–73.
6. Dalmau J, Lancaster E, Martinez-Hernandez E, et al. Clinical experience and laboratory investigations in patients with anti NMDAR encephalitis. Lancet Neurol 2011;**10**:63–74.

CASE 35

A Recurring Pain in the Neck

Fiona McGill

History

A 38-year-old female presented to an accident and emergency department with a 2-day history of headache and neck pain. She had a past medical history of chronic fatigue syndrome and a family history of subarachnoid haemorrhage. She denied any fevers or chills. She took no regular medications and had no allergies. She had recently been prescribed some antibiotics by her general practitioner for an upper respiratory tract infection.

Examination

On examination she looked well. She was speaking normally and had a Glasgow coma score of 15. She was afebrile and haemodynamically stable with a blood pressure of 100/55 and a heart rate of 70. She had mild photophobia and mild neck stiffness. Her cardiovascular, respiratory, gastrointestinal and neurological examinations were all completely normal. She had a crusting rash on her hand and buttock.

Initial Differential Diagnosis

Due to her family history and presentation, the initial diagnosis was felt most likely to be a subarachnoid haemorrhage. Other diagnoses considered were migraine and a simple tension headache.

Results of Initial Investigations

Her full blood count, urea, creatinine and electrolytes were all normal. Liver enzymes and clotting tests were also normal. She went on to have an urgent computed tomography (CT) scan of her head to rule out a subarachnoid haemorrhage. This was reported as showing no sign of an acute bleed, but the radiologist suggested performing a lumbar puncture (LP) to completely exclude a subarachnoid haemorrhage.

The LP was done and initial results were as follows: white cell count 500×10^9 cells/ml, 98% lymphocytes, red cell count 26×10^6 cells/ml; no organisms were seen on Gram staining. The cerebrospinal fluid (CSF) protein was 4.2 g/l and CSF glucose was 2.8 mmol/l (serum glucose 5.4 mmol/l).

Refined Differential Diagnosis

Given the high percentage of lymphocytes in the CSF, the differential diagnosis was now considered to be either viral meningitis or partially treated bacterial meningitis.

Results of Definitive Investigations

The final CSF results came back a few days later. The CSF had no bacterial growth. The polymerase chain reaction (PCR) was used to test for a panel of viruses and herpes simplex virus (HSV) type 2 was positive. All other viruses (enteroviruses, HSV type-1 and varicella zoster virus) were negative.

Diagnosis

Herpes simplex virus type 2 meningitis.

Management and Outcome

She was treated with intravenous aciclovir for 1 week, but then refused any further cannulation and was discharged home. She was seen in clinic twice over the next 6 months where she continued to complain of headaches and neck pain, which eventually settled.

Two years after her first admission she presented to the accident and emergency department again with a headache and neck pain. She again had a CT scan to rule out a subarachnoid haemorrhage and then went on to have an LP. The LP showed: 170×10^9 white cells/ml, 95% lymphocytes with no red cells; protein of 8.2 g/l and a CSF glucose of 3.4 mmol/l (plasma 5.6 mmol/l). The CSF PCR was again positive for HSV-2.

This time she had concurrent genital lesions and was treated with oral valaciclovir for a week.

She had three further admissions with similar symptoms over the next few years. During these she refused further LPs and would not accept intravenous aciclovir, and could not tolerate oral valaciclovir, as she suffered constipation while on it. She continued to complain of headaches in between episodes.

Diagnosis

Recurrent herpes simplex virus type 2 meningitis, also known as Mollaret's meningitis.

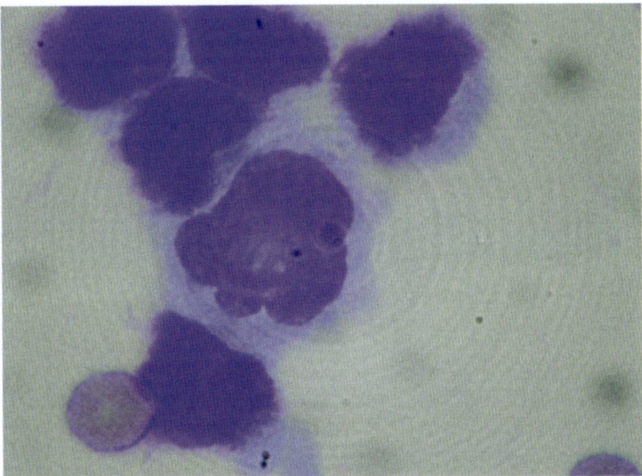

Figure 35.1. Mollaret's cells.

Prevention

Work is ongoing to develop a vaccine to protect against primary infection with HSV-2. There has been one randomised controlled trial looking at oral valaciclovir as prevention for recurrent HSV-2 meningitis, but this was not effective, possibly because the dose of valaciclovir chosen was too low [1].

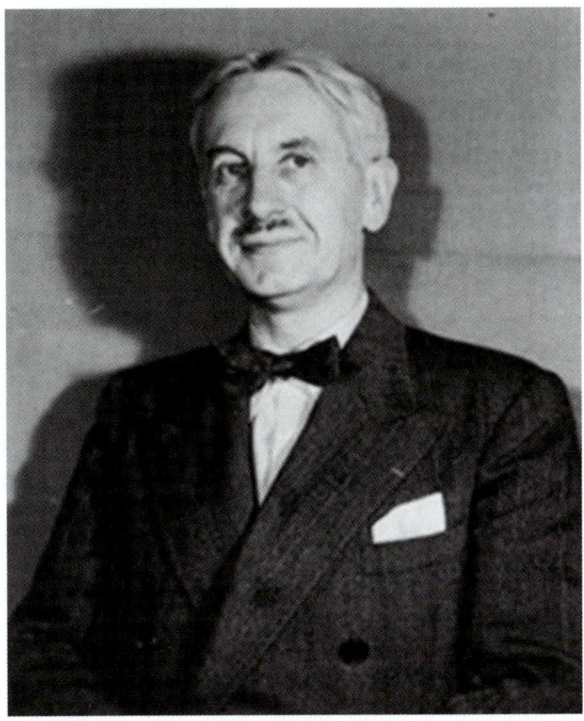

Figure 35.2. Pierre Mollaret. (Reprinted by permission of Springer Nature from [5] in the *Journal of Neurology*.)

Discussion

In 1944 a French microbiologist, Pierre Mollaret, described three patients with recurrent meningitis (**Figure 35.1**). Examination of the CSF of these patients revealed large mononuclear cells, which he termed Mollaret cells, and the disease known subsequently as Mollaret's meningitis (**Figure 35.2**) [2]. Mollaret cells have since been discovered to be monocytes. Mollaret also described a CSF pleocytosis that was initially predominantly polymorphic but rapidly changed to become predominantly lymphocytic. The terms recurrent lymphocytic meningitis, recurrent benign lymphocytic meningitis or recurrent aseptic meningitis are often used now in preference to Mollaret's meningitis, as many cases do not fit Mollaret's exact description.

Recurrent lymphocytic meningitis is most commonly caused by HSV-2 [3,4], although numerous other viruses have also been documented to cause recurrent episodes of meningitis. The prevalence of HSV-2 associated recurrent lymphocytic meningitis has been estimated to be 2.2/100,000 in one study carried out in Finland [5].

The classical description is recurrent episodes of headache and meningism, accompanied by a CSF pleocytosis (polymorphic in the first 24 hours but rapidly changing to a lymphocytic picture); the episodes are weeks, months or years apart, and are separated by periods of complete recovery. Often attacks get less frequent and less severe as a patient gets older, and may eventually cease altogether. Traditionally, the definition of Mollaret's meningitis also required the lack of evidence of an aetiological agent. However, with the improvement of diagnostic techniques it has become clear that HSV-2 is probably responsible for the majority of what was previously called Mollaret's meningitis. CSF PCR for HSV-2 (and other viruses) should be requested in cases of recurrent lymphocytic meningitis. Nowadays the Mollaret cell is seldom seen in practice, possibly due to delays in performing a lumbar puncture.

Recurrent lymphocytic meningitis occurs most commonly in females, often young sexually active females [3,4,6]. Despite HSV-2 being the causative agent in most cases of genital herpes, most episodes of meningitis due to HSV-2 are not associated with concurrent genital lesions (**Figure 35.3**) [7].

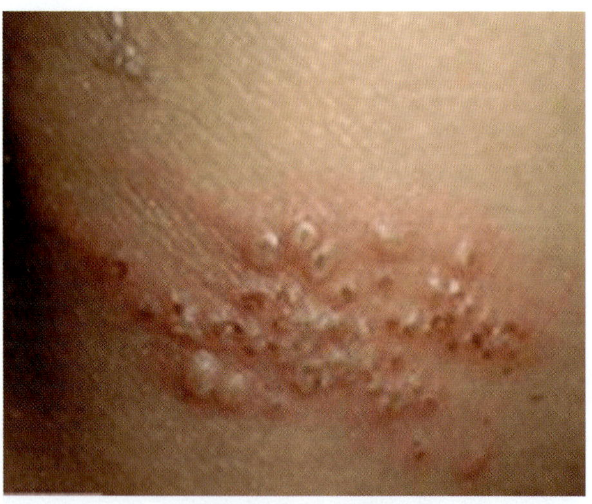

Figure 35.3. Typical eruption of HSV-2 on the buttocks.

Looking Back

Mollaret was decorated with the French Croix de Guerre after the First World War. He then studied under Professor Georges Charles Guillain (of Guillain–Barré syndrome) and worked at the famous French hospital the Pitié-Salpêtrière.

Did You Know?

Pierre Mollaret's first description actually described patients with a polymorphic CSF, not a lymphocytic CSF.

Recurrent lymphocytic meningitis is difficult to treat as there is little evidence to guide treatment or prophylaxis. Most people who have an episode of HSV-2 meningitis do not get recurrent episodes. However, those who do can have several episodes several years apart, or a few months apart. Aciclovir or valaciclovir are often given for both treatment and prophylaxis, but whether either is truly beneficial is not known [1].

Key Points

- Most cases of HSV-2 meningitis are single episodes, but a small number of people develop recurrent HSV-2 meningitis (Mollaret's syndrome).
- HSV-2 meningitis occurs most commonly in sexually active young females.
- Although the virus also causes genital lesions, in most cases of HSV-2 meningitis there are no apparent lesions, or previous history of lesions.
- There is no established treatment, although aciclovir or valaciclovir may help in acute attacks or as prophylaxis.

References

1. Aurelius E, Franzen-Rohl E, Glimaker M, et al. Long term valacyclovir suppressive treatment after herpes simplex virus type-2 meningitis: a double blind, randomized controlled trial. Clin Infect Dis 2012;**54**:1304–13.
2. Mollaret P. La meningite endothelio-leukocytaire multi-recurrente benigne. Rev Neurol (Paris) 1944;**76**:57–67.
3. Tedder DG, Ashley R, Tyler KL, Levin MJ. Herpes simplex virus infection as a cause of benign recurrent lymphcytic meningitis. Ann Intern Med 1994;**121**:334–8.
4. Kupila L, Vainionpaa R, Vuorinen T, Marttila RJ, Kotilainen P. Recurrent lymphocytic meningitis. Arch Neurol 2004;**61**:1553–7.
5. Vitturi BK, Sanvito WL. Pierre Mollaret (1898–1987). J Neurol 2018;1-2 .
6. Kallio-Laine K, Seppanen M, Kautiainen H, et al. Recurrent lymphocytic meningitis positive for herpes simplex virus type 2. Emerg Infect Dis 2009;**15**:1119–22.
7. Landry ML, Greenwold J, Vikram HR. Herpes simplex type-2 meningitis: presentation and lack of standardized therapy. Am J Med 2009;**122**:688–91.

CASE 36

History Repeating?

Anand Iyer and Rachel Kneen

History

A 6-year-old boy presented with an acute onset weakness of the right side of his face and nasal speech, followed 2 days later by right-sided shoulder pain and right upper limb weakness. Five days before the facial weakness he had a '24-hour bug' with diarrhoea, vomiting and fever. He had taken paracetamol and ibuprofen for fever at the time he was unwell with gastroenteritis, but was no longer taking any medication.

His mother's pregnancy and delivery were normal with no complications. The child's developmental progress was normal and immunisations were up to date. There was no history of foreign travel, and no reason to suspect he was immunocompromised. His younger sister had also had the gastroenteritis illness, but she had made a full recovery.

Examination

On examination, he had a flaccid paralysis affecting the whole of the right upper limb, predominantly affecting proximal movements with decreased deep tendon reflexes and normal sensation. Examination of the left upper limb and both lower limbs was normal. He also had an abnormal facial appearance (**Figure 36.1**). In addition, the right side of the soft palate did not elevate on phonation and there was objective weakness of the right sternocleidomastoid muscle, due to paralysis of cranial nerves 10 and 11, respectively. The other cranial nerves were intact and funduscopy was normal.

Differential Diagnosis

He had multifocal lower motor neuron weakness involving three cranial nerves (7, 10 and 11) and nerves of the brachial plexus. The former may represent either a polyneuropathy involving multiple cranial nerves or brainstem parenchymal pathology and the latter may represent a polyradiculopathy, brachial plexopathy or anterior horn cell lesions. Potential aetiologies include post-infectious phenomena (e.g. Guillain–Barré syndrome with cranial involvement, or a Miller Fisher syndrome variant), infectious basal meningeal and brachial leptomeningeal infiltration, anterior horn cell infection, or mononeuritis multiplex.

Initial Investigations

All initial blood tests were normal except a slight elevation of the erythrocyte sedimentation rate (12 mm/hour) and a low peripheral lymphocyte count of 2.12 cells/mm^3. A lumbar puncture on day 3 of the weakness revealed a pleocytosis with white cell count 18 cells/mm^3 (16 monocytes), normal glucose ratio, lactate and protein. Cerebrospinal fluid (CSF), polymerase chain reaction (PCR) for herpes simplex virus, varicella zoster virus and enteroviruses was negative.

Nerve conduction studies of the right median and ulnar motor nerves showed reduced motor response amplitudes (1.74 mV in abductor policis brevis and 1.63 mV in adductor digiti minimi) with normal conduction velocities (45.8 m/s cubital fossa; 53.6 m/s below epicondyle). He also had electromyography (**Figure 36.2**).

Figure 36.1. Picture of a 6-year-old boy who presented with diarrhoea and vomiting, followed by nasal speech. He has been asked to raise his eyebrows.

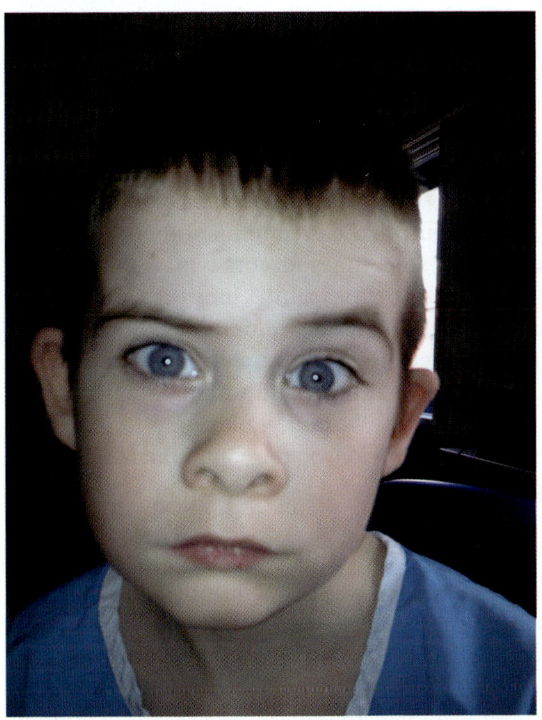

This demonstrates weakness of the frontalis on the right corresponding to a partial lower motor neuron VIIth palsy. (Photo: Rachel Kneen, reproduced with the permission of his parents.)

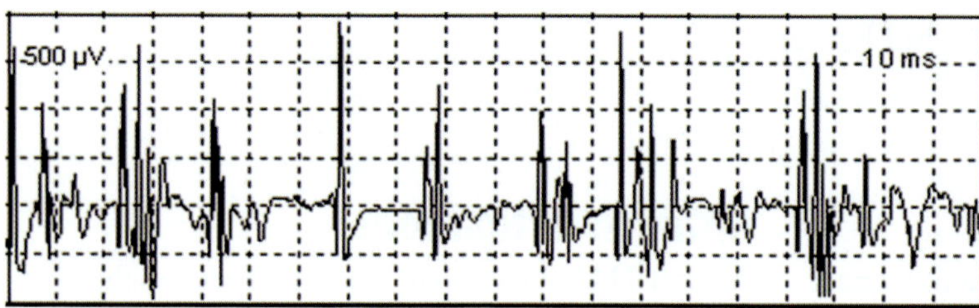

Figure 36.2. Electromyography of the right deltoid in the same child.
This shows no spontaneous activity and reduced interference pattern with some rapidly firing, but otherwise normal, motor units. These changes suggested anterior horn cell involvement in the right upper limb.

Definitive Investigations

Stool and throat swab samples were sent for PCR, and enterovirus was detected in both. This was subsequently confirmed to be echovirus 18 on genetic sequencing of the *VP1* gene.

Diagnosis

Acute flaccid paralysis due to myelitis caused by echovirus 18.

Management and Outcome

Without any specific therapy he began to improve over the next 4 weeks (**Figure 36.3**). However, he was left with some residual weakness and wasting of the right upper limb, which was still apparent 2 years after the illness.

Figure 36.3. Picture of the same child 4 weeks after the onset of neurological symptoms.

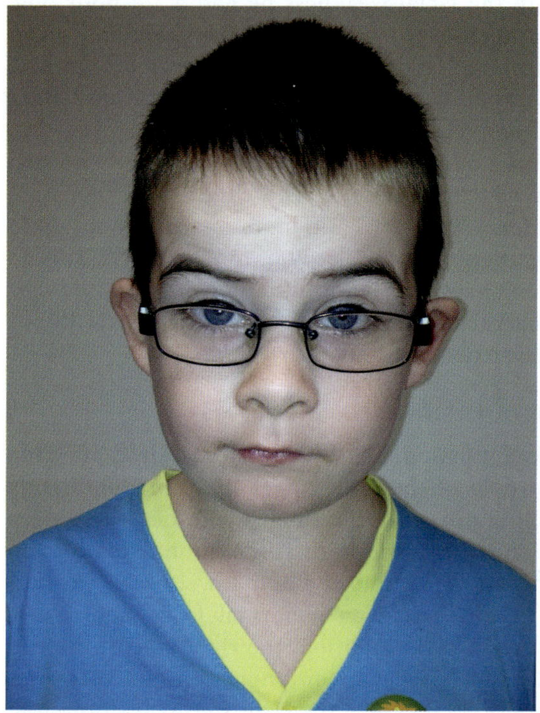

This shows complete resolution of the partial right cranial nerve VIIth palsy. (Photo: Rachel Kneen, reproduced with the permission of his parents.)

Prevention

There is no vaccine against echovirus 18. Like other enteroviruses, echoviruses are transmitted predominantly by the faeco-oral route, and so personal hygiene is key to limiting their spread.

Echoviruses are transmitted person-to-person; the faecal–oral route is the predominant mode, although transmission sometimes occurs via respiration of oral secretions such as saliva. Indirect transmission occurs through numerous routes, including via contaminated water, food and fomites (inanimate objects). Contaminated swimming and wading pools can also transmit the virus. Also, there are well-documented reports of transmission via the contaminated hands of hospital personnel.

Discussion

Non-polio enteroviruses are frequently detected as the causative agent in acute flaccid paralysis surveillance. However, echovirus 18 has not been reported to cause acute flaccid paralysis, being more commonly associated with viral exanthematous illness and aseptic meningitis [1]. Therefore, it is not clear if this virus was the cause of this child's polio-like acute flaccid paralysis, although it seems possible. The alternative is that he had been infected with the virus, and now was continuing to carry it in his throat swab and stool, but it was coincidental to his acute flaccid paralysis. If this child had visited South-East Asia, the concern would be that the polio-like illness was due to enterovirus 71, which is associated with huge outbreaks of acute flaccid paralysis [2]. Another potential cause to consider would be a flavivirus such as Japanese encephalitis or West Nile virus in the context of the appropriate geographical exposure.

Enterovirus infection can manifest as hand, foot and mouth disease, poliomyelitis-like acute flaccid paralysis, aseptic meningitis, or rhombencephalitis

[3]. Infection predominantly affects children, particularly in East Asia. Severe systemic complications such as cardiorespiratory collapse and pulmonary oedema can occur, particularly with enterovirus 71 infection [3]. PCR of throat and vesicle swabs and/or of stool are particularly useful in establishing the diagnosis, although clearly samples from otherwise sterile sites, such as vesicle swabs, or CSF, are of greatest utility in confirming enterovirus infection as the cause of the acute neurological presentation [4]. Although CSF PCR is useful for many enteroviruses, for enterovirus 71 it is often negative. On magnetic resonance imaging, inflammation of the anterior horns of the spinal cord may be seen along with inflammation of the dorsal pons and medulla. No direct antiviral therapy is established and treatment is currently supportive [3,4].

Key Points

- Enterovirus infection can cause a range of manifestations including aseptic meningitis, brainstem encephalitis, or an acute flaccid paralysis due to anterior horn cell involvement.
- Enterovirus infection can often be established by PCR of throat swab, rectal swab and vesicles, if present.
- Management is supportive.

Looking Back

Enteroviruses, to a large extent identified by Albert Sabin, are now recognised to be one of the genera of the 'picornavirus' family, so termed for being small 'pico-' RNA viruses [5].

Did You Know?

The name echovirus comes from 'enteric cytopathic human orphan' virus; these viruses were first identified in the 1950s in faeces, hence 'enteric', and damaged cells in tissue culture, 'cytopathic', but they were not associated with any disease, hence 'orphan viruses'.

References

1. Tsai H-P, Huang S-W, Wu F-L, et al. An echovirus 18-associated outbreak of aseptic meningitis in Taiwan: epidemiology and diagnostic and genetic aspects. J Med Microbiol 2011;**60**:1360–5.
2. Solomon T, Lewthwaite P, Perera D, et al. Virology, epidemiology, pathogenesis, and control of enterovirus 71. Lancet 2010;**10**:778–90.
3. Ooi MH, Wong SC, Lewthwaite P, Cardosa MJ, Solomon T. Clinical features, diagnosis and management of enterovirus 71. Lancet Neurol 2010:**9**;1097–105.
4. Solomon T, Michael BD, Smith PE, et al. Management of suspected viral encephalitis in adults: Association of British Neurologists and British Infection Association National Guideline. J Infect 2012;**64**:347–3.
5. Melnick JL. The discovery of the enteroviruses and the classification of poliovirus among them. Biologicals 1993;**21**:305–9.

CASE 37 A Little Light-headed

Fiona McGill

History

A 70-year-old man was admitted with an acute onset of confusion. He had a preceding 5-day history of a headache, sore throat and coryzal symptoms. In the afternoon of the day of admission he became acutely confused and his wife said he appeared vacant. His past medical history included non-insulin-dependent diabetes for which he took Metformin. He was otherwise fit and well and had no other significant past medical history. He lived with his wife and was independent at home.

Examination

In the accident and emergency department he was found to be febrile with a temperature of 39.4°C. He was tachycardic with a heart rate of 140 beats per minute and his blood pressure was 110/60 mmHg. On examination he had some basal crepitations on the right side of his chest and some mild neck stiffness. There was no photophobia and Kernig's test was negative. He was mildly confused, being disoriented in time, but not person or place.

Initial Differential Diagnosis

- Systemic sepsis
- Pneumonia
- Meningitis
- Encephalitis

Results of Initial Investigations

Bloods taken on admission returned showed a mildly raised white cell count at 12.1 × 10^9/l with a neutrophilia and an elevated C-reactive protein of 136 mg/l. Renal and liver function was normal. Chest X-ray revealed some patchy consolidation at the right base.

An urgent computer tomography (CT) scan of the head was performed (**Figure 37.1**).

Refined Differential Diagnosis

1. Pneumocephalus secondary to chronic sinusitis
2. Potential for underlying carcinoma with bony erosion

Results of Definitive Investigations

In view of the altered mental state a lumbar puncture was also performed. This had an opening pressure of 28 cm H_2O, the appearance was cloudy and the cerebrospinal fluid (CSF) white cell count was 4170 × 10^6 cells/ml (82% polymorphonuclear cells). The CSF protein was 3.99 g/l, the CSF glucose was 1.1 mmol/l and serum was 8.6 mmol/l (ratio: 13%). The CSF Gram stain was abnormal (**Figure 37.2**).

The pneumococcal latex antigen test was also positive. Blood cultures, performed before starting antibiotics, grew a fully sensitive *Streptococcus pneumoniae*.

Diagnosis

Pneumocephalus secondary to pneumococcal meningitis caused by sinusitis.

Figure 37.1. CT scan of the head of a 70-year-old man presenting with acute confusion.

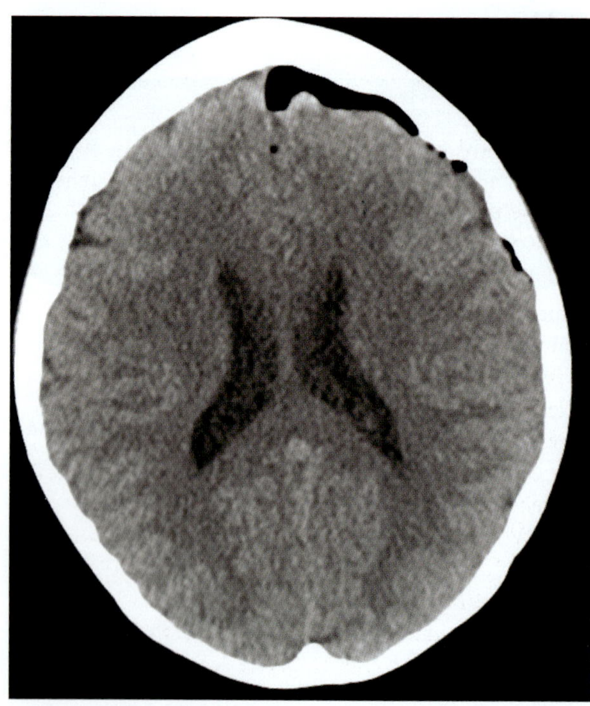

This shows air in the left subdural area around the left cerebral hemisphere (pneumocephalus around the left subdural area) with mucosal thickening of the frontal, ethmoid and sphenoid sinus and associated mucosal thickening of the middle ear.

Figure 37.2. The patient's Gram stain

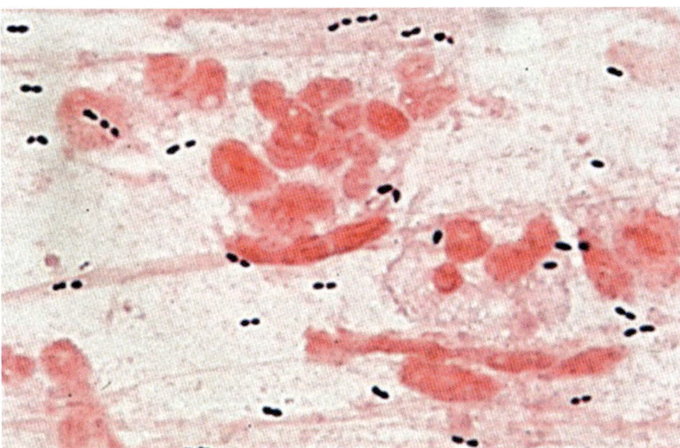

This shows the typical Gram-positive diplococci of *Streptococcus pneumoniae.*

Management and Outcome

The patient was commenced on broad-spectrum antibiotics swiftly after admission; initially this was ceftriaxone, but ciprofloxacin was later added to cover the potential of *Pseudomonas* infection from the ear. The ciprofloxacin was stopped when *Streptococcus pneumoniae* was cultured from the blood cultures. The patient initially improved but after a week of treatment he developed an acute expressive dysphasia. A second CT scan of the head was performed (**Figure 37.3**). He was transferred to the regional neurocentre where frank pus was drained from the collection by the neurosurgeons. No organisms were grown from the pus. The patient was treated with 4 weeks of intravenous antibiotics and made a good recovery.

Prevention

Some pneumococcal disease can be prevented with vaccination. There are two types of vaccination: 13-valent pneumococcal conjugate vaccine (PCV) covers 13 different serotypes of *Streptococcus pneumoniae* and 23-valent pneumococcal polysaccharide vaccine (PPV), which covers 23 serotypes. In the UK, the PCV vaccine is given as part of the childhood immunisation schedule; the PPV is given to at-risk individuals, i.e. those over 65, people who are asplenic, have chronic respiratory, heart, liver or kidney disease, or diabetes, those with immunodeficiency, including HIV, individuals with cochlear implants and individuals with CSF leaks [1].

Discvussion

Pneumococcal meningitis is caused by the Gram-positive bacterium *Streptococcus pneumoniae. S.*

Figure 37.3. A second CT performed on the same patient, who developed acute dysphasia one week into treatment.

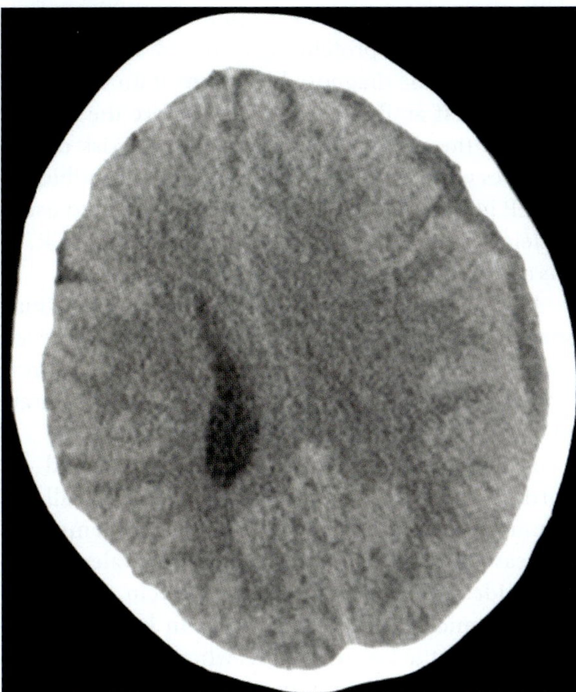

This shows a subdural collection with oedema and midline shift.

pneumoniae normally lives as a commensal bacteria in the upper respiratory tract and does not invade; however, the bacterium contains certain virulence factors which may lead to invasive disease, one of the most important being the capsule.

Streptococcus pneumoniae is the commonest bacterial cause of meningitis in adults and school-aged children, although the incidence has decreased since the introduction of vaccination. Pneumococcal meningitis carries a higher mortality and morbidity rate than other forms of bacterial meningitis [2,3], with a case fatality rate of between 18% and 30%.

Pneumococcal meningitis can present with meningism or it may present with a more encephalitic-type illness with reduced consciousness. Ninety-five percent of patients have at least two of: headache, fever, neck stiffness or altered mental state [2].

Blood cultures before antibiotics are essential to enhance the chances of growing the organism and obtaining antibiotic sensitivities. A lumbar puncture is also essential, where it is not contraindicated, to confirm meningitis as the cause of the illness.

As in this case, lumbar puncture will commonly show a moderately raised white cell count, normally with a predominance of neutrophils. The CSF glucose will be low and the protein will be raised. The causative organism can be diagnosed by Gram stain or culture of the CSF. If antibiotics are given before the lumbar puncture the CSF may well be sterile; the risk of this increases with the amount of time between antibiotics and LP [4]. Therefore, CSF should also be tested using nucleic acid amplification techniques such as PCR, as this can increase the yield [5].

Latex agglutination tests for bacterial antigens may be also used as they provide a rapid diagnosis. However, they have poor sensitivity and do not provide antimicrobial susceptibilities; therefore, treatment is rarely altered on the basis of this test.

Initial antibiotics should comprise a second- or third-generation cephalosporin, which cover all the common causes of community-acquired meningitis. In areas where penicillin resistance is prevalent a glycopeptide antibiotic, such as vancomycin, should be added. Penicillin resistance occurs in less than 10% of isolates in the UK. Therefore, when the organism is cultured and the sensitivities known, antibiotics can often be rationalised to penicillin alone.

Antibiotics should be given for 10–14 days in pneumococcal meningitis. Duration should be lengthened in patients with pyogenic collections. Steroids have been shown to reduce mortality in adult patients with pneumococcal meningitis and reduce hearing loss in others, especially *Haemophilus* meningitis in children.

Complications and consequences of pneumococcal meningitis include death, deafness, cognitive dysfunction, cerebral infarction, seizures and suppurative collections, as was seen in this case. Complications are significantly more common in pneumococcal than in meningococcal meningitis, which is the other common cause in western settings [2].

Pneumocephalus (air in the cranial cavity) is a rare complication of meningitis and when it occurs with pneumococcal meningitis is normally always associated with sinusitis or mastoiditis.

Key Points

- Pneumococcal meningitis occurs in older adults.
- The common serotypes can be prevented by vaccination, but this does not eliminate the risk of less-common serotypes.
- Preceding or concurrent respiratory tract infections can be a clue to the aetiology.
- Pneumocephalus (air in the cranial cavity) is a rare complication of meningitis.
- Treatment should be started without delay and refined on the basis of cultures.
- Blood cultures are essential to enhance the chance of isolating the bacteria.
- CSF PCR should be considered in cases where antibiotics have been started prior to lumbar puncture.

Looking Back

The *Streptococcus pneumoniae* bacterium was first discovered in 1881 by Louis Pasteur and named because of its association with pneumonia.

Did You Know?

When grown in culture medium *Streptococcus pneumoniae* forms a colony with a depressed centre, which is known as a draughtsman colony (**Figure 37.4**).

A

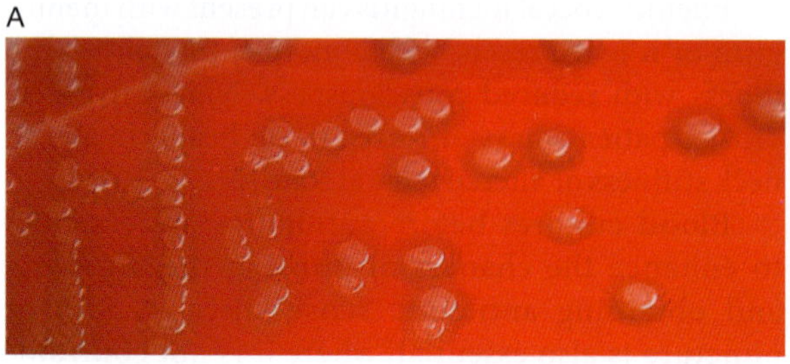

B

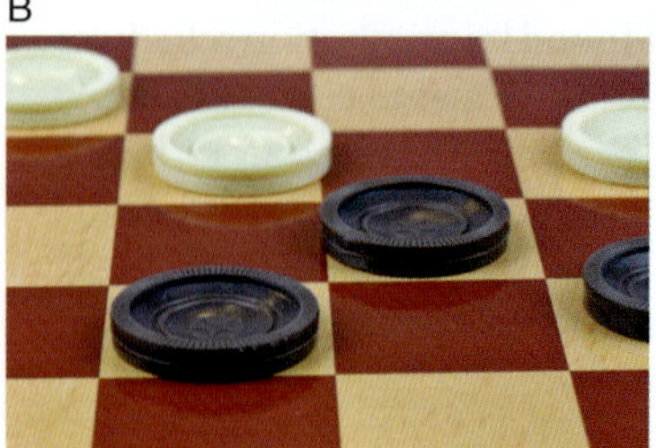

Figure 37.4. (A) *Streptococcus pneumoniae* growing on agar showing typical 'draughtsman' colonies (B). (Source of (B): Douglas Sacha via Getty Images)

References

1. Department of Health. Immunisation against Infectious Diseases: "The Green Book". www.gov.uk/government/publications/pneumococcal-the-green-book-chapter-25 (accessed May 30, 2018).
2. van de Beek D, de Gans J, Spanjaard L, et al. Clinical features and prognostic factors in adults with bacterial meningitis. N Engl J Med 2004;**351**:1849–59.
3. Thigpen MC, Whitney CG, Messonnier NE, et al. Bacterial meningitis in the United States, 1998–2007. N Engl J Med 2011;**364**:2016–25.
4. Michael B, Menezes B, Cunniffe J, et al. Effect of delayed lumbar punctures on the diagnosis of acute bacterial meningitis in adults. Emerg Med J 2010;**27**:433–8.
5. Chiba N, Murayama SY, Morozumi M, et al. Rapid detection of eight causative pathogens for the diagnosis of bacterial meningitis by real-time PCR. J Infect Chemother 2009;**15**:92–8.

CASE 38

Coma in the Family?

Jennifer Lemon, Anu Goenka and Rachel Kneen

History

A 4-year-old Caucasian boy presented with a 3-day history of being unwell with fevers up to 39°C, coryza, abdominal pain, vomiting, sore throat and a brief generalised tonic–clonic seizure. The day before admission he had become increasingly drowsy with intermittent confusion and his mother reported that he had been complaining that he could not see properly. There was no rash or headache. There was no significant past medical history and he had normal neurological development. He was fully vaccinated and there was no history of recent foreign travel.

Examination

He was encephalopathic with a fluctuating Glasgow coma score of 13–14/15; he was intermittently responsive, appearing confused when woken to voice and then becoming unresponsive again. Neurological examination revealed normal tone with brisk reflexes and bilateral up-going plantar responses. Pupils were equal and reactive but he was photophobic and complained of poor vision when roused. There was no meningism or abnormal movements. His throat was inflamed but with no evidence of tonsilar exudate and systemic examination was otherwise unremarkable.

Initial Differential Diagnosis

- Meningoencephalitis
  - Infectious, para-/post-infectious or autoimmune cause (including acute disseminated encephalomyelitis)
- Encephalopathy of another cause including toxic, metabolic, genetic, e.g. Leigh syndrome, a mitochondrial cytopathy

Results of Initial Investigations

Blood tests showed that the C-reactive protein was 16 mg/l, white cell count (WCC) 4 cells/mm^3, neutrophils 1.6 cells/mm^3, with an elevated urea of 8.3 mmol/l and blood glucose of 4.8 mmol/l. Blood gas showed a metabolic acidosis with pH of 7.31. Liver function tests were markedly abnormal with alanine aminotransferase of 1452 iu/l, with normal ammonia. The chest X-ray showed peri-hilar changes but no focal consolidation.

On lumbar puncture, clear colourless cerebrospinal fluid (CSF) was obtained with WCC 3×10^6 cells/mm^3 with no organisms seen on Gram stain. CSF protein was mildly elevated at 0.63 g/l and glucose was 3.5 mmol/l (CSF to serum ratio 0.7). A computed tomography (CT) brain scan was normal. Cranial magnetic resonance imaging (MRI) was performed

Figure 38.1. Axial T2-weighted MRI brain scan of a 4-year-old Caucasian boy who presented with a 3-day history of fevers.

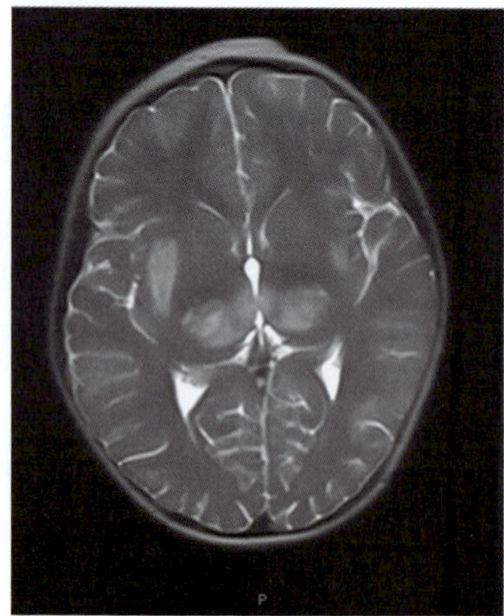

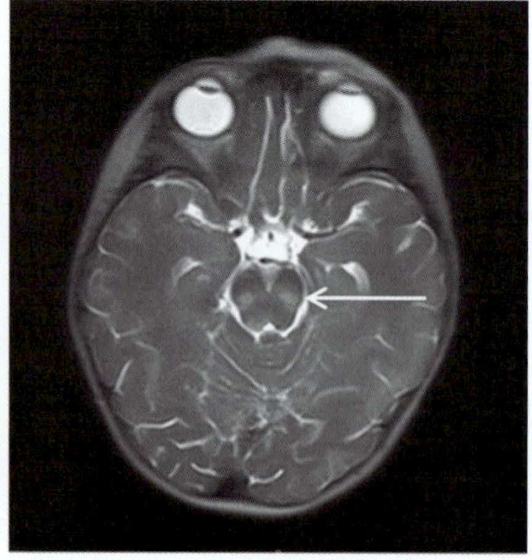

The images show bilateral symmetrical signal changes in the thalami, internal capsule, tegmentum and limbic structures (A) and brainstem (arrow; B) consistent with acute necrotising encephalopathy

(**Figure 38.1**). Blood and CSF cultures were negative, and CSF viral polymerase chain reaction (PCR) was negative for herpes simplex virus, varicella zoster virus, enteroviruses and influenza A and B. Serum and CSF voltage-gated potassium channel (VGKC) and *N*-methyl-D-aspartate (NMDA) receptor antibodies also later came back as negative.

Results of Definitive Investigations

PCR of respiratory secretions was positive for influenza A: H1N1.

Diagnosis

The clinical picture and MRI changes were consistent with acute necrotising encephalopathy in association with influenza A, H1N1.

Management and Outcome

Initial treatment included intravenous (IV) ceftriaxone, aciclovir and oral clarithromycin as well as IV methylprednisolone. However, he deteriorated a few hours after admission with falling Glasgow coma score and further generalised seizures. He was transferred to the intensive care unit and was ventilated for 3 days. The confusion improved over the next few days. Ongoing treatment included 3 days of IV methylprednisolone followed by a tapering course of prednisolone and intravenous immunoglobulin given over 2 days on day 4 and 5 of admission. Ophthalmological assessment showed decreased visual acuity and abnormal visual evoked responses, in the absence of any evidence of ocular pathology, reflecting cortical visual impairment. Following intensive neuro-rehabilitation the child was discharged 6 weeks later. Ongoing problems at discharge included reduced visual acuity, short-term memory loss and a mild left hemiparesis. Follow up neuropsychology assessments have revealed significant cognitive deficits including memory problems.

Prevention

Acute necrotising encephalopathy is a rare form of acute encephalopathy and there is no known prevention. Some cases with recurrent or familial acute necrotising encephalopathy have been reported in association with a mutation in the Ran-binding Protein 2 (*RANBP2*) gene (**Figure 38.2**). Immunisation for seasonal influenza is available, particularly for high-risk groups.

Discussion

Acute necrotising encephalopathy is characterised by an acute encephalopathic illness on a background of suspected viral infection, most often influenza A (Box 38.1).

Box 38.1. Diagnostic criteria for acute necrotising encephalopathy, adapted from Mizuguchi et al.[1,2].

1. Clinical: acute encephalopathy following a viral febrile illness with alteration in level of consciousness and seizures.
2. Laboratory: CSF leucocyte count less than 8/mm^3 with elevated protein is commonly observed. Variable elevation in transaminases with normal ammonia.
3. Imaging: CT/MRI findings of symmetrical multifocal brain lesions with involvement of the thalami. Lesions may also be found in the cerebral periventricular white matter, internal capsule, putamen, upper brainstem tegmentum and cerebellar medulla.
4. Exclusion of differential diagnoses:
   a. Clinical: overwhelming bacterial/viral infection, fulminant hepatitis, toxic shock syndrome, haemolytic uraemic syndrome, Reye syndrome, haemorrhagic shock and encephalopathy syndrome and heat stroke.
   b. Radiological/pathological: Leigh encephalopathy, glutaric acidaemia, methylmalonic acidaemia, Wernicke encephalopathy, carbon monoxide poisoning, ADEM, acute haemorrhagic leukoencephalitis, cerebral infarction, trauma.

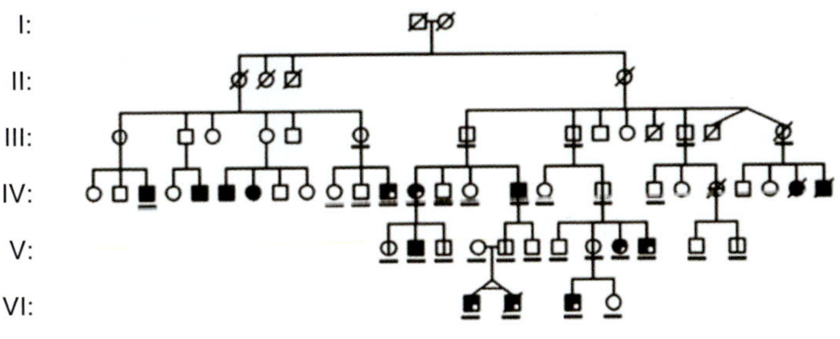

Figure 38.2. Pedigree of a family with acute necrotising encephalopathy (ANE) due to a *RANBP2* mutation, which shows the variable penetrance of the mutation. Symbol notations: filled, carrier affected with ANE; filled with white lower right quadrant, carrier with recurrent ANE; horizontal bar, encephalopathy unconfirmed as ANE; diagonal bar, carrier not affected with ANE; underline symbol, DNA studied). (Reproduced with permission from [3].)

Acute necrotising encephalopathy was first identified in Japan and has been most commonly, but not always, reported in East Asia. It is a paediatric illness, predominantly affecting children less than 5 years of age. It is very rare, with less than 100 cases reported. The pathogenesis is unknown but studies have shown evidence of increased pro-inflammatory cytokine levels in the serum and CSF of acute necrotising encephalopathy patients leading to the hypothesis that a 'cytokine storm' may play an important role [4]. Post-mortem examination has shown symmetrical multifocal acute necrosis and oedema involving grey and white matter with evidence of blood–brain barrier disruption [2]. Acute necrotising encephalopathy usually occurs soon after an upper respiratory tract infection; the most commonly isolated virus is influenza, but cases have been reported following many other infectious agents [5]. Some cases may be recurrent or familial and a recent study which reported 16 such cases found an autosomal dominant genetic mutation in *RANBP2* in 12 [3]. *RANBP2* is a nuclear pore protein with complex roles within the cell cycle. The mechanism by which it may predispose individuals to developing acute necrotising encephalopathy is not understood and the genetic defect shows variable penetrance, with some carriers never displaying symptoms (**Figure 38.2**). The mutation has not been found in sporadic cases [3,6].

Acute necrotising encephalopathy classically presents with high fever, lethargy and seizures on a background of viral symptoms. The child may be delirious and coma progresses rapidly. Other common neurological findings include decerebrate/decorticate posturing, hyper-reflexia, miosis and papilloedema. Shock and other signs of systemic compromise may be present [2]. Blood tests commonly reveal variable elevations in serum amino transaminases, lactate dehydrogenase, creatine kinase and urea with a metabolic acidosis. Normal ammonia and blood glucose can help to distinguish acute necrotising encephalopathy from Reye's syndrome, an important differential diagnosis [2,5]. Thrombocytopaenia and deranged clotting studies are reported in severe cases. CSF analysis often reveals mildly elevated protein with no pleocytosis [2,5]. EEG is non-specific, showing diffuse slow waves, typical of any encephalopathy. Neuroimaging reveals bilateral symmetrical lesions, which invariably affect the thalami in addition to the cerebral white matter, brainstem and cerebellum; however, CT can be normal, particularly early in the disease [2].

The evidence base to guide the treatment of ANE is limited to anecdotal reports variably describing the use of steroids, IVIG, antiviral therapy, anti-cytokine therapy and plasmapheresis [5]. Some have also attempted therapeutic hypothermia [7]. There is some limited retrospective data describing a better outcome in those who had received steroid treatment early and those without brainstem lesions on imaging [8].

Classically the disease peaks in severity after a few days with gradual recovery over a period of several weeks. Prognosis is variable and young age, brainstem lesions and high aminotransferases have been associated with a worse outcome. The majority of survivors have neurological impairment of varying degrees [9].

Key Points

- Acute necrotising encephalopathy is a rare acute para-/post-infectious encephalopathy
- Think of it in an encephalopathic child with metabolic acidosis, and abnormal liver function tests, but normal ammonia and glucose (unlike Reye's syndrome)
- Characteristic imaging findings include bilateral symmetrical thalamic lesions, and sometimes involvement of the cerebral white matter, brainstem and cerebellum.
- Acute necrotising encephalopathy may be more common in East Asian populations, and in familial cases is associated with mutations in the *RANBP2* gene.

Looking Back

In 1979, the first case report of a child with acute encephalopathy and multifocal symmetrical brain lesions was published. However, it was not until 1995 that Japanese paediatrician Mizuguchi identified acute necrotising encephalopathy as a separate disease entity, by examining features of cases with similar clinical, radiological and pathological features.

Did You Know?

The word influenza is thought to derive from the Latin term *influentia*, used to convey the belief in the fifteenth and sixteenth centuries that the epidemics occurred due to unfavourable astrological 'influence' [10] (**Figure 38.3**)

LVCAS GAVRICVS GEOPHO: NESIS EP.
Dum coeli arcanos motus et ſidera tractas,
Eſt data Pontificis munere mitra tibi.

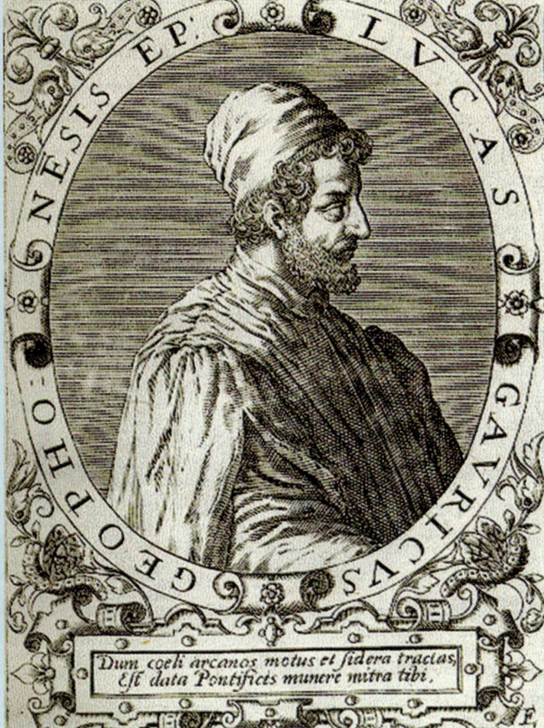

Figure 38.3. Luca Gaurico, a sixteenth-century Italian Astrologer who believed that the fate of man was influenced by the stars. (Artwork held at Université de Mannheim.)

References

1. Mizuguchi M, Yamanouchi H, Ichiyama T, Shiomi M. Acute encephalopathy associated with influenza and other viral infections. Acta Neurol Scand 2007;**115**:45–56.
2. Mizuguchi M, Abe J, Mikkaichi K, et al. Acute necrotising encephalopathy of childhood: a new syndrome presenting with multifocal, symmetric brain lesions. J Neurol Neurosurg Psychiatry 1995;**58**:555–61.
3. Neilson DE, Adams MD, Orr CMD, et al. Infection-triggered familial or recurrent cases of acute necrotizing encephalopathy caused by mutations in a component of the nuclear pore, *RANBP2*. Am J Human Gene 2009;**84**:44–51.
4. Kansagra SM, Gallentine WB. Case report: cytokine storm of acute necrotizing encephalopathy. Pediatr Neurol 2011;**45**:400–2.
5. Fung S, Lau K, Cherk S, Kan E. Parainfluenza infection associated acute necrotising encephalopathy: survival despite initial fulminant neurological presentation. Hong Kong J Paediatr 2011;**16**:278–84.
6. Loh N, Appleton DB. Untreated recurrent acute necrotising encephalopathy associated with *RANBP2* mutation, and normal outcome in a Caucasian boy. Eur J Pediatr 2010;**169**:1299–302.
7. Munakata M, Kato R, Yokoyama H, et al. Combined therapy with hypothermia and anticytokine agents in influenza A encephalopathy. Brain Dev 2000;**22**:373–7.
8. Okumura A, Mizuguchi M, Kidokoro H, et al. Original article: Outcome of acute necrotizing encephalopathy in relation to treatment with corticosteroids and gammaglobulin. Brain Dev 1999;**31**:221–7.
9. Mizuguchi M. Acute necrotizing encephalopathy of childhood: a novel form of acute encephalopathy prevalent in Japan and Taiwan. Brain Dev 1997;**19**:81–92.
10. DeLacy M. The conceptualization of influenza in eighteenth century Britain: specificity and contagion. Bull Hist Med 1993;**67**;74–118.

CASE 39

A Travelling Salesman, Slowing Down

Sam Nightingale

History

A 56-year-old man presented to a hospital in the USA with memory problems. He was born in the UK, but in his role as a deputy director of an international company he had travelled extensively in Asia and the Americas and now lived in California. Over the past 2–3 months he had become increasingly forgetful. He had been finding it difficult to concentrate at work and his colleagues commented his work rate had slowed down. They also felt his personality had changed, becoming apathetic and withdrawn. He had stopped socialising after work and friends felt he may be depressed.

He had no significant past medical history other than two episodes of shingles over the past three years. In the past few months he had had several episodes of loose stool, and had lost around a stone in weight. There were no urinary symptoms.

Examination

He had a flat affect but conversed normally with no dysphasia. He scored 24/30 on the mini-mental state examination, losing points on attention and calculation, orientation and recall.

His gait was a little slow and broad-based, although there was no clinical evidence of limb ataxia or bradykinesia. The rest of the neurological examination was recorded as unremarkable.

General examination revealed dry flaky skin, and two scars in thoracic dermatomes corresponding to previous shingles. There were multiple small non-tender lymph nodes palpable in the cervical and inguinal regions.

Results of Initial Investigations

His haemoglobin was slightly low at 115 g/l, with a mean corpuscular volume of 85 fl, his white cell count (WCC) was 3.5×10^9/l and platelets were 120×10^9/l. His initial renal and hepatic biochemistry were normal. His inflammatory markers were slightly raised with a C-reactive protein of 15 mg/l and erythrocyte sedimentation rate of 22 mm/hour. Thyroid function, vitamin B12, VDRL and TPHA were all normal. He was ANA-positive 1:160 (low titre) and ANCA-negative. A urine dipstick examination was normal.

A lumbar puncture (LP) showed an opening pressure of 18 cm H_2O, the WCC was 5×10^6/l (100% lymphocytes), protein 0.6 g/l, glucose 3.4 mmol/l (plasma glucose 5.6 mmol/l) and there were matched oligoclonal bands in the cerebrospinal fluid (CSF) and blood. The CSF was both Gram stain and culture negative; viral polymerase chain reaction was negative for herpes simplex virus types 1 and 2, varicella zoster virus (VZV), parechovirus, enterovirus, Epstein–Barr virus (EBV), cytomegalovirus (CMV); CSF VDRL and TPHA were also negative. It was not recorded whether his cognitive impairment or gait improved with the LP.

A magnetic resonance imaging (MRI) of his brain was performed (**Figure 39.1**). Electroencephalography showed non-specific slowing.

Initial Differential Diagnosis

Due to the cognitive problems, gait disturbance and MRI abnormalities he was initially diagnosed with normal pressure hydrocephalus, although no urinary symptoms were present. Repeat LP was arranged to see if there was therapeutic response to CSF removal. Due to the abnormalities in full blood count he was due to undergo investigation for haematological malignancy; however, he did not attend this appointment for further investigation or repeat lumbar puncture and was lost to follow-up.

Further History and Examination

His memory problems worsened and he lost his job. He became withdrawn and lost all interest in hobbies and social activities. He had difficulties with fine movements and needed help doing up buttons. His gait slowed down and became shuffling. He was unsteady with frequent falls. As he now required care he returned to the UK to live with his sister. At this point, 3 months after initial presentation in the USA, he re-presented to medical care in the UK.

He now had marked cognitive impairment, particularly in learning of new information, information processing and attention/concentration. Mini-mental state examination was now 11/30. He was withdrawn and minimally conversant, rarely making eye contact.

There was significant bradykinesia and his gait was slow and shuffling. Limb power was normal but tone

Figure 39.1. (A) T1-weighted- and (B) T2-weighted saggital MRI images of a 56-year-old man with 2–3 months cognitive decline.

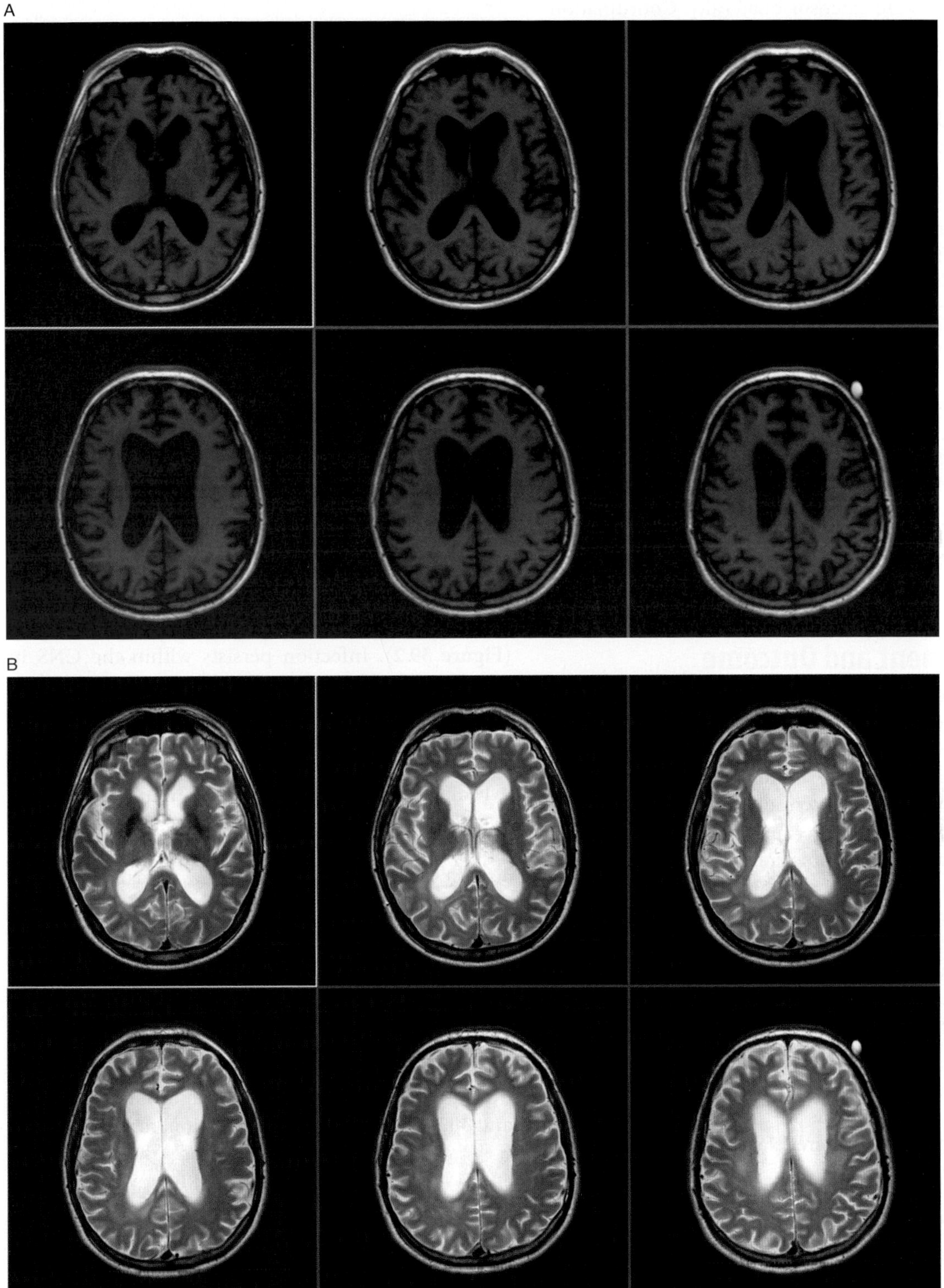

This reveals enlarged lateral ventricles, and sulci, without evidence of obstructive hydrocephalus. No intra- or extra-parenchymal lesion is identified. There is no abnormal enhancement with gadolinium.

was increased throughout, reflexes were brisk and plantar responses were extensor bilaterally. Coordination was normal. There was loss to pin-prick sensation in the toes bilaterally, vibration sense was present at the ankles. Frontal release signs were present.

He underwent further investigations. Lumbar puncture was repeated: WCC 7 × 10^6/l (100% lymphocytes), protein 1.03 g/l, glucose 2.3 mmol/l (plasma 4 mmol/l); Gram stain, India ink and Ziehl–Neelsen stains were negative. MRI appearances were essentially unchanged from earlier.

Results of Definitive Investigations

HIV antibody test was positive. Further tests revealed his CD4+ve T cell count was 9 c/ml; the HIV viral load was 140,000 c/ml; and his hepatitis C antibody was negative.

CSF cryptococcal antigen was negative, as was viral PCR for CMV, EBV, VZV, JC virus. CSF HIV was positive with a viral load of 200,000 copies/ml.

Diagnosis

HIV-associated dementia.

Management and Outcome

He was treated with combination antiretroviral therapy (efavirenz, tenofovir, entricitabine) with good immune recovery. CD4+ve T-cell count increased to 220 copies/ml over 3 months. He became more responsive and less withdrawn. His memory improved, although he remained impaired with mini-mental state examination of 21/30. His bradykinesia and gait improved, although he remained slow and required assistance for complex fine tasks. He was discharged to live with his sister with the help of carers once a day.

Prevention

Prevention of HIV-associated dementia is by early recognition and antiretroviral treatment. In those for whom cognitive problems are the first presentation of HIV the diagnosis is often delayed as a HIV test was not done earlier.

Discussion

HIV-associated dementia describes a syndrome of marked cognitive impairment that occurs in advanced HIV disease, usually at CD4 counts less than 200 copies/ml, and is an AIDS-defining illness. It is due to HIV

Figure 39.2. A high-power microscopic view of a section of brain from a child with HIV encephalitis, the histopathological correlate of HIV-associated dementia. A multinucleate giant cell is arrowed. (Image W0043194 from the Wellcome Library (reproduced under CC0).)

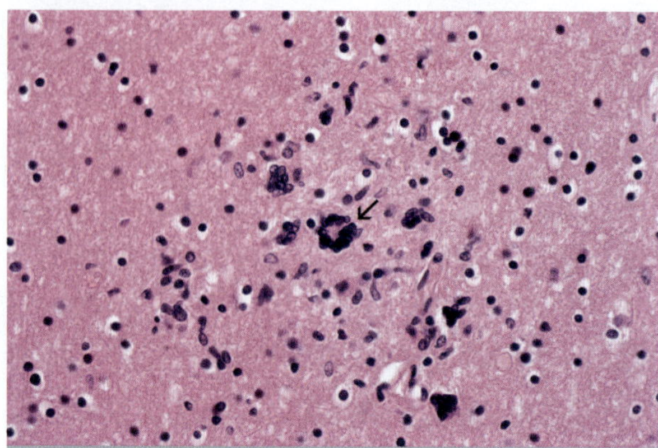

infection itself, rather than the effect of opportunistic infections.

HIV enters the brain early in infection via infected macrophages and monocytes. Pathologically, activated macrophages and astrocytes, sometimes with multinucleated giant cells, are seen in the brain parenchyma (**Figure 39.2**). Infection persists within the CNS in perivascular macrophages and microglia, although direct neuronal infection is rare [1]. Pro-inflammatory cytokines and toxic viral products cause blood–brain barrier breakdown, rarefaction of white matter, astrocyte apoptosis, dendritic simplification, and neuronal loss [2]. Subcortical structures such as basal ganglia and the hippocampus appear to be the most vulnerable and the clinical phenotype of HIV-associated dementia is that of subcortical dementia with a combination of cognitive and motor impairment (**Table 39.1**).

There may be clues in the history that someone with cognitive impairment has HIV, such as recurrent herpes zoster, weight loss and diarrhoea, as there was in this case. Other clues may come from routine investigations: normocytic anaemia, lymphopaenia and thrombocytopaenia are present in around 65%, 80% and 30% of those with HIV infection, respectively [3]. HIV is an important treatable cause of dementia and an HIV test should be performed in anyone presenting with cognitive problems, regardless of age, race or sexual orientation [4].

The case described above illustrates the typical progression and clinical features of the disease. Initially motor features were minimal and cognitive impairment was the prominent complaint. Early symptoms

Table 39.1 International HIV Dementia Scale.
A tool to help classify HIV patients with dementia, used especially in research.

Memory Registration: Give four words to recall (dog, hat, bean, red) – 1 second to say each. Then ask the patient to say all four words after you have said them.

Repeat words if the patient does not recall them all immediately. Tell the patient you will ask for recall of the words again a bit later.

1. Motor speed

Have the patient tap the first two fingers of the non-dominant hand as widely and as quickly as possible.

4 = 15 in 5 seconds

3 = 11–14 in 5 seconds

2 = 7–10 in 5 seconds

1 = 3–6 in 5 seconds

0 = 0–2 in 5 seconds

2. Psychomotor speed

Have the patient perform the following movements with the non-dominant hand as quickly as possible.

- Clench hand in fist on flat surface
- Put hand flat on surface with palm down
- Put hand perpendicular to the flat surface on the side of the 5th digit
- Demonstrate and have patient perform twice for practice

4 = 4 sequences in 10 seconds

3 = 3 sequences in 10 seconds

2 = 2 sequences in 10 seconds

1 = 1 sequence in 10 seconds

0 = unable to perform

3. Memory-recall

Ask the patient to recall the four words. For words not recalled, prompt with a semantic clue as follows:

Animal (dog); piece of clothing (hat); vegetable (bean); colour (red).

Give 1 point for each word spontaneously recalled. Give 0.5 points for each correct answer after prompting.

Maximum 4 points.

Total International HIV Dementia Scale Score: this is the sum of the scores on items 1–3. The maximum possible score is 12 points.

A patient with a score of less than or equal to 10 should be evaluated further for possible dementia.

include forgetfulness and inability to concentrate, as well as personality changes such as apathy, diminished libido, emotional lability and depression. Individuals may withdraw from social activities or have difficulty managing the financial and administrative aspects of their life. In moderate disease motor abnormalities become more prominent, particularly slowing and impairment of fine movements, for example doing up buttons. In this case there was significant progression over weeks to months with bradykinesia, spasticity, pyramidal signs, gait disturbance and frontal release signs. Late features include psychiatric disturbances, mutism, paraplegia, seizures, incontinence and myoclonus.

HIV-associated dementia is a diagnosis of exclusion because multiple central nervous system (CNS) pathologies occur in people with HIV. Rapidly developing symptoms should warrant investigation for a different aetiology, particularly if associated with impairment of consciousness, headache or neck stiffness, which are not features of HIV-associated dementia. There should be a low threshold for LP to exclude CNS infections such as neurosyphilis, cryptococcal meningitis, tuberculous meningitis, EBV-related primary CNS lymphoma, or encephalitis due to VZV, CMV or EBV. In HIV-associated dementia the CSF is usually unremarkable, although there may be a mild pleocytosis, rarely exceeding 50×10^6/l and matched oligoclonal bands are often present. In the pre-antiretroviral therapy era greater levels of HIV RNA in the CSF were seen [5].

MRI may show large confluent periventricular lesions, hyperintense and relatively symmetrical in the white matter with atrophy representing leukoencephalopathy. None of these findings are specific for HIV-associated dementia and the disease may be present with a normal MRI. In this case ex-vacuole hydrocephalus, caused by volume loss from significant white matter atrophy rather than changes in CSF flow, was initially mistaken for normal pressure hydrocephalus.

Many individuals with HIV-associated dementia improve when commenced on antiretroviral medications [6]. This can be quite marked and some individuals return to independence following treatment; however, response is variable and others may show only modest improvement. Some antiretroviral drugs achieve higher levels in the CSF than others; however, opinions vary as to whether to choose antiretroviral treatment for patients with HIV-associated dementia on the basis of the drugs' CNS penetration [7,8].

Since combination antiretroviral therapy has been widely available in the West the incidence of HIV-associated dementia has declined; however, more subtle neurocognitive impairments remain. Several cross-sectional studies in the antiretroviral era have estimated the prevalence of HIV-associated neurocognitive disorders in the region of 20–50% [9]. This is thought to be due to a combination of demographic factors, comorbidities, antiretroviral neurotoxicity and substance misuse, as well as the potential impact of limited CNS penetration of antiretrovirals leading to loss of control of HIV replication in the CNS.

Key Points

- HIV is an important treatable cause of dementia. All patients presenting with acquired cognitive impairment should have an HIV test [10,11].
- HIV-associated dementia is typically a subcortical dementia presenting with a combination of motor and cognitive features, including bradykinesia, spasticity, poor attention and concentration, apathy, social withdrawal and depression.
- HIV-associated dementia is a diagnosis of exclusion. Other HIV-related CNS infections must be ruled out, particularly if there is rapid progression, headache, or signs of meningism.
- Although the incidence of HIV-associated dementia has declined with antiretroviral treatment, milder forms of cognitive impairment appear to be common.

Looking Back

In the pre-antiretroviral era, up to 40% of those with AIDS developed HIV-associated dementia before death.

Did You Know?

In the pre-antiretroviral drug era, HIV testing required all sorts of rather complicated counselling, requiring specially trained nurses. Now that the disease is treatable, testing for HIV should be performed as readily as testing for syphilis.

In the UK, 90,000 people are infected with HIV, a quarter of whom are unaware of their diagnosis [10].

References

1. Budka H. Neuropathology of human immunodeficiency virus infection. Brain Pathol 1991;**1**:163–75.
2. Navia BA, Cho ES, Petito CK, Price RW. The AIDS dementia complex: II. Neuropathology. Annals Neurol 1986;**19**:525–35.
3. Das G, Baglioni P, Okosieme O. Primary HIV infection. BMJ 2010;**341**:c4583.
4. Palfreeman A, Fisher M, Ong E, et al. Testing for HIV: concise guidance. Clin Med 2009;**9**:471–6.
5. Sonnerborg AB, Ehrnst AC, Bergdahl SK, et al. HIV isolation from cerebrospinal fluid in relation to immunological deficiency and neurological symptoms. AIDS 1988;**2**:89–93.
6. Cysique LA, Vaida F, Letendre S, et al. Dynamics of cognitive change in impaired HIV-positive patients initiating antiretroviral therapy. Neurology 2009;**73**:342–8.
7. Williams I, Churchill D, Anderson J, et al. British HIV Association guidelines for the treatment of HIV-1-positive adults with antiretroviral therapy 2012. HIV Med 2012;**13**:1–85.
8. Letendre S, Marquie-Beck J, Capparelli E, et al. Validation of the CNS Penetration-Effectiveness rank for quantifying antiretroviral penetration

into the central nervous system. Arch Neurol 2008;**65**:65–70.

9. Heaton RK, Clifford DB, Franklin DR Jr, et al. HIV-associated neurocognitive disorders persist in the era of potent antiretroviral therapy: CHARTER Study. Neurology 2010;**75**:2087–96.

10. Health Protection Agency. HIV in the United Kingdom: 2011 Report. London: Health Protection Services; 2011.

11. Nightingale S, Michael BD, Defres S, Benjamin LA, Solomon T. Test them all; an easily diagnosed and readily treatable cause of dementia with life-threatening consequences if missed. Pract Neurol 2013;**13**:354–6.

CASE **40** # A Nasty, Rare and Ironic Unwanted Effect

Hema Bentur and Rachel Kneen

History and Examination

A 6-year-old girl with idiopathic thrombocytopaenia purpura (ITP) was being treated as a day case with intravenous immunoglobulin (IVIG) at a total dose of 2 g/kg over 2 days. On day 2 of treatment she represented to hospital, 6 hours after completion of the infusion, with severe headache, vomiting, fever and neck stiffness. On examination, her temperature was 38°C and her vital signs were stable. She had signs of meningeal irritation in the form of marked neck stiffness and photophobia, in addition to positive Kernig's and Brudzinski's signs. Fundus examination was normal and there was no focal neurological deficit. Other systems were normal and a diagnosis of meningitis was felt to be most likely.

Differential Diagnosis

The differential diagnosis included meningitis, which may have been viral, bacterial, mycobacterial, fungal or aseptic, such as due to IVIG therapy. Although she did not present with the classical thunderclap headache, meningeal irritation could also have been caused by a subarachnoid haemorrhage secondary to ITP.

Investigations

Baseline bloods revealed: C-reactive protein 44 mg/l, white cell count (WCC) 11.5 cells/mm^3, platelets 90/mm^3, urea, electrolytes and liver function tests were normal.

A lumbar puncture was performed and, although the opening pressure was not measured, the cerebrospinal fluid (CSF) had a clear and colourless appearance. The CSF WCC was 610 cells/mm^3 with 92% neutrophils. The CSF and serum glucose were 3.4 and 6.5 mmol/l, respectively, giving a ratio of 0.52 and the protein was 0.25 g/l. CSF Gram stain was negative and bacterial cultures of CSF and blood were negative. A computer tomography brain scan was normal, with no intracranial bleed. Subsequently, polymerase chain reaction (PCR) testing of CSF was negative for herpes simplex virus, varicella zoster virus, enterovirus, parechovirus, *Meningococcus* and *Pneumococcus*.

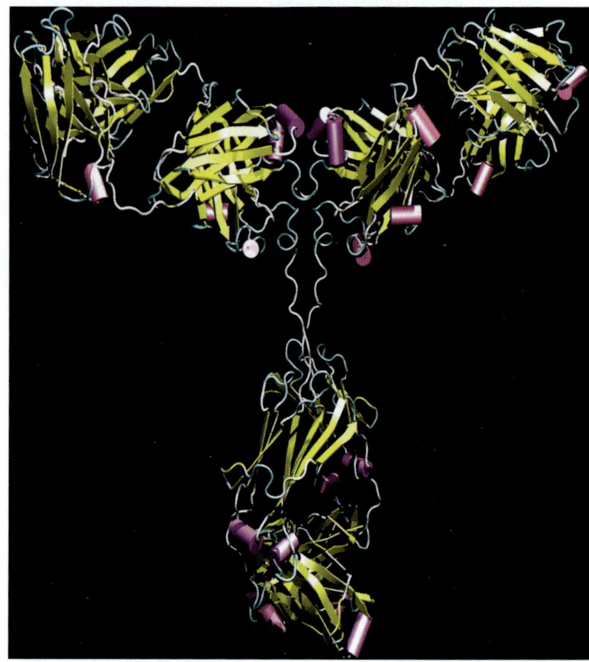

Figure 40.1. A molecular model of a single immunoglobulin G (IgG) antibody showing the two long heavy chains and the two shorter light chains. (Image by Dr Tim Evans/Science Photo Library.)

Progress

She was treated with analgesia and intravenous (IV) fluids, which led to a rapid improvement in her symptoms. She was also initially treated with IV cefotaxime for 48 hours, which was discontinued when the CSF cultures and bacterial PCR results were found to be negative. She made an excellent recovery over the next 48 hours.

Diagnosis

Aseptic meningitis secondary to immune reaction to intravenous immunoglobulin therapy.

Discussion

IVIG is an immunomodulatory agent with a spectrum of proposed mechanisms of action including direct neutralisation of antigens and toxins, blockade of Fc receptors on immune system cells, and suppression of synthesis of cytokines and autoantibodies (**Figure 40.1** and **Table 40.1**) [1]. It is used in the treatment of various disorders

Table 40.1 Hypothesised modes of action of intravenous immunoglobulin (from [2] with permission of Elsevier).

- Saturation and modulation of the expression of Fc receptors
- Binding of sialylated-IgG to DC-Sign
- Saturation of neonatal Fc receptors
- Modulation of dendritic cells
- Expansion of regulatory T cells
- Decreasing pro-inflammatory effects of monocytes
- Decreasing the interferon-response
- Inhibition of the complement activation cascade
- Neutralisation of chemokines and/or cytokines
- Inhibition of apoptosis
- Neutralisation of auto-antibodies

Ig, immunoglobulin; DC-Sign, dendritic cell-specific intercellular adhesion molecule-3-grabbing non-integrin.

including primary immune deficiencies, ITP, Kawasaki disease, Guillain–Barré syndrome and other demyelinating polyneuropathies, autoimmune encephalitis, autoimmune haemolytic anaemia, autoimmune neutropaenia, acquired haemophilia A, systemic lupus erythematosus, rheumatoid arthritis, myasthenia gravis, paediatric acquired immunodeficiency syndrome, bone marrow transplantation, and an expanding range of medical conditions; for some of these there is good evidence of efficacy, for others it is less clear (**Table 40.2**) [1,3].

IVIG is produced from the pooled plasma of healthy donors. Differences in manufacturing and the stabilisers, diluents and concentrations used in the various commercial preparations lead to variations in side effect profile and tolerability [4]. The effectiveness of IVIG is well-documented for many of the conditions described, and it is generally considered as a safe therapy. Most frequent adverse effects are mild and transient, which include headache, flushing, fever, chills, myalgia, fatigue, dyspnoea, back pain, nausea, vomiting, diarrhoea, blood pressure changes and tachycardia [5,6]. One study reported mild to moderate headache in just over half of their patients following IVIG therapy [3]. Most symptoms resolve within an hour of stopping or slowing of infusion, and respond to simple symptomatic treatment. More serious effects are rare and include anaphylaxis, haemolysis, hepatitis, thrombosis, arthritis and renal failure [5,6].

Aseptic meningitis has been reported as a serious complication following IVIG therapy, with some studies reporting this in up to11–17% of patients, but routine clinical risk quoted in UK guidelines is < 5% [3,7]. It is a self limiting condition and the exact mechanism is not understood. The possible mechanisms include a hypersensitivity reaction to the direct entry of IgG into the CSF, sensitivity to the stabilising products, cytokine

Table 40.2 Association of British Neurologists Guidelines for the use of IVIG. (Reproduced from [8] with permission of Elsevier.)

Group A. IVIG use supported by randomised controlled trials:

- Guillain–Barré syndrome
- Chronic inflammatory demyelinating polyradiculoneuropathy
- Multifocal motor neuropathy with conduction block
- Paraprotein-associated demyelinating neuropathy
- Myaesthenia gravis
- Lambert–Eaton myaesthenic syndrome
- Dermatomyositis and polymyositis

Group B. IVIG may be considered under special circumstances (specific details in guidelines)

- Acute disseminated encephalomyelitis
- CNS vasculitis
- Intractable epilepsy
- Multiple sclerosis
- Neuromyotonia
- Paraneoplastic disorders
- Potassium-channel antibody-associated, non-neoplastic limbic encephalitis
- Stiff person syndrome

Group V. There is no evidence to support the use of IVIG

- Chronic fatigue syndrome
- Inclusion body myositis
- Peripheral neuropathy (other than those above)

The UK Department of Health introduced a Demand Management Programme with colour coding to reflect the prioritisation of immunoglobulin treatment in times of shortage, based on the availability of alternative treatments and strength of clinical evidence.

release triggered by the therapy, increased sensitivity of the meningeal vasculature to exogenous IgG and direct meningeal irritation [3]. In the majority of patients developing meningitis, symptoms are reported to occur within 48 hours of IVIG infusion, but some cases have presented as late as 7 days after the infusion [9]. Patients with a history of migraine are reported to be more likely to develop aseptic meningitis, but there does not appear to be a link to different preparations of immunoglobulins [3,10]. The risk has been reported as higher in those receiving high-dose treatment [10]. Aseptic meningitis has also been reported following administration of other treatments including anti-inflammatory drugs (e.g. ibuprofen, naproxen), sulphonamides, allopurinol and methotrexate [10,11].

Occasionally, recurrence has been reported after repeated IVIG, but no long-term sequelae have been reported. Several approaches have been suggested to attempt to reduce the risk of aseptic meningitis in those receiving IVIG, for those who are either considered at particular risk or who have had previous aseptic meningitis in response to IVIG, but the evidence is anecdotal.

These include slow infusion of low-concentration IVIG products with hydration [10,11]. Once aseptic meningitis has developed, and infectious causes have been excluded, symptomatic treatment alone is usually sufficient [11]. There is no evidence to support the use of corticosteroids [3,11].

Key Points

- Aseptic meningitis is a recognised complication of IVIG therapy and clinicians should be vigilant for the signs and symptoms.
- The risk/benefit of further doses of IVIG in a patient with previous aseptic meningitis should be weighed up.

Looking Back

Processes to fractionate human plasma, the initial step for IVIG production, were first developed in the 1940s by American scientists to create a stable blood derivative, albumin, that could be stockpiled for treating soldiers with blood loss in World War II.

Did You Know?

IVIG was initially developed to prevent and treat infectious diseases, such as measles and polio, through passive transfer of antibodies, before being used as replacement therapy in the primary immune deficiencies. Later its role in autoimmune and inflammatory conditions was established, though quite how it works in these conditions is not known.

References

1. Ramasubramanian KV, Kumar A, Kabra SK, Seth V. The role of intravenous immunoglobulins in pediatric diseases. Indian Pediatr 1999;**36**:51–63.
2. Chaigne B, Mouthon L. Mechanisms of action of intravenous immunoglobulin. Transfus Apheresis Sci 2017;**56**:45–9.
3. Sekul EA, Cupler EJ, Dalakas MC. Aseptic meningitis associated with high-dose intravenous immunoglobulin therapy: requency and risk factors. Ann Intern Med 1994;**121**:259–62.
4. Cherin P, Cabane J. Relevant. Criteria for selecting an intravenous immunoglobulin preparation for clinical use. Biodrugs 2010;**24**:211–23.
5. Duhem C, Dicato MA, Ries F. Side-effects of intravenous immune globulins. Clin Exp Immunol 1994;**97**(Suppl 1):79–83.
6. Scribner CL, Kapit RM, Phillips ET, Rickles NM. Aseptic meningitis and intravenous immunoglobulin therapy. Ann Intern Med 1994;**121**:305–6.
7. Schiavotto C, Ruggeri M, Rodeghiero F. Adverse reactions after high-dose intravenous immunoglobulin: incidence in 83 patients treated for idiopathic thrombocytopenic purpura (ITP) and review of the literature. Haematologica 1993;**78**: 35–40.
8. Solomon T, Michael BD, Smith PE, et al. Management of suspected viral encephalitis in adults – Association of British Neurologists and British Infection Association National Guidelines. J Infect 2012;**64**:347–73.
9. Picton P, Chisholm M. Aseptic meningitis associated with high dose immunoglobulin: ase report. BMJ 1997;**315**:1203–4.
10. Jolles S, Sewell WA, Leighton C. Drug-induced aseptic meningitis: diagnosis and management. Drug Saf 2000;**22**:215–26.
11. Jolles S, Hill H. Management of aseptic meningitis secondary to intravenous immunoglobulin. BMJ 1998;**316**:936.

CASE **41** A Rash Diagnosis

Fiona McGill

History

A 17-year-old male was admitted to an accident and emergency department with a 24-hour history of fevers, headache and vomiting. He had had an upper respiratory tract infection for 24 hours prior to admission with a sore throat and coryzal symptoms. He was otherwise fit and well and preparing for A levels at school. He smoked socially and drank alcohol at weekends. He did not take any illegal drugs. He lived at home with his parents and six siblings. Most members of the family had recently had what was thought to be viral gastroenteritis and his youngest brother had been admitted to the children's ward the preceding day with a febrile illness.

Examination

On examination his temperature was 38.2°C, heart rate was 85 beats per minute and his blood pressure was 110/62 mmHg. He was not requiring any supplemental oxygen. Cardiovascular, respiratory and gastrointestinal examinations were all normal. His tonsils and pharynx were erythematous but with no signs of pus or quinsy. He was obviously photophobic and had mild neck stiffness on examination. He also had a rash over his torso and legs (**Figure 41.1**).

Figure 41.1. A 17-year-old patient presenting with headache and fever had a rash similar to this.

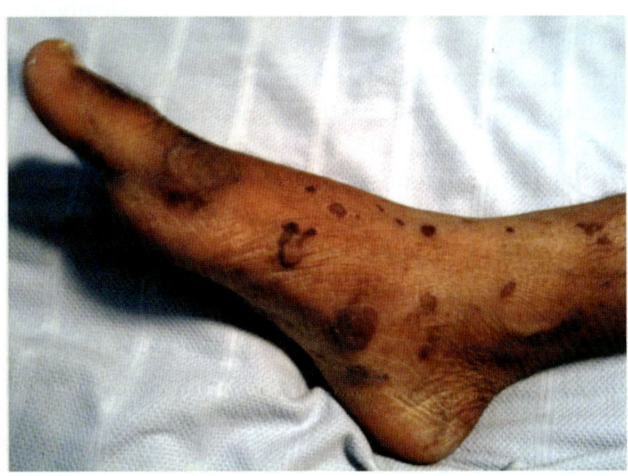

This shows a maculopapular, non-blanching rash. (Photo: Tom Solomon.)

Initial Differential Diagnosis

- Tonsillitis
- Meningitis
- 'Viral illness'
- Norovirus infection

Results of Initial Investigations

Blood tests revealed a peripheral white cell count of 18.2 × 10^9/l with a neutrophil count of 14.34 × 10^9/l and a lymphocyte count of 2.02 × 10^9/l. His C-reactive protein was 184 mg/l. Renal and liver function were normal.

A computer tomography (CT) head scan showed a small amount of cerebral oedema, but no shift of brain compartments.

A lumbar puncture (LP) was performed and found clear and colourless cerebrospinal fluid (CSF), with an opening pressure of 31 cm H_2O; the CSF white cell count was 1403 × 10^6 cells/ml (84% polymorphs), glucose was 1.6 mmol/l (serum 11.6 mmol/l) and protein 6.73 g/l; microscopy confirmed the diagnosis (**Figure 41.2**).

Results of Definitive Investigations

Blood cultures grew *Neisseria meningitidis* within 10 hours.

CSF cultures were negative.

CSF polymerase chain reaction (PCR) was positive for *Neisseria meningitidis.*

Figure 41.2. Microscopy of CSF from a similar patient with fever and meningism.

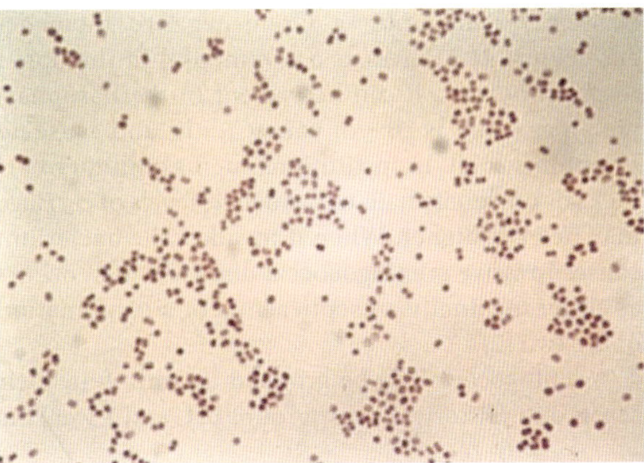

This shows Gram-negative diplococci.

Diagnosis

Meningococcal meningitis and septicaemia.

Management and Outcome

The patient was commenced on intravenous ceftriaxone as soon as he was admitted to hospital. Although he appeared stable on admission he quickly developed septic shock and deteriorated with a drop in conscious level and cardiorespiratory collapse. He was intubated and ventilated for 24 hours and received inotropic support. He had a magnetic resonance imaging (MRI) scan which excluded a venous sinus thrombosis. He improved after 48 hours of cardiorespiratory support and specific antibiotics and he was transferred back to the ward. He received 7 days of intravenous antibiotics in total and was discharged home.

It was also discovered that the patient's younger brother, who had been admitted to the paediatric ward, also had meningococcal meningitis. The rest of the family received prophylaxis.

Prevention

Meningococcal vaccines are available for many serogroups of *Meningococcus*, namely A, C, W135 and Y. Currently in the UK, serogroup C is routinely used in the childhood immunisation schedule and is also given to others at risk, e.g. those who are asplenic or have complement deficiency. There is also a quadrivalent vaccine (ACWY) which should be given to certain risk groups, including travellers to endemic areas [1]. A vaccine against serogroup B has recently been introduced for young children in several countries, including the UK.

Discussion

Neisseria meningitidis, a Gram-negative diplococcus (**Figure 41.3**), lives as a commensal in the upper respiratory tract. It can be present in the nasopharynx in as many as 20% of young adults and cause no symptoms at all. In institutions such as military barracks or university halls of residence, levels of carriage may be even higher. When it invades, the bacterium causes invasive meningococcal disease which occurs as either meningitis or septicaemia or a combination of the two [2].

Meningococci can be grouped according to their serogroup. Historically, serogroups B, C and Y were the commonest in the UK. Following successful vaccination campaigns against serogroup C, the majority of invasive meningococcal disease in the UK is now caused by serogroup B. Other serogroups are common in other parts of the world, such as A in the meningitis belt in Africa, and W135, which has been associated with pilgrimage to Saudi Arabia for the Hajj.

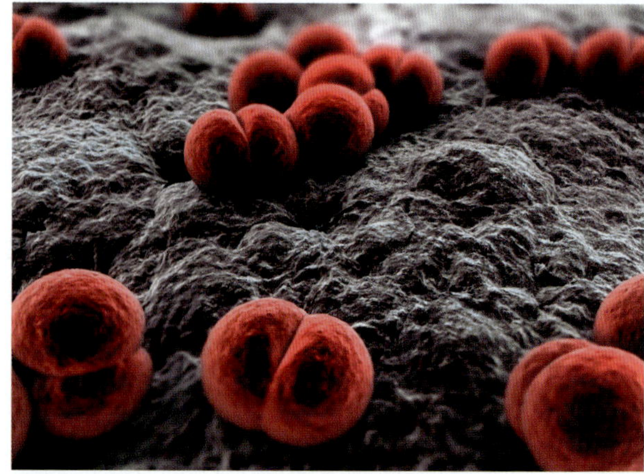

Figure 41.3. Scanning electron micrograph of the Gram-negative diplococci of *Neisseria meningitides*.

Meningococcal disease mainly affects young children (aged 0–5 years) and young adults (15–19 years). In adults *Neisseria meningitidis* is the second most common cause of bacterial meningitis, after *Streptococcus pneumoniae* [3,4].

Meningococcal meningitis is less likely to present with the classic triad of symptoms (neck stiffness, fever and altered consciousness) than pneumococcal meningitis. However, if a rash is present in a patient with meningism, the pathogen is significantly more likely to be *Neisseria meningitidis*. The rash of meningococcal disease can take many forms, but classically it is petechial and non-blanching, as demonstrated by the 'glass test' (**Figure 41.4**). Case fatality rates are lower in meningococcal disease than pneumococcal disease, but increase with age [5].

Definitive diagnosis is made by culturing or identifying the bacteria from CSF or blood. CSF will become sterile rapidly after antibiotics are given (as quickly as 2 hours); therefore, pre-antibiotic blood cultures and non-culture diagnostic methods, such as nucleic acid amplification, are important to isolate or identify the organism [6]. The CSF will normally show a raised white cell count with a predominance of neutrophils, as it did for the patient described here, although if

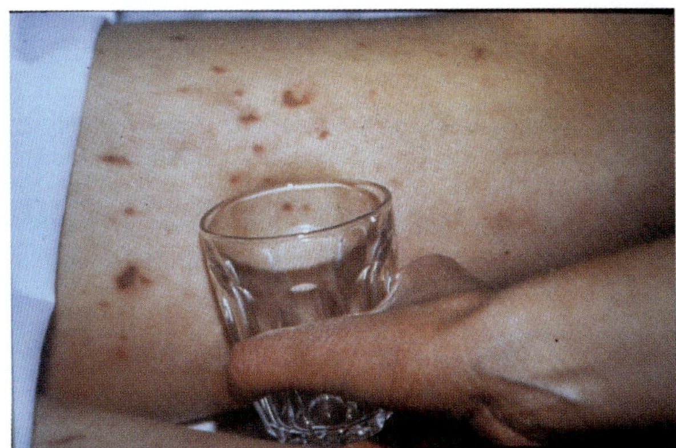

Figure 41.4. Glass test showing the non-blanching petechial rash of meningococcal disease, which persists despite the pressure of the glass. (Figure kindly provided by the Meningitis Research Foundation.)

antibiotics have been given before the LP the predominant cell type may be lymphocytes.

Broad-spectrum antibiotics should be initiated on suspicion of meningitis (after blood cultures have been taken). If a LP can be done within half an hour then ideally antibiotics could wait until after the lumbar puncture [7]. Practically, this is rarely possible and so they should be initiated as soon as possible after the blood cultures have been taken. Second- or third-generation cephalosporins are usually the treatment of choice [8].

The duration of treatment has not been determined definitively, but it is likely that 5–7 days is adequate [9].

Neisseria meningitidis is transmitted via the respiratory route and so chemoprophylaxis is recommended for close contacts of patients with invasive meningococcal disease. Meningitis is a notifiable disease in the UK and in many other countries.

Key Points

- *Neisseria meningitidis* can cause meningitis, septicaemia, or both, and predominantly affects children and young adults.
- Blood cultures and a lumbar puncture are essential in the diagnosis of the disease.
- Antibiotics should be given immediately after blood cultures are taken, because patients can deteriorate rapidly.
- Non-culture methods, such as polymerase chain reaction, can be helpful in culture-negative cases.
- Prophylaxis should be given to contacts.

Did You Know?

British Paralympian Jonnie Peacock, who won Gold at the 2012 Paralympics (**Figure 41.5**), had his right leg amputated when he contracted meningococcal meningitis and septicaemia aged 5.

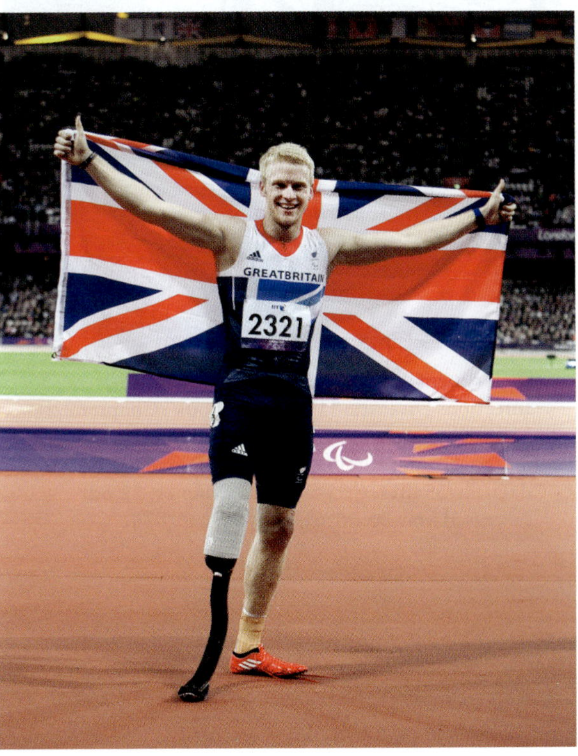

Figure 41.5. British Paralympian Jonnie Peacock had meningococcal meningitis and septicaemia aged 5, and lost his right leg. (Photo courtesy of Helene Wiesenhaan.)

Looking Back

Swiss physician Gaspard Vieusseux first described meningococcal disease in 1805, following an epidemic in Geneva, Switzerland. In 1884, Ettore Marchiafava and Angelo Celli first observed the bacterium inside cells in the CSF and three years later Anton Weichselbaum (**Figure 41.6**) isolated it from the CSF of patients with bacterial meningitis.

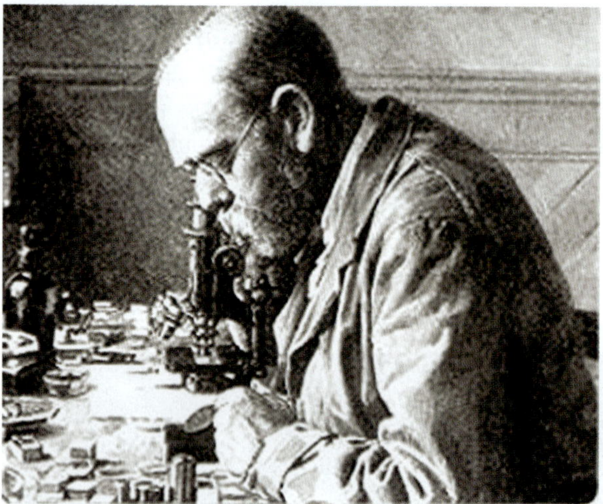

Figure 41.6. Austrian pathologist and bacteriologist Anton Weichselbaum, who cultured *Neisseria meningitidis* from CSF and blood, thus showing the organism causes meningococcal disease.

References

1. Department of Health. Immunisation against Infectious Diseases: "The Green Book". Chapter 22: Meningococcal. https://assets.publishing.service.gov.uk/government/uploads/system/uploads/attachment_data/file/554011/Green_Book_Chapter_22.pdf (accessed May 30, 2018).
2. McGill F, Heyderman RS, Panagiotou S, Tunkel AR, Solomon T. Acute bacterial meningitis in adults. Lancet 2016;**388**:3036–47.
3. Schuchat A, Robinson K, Wenger JD, et al. Bacterial meningitis in the United States in 1995. N Engl J Med 1997;**337**:970–6.
4. Thigpen MC, Whitney CG, Messonnier NE, et al. Bacterial meningitis in the United States, 1998–2007. N Engl J Med 2011;**364**:2016–25.
5. van de Beek D, de Gans J, Spanjaard L, et al. Clinical features and prognostic factors in adults with bacterial meningitis. N Engl J Med 2004;**351**:1849–59.
6. Kanegaye JT, Soliemanzadeh P, Bradley JS. Lumbar puncture in pediatric bacterial meningitis: defining the time interval for recovery of cerebrospinal fluid pathogens after parenteral antibiotic pretreatment. Pediatrics 2001;**108**:1169–74.
7. Heyderman RS, Lambert HP, O'Sullivan I, et al. Early management of suspected bacterial meningitis and meningococcal septicaemia in adults. J Infection 2003;**46**:75–7.
8. McGill F, Heyderman RS, Michael BD, et al. The UK joint specialist societies guideline on the diagnosis and management of acute meningitis and meningococcal sepsis in immunocompetent adults. J Infect 2016;**72**:405–38.
9. Tunkel AR, Hartman BJ, Kaplan SL, et al. Practice guidelines for the management of bacterial meningitis. Clin Infect Dis 2004;**39**:1267–84.

CASE 42

Seizure in a Seasoned Traveller

Alastair Miller

History

A 47-year-old, right-handed man presented at his local hospital following a first generalized tonic–clonic seizure. This had been preceded by some abnormal sensations of the right side of the face and right arm, but there were no other focal features. He made a spontaneous recovery and there was no recurrence of seizures.

He was self-employed as a mountaineering instructor and trek leader, so had an extensive travel history, having visited many countries in Southeast Asia, South America and Africa over the previous few years. He had returned from a trip to Thailand 5 weeks prior to the presentation. Much of his time was spent trekking so he had close contact with the local people and had lived extensively in rural and resource-poor areas. He was a non-smoker who drank about 8 units of alcohol a week and did not use recreational drugs. He had never had a head injury and had never previously lost consciousness. He had not had any previous neurological or cardiological history.

Examination

Neurological examination and general physical examination when he had recovered from the seizure were entirely normal.

Investigations

Full blood count, including eosinophil count, was entirely normal. Biochemistry was normal with the exception of a mild elevation in his liver enzymes, which was thought to be due to increased alcohol use while on his trip to Thailand.

Serology for HIV, viral hepatitis, syphilis, toxoplasma and shistosomiasis were all negative. Stool examination demonstrated no ova, cysts or parasites.

A routine non-ictal electroencephalogram was normal.

Initial Differential Diagnosis

The preceeding sensory symptoms indicate that this was a partial seizure with secondary generalisation. The differential diagnoses of a focal-onset seizure, particularly in a traveller include:

- Encephalitis, often viral, although this is usually associated with a febrile prodrome, and altered consciousness
- Toxoplasmosis (if immunocompromised)
- Cerebral abscess
- Other infections, including neurocysticercosis, syphilis, trypanosomiasis or schistosomiasis
- Neoplasia (primary or secondary)
- Cerebrovascular disease
- Adult-onset ideopathic epilepsy

Results of Definitive Investigations

Cerebral imaging with computer tomography (CT) and magnetic resonance imaging (MRI) were performed (**Figure 42.1A,B**).

Following this, a plain radiograph of the thighs was performed (**Figure 42.2**).

Diagnosis

The combination of the travel history, the focal symptoms preceding the seizure, and the characteristic imaging (both cerebral and musculoskeletal) was strongly suggestive of neurocysticercosis.

Serology for *Taenia solium* was strongly positive. One might have anticipated an eosinophilia secondary to the helminthic infection of the tissues, but this is by no means invariable.

Management and Outcome

The diagnosis was explained to him and he was started on dexamethasone 4 mg once daily and then albendazole was started and given for 10 days. This was followed by a single dose of praziquantel. He was also started on carbamazepine to reduce the risk of further seizures.

Figure 42.1. A CT (A), T2-weighted MRI (B), and gadolinium-enhanced T1-weighted MRI (C) similar to those of a 47-year-old gentleman who presented with a single generalised tonic–clonic seizure after returning from Thailand.

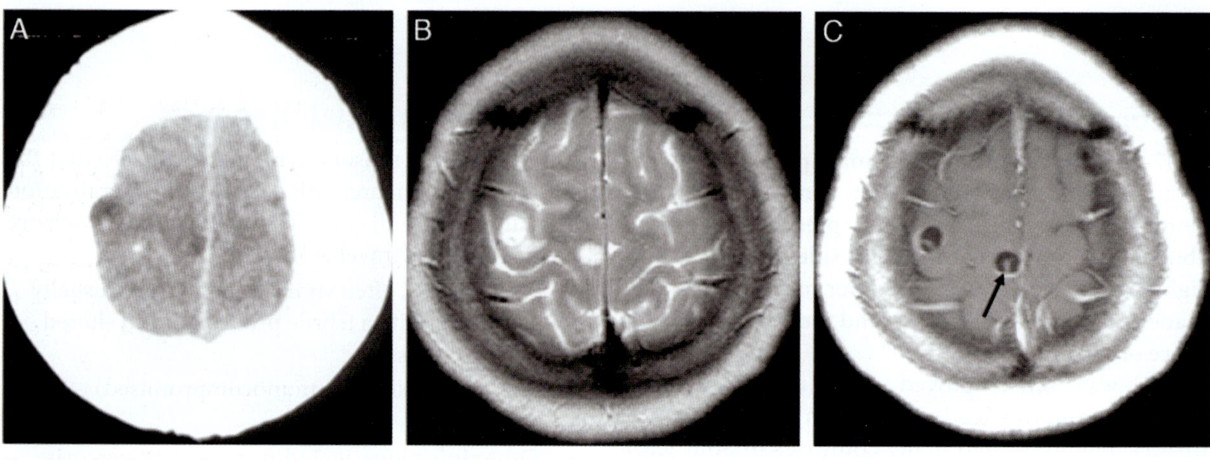

The CT and MRI scans show several small ring-enhancing cysts; one is arrowed in (C).

Figure 42.2. Plain radiograph of the thighs similar to those seen in the same patient.

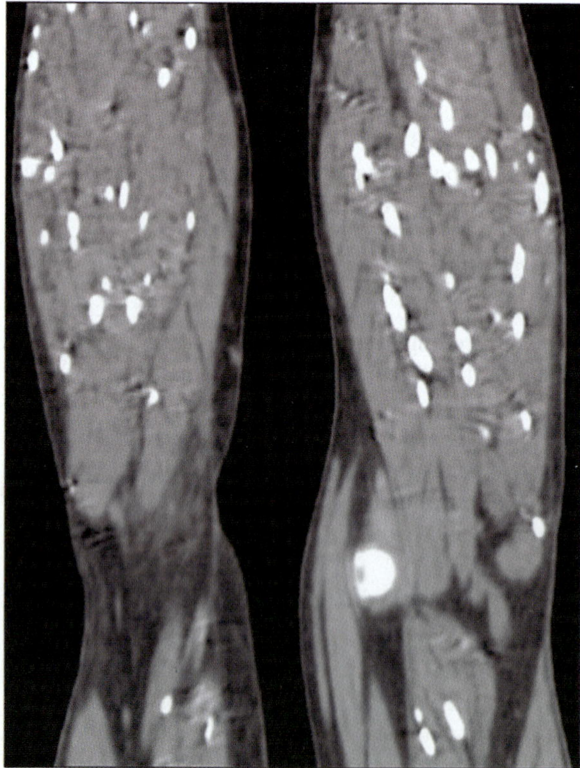

This demonstrates multiple radio-opaque lesions present in both lower limbs, predominantly in muscular tissue, as did a radiograph of the clavicle taken 2 years previously. (Reproduced with permission from: Banu A, Veena N. A rare case of disseminated cysticercosis: case report and literature review. Ind J Med Microbiol 2011;29(2):180–3.)

He was told that he should not drive or rock climb, or do other activities that would expose him to risk of harm were he to have another seizure. It was explained to him that the treatment was likely to have killed all the larvae and that his overall prognosis was very good, although there remained the possible risk of further seizures.

Discussion

In the lifecycle of *Taenia solium* man becomes the definitive host by ingesting inadequately cooked pork that contains encysted immature larvae (cysticerci) (**Figure 42.3**). These then mature to produce an adult tapeworm in the human gut. During this period, called taeniasis, the patient is usually asymptomatic, but this still results in infective ova being produced and excreted in the faeces. In the parasite's lifecycle, infected faeces are then eaten by pigs, which are intermediate hosts; the parasite hatches, penetrates into muscle, and develops here into cysticerci, to complete the cycle.

Humans develop cysticercosis through eating human faeces contaminated with ova, so that they become intermediate hosts.

The ova hatch in the stomach and duodenum, releasing oncospheres that penetrate through the gut wall and are disseminated in the blood vessels. In most tissues the resulting cysts are eliminated by a host immune response, but in central nervous system tissue and the eye they are protected from the immune response; in both striated and cardiac muscle tissues

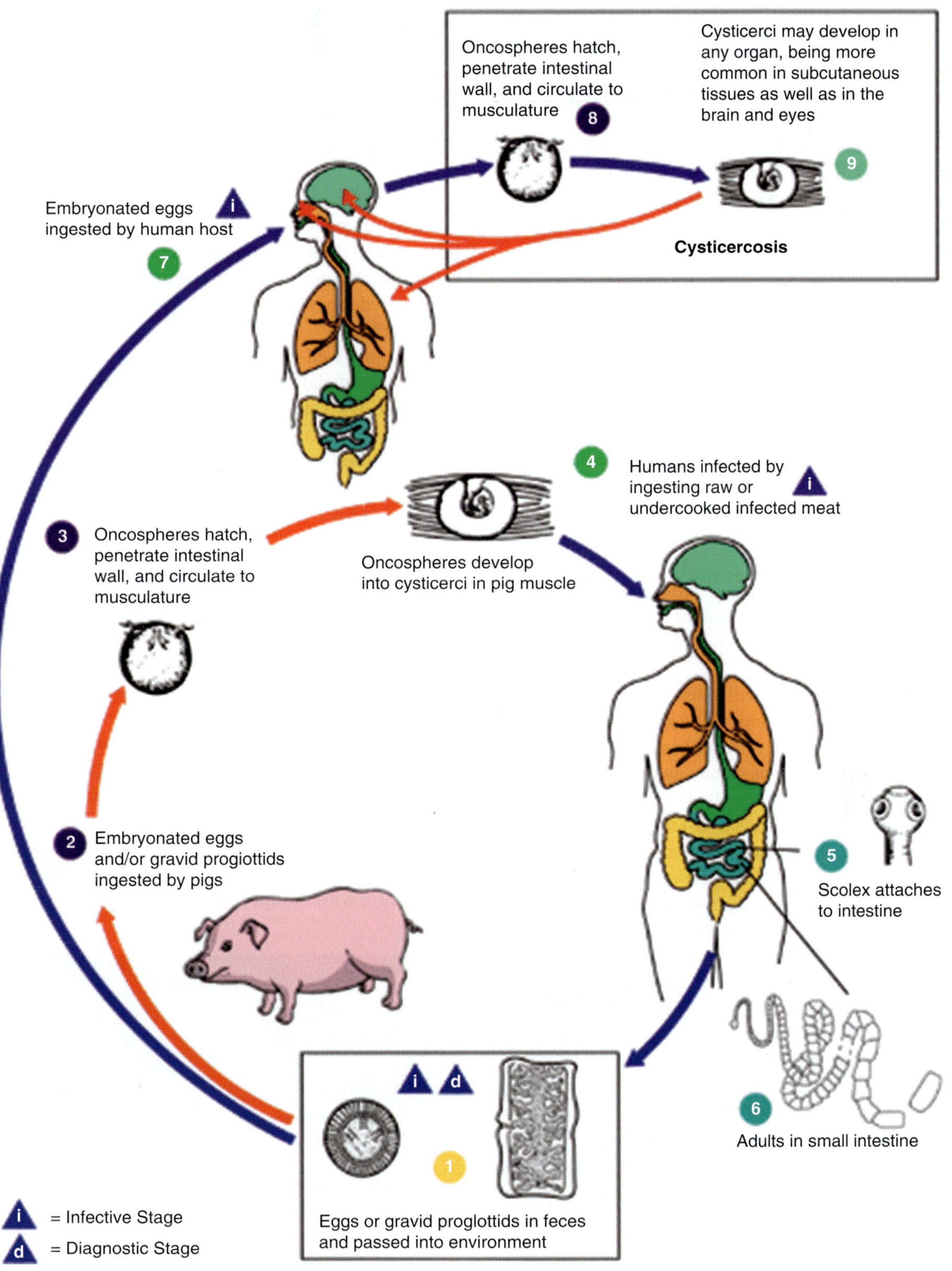

Figure 42.3. Lifecycle of *T. solium*. (From: www.cdc.gov/parasites/images/cysticercosis/cysticercosis_lifecycle.gif)

they grow too quickly to be overcome by host immunity (**Figure 42.3**). If a human has tissue cysts of *T. solium* then this is termed 'cysticercosis' and if the cysts are present in the central nervous system then it is termed 'neurocysticercosis'.

Humans can also develop cysticercosis if they have taeniasis and then ingest the ova of their own adult tapeworms, 'auto-infection', although this is thought to be less common.

Cysts are generally about 1 cm in diameter, consisting of the head, or 'scolex', of the tapeworm surrounded by a vesicle consisting of the embryonic body of the worm and all enclosed in a host-derived capsule. After some years as a viable cyst, the immune system will damage it to cause death of the worm and involution of the cyst. As this immunological activity continues, it may be associated with thickening of the cyst wall and an increase in surrounding cerebral oedema. There may therefore be an increased likelihood of clinical neurological events, such as seizures, at this stage of the natural history. Subsequently, as the cyst dies it may calcify.

Cysticercosis is common wherever adult tapeworms are prevalent and therefore is endemic in many low-income countries but especially in Latin America and Southeast Asia.

An adult tapeworm will cause virtually no symptoms and may only be incidentally identified when segments of the worm are observed in faeces. Cysticerci other than in the nervous system again give rise to few symptoms, but may be identified as a result of an individual becoming aware of non-tender subcutaneous nodules in affected muscle. They may also be identified if an affected area of muscle undergoes an X-ray coincidentally. Occasionally cysticerci may develop in the eye, and this can give rise to uveitis and/or retinitis with the potential for visual damage.

Neurocysticercosis may cause elevated intracranial pressure; however, seizures are the most common presentation and they may occur at any time once the cysts have developed. In the developing world, neurocysticercosis is the single most common cause of acquired epilepsy [1]. The diagnosis should be considered in anyone with adult-onset epilepsy, especially if there is an appropriate travel or exposure history. The diagnosis is confirmed by appropriate neuroimaging, by CT or MRI, as in the case described here. This may not only identify the cysts but also give some information regarding their current viability or immunological activity. Diagnosis can be further confirmed by positive serology for *T. solium*. Western blot is approximately 98% sensitive if there is more than 1 active lesion present and up to 100% specific [2].

Seizures associated with neurocysticercosis should be treated in the same approach as focal epilepsy of any cause. Sometimes ventriculoperitoneal shunting may be required if neurocysticercosis results in obstructive hydrocephalus.

It is now well-established that antiparasitic treatment is beneficial. As in this case, albendazole, often combined with dexamethasone, is often used [3]. If albendazole cannot be used because of toxicity then praziquantel also has anti-cyst activity.

Key Points

- Neurocysticercosis occurs mostly as a consequence of consuming the ova of *taenia solium* through faeco-oral transmission, rather than through the consumption of pork.
- Cysticerci may be identified on an X-ray of the affected muscle, which may be asymptomatic or have palpable non-tender nodules.
- Neurocysticercosis is the most common cause of acquired epilepsy in the developing world.
- As serology is highly sensitive and specific, and as there is effective antiparasitic and adjunctive anti-inflammatory therapy, neurocysticercosis is an important differential in those presenting with seizures with the appropriate travel history.

Looking Back

As far back as the ancient Egyptians at almost 2000 BC, there have been references to tapeworms. Moreover, descriptions of 'measled pork' were noted by Aristotle (**Figure 42.4**).

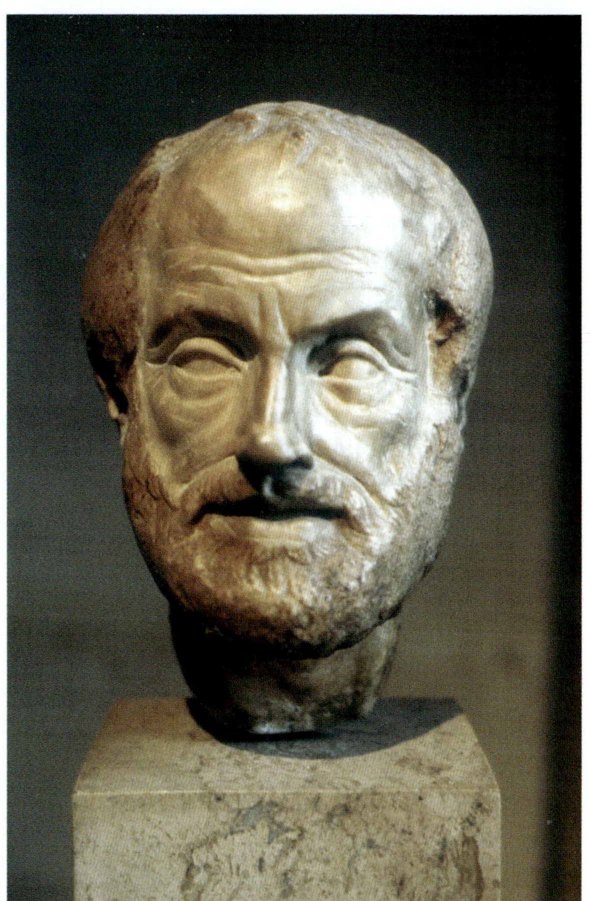

Figure 42.4. Aristotle's description of 'measled pork' is thought to be an early descripton of pig infected with *Taenia solium*. (From: photos.com)

Did You Know?

Infectivity was proven in 1850 by Kuchenmeister in a study in which he fed pork containing cysticerci to prisoners on death row and recovered the developed tapeworms from their intestines after execution [4].

References

1. Singh G, Burneo JG, Sander JW. From seizures to epilepsy and its substrates: neurocysticercosis. Epilepsia 2013;**54**:783–92.
2. Del Brutto OH. Diagnostic criteria for neurocysticercosis revisted. *Pathogen Global Health* 2012;**106**:299–304.
3. Otte WM, Singla M, Sander JW, Singh G. Drug therapy for solitary cysticercus granuloma: a systematic review and meta-analysis. Neurology 2013;**80**:152–62.
4. Küchenmeister, F. The Cysticercus cellulosus transformed within the organism of man into *Taenia solium*. Lancet 1861;**i**:39.

CASE 43

Stiff and Stuporous

Stephen Ray and Rachel Kneen

History

A 4-year-old, previously healthy and fully immunised girl presented to hospital with a 4-day history of feeling generally unwell, with myalgia, lethargy and a fever of up to 38°C.

Over the 48 hours leading up to admission, she had developed headache, lethargy and drowsiness. The parents informed the medical team that she was unable to walk and did not recognise them. On the day of admission she had two brief, right-sided focal seizures.

Two weeks prior to presentation, she had complained of a sore throat, myalgia, coryzal symptoms and fever lasting 4 days. At this time, the parents had taken her to their primary care general practitioner and she had received a course of penicillin V for tonsillitis.

Examination

On the admission examination, she was afebrile and her heart rate, blood pressure and oxygenation were within acceptable limits. She was encephalopathic with a Glasgow coma score of 13/15 and she had a stiff neck. No rashes or lymphadenopathy were present.

Neurological examination revealed generalised hypertonia, but normal power throughout the lower and upper limbs bilaterally. She was able to bear weight on her feet and sit up if supported, but could not walk. All deep tendon reflexes were brisk and the plantar responses were extensor bilaterally. Sensory testing was difficult to perform due to confusion, but appeared to be normal. Her pupil responses and eye movements were normal. Testing of the other cranial nerves was also normal. No cerebellar signs were present.

Initial Differential Diagnosis

- Acute encephalitis syndrome
  - Viral
  - Bacterial
  - Autoimmune (post- or para-infectious), e.g. Acute disseminated encephalomyelitis (ADEM)
- Other non-infectious or inflammatory encephalopathy, e.g. toxic, metabolic

Results of Initial Investigations

Serum analysis showed a white cell count (WCC) 14 × 10^6/l, erythrocyte sedimentation rate 15 mm in 1 hour and normal C-reactive protein and routine biochemistry. Serum antibodies for a vasculitis screen were negative. Additional serum analysis for VGKC-complex, NMDA receptor, thyroid peroxidase and paraneoplastic antibodies were also negative.

A throat swab did not identify any growth on bacterial culture.

She underwent a lumbar puncture and the cerebrospinal fluid (CSF) WCC was 22 × 10^6/l (neutrophil 14 × 10^6/l), red cell count 6 × 10^6/l, Gram stain negative, glucose ratio 56% (CSF glucose 2.2: plasma glucose 3.9) and oligoclonal bands were not detected. Subsequent tests for herpes simplex virus, varicella zoster virus and enterovirus was negative.

A computer tomography brain scan was normal.

Results of Definitive Investigations

A magnetic resonance imaging (MRI) scan was performed (**Figure 43.1**).

Serum anti-streptolysin O titres were positive at 800 units, and serum basal ganglia antibodies were present.

Diagnosis

Post-streptococcal acute disseminated encephalomyelitis.

Management and Outcome

Intravenous (IV) methylprednisolone was given once a day for 3 days. Treatment was then changed to oral prednisolone and a tapering course was given over 4 weeks. She was discharged on day 10 with normal sensorium and no gait disturbance but with residual mild hypertonia that was causing fatigue. At 3-month follow-up she was back to baseline.

Prevention

ADEM is most often a post-infectious process following a viral illness (**Table 43.1**); immunisation against a potential triggering virus, where available, thus lowers the incidence of ADEM from that cause. ADEM can also be triggered following vaccinations, but this is much rarer. For example, the incidence of ADEM following primary measles virus infection is 1/1000, but the incidence of ADEM following measles vaccination is 1–2/million [1].

Table 43.1 Types of infections and vaccinations associated with acute disseminated encephalomyelitis (data from [3]).

Infections and vaccinations associated with ADEM		
Infections		
	Virus	
		Cytomegalovirus
		Coronavirus
		Coxsackievirus
		Epstein–Barr virus
		Hepatitis A and B
		Human herpes virus 6
		HIV
		Herpes simplex virus
		Human T-cell lymphotrophic virus
		Influenza A and B
		Mumps
		Rubella
		Smallpox
		Varicella zoster
	Bacteria	
		Borrelia burgdorferi
		Campylobacter
		Chlamydiae
		Legionella
		Leptospira
		Mycoplasma pneumoniae
		Streptococcus
		Rickettsia rickettsii
	Parasite	
		Malaria
Vaccinations		
		Diphtheria
		Hepatitis B virus
		Influenza
		Japanese encephalitis virus
		Poliomyelitis
		Rabies
		Smallpox
		Tetanus
		Varicella zoster
		Yellow fever

Figure 43.1. T2-weighted axial and coronal MRI brain scan of a 4-year-old girl who presented with confusion and generalised hyper-reflexia.

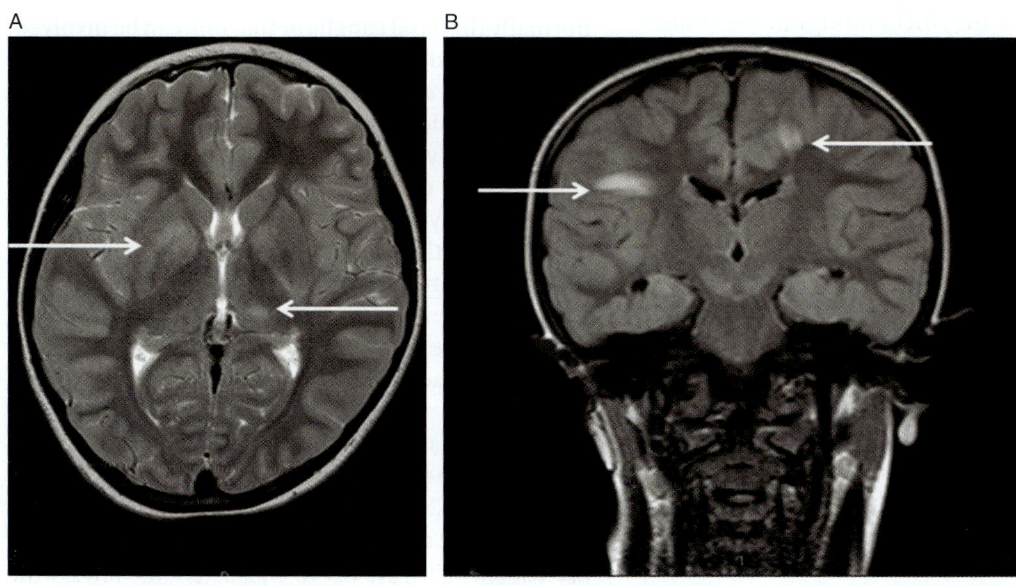

The images show high signal in the basal ganglia and asymmetrical high signal in the deep white matter consistent with ADEM (arrows).

Table 43.2 Consensus definitions for different categories of ADEM as defined by The International Paediatric Multiple Sclerosis Study Group [7].

Type of ADEM	Inclusion criteria

Monophasic ADEM	• A first polyfocal clinical CNS event with presumed inflammatory cause that must include encephalopathy (that cannot be explained by fever) is present, defined as:
	  • Behavioural change, e.g. confusion, excessive irritability
	  • Alteration in consciousness, e.g. lethargy, coma
	• Event should be followed by improvement, either clinically, on MRI, or both, but there may be residual deficits
	• No history of a clinical episode with features of a prior demyelinating event
	• No other aetiologies can explain the event
	• New or fluctuating symptoms, signs or MRI findings occurring within 3 months of the inciting ADEM event are considered part of the acute event
	• Neuroimaging shows focal or multifocal lesion(s), predominantly involving white matter, without radiologic evidence of previous destructive white matter changes:
	  • Brain MRI, with FLAIR or T2-weighted images, reveal diffuse, poorly demarcated, large, > 1–2 cm lesions involving predominantly the cerebral white matter; T1 hypointense white matter lesions are rare; deep grey matter lesions (e.g. thalamus or basal ganglia) can be present
	  • In rare cases, brain MR images show a large single lesion (> 1–2 cm), predominately affecting white matter
	  • Spinal cord MRI may show confluent intramedullary lesions(s) with variable enhancement, in addition to abnormal brain MRI findings above specified

Multiphasic ADEM	• ADEM followed by a new clinical event also meeting the criteria for ADEM, associated with new or re-emergence of prior clinical and MRI findings • The subsequent event must occur at least 3 months after the onset of the initial ADEM event

Discussion

Acute disseminated encephalomyelitis is classically a monophasic inflammatory demyelinating disorder of the central nervous system (CNS) with multiple lesions developing weeks after a typically benign viral or bacterial illness [1,2]. Patients may also have lesions in the spinal cord that may or may not cause symptoms of a transverse myelitis. The diagnosis is essentially based on the MRI findings in the context of an appropriate history. When associated with a predisposing infection this is usually peripheral, rather than in the CNS. Blood samples, throat and rectal swabs are thus needed to establish such infections.

ADEM is predominantly a paediatric disorder, with an incidence of 0.4–0.9/100,00 [3]. There is a seasonal distribution, with the majority of cases occurring in the winter and early spring months. The presentation of ADEM is dependent on the location and severity of the demyelinating inflammatory process. Non-specific symptoms of systemic upset, such as headache and fever, are common. Other features include meningism, seizures, coma, motor deficits, involuntary movements and optic neuritis [2,4–6]. Patients may need intensive or high-dependency care.

In 2007, The International Paediatric Multiple Sclerosis Study Group published consensus definitions of paediatric CNS inflammatory demyelinating disorders (**Table 43.2**) [7]. Whereas ADEM in children requires there to be encephalopathy, up to 50% of adults have ADEM without encephalopathy [8].

ADEM is considered to be an autoimmune disease. It is a predominately inflammatory process, with minor demyelination, normally of small perivenous areas (**Figure 43.2**) [9,10]. Lesions containing lymphocytes and monocytes in small vessels of white matter and the brain stem are classical [2,11]. Grey matter, normally the basal ganglia or thalami, can be involved, as in the case described here. The immune response is thought to be driven by molecular mimicry, whereby there is homology between myelin sheath and pathogen surface glycoproteins leading to a T cell-initiated autoimmune response [3,5]. Antibodies to myelin oligodendrocyte glycoprotein (MOG) are thought to contribute to the demyelination process. MOG is present on the outmost surface of the myelin sheath in the CNS, making it vulnerable to autoantibodies. MOG antibodies are present in over 40% of children presenting with acute demyelination [12]. The presence of antibodies to MOG do not distinguish between monophasic and chronic disease, e.g. multiphasic ADEM (**Table 43.2**); this form occurs in 0–25% of paediatric cases [2,10,14].

Due to the relative rarity of ADEM, pharmacological management is based on reports of successful corticosteroid treatment of single cases or small case series

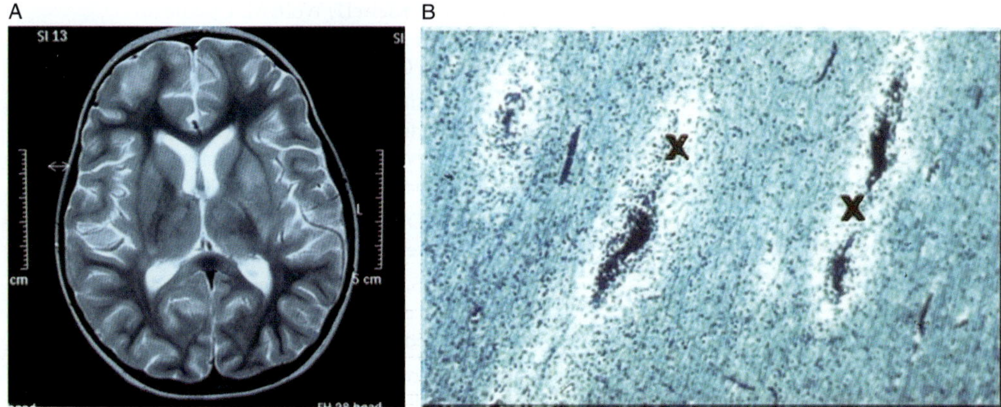

Figure 43.2. A histological slide from a case of ADEM. Myelin basic protein is dyed blue. White areas represent areas of demyelination surrounding venules, in keeping with perivenular demyelination.

[13] High-dose IV methylprednisolone is typically used as first-line treatment, which may be followed by a tapering of oral steroids. Plasmapheresis and IV immunoglobulins are usually reserved for resistant cases. Neurorehabilitation is also central to the care of patients with ADEM, both in the acute disease and ongoing in follow-up after discharge.

The prognosis of ADEM is generally good both in children and adults: the survival was 100% in three separate paediatric studies [2,10,14]. Mortality is higher in adults, particularly those admitted to intensive therapy units, and is reported to be between 8% and 25% [3]. Residual deficits are reported in 17–43% in children, with symptoms including gait disturbance, urinary symptoms or paraplegia secondary to spinal cord involvement [2,10,14].

Key Points

- Acute disseminated encephalomyelitis (ADEM) predominately affects children, most commonly in the winter and spring.
- In children, it typically presents with an acute febrile encephalopathy, with or without focal neurological disease. Adults with ADEM are often not encephalopathic.
- Abnormal T2-weighted and T2 FLAIR MRI signal changes establish the diagnosis of ADEM, but analysis of peripheral samples, such as throat swabs, are more likely to determine the precipitating infection rather than CSF analysis.
- The outcome is generally good with low mortality rates, although some children may have ongoing neurological problems.
- ADEM is usually a monophasic illness, but in some series up to a quarter may have a subsequent event.

Looking Back

The term ADEM was first used in 1946 to describe any immune-mediated encephalomyelitis [15]. In 1986, MRI studies were performed on a case series of patients with ADEM, first describing the characteristic lesions that now support an earlier and more robust diagnosis [16].

Did You Know?

In 1790, James Lucas of Leeds General Infirmary described a case of neurological disease following measles now thought to be the first published description of ADEM (**Figure 43.3**) [17]. He wrote about a 23-year-old woman who, 8 days after fever and *'the measles … perceived that she was deprived of the use of her lower limbs … She could not pass any urine … and an obstinate constipation succeeded'.*

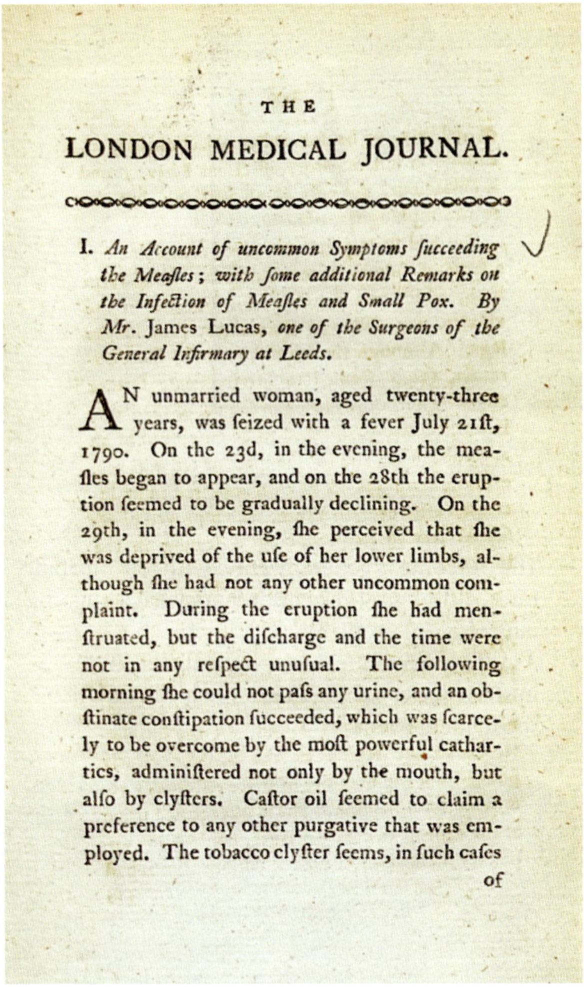

THE

LONDON MEDICAL JOURNAL.

I. *An Account of uncommon Symptoms ſucceeding the Meaſles; with ſome additional Remarks on the Infection of Meaſles and Small Pox. By Mr.* James Lucas, *one of the Surgeons of the General Infirmary at Leeds.*

AN unmarried woman, aged twenty-three years, was ſeized with a fever July 21ſt, 1790. On the 23d, in the evening, the meaſles began to appear, and on the 28th the eruption ſeemed to be gradually declining. On the 29th, in the evening, ſhe perceived that ſhe was deprived of the uſe of her lower limbs, although ſhe had not any other uncommon complaint. During the eruption ſhe had menſtruated, but the diſcharge and the time were not in any reſpect unuſual. The following morning ſhe could not paſs any urine, and an obſtinate conſtipation ſucceeded, which was ſcarcely to be overcome by the moſt powerful cathartics, adminiſtered not only by the mouth, but alſo by clyſters. Caſtor oil ſeemed to claim a preference to any other purgative that was employed. The tobacco clyſter ſeems, in ſuch caſes

of

Figure 43.3. Lucas' original 1790 account of a widespread neurological dysfunction following measles infection, now known to be ADEM. (From: www.ncbi.nlm.nih.gov/pmc/articles/PMC5550207/)

References

1. Bennetto L, Scolding N. Inflammatory/post-infectious encephalomyelitis. J Neurol Neurosurg Psychiatry 2004;**75**:i22–8.
2. Murthy SN, Faden HS, Cohen ME, Bakshi R. Acute disseminated encephalomyelitis in children. Pediatrics 2002;**110**:e21.
3. Sonneville R, Klein IF, Wolff M. Update on investigation and management of postinfectious encephalitis. Curr Opin Neurol 2009;**23**:300–4.
4. Dale RC, Church AJ, Cardoso F, et al. Poststreptococcal acute disseminated encephalomyelitis with basal ganglia involvement and auto-reactive antibasal ganglia antibodies. Ann Neurol 2001;**50**:588–95.
5. Wingerchuk DM. The clinical course of acute disseminated encephalomyelitis. Neurol Res 2006;**28**:341–7.
6. Tenembaum S, Chamoles N, Fejerman N. Acute disseminated encephalomyelitis: a long-term follow-up study of 84 pediatric patients. Neurology 2002;**59**:1224–31.
7. Krupp LB, Tardieu M, Amato MP, et al. International Pediatric Multiple Sclerosis Study Group criteria for pediatric multiple sclerosis and immune-mediated central nervous system demyelinating disorders: revisions to the 2007 definitions. Mult Scler 2013;**19**:1261–7.
8. Koelman DL, Chahin S, Mar SS, et al. Acute disseminated encephalomyelitis in 228 patients: a retrospective, multicenter US study. Neurology 2016;**86**:2085.
9. Wingerchuk DM. Postinfectious encephalomyelitis. Curr Neurol Neurosci Rep 2003;**3**:256–64.
10. Dale RC, de Sousa C, Chong WK, et al. Acute disseminated encephalomyelitis, multiphasic disseminated encephalomyelitis and multiple sclerosis in children. Brain 2000;**123**:2407–22.
11. Lassmann H. Acute disseminated encephalomyelitis and multiple sclerosis. Brain 2010;**133**:317–19.
12. Probstel AK, Dornmair K, Bittner R, et al. Antibodies to MOG are transient in childhood acute disseminated encephalomyelitis. Neurology 2011;**77**:580–8.
13. Tselis A. Acute disseminated encephalomyelitis. Curr Treat Options Neurol 2001;**3**:537–42.
14. Hynson JL, Kornberg AJ, Coleman LT, et al. Clinical and neuroradiologic features of acute disseminated encephalomyelitis in children. Neurology 2001;**56**:1308–12.
15. Margulis MS, Soloviev VD, Shubladze AK. Aetiology and pathogenesis of acute sporadic disseminated encephalomyelitis and multiple sclerosis. J Neurol Neurosurg Psychiatry 1946;**9**:63–74.
16. Atlas SW, Grossman RI, Goldberg HI, et al. MR diagnosis of acute disseminated encephalomyelitis. J Comput Assist Tomogr 1986;**10**:798–801.
17. Lucas J. An account of uncommon symptoms succeeding the measles: with additional remarks on the infection of measles and smallpox. London Med J 1790:325–31.

CASE 44

Just Unlucky?

Rachel Kneen and Jennifer Lemon

History

A 4-year-old boy presented to hospital with a 24-hour history of headache, lethargy, reduced oral fluid intake, vomiting and fever, on a background of a coryzal illness. There was no history of photophobia or a stiff neck. The child had not been travelling overseas and there was no known recent contact with anyone with an infectious disease, or a history suggesting susceptibility to infections. He had been seen in outpatients aged 2 years for constipation and poor weight gain (weight 2nd–9th centile). Investigations for failure to thrive revealed a low immunoglobulin (Ig) A. He was fully vaccinated, including the seven-valent pneumococcal conjugate vaccine (PCV7).

Examination

On admission, he was febrile (39.5°C) and tachycardic (heart rate 140 beats per minute). He was miserable but alert. He had bilateral enlarged, red tonsils but systemic examination was otherwise unremarkable. There were no signs of meningism and no focal neurological signs. A few hours after admission, he deteriorated with increasing lethargy and at this stage, neck stiffness was noted.

Initial Differential Diagnosis

- Acute meningitis, bacterial, or viral
- Upper-lobe pneumonia with associated neck stiffness
- Tonsillar or peritonsillar abscess

Results of Initial Investigations

Blood tests revealed a C-reactive protein of 137 mg/l, white cell count (WCC) 14.7 cells/mm^3 with a neutrophil predominance. Chest X-ray showed bilateral perihilar infiltrates. The cerebrospinal fluid (CSF) appeared cloudy with WCC 5230 cells/mm^3 (96% neutrophils), red cell count 3 cells/mm^3, glucose 1.4 mmol/l (plasma level 4.6, ratio = 0.3) and elevated protein 0.6 g/l.

Progress and Further Investigations

With this picture suggestive of bacterial meningitis, he was commenced on intravenous (IV) fluids, IV cefotaxime and IV dexamethasone for 4 days. CSF cultures grew a fully sensitive *Streptococcus pneumoniae* and blood and CSF were also positive for *Streptococcus pneumoniae* antigen. He made good progress and received a total of 17 days IV treatment. There were no neurological sequelae from this episode. Serotyping revealed *S. pneumoniae*, type 23B, which is not covered by the 7- or 13-valent PCV. Vaccine responses to PCV7 were tested and showed diminished responses to five of the serotypes so he was revaccinated with the 13-valent vaccine (PCV13). Subsequent vaccine responses were normal. Immunoglobulin levels including IgA were retested and were all normal.

He remained well for over a year until he presented with a further episode of pneumococcal meningitis with bacteraemia. He was treated with a full course of IV antibiotics and recovered with no sequelae. He was commenced on prophylactic amoxicillin. Hearing screening post-meningitis was normal.

Refined Differential Diagnosis

At this stage he clearly had recurrent bacterial meningitis, causes of which include immunodeficiencies, structural causes, including abnormal CSF connection (congenital or acquired), or para-meningeal infection.

Further immunological investigations including complement levels, were normal.

Results of Definitive Investigations

Computer tomography (CT) scan and subsequent magnetic resonance imaging (MRI) were performed on this occasion (**Figures 44.1** and **44.2**).

Diagnosis

Recurrent pneumococcal meningitis, secondary to persistent craniopharyngeal canal: an abnormal embryonic bony channel between the floor of the sella turcica and the nasopharynx.

Management and Outcome

The neurosurgical team undertook further detailed views of the canal and he underwent endoscopic surgery to repair the defect and reconstruct the sella floor. The surgery was successful and he has remained well post-operatively with no further episodes of meningitis.

Prevention

Vaccination is central to primary prevention of invasive pneumococcal disease including meningitis. PCV7 was introduced into the UK childhood vaccination programme in 2006 and replaced by PCV13 in 2010, which protects against 13 serotypes. At-risk groups (all adults over 65, children over 2 years, and adults with long-term illnesses) are offered vaccination with the pneumococcal polysaccharide vaccine [1]. Following introduction of PCV7 in the USA, the incidence of vaccine serotype pneumococcal meningitis across all ages fell by 73%. However, the non-vaccine serotype incidence rose by 60.5% [2]. Data from the Health Protection Agency (now Public Health England) has also shown this serotype replacement. Invasive pneumococcal disease secondary to PCV7 serotypes fell markedly after introduction of PCV7; however, non-vaccine serotypes increased, predominantly those in PCV13 [1] (**Figure 44.3**).

Prevention of recurrent meningitis involves investigation and management of the underlying cause [3]. Prophylactic antibiotics should be given until a definite cause has been found and effectively treated.

Figure 44.1. Sagittal CT scan of a 4-year-old boy with recurrent bacterial meningitis.

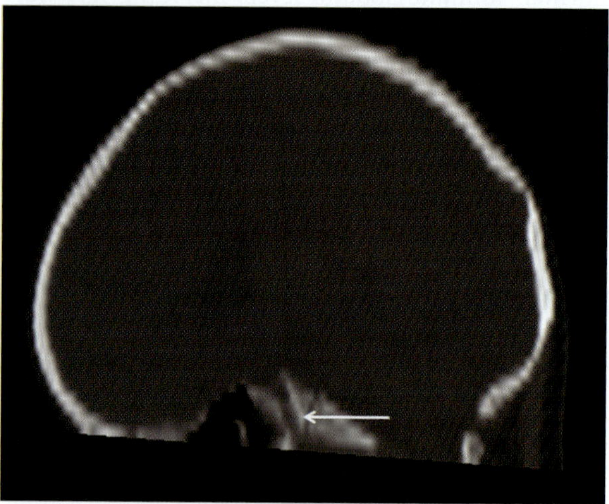

This shows a craniopharyngeal canal - an abnormal bony canal from the floor of the sella turcica to the posterior wall of the nasopharynx (arrow).

Discussion

The definition of recurrent bacterial meningitis is generally agreed to include: either two or more episodes of meningitis with isolation of different causative organisms, or a second episode by the same organism > 3 weeks after completion of therapy for the first [3]. It has been reported in up to 6% of adults [4] and 1.3% of children [5] with a previous episode of community-acquired bacterial meningitis.

A review of 363 adults and children with an identified cause for recurrent bacterial meningitis found 59% were due to anatomical problems, 36% due to immunodeficiency and 5% due to para-meningeal infections including otitis media and sinusitis [3]. A cause can often be identified and, although this may reflect publication bias, one review found only 6% of published cases had no cause found [6].

Most anatomical abnormalities are due to lesions in the cranial or cervical region. Rhinorrhoea or otorrhoea on a background of significant head injury is the classical presentation of a traumatic fistula.

Figure 44.2. Sagittal and axial T2-weighted MRI in the same child.

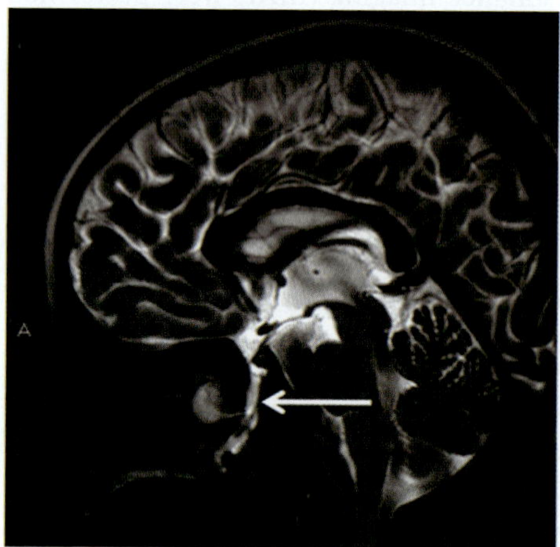

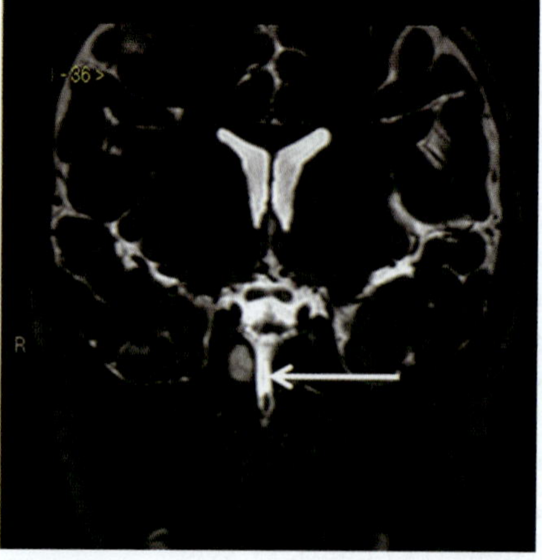

The scan shows high signal in the region of the craniopharyngeal canal reflecting a persistent craniopharyngeal canal (arrows).

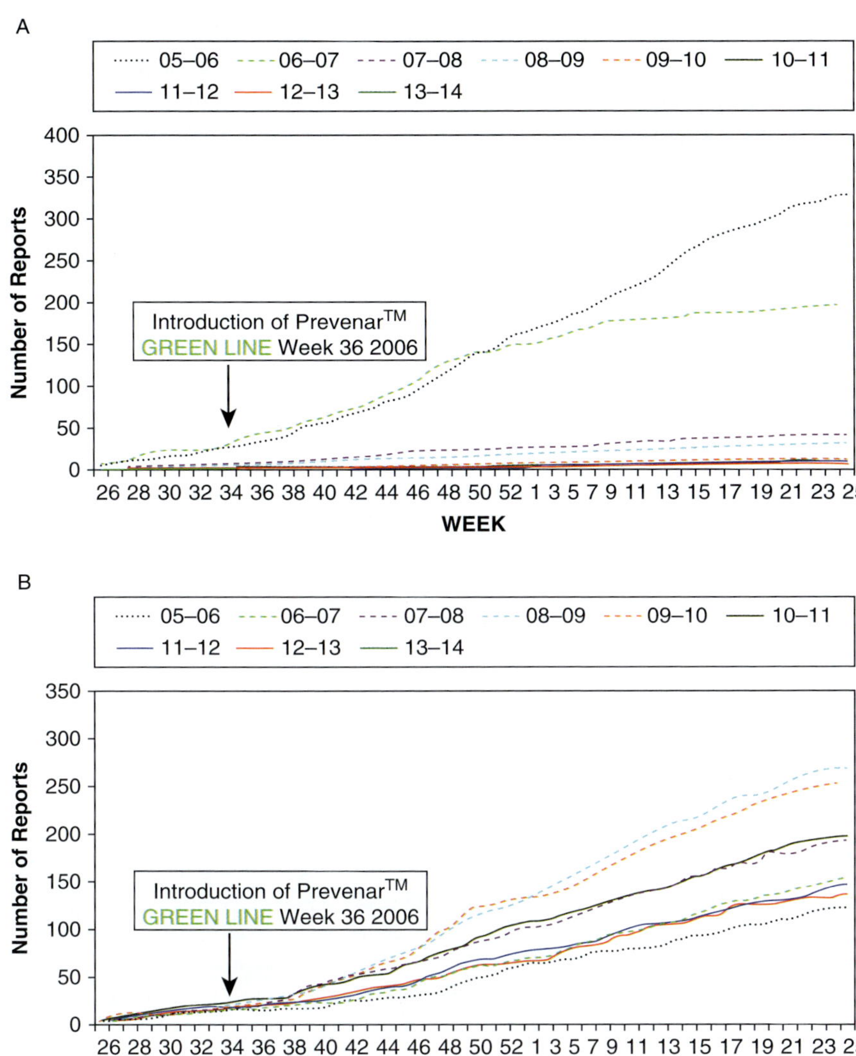

Figure 44.3. Data from the Health Protection Agency (now Public Health England) showing cumulative weekly numbers of reported invasive pneumococcal disease in children < 2 years in England and Wales by year: July–June (2005–2013). Pneumococcal/ EpidemiologicalDataPneumococcal/CurrentEpidemiologyPneumococcal/ (last accessed October 1, 2013). (A) Invasive pneumococcal disease due to any of the seven serotypes in Prevenar 7™. (B) Invasive pneumococcal disease due to non Prevenar 7™ serotypes (note PCV 13 was introduced in April 2010). (Graphs reproduced from the Health Protection Agency, subject to Public Health England copyright protection. www.hpa.org.uk/Topics/InfectiousDiseases/InfectionsAZ/)

However, CSF leakage may be occult and meningitis can occur several decades after trauma [3,6]. A variety of congenital malformations that cause an abnormal connection to the CSF can predispose to recurrent meningitis. These include heterotrophic brain tissue (meningocoele or encephalocoele), epidermoid cysts, dermoid cysts, dermal sinus tracts, neuroenteric cysts and inner ear defects, including Mondini dysplasia, a congenital inner ear dysplasia, with underdevelopment of the cochlear and CSF fistula to the middle ear [3]. A clue to congenital middle ear defects is sensorineural hearing loss, which may be falsely attributed to post-meningitic sequelae [6]. The persistent craniopharyngeal canal seen in this case is a rare cause of recurrent meningitis. The defect can be small, as in this case, or large with other associated midline facial defects and skull base malformations including encephalococles. Recurrent meningitis appears to be an uncommon presentation and symptoms of pituitary malfunction are more commonly reported. In cases where there is recurrent meningitis or CSF leakage, surgery is warranted [7].

A variety of immunodeficiency syndromes have been implicated in patients with recurrent meningitis. In particular, immunological susceptibility occurs particularly where there is reduced defence against encapsulated organisms, as in patients with asplenia and complement deficiencies [3].

The causative organism may help indicate the underlying cause. Recurrent meningitis due to *Neisseria meningitidis* occurs predominantly in those with complement deficiency. *Staphylococcus aureus* meningitis is uncommon but almost always associated with an underlying cause. *Escherichia coli* and enteric organisms predominantly cause neonatal meningitis and recurrent episodes may be associated with lower spinal CSF fistulas [3]. Nevertheless, *S. pneumoniae* is the most commonly isolated organism overall, present in > 60% of episodes [3,6]. It is particularly common in patients with abnormal cranial CSF connection, as in this case [3].

Assessment of recurrent meningitis requires a systematic approach. History should include questions regarding head trauma, CSF leakage, hearing impairment, speech and language delay, failure to thrive and personal or family history of recurrent or severe infections. Careful examination is required to detect a sinus or occult spinal lesion: examination of the whole of the midline externally should be undertaken, including searching through the hair. Stigmata of immunodeficiency should be specifically looked for [2]. Audiological examination, screening for anosmia and involvement of an ear, nose and throat specialist is important. CSF leakage, may be induced by the Valsalva manoeuvre and can be confirmed by the presence of Beta 2 transferrin in the fluid obtained [3,5].

One diagnostic algorithm that has been proposed is that by Tebrugge and Curtis in 2008. They advise that first-line investigations involve baseline tests of immune function including full blood count, blood film, immunoglobulins, IgG subsets, total haemolytic complement, HIV test (depending on risk factors) and abdominal ultrasound to detect asplenia. Indeed, UK meningitis guidelines recommend an HIV test in all patients with suspected bacterial meningitis. Further investigations are targeted according to findings [3]. Detailed cranial imaging including high-resolution CT or MRI is essential, although it remains important to discuss the appropriate imaging modality with a neuroradiologist [3,5,8]. Radionucleotide cisternography, which involves intrathecal injection of contrast material and interval imaging for up to 72 hours, is another technique for detecting CSF leaks. However, it does not allow exact localisation of the lesion and is limited by side effects and a sensitivity of 55–76% [3]. Intrathecal fluorescein may also be used for diagnosis and intraoperatively during surgery to repair CSF leaks [9]. Management involves treatment of the underlying cause, which in the case of communicating CSF lesions involves surgical repair [5,8].

Key Points

- Recurrent bacterial meningitis almost always has an underlying cause that can be determined, either structural or immunological.
- Diagnostic work-up involves assessment of immune function and a careful search for a congenital or acquired anatomical CSF communication.
- The pathogen involved may provide some clue as to the underlying aetiology. *S. pneumoniae*, the most commonly isolated organism, suggests a cranial CSF leak; *Neisseria meningitidis* occurs predominantly in those with complement deficiency; *Escherichia coli* and enteric organisms may be associated with lower spinal CSF fistulas.

Looking Back

The craniiopharyngeal canal marks the original position of Rathke's pouch, named after Martin Heinrich Rathke (1793–1860), a German anatomist recognised as one of the founders of modern embryology.

Did You Know?

Sella turcica, the saddle-shaped depression in the body of the sphenoid bone, is also the name of a 2010 horror movie.

References

1. Salisbury D, Ramsay M, Noakes K, eds. Chapter 10: Pneumococcal. In: Department of Health Green Book; *Immunisation Against Infectious Disease*. 3rd ed. Norwich: The Stationary Office; 2006 (chapter updated 2012). www.wp.dh.gov.uk/immunisation/

files/2012/07/Green-Book-Chapter-25-v4_0.pdf.pdf (accessed May 11, 2018).

2. Tan TQ. Pediatric invasive pneumococcal disease in the United States in the era of pneumococcal conjugate vaccines. Clin Microbiol Rev 2012;**25**:409–19.
3. Tebruegge M, Curtis N. Epidemiology, etiology, pathogenesis, and diagnosis of recurrent bacterial meningitis. Clin Microbiol Rev 2008;**21**:519–37.
4. Durand ML, Calderwood SB, Weber DJ, et al. Acute bacterial meningitis in adults. A review of 493 episodes. N Engl J Med 1993;**328**:21–8.
5. Drummond DS, de Jong A, Giannoni C, Sulek M, Friedman EM. Recurrent meningitis in the pediatric patient – the Otolaryngologist's role. Int J Pediatr Otorhinolaryngol 1999;**48**:199–208.
6. Kline MW. Review of recurrent bacterial meningitis. Pediatr Infect Dis J 1989;**8**:630–4.
7. Pinilla-Arias D, Hinojosa J, Esparza J, Muñoz, A. Recurrent meningitis and persistence of craniopharyngeal canal: case report. Neurocirugia 2009;**20**:50–3.
8. Lieb G, Krauss J, Collmann H, Schrod L, Sorensen N. Recurrent bacterial meningitis. Eur J Pediatr 1996;**155**:26–30.
9. Seth R, Benninger MS, Rajasekaran K, Batra PS. The utility of intrathecal fluorescein in cerebrospinal fluid leak repair. Otolaryngology 2010;**143**:626–32.

CASE **45** Missing the Point

Benedict D. Michael

History

A 73-year-old retired female presented with an 8-day history of a gradually progressive incoordination of her upper limbs, which she described as 'clumsy' and had resulted in her misjudging the distance of objects, such as cups. Also, over the last 2 days she had increasing difficulty walking, although there had been no falls. Her husband described her walking 'as if she had had a few too many sherries'. He also thought that on occasion her speech had been abnormal and possibly slightly slurred. However, both the patient and her husband denied her having excessive alcohol consumption. Over the preceding 3 days leading up to the admission, the husband reported that she had been behaving oddly, often seeming drowsy and 'muddled' at times; however, there had been no clear evidence of loss of consciousness or stereotyped movements to suggest seizure activity.

There was a mild non-specific global headache during this period but there was no nausea or vomiting. There was no history of fever, rigors or meningism and she did not have any significant travel history. There was no neck pain or trauma, and nothing to suggest an underlying malignancy.

She had undergone a recent mammogram, which was normal, and there had been no change in bowel habit, no weight loss or night sweats. She was a lifelong non-smoker. She had a past medical history of type 2 diabetes mellitus and hypertension, which were well-controlled on metformin and ramipril, respectively.

Figure 45.1. The patient had a rash similar to that shown here.

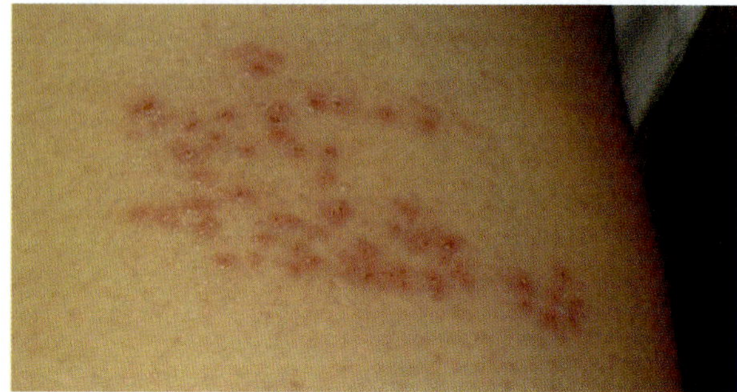

This shows a dermatomal eruption of varicella zoster. (Image courtesy of Marie Griffiths, reproduced under CC BY-SA 3.0 license.)

Examination

On examination she was apyrexial, but noted to have a rash (**Figure 45.1**). Neither she nor her husband had mentioned this. She had normal power in both upper and lower limbs and tone, and reflexes were normal throughout with flexor plantars bilaterally. Pin-prick, vibration and proprioception were normal throughout. Her gait was abnormal with wide-set feet and instability, veering particularly towards the left side. There was dysmetria (past-pointing) and tremor, worst at the point of intention, of her upper limbs, which was most severe on the left. There was no truncal ataxia. Her speech was abnormal with a scanning nature.

Initial Differential Diagnosis

The neurological signs were those of a cerebellar syndrome most marked on the left; the shingles could indicate varicella zoster virus (VZV) as a cause, or could be a sign of underlying disease for example malignancy.

- Cerebellar syndrome
    - Post-infectious cerebellitis
    - Infectious cerebellitis
    - Neoplasia (primary or secondary)
    - Paraneoplastic cerebellitis
    - Vascular (infarction secondary to thromboembolism, haemorrhage or dissection)

Results of Initial Investigations

Finger-prick glucose, renal and liver functions were normal. She had a mildly raised C-reactive protein (8.1 mg/l) and erythrocyte sedimentation rate (22 mm/hour). She had an elevated glucose level although her HbA1c was within normal limits. Onconeuronal antibodies for paraneoplastic processes were requested.

A computer tomography (CT) brain scan demonstrated bilateral but asymmetrical oedema of the cerebellum, which was most extensive on the left. There was no evidence of hydrocephalus.

A lumbar puncture was performed; the opening pressure was normal (18 cm H_2O), the cerebrospinal fluid (CSF) had a white cell count of 42 cells/mm^3 with a lymphocyte predominance, there were 3 red blood cells/mm^3, the protein was elevated at 7.9 mg/l and the CSF to serum glucose ratio was normal (4.1/7.8 mg/l).

Progress and Further Investigations

Viral polymerase chain reaction (PCR) of the CSF was negative for herpes simplex virus types 1 and 2, VZV, enterovirus, parechovirus, Epstein–Barr virus, cytomegalovirus and human herpes virus types 6 and 7. Plasma serology was negative for *Treponema pallidum* and plasma HIV types 1 and 2 antibody and P24 antigen were negative.

A magnetic resonance imaging (MRI) scan of the head was performed (**Figure 45.2**).

It demonstrated bilateral high signal of the cerebellar hemispheres, predominantly involving the cortices, which was most severe and extensive on the left; there was also early evidence of hydrocephalus, with slight effacement of the sulci and early enlargement of the ventricles.

A CT of her chest, abdomen and pelvis demonstrated several inguinal lymph nodes, the largest of which was 6 cm in diameter. A fine-needle aspiration of one of the lymph nodes was performed under ultrasound guidance and only demonstrated reactive changes, with no evidence of malignancy.

Definitive Investigation Results

Antibody testing was performed on the CSF for anti-VZV immunoglobulin (Ig) G, which was positive; anti-VZV IgG was also positive in the serum; however, Reiber's formula, which uses the CSF:serum albumin ratio, indicated that there was intrathecal production of VZV antibody (Box 45.1). She also had PCR performed on one of the vesicles from her back, which was positive for VZV.

Box 45.1. Reiber's Formula for the Detection of Intrathecal Synthesis of Antibody [1].

$$\text{Antibody Index} = \frac{\text{CSF IgG/serum IgG}}{\text{CSF albumin/serum albumin}}$$

Diagnosis

Post-varicella zoster cerebellitis.

Management and Outcome

Because the PCR of the CSF was negative for varicella zoster, this was felt to be in keeping with a post-infectious cerebellitis, rather than an acute VZV cerebellitis, even though she actually had the skin rash at the time. The decision was taken not to treat with aciclovir. Given the MRI findings she was started on steroids; she was given 1 g of methylprednisolone intravenously per day for 5 days. She did not require mannitol or glycerol therapy and did not require neurosurgical intervention. She was also given a glucose–potassium–insulin infusion to manage her elevated serum glucose levels. She made a

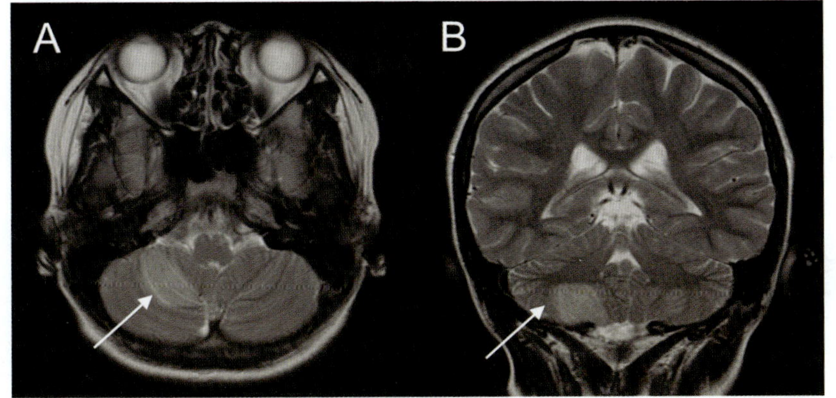

Figure 45.2. The patient's MRI scan was similar to this one.
It shows high signal intensity in the cerebellar white matter on T2-weighted images particularly on the right (A, axial and B, coronal; arrows), although these changes were more prominent on the patient's left. (Reproduced from [2] with permission of Elsevier.)

gradual recovery with steroids and neurorehabilitation and returned to her baseline level of functioning.

Prevention

There are live attenuated vaccines which protect against primary VZV infection. In the USA they are recommended for everyone. In the UK they are recommended for certain groups only, e.g. non-immune healthcare workers, and contacts of susceptible immunocompromised individuals. This is to protect those individuals; it is not given to the immunocompromised themselves because it is a live vaccine. The vaccines are not thought to protect those already infected with VZV from developing shingles.

Discussion

This case highlights the importance of thorough examination of the patient, not only focusing on the neurological signs. In this case the patient and husband had not known that shingles might be related to her presenting problems. Therefore, they did not mention it to the clinical team and it was only on examination that the resolving vesicular dermatomally distributed rash was identified.

VZV can affect all aspects of the neuroaxis. Acute cerebellar ataxia is the most common manifestation in children, occurring in approximately 1/4000 [3], but it can also occur in adults. It should thus be considered in adults with acute cerebellitis, particularly if following an episode of shingles [4]. The development of zoster before the age of 60 years may also be more common in those who acquired the primary VZV infection when they were aged under 4 years; this may parallel the increased risk of sub-acute sclerosing panencephalitis, which is more common in patients who acquired the primary measles infection at a younger age (< 2 years) [5]. However, VZV may even cause an acute cerebellitis without development of the classical zoster rash in some cases and, in such situations, a history of early chickenpox may encourage investigation [5].

Unlike acute VZV encephalitis in which aciclovir therapy is indicated, in post-infectious VZV cerebellitis, as the virus is thought to have been cleared from the CSF and as the course is usually self-limiting, many cases will not require any specific treatment [6]. In this case, intravenous methylprednisolone was prescribed for the acute cerebellar oedema, although the evidence for its benefit is limited; patients also require supportive therapy, including access to neurological rehabilitation [6].

Key Points

- VZV can cause an acute cerebellitis syndrome in adults as well as children.
- In acute cerebellitis, take a thorough history, including the age of development of previous chickenpox.
- Always examine the patient thoroughly, as some may not mention a rash.

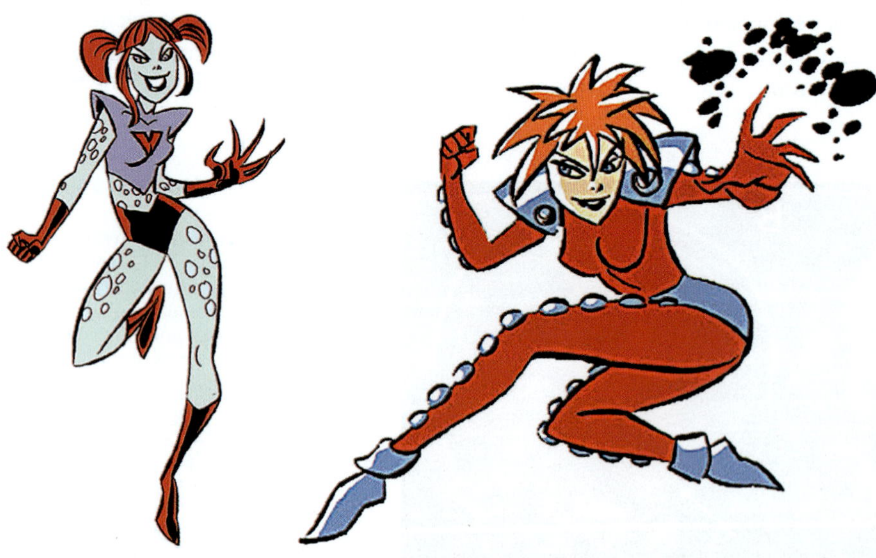

Figure 45.3. The 'Blister Sisters', the Centre for Disease Control and Prevention , USA, mascots for VZV vaccination.

Looking Back

The dermatological manifestation of zoster has been described since ancient times, and it was for a long time considered to be a variant of smallpox or 'variola'. It was not until William Osler (**Figure 45.4**), in 1892, documented a case in which he demonstrated that *'an attack of one does not confer immunity from an attack of the other'* that there was clinical evidence that zoster was a distinct entity from variola [7].

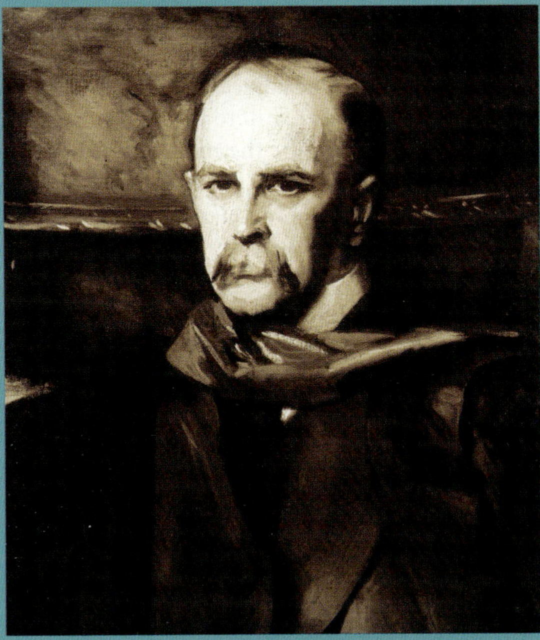

Figure 45.4. Sir William Osler, who demonstrated that chickenpox is not a variant of smallpox, because one did not confer immunity from the other. (From: Wellcome Collection, reproduced under CC BY 4.0 license.)

Did You Know?

Some medical historians have traced the nomenclature of the term 'chickenpox' back to a small chickpea, which the early rash of varicella is purported to resemble [5].

References

1. Reiber H. Flow rate of cerebrospinal fluid (CSF) – a concept common to normal blood-CSF barrier function and to dysfunction in neurological diseases. J Neurol Sci 1994;**122**:189–203.
2. Suzuki S, Kaga A, Lusaka N, et al. A case of acute cerebellitis with a unique sequential change on magnetic resonance imaging. Pediatr Neurol 2014;**51**:279–81.
3. Paul R, Singhania P, Hashmi MA, Bandyopadhyay R, Banerjee AK. Post chicken pox neurological sequelae: the distinct presentations. J Neurosci Rural Pract 2010;**1**:92096.
4. Gilden DH, Kleinschmidt-DeMasters BK, LaGuardia JJ, Mahalingam R, Cohrs RJ. Neurologic complications of the reactivation of varicella-zoster virus. N Engl J Med 2000;**342**:635.
5. Gilden D, Cohrs RJ, Mahalingam R, Nagel MA. Neurological disease produced by varicella zoster virus reactivation without rash. Curr Top Microbiol Immunol 2010;**342**:243–53.
6. Solomon T, Michael BD, Smith PE, et al. Management of suspected viral encephalitis in adults: Association of British Neurologists and British Infection Association National Guideline. J Infect 2012;**64**:347–73.
7. Arvin AM, Gershon AA. Varicella Zoster Virus: Virology and Clinical Manifestations. Cambridge: Cambridge University Press; 2000: 9–11.

CASE 46

A Monster in my Body?

Jennifer Lemon and Rachel Kneen

History

A 14-year-old Caucasian girl presented to outpatients following two probable complex partial seizures, affecting the right hand, arm and leg. These occurred on a background of a year-long history of non-specific headaches over the right fronto-temporal region, which had increased in intensity over the past 2 months. There were no associated neurological or systemic symptoms and the headaches did not have any features suggestive of raised intracranial pressure.

She was otherwise fit and well with no significant past medical history. She had travelled widely with her family to Asia and Africa.

Examination

She had papilloedema and mild left-sided intention tremor. Neurological examination was otherwise entirely normal.

Initial Differential Diagnosis

- Space-occupying intracranial lesion(s)
    - Tumour: malignant or benign
    - Abscess
- Neurocystercicosis (in view of the travel history)

Initial Investigations

Full blood count, renal and liver function tests, coagulation screen and lactate dehydrogenase were within normal limits. C-reactive protein was 23 mg/l and erythrocyte sedimentation rate 49 mm in 1 hour. A magnetic resonance imaging (MRI) scan was performed (**Figure 46.1**).

This revealed a broad-spaced enhancing extra-axial mass affecting the meninges of the right frontal and temporal lobes. There was underlying mass effect with compression of the adjacent right lateral ventricle and 6 mm of midline shift to the left. A meningeal tumour was thought to be the most likely diagnosis. The teenager was concerned she had picked up a rare infectious disease on her travels and asked if she may have a 'monster in her body', as she had been watching a programme about this on the television.

Infectious work-up included tests for *Mycobacteria* spp., *Bartonella henselae* and *B. quitana, Brucella* spp., *Borrelia burgdorferi*, tick-borne encephalitis virus, sindbis virus, sandfly fever virus, spotted fever, epidemic typhus, *Coxiella burnetii, Toxoplasma gondii*, HIV, varicella, hydatid disease and neurocysticercosis. All were negative.

A dural biopsy was performed (**Figure 46.2**).

Other investigations: liver function tests, renal function, thyroid function tests, ferritin were normal. Serum angiotensin converting enzyme (ACE) was normal at 22 units/l. pANCA/cANCA, autoantibodies, voltage-gated potassium channel antibodies, *N*-methyl-D-aspartate receptor antibodies and thyroid peroxidise antibodies were all negative. Cerebrospinal

Figure 46.1. MRI scan of a 14-year-old girl with a long history of headache and two complex partial seizures.

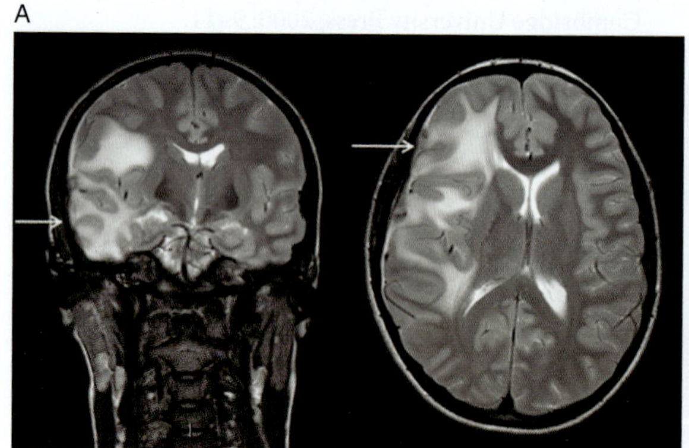

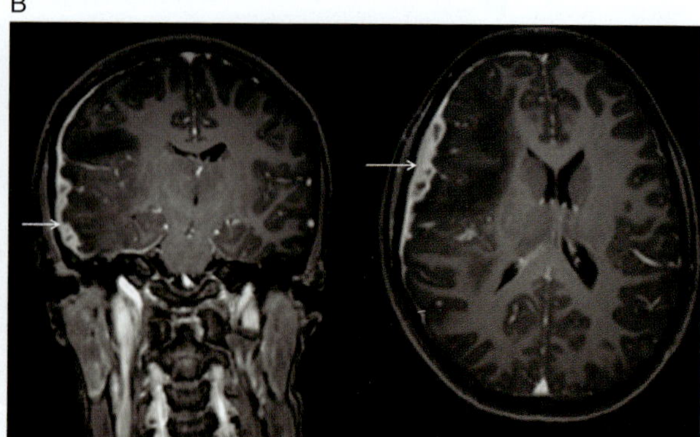

These demonstrate: (A) Cortical and white matter signal abnormality in the right temporal and frontal lobes (arrows) with midline shift and oedema. (B) T1-weighted with gadolinium demonstrating meningeal enhancement over the right cerebral hemisphere (arrows).

Figure 46.2. A dural biopsy of the same child.

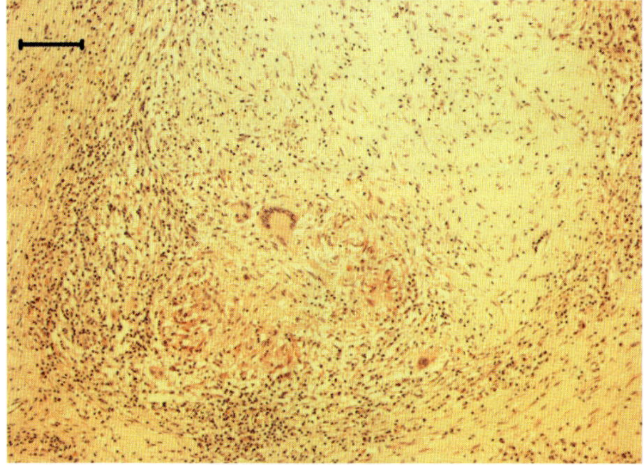

The biopsy shows multinucleated giant cells (Langhans type) and epithelioid cells (centre) surrounded by loose aggregate of T cells within dense fibrous tissue (of the biopsied meninges). The appearances are those of a granulomatous inflammation consistent with neurosarcoidosis. Bar = 100 μm. (Courtesy of Dr Atik Baborie.)

fluid (CSF) analysis taken at the time of the dural biopsy was normal; oligoclonal bands were not detected and ACE levels were normal.

A chest X-ray was normal.

Differential Diagnosis

- Meningeal neoplasia
- Granulomatous pachymeningitis

Management and Outcome

She was commenced on a tapering dose of prednisolone, starting dose 30 mg daily for 2 weeks. Cranial imaging improved at 3 months, but the appearances had returned to those seen at presentation 3 months later. A repeat biopsy containing brain parenchyma (to rule out a lymphoma) showed identical findings to the original biopsy. She was commenced on a 6-month course of intravenous cyclophosphamide using the local central nervous system (CNS) vasculitis protocol. Improvement in the imaging was noted and her treatment was converted to mycophenolate mofatil (1 g three times daily) as maintenance orally. Improvement was not sustained and she started to complain of headaches again. After 4 months, treatment was changed to monthly infliximab infusions which led to a resolution of symptoms and an improvement on MRI imaging.

Diagnosis

Inflammatory pachymeningitis, likely secondary to neurosarcoidosis.

Discussion

This is a rare clinical scenario in children and adults. The initial diagnosis was felt likely to be a meningeal tumour; therefore, only a dural biopsy was taken. However, there is a wide differential diagnosis for lesions affecting the dura. This includes meningiomas, other CNS neoplasms, metastases, and non-neoplastic granulomas [1].

The term 'pachymeningitis' describes inflammation of the dura mater and is characterised by diffuse or localised meningeal thickening and gadolinium enhancement on MRI. The lesions can be difficult to differentiate on imaging alone as they have similar characteristics to meningiomas. Neuropathology is therefore essential for accurate diagnosis.

Headache is present in almost all cases and ophthalmological symptoms and signs are common. Other clinical manifestations depend on the location of meningeal involvement. The main causes include neurosarcoid, tuberculosis, intracranial hypotension and rheumatoid arthritis, but many cases are idiopathic. Rare causes include systemic lupus erythematosus, Wegner's granulomatosis, plasma cell granulomas, sinus histiocytosis, listeriosis, syphilis, *Borrelia* spp., fungal infections and neoplasm. In HIV-positive patients a variety of opportunistic infections have been implicated [2,3].

Sarcoidosis is an idiopathic granulomatous disorder which can affect multiple body systems. It typically presents in young and middle-aged adults and has a female predominance. The commonest manifestations are pulmonary and skin manifestations including erythema nodosum. Neurosarcoidosis can affect any part of the central or peripheral nervous system with a wide range of clinical manifestations. It is identified in about 5% of patients with established sarcoidosis, but post-mortem studies show that a quarter of sarcoidosis patients have histological CNS involvement. It can also occur as the initial presentation of systemic sarcoidosis or less commonly as an isolated pathology. The characteristic histopathology seen in sarcoidosis is a non-caseating epithelioid granuloma with highly differentiated phagocytes and lymphocytes, as seen in this case. The disease process in the CNS is thought to start with a granulomatous inflammatory meningitis, which then spreads to involve the brain parenchyma [4,5].

Neurosarcoidosis can present with cranial nerve palsies, aseptic meningitis, headaches, seizures, peripheral neuropathies, myopathies, neuropsychiatric and neuroendocrine problems [4]. In adults, cranial neuropathies are seen most frequently; however, in prepubertal children, seizures have been reported as the most common presenting feature [6]. The diagnosis of neurosarcoid can be challenging as there is no specific test. Diagnosis depends on typical clinical features, including looking for evidence of systemic sarcoidosis, exclusion of other disease and supportive histology; however, there are no universally accepted and validated diagnostic criteria. Histology demonstrating non-caseating granulomas is the gold standard, although other causes of granulomatous inflammation, predominantly infectious need to be excluded. The commonest imaging finding in neurosarcoidosis is gadolinium-enhancing leptomeningeal involvement. Typical CSF findings include elevated protein levels with pleocytosis; however, normal CSF, as seen in this case, does not exclude neurosarcoid. Sarcoid granulomas produce ACE and therefore high levels are often seen in sarcoidosis. CSF ACE is more useful than serum ACE in neurosarcoidosis. Studies have shown CSF ACE to have a sensitivity of 24–55% and a specificity of 94–95% for the diagnosis of neurosarcoidosis. Nozaki and Judson provide a very detailed review of the diagnostic work-up required for suspected neurosarcoid [4].

Corticosteroids are first-line therapy for neurosarcoidosis and high-dose steroids usually produce a good response. However, several patients fail to show remittance or relapse when steroids are tapered and require maintenance steroids with additional cytotoxic/immunomodulatory agents. Chloroquine may also be used as an alternative/adjuvant to steroids. Radiotherapy and other pharmacological agents including infliximab have been rarely used, with some reported success. Surgery is reserved for life-threatening lesions or failure of medical therapy [4]. Resolution has been reported in up to 46% of cases, but many studies report a much lower rate of success. In CNS disease, studies have shown a chronic course in one- to two-thirds of patients [5].

Looking Back

Sarcoid was first described by the English doctor, Sir Jonathan Hutchinson (**Figure 46.3**) (1828–1913), who described a 'Case of livid papillary psoriasis' in his book *Illustrations of Clinical Surgery* in 1877.

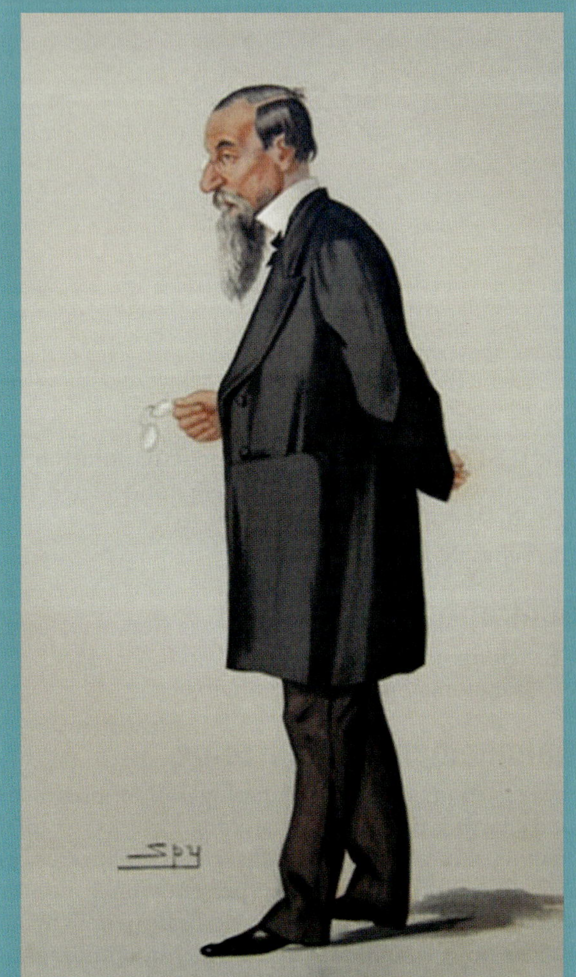

Figure 46.3. Sir Jonathan Hutchinson was an international medical personality sketched here by Spy (Sir Lesley Ward) for Vanity Fair magazine 27 Sep 1890.

Key Points

- Pachymeningitis is inflammation of the dura mater, characterised by meningeal thickening and gadolinium enhancement on MRI.
- Common causes include neurosarcoid, tuberculosis, intracranial hypotension and rheumatoid arthritis.
- Rarer causes include other granulomatous conditions, infections and tumours, but many cases are idiopathic.
- Neurosarcoid is treated with corticosteroids, followed by other immunosuppressives.

Did You Know?

Pulmonary sarcoidosis is one of the few lung diseases that is more common in non-smokers.

References

1. Chourmouzi D, Potsi S, Moumtzouoglou A, et al. Dural lesions mimicking meningiomas: a pictorial essay. World J Radiol 2012;**4**:75.
2. Bonnin N, Chiambaretta F, Ulla M, et al. Toxoplasmic pachymeningitis with visual field impairment in a single-eyed patient and a literature review. Oman J Ophthalmol 2012;**5**:46–50.
3. Ranoux D, Devaux B, Lamy C, et al. Meningeal sarcoidosis, pseudo-meningioma, and pachymeningitis of the convexity. J Neurol Neurosurg Psychiatry 1992;**55**:300–3.
4. Nozaki K, Judson MA. Sarcoidosis: neurosarcoidosis: clinical manifestations, diagnosis and treatment. Presse Med 2012;**41**:e331–48.
5. Gascón-Bayarri J, Mañá J, Martínez-Yélamos S, et al. Neurosarcoidosis. Report of 30 cases and a literature survey. Eur J Intern Med 2011;**22**:e125–32.
6. Baumann RJ, Robertson WC. Neurosarcoid presents differently in children than in adults. Pediatrics 2003;**112**:E480–6.

CASE **47** # Not Quite So Reserved Anymore

Sam Nightingale

History

A 59-year-old male IT programmer presented with confusion and altered behaviour . Over the past 3–5 weeks his short-term memory had deteriorated; for example, he had been having problems remembering his tablets and was unable to concentrate at work. His wife commented that his personality had changed; he quickly became angry or unhappy and despite normally being quite a reserved gentleman, he had also made several inappropriate sexual comments about a neighbour. He was otherwise well and had no headache, meningism or fever. There were no locomotive symptoms.

He had a 10-year history of type 2 diabetes complicated by diabetic neuropathy, nephropathy and retinopathy. He had developed end-stage renal failure and 2 years previously underwent a renal transplant. He remained on maintenance immunosuppression with mycophenolate and tacrolimus to prevent rejection. There was no other significant past medical history and he denied the use of illicit substances or excessive alcohol.

Examination

The mini-mental test score was high, 28/30 (losing points on the date and drawing overlapping pentagons). Nevertheless, he appeared slow of thought and there was evidence of perseveration and reduced abstraction but no frontal release signs. There was impaired sensation to the mid shin and areflexia at the ankles (this was longstanding and due to diabetic neuropathy). The rest of the neurological examination was normal at this time.

Initial Differential Diagnosis

This was a middle-aged gentleman with known immunosuppression who had several weeks' history of cognitive decline and disinhibition, but no other focal neurological signs. The differential included infections such as tuberculosis, syphilis, herpes simplex virus (HSV), JC virus, fungal infections; neoplastic causes, including gliomas and metastases; causes unrelated to his immune status were considered such as prion disease and vascular causes.

Results of Initial Investigations

Routine blood tests, including tumour markers, were normal. His renal function was stable – urea 6.6 mmol/l and creatinine 104 mmol/l.

A magnetic resonance imaging (MRI) head scan was performed (**Figure 47.1**).

A lumbar puncture (LP) was performed and showed an opening pressure of 20 cm H_2O, white cell count 6×10^6/l, red cell count 64×10^6/l, protein 0.7 g/l, glucose 8 mmol/l (plasma 14 mmol/l). No organisms were identified on Gram stain or culture and viral polymerase chain reaction (PCR) was negative for HSV, cytomegalovirus, Epstein–Barr virus, varicella zoster virus and enterovirus.

Results of Definitive Investigations

The clinical picture and MRI were consistent with a sub-acute sub-cortical progressive cognitive impairment with associated changes in personality and behaviour.

In the context of immunosuppression, due to renal transplant therapy, JC virus was assessed by PCR of the cerebrospinal fluid (CSF). The PCR for JC virus was positive at 230,000 copies/ml.

Diagnosis

The high JC virus titre in the CSF supported the diagnosis of progressive multifocal leukoencephalopathy (PML) secondary to immunosuppression. The findings were felt to be diagnostic and therefore a brain biopsy was not performed.

Management and Outcome

Following discussion with the renal transplant team, his mycophenolate was stopped but he remained on tacrolimus 1 mg bd. Despite this, he continued to deteriorate. He had difficulty dressing and was becoming increasingly unsteady on his feet. On examination he had evidence of pyramidal weakness of the left upper and lower limbs, a right homonymous hemianopia and apraxia.

A repeat MRI brain scan at this time showed interval progression with new lesions in the left occipital and

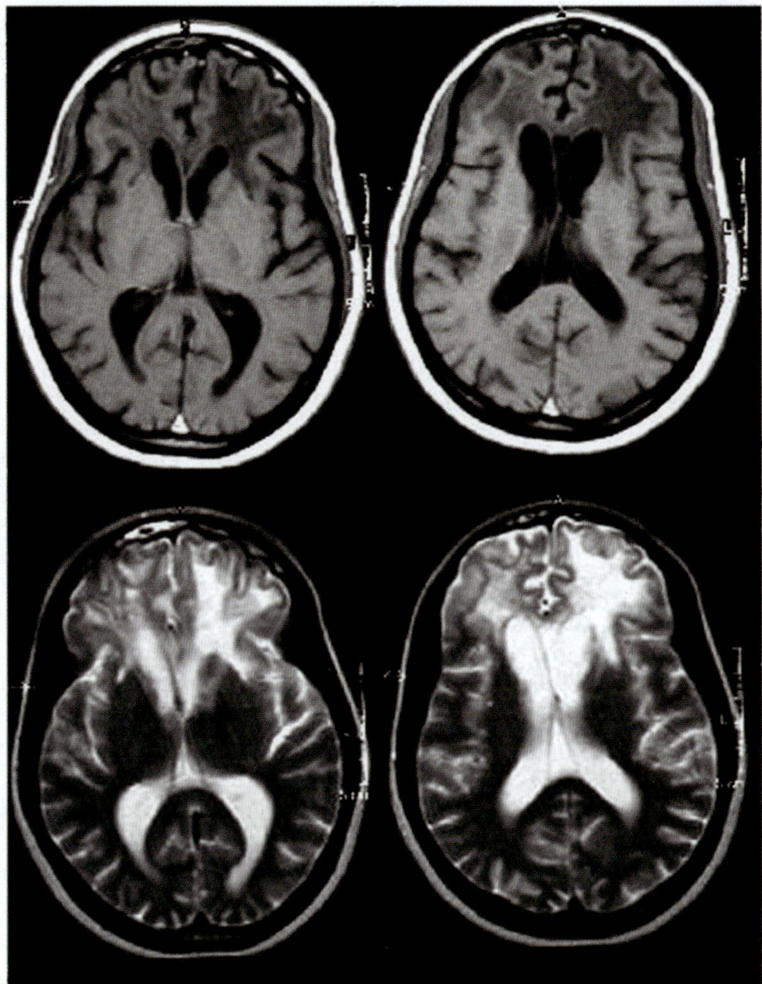

Figure 47.1. T1-weighted (upper) and T2-weighted (lower) axial MRI scan images in a 59-year-old with sub-acute personality, behaviour and cognition change.
This demonstrates large areas of white matter signal abnormality within both frontal lobes, more pronounced on the left than right. There is no mass effect or contrast enhancement. The cortical grey matter is not involved.

right parietal lobes, involving the splenium of the corpus callosum. As previously, there was no enhancement or mass effect and the abnormalities were restricted to the cerebral white matter. Perfusion-weighted sequences did not demonstrate any areas of hypoperfusion. Diffusion-weighted sequences revealed areas of relatively restricted diffusion along the margins of the lesion. The MR spectroscopy demonstrated reduced *N*-acetylaspartate with no significant lactate peak and choline was elevated. These findings were consistent with PML, rather than a malignant process such as glioma and lymphoma.

Tacrolimus was stopped and he was maintained on prednisolone 10 mg daily. He was started on mefloquine 250 mg base (equivalent to 275 mg salt) for 3 days and then once weekly for potential anti-PML properties.

He initially appeared to stabilise, but after 3 weeks neurological deterioration continued and he developed generalised seizures. He died 2 months later.

Discussion

PML is a demyelinating condition due to JC virus infection and occurs in association with immunosuppression. JC virus causes central demyelination through destruction of oligodendrocytes and myelin processes. Damage to these cells results in a failure of the natural turnover of myelin. Typically this process is characterised by only a very limited inflammatory infiltrate in the CSF and brain parenchyma, although florid, inflammatory forms do occur, particularly in association with immune reconstitution following treatment for HIV [1]. JC virus is a ubiquitous DNA virus and by adulthood 50–80% of immunologically normal people in the UK are seropositive [1]. The route of infection is unclear, but contaminated food and water are the proposed mechanisms as the virus has been isolated from sewage.

Most cases of PML are in HIV-positive individuals and PML is an AIDS-defining condition. Prior to antiretroviral therapy PML occurred in around 5% of people with HIV prior to death [2]. Incidence has decreased in areas where antiretroviral treatment is available; however, prevalence has increased with improved survival. PML occurs disproportionately in HIV compared to other forms of immunosuppression [3], but can occur in those with severe immunodeficiency such as transplant recipients, as demonstrated in this case [4]. PML can occur as a complication of certain monoclonal immune-suppressive therapies. For example, patients starting nataluzimab (tysabri) therapy for multiple sclerosis should be warned of the risk of PML, currently thought to be around 1 in 1000 cases [5]; in addition, the JC virus serostatus and urine JC virus PCR can be used to stratify the risk of developing PML on this therapy. Other risk factors include duration of therapy and prior use of certain immunosuppressive therapies [6,7]. Other monoclonal therapies associated with PML include efalizumab (Raptiva), which has now been withdrawn as a treatment for psoriasis because of the risk. There also appears to be an increased risk in association with rituximab (Maptera).

The clinical presentation of PML is typically one of an insidious onset of a focal neurological deficit, dependent on the site of the lesion or lesions. For example, a hemiparesis, frontal lobe syndromes and cortical blindness. Cognitive deficits, typically of a subcortical nature, occur in around a third of cases, usually alongside focal neurology, but they may be the sole presenting feature, particularly in those with bifrontal lesions such as in this case. Although primarily a subcortical process, seizures can occur in around 20% [2]. Headache, fever or meningism are usually absent and, if present, raise suspicion of an alternative central nervous system infection.

Demonstration of JC viral DNA in the CSF in those with an appropriate clinical syndrome is highly specific for PML. The sensitivity of viral PCR is greater than 70% and this increases with progression of disease. Therefore, if the initial CSF PCR is negative but the clinical suspicion remains high, a repeat LP should be performed and the CSF tested again. The MRI scan may show characteristic multifocal white matter lesions corresponding to the areas of clinical deficits. Typically there is no mass effect or contrast enhancement, reflecting the fact that there is little inflammation. The lesions found on MRI of patients with PML can be distinguished from the white matter changes of HIV-associated dementia by the asymmetry, lack of atrophy and the involvement of the subcortical U-fibres. Diffusion-weighted imaging and MRI spectroscopy can also be useful to distinguish PML from malignancy, as in this case. Often the definitive diagnosis is established by histopathological assessment of brain biopsy tissue, which demonstrates demyelination, bizarre astrocytes and enlarged oligodendroglial nuclei in association with JC virus (**Figures 47.2** and 47.3). However, brain biopsy is not always required, as in the case described, as clinical and imaging manifestations consistent with PML in a patient in whom JC virus is detected by PCR of the is also considered diagnostic [8].

There is currently no specific treatment of PML other than reversal of immune suppression, when possible [6]. In addition to partial reversal of immune suppression in this case, mefloquine was tried on the basis of *in vitro* efficacy and case reports [9]. However, mefloquine, along with a number of other agents with promising *in vitro* effect against JC virus, have not proved efficacious in clinical trials [10]. Without reversal of immune suppression PML is invariably fatal, usually within months of diagnosis. In this case

Figure 47.2. High-power microscopic view of a section of white matter from the brain of an adult with PML, which shows a large astrocyte near the centre. Many of the other small cells have eosinophilic, pink-staining, intranuclear inclusions which are collections of JC virus. The arrow indicates an infected oligodendrocyte. (From: Wellcome images (W0043178).)

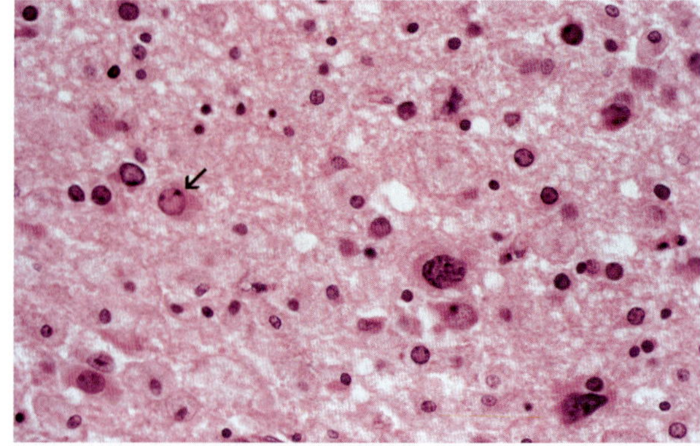

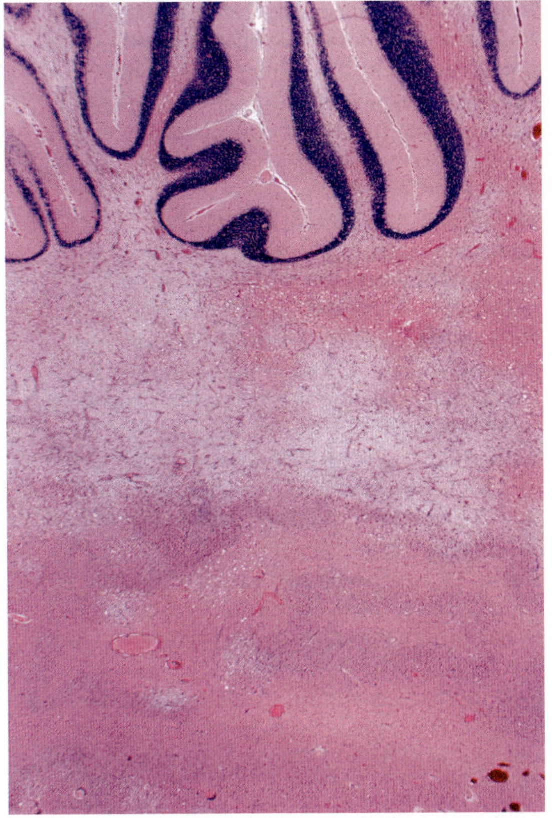

Figure 47.3. Low-power microscopic view of a section of cerebellum from the brain of an adult with PML. The white matter beneath the nuclear layer of the cortex is paler than the lower white matter, due to myelination. (From: Wellcome images (W0043175).)

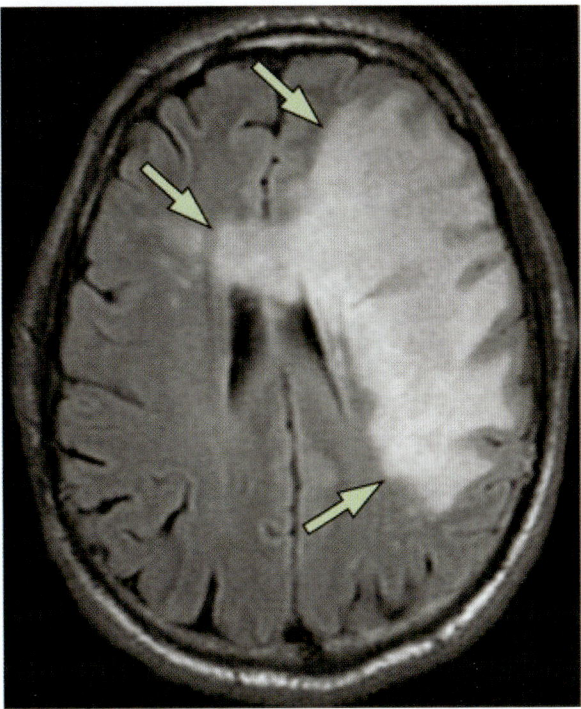

Figure 47.4. Axial T2 FLAIR MRI from a patient with PML IRIS showing lesions in the left hemispheric white matter and the corpus callosum. (Reproduced from [13] by permission of Elsevier.)

immunosuppressive treatment was ultimately stopped, although this must be balanced against the risks of transplant rejection. In those with PML secondary to HIV infection, antiretroviral treatment can stabilise disease, sometimes for months or years [11]. Cases of PML secondary to monoclonal antibody treatment should receive plasma exchange [5].

Rapid improvements in immune function following the above measures may lead to a paradoxical worsening of clinical disease associated with inflammation and swelling of lesions; termed immune reconstitution inflammatory syndrome (IRIS) (**Figure 47.4**). This may occur following plasma exchange for nataluzimab-associated PML, as well as for those receiving antiretroviral therapy for HIV. In some patients commencing antiretroviral therapy previously asymptomatic disease may be unmasked. IRIS associated with PML can be managed with corticosteroids [12].

Key Points

- PML is characterised by CNS demyelination due to JC virus in association with immunosuppression.
- Most cases are seen in advanced HIV infection; however, PML can occur with immunosuppression from other causes, e.g. transplant recipients and those receiving some monoclonal antibody treatments.
- There is no specific anti-JC virus treatment for PML; instead, immune function should be improved if possible.
- If immune function can be restored, PML may stabilise for several years; without this PML is universally fatal.
- Rapid improvements in immune function may lead to a paradoxical worsening of PML as part of an IRIS.

Looking Back

Pathological cases similar to PML were described as early as 1930 by German pathologist Hallervorden; however, PML was not crystallised as a distinct term until the late 1950s. Astrom and colleagues first described the illness in 1958 on the basis of its unique pathological features, including demyelination, abnormal oligodendroglial nuclei and giant astrocytes.

Did You Know?

In 1970 an American war veteran named John Cunningham developed PML as a complication of Hodgkin's disease. A new polyoma virus was isolated from his brain tissue at post mortem and subsequently named with his initials – JC virus [14].

References

1. Major EO, Amemiya K, Tornatore CS, Houff SA, Berger JR. Pathogenesis and molecular biology of progressive multifocal leukoencephalopathy, the JC virus-induced demyelinating disease of the human brain. Clin Microbiol Rev 1992;**5**:49–73.
2. Saribas AS, Ozdemir A, Lam C, Safak M. JC virus-induced progressive multifocal leukoencephalopathy. Future Virol 2010;**5**:313–23.
3. Berger JR. Progressive multifocal leukoencephalopathy in acquired immunodeficiency syndrome: explaining the high incidence and disproportionate frequency of the illness relative to other immunosuppressive conditions. J Neurovirol 2003;**9**(Suppl 1):38–41.
4. Mateen FJ, Muralidharan R, Carone M, et al. Progressive multifocal leukoencephalopathy in transplant recipients. Annals Neurol 2011;**70**:305–22.
5. Yousry TA, Major EO, Ryschkewitsch C, et al. Evaluation of patients treated with natalizumab for progressive multifocal leukoencephalopathy. N Engl J Med 2006;**354**:924–33.
6. Sorensen PS, Bertolotto A, Edan G, et al. Risk stratification for progressive multifocal leukoencephalopathy in patients treated with natalizumab. Mult Scler 2012;**18**:143–52.
7. Hunt D, Giovannoni G. Natalizumab-associated progressive multifocal leucoencephalopathy: a practical approach to risk profiling and monitoring. Pract Neurol 2012;**12**:25–35.
8. Berger JR, Aksamit AJ, Clifford DB, et al. PML diagnostic criteria: consensus statement from the AAN Neuroinfectious Disease Section. Neurology 2013;**80**:1430–8.
9. Gofton TE, Al-Khotani A, O'Farrell B, Ang LC, McLachlan RS. Mefloquine in the treatment of progressive multifocal leukoencephalopathy. J Neurol Neurosurg Psych 2011;**82**:452–5.
10. Brew BJ, Davies NW, Cinque P, Clifford DB, Nath A. Progressive multifocal leukoencephalopathy and other forms of JC virus disease. Nature Rev Neurol 2010;**6**:667–79.
11. Antinori A, Cingolani A, Lorenzini P, et al. Clinical epidemiology and survival of progressive multifocal leukoencephalopathy in the era of highly active antiretroviral therapy: data from the Italian Registry Investigative Neuro AIDS (IRINA). J Neurovirol 2003;**9**(Suppl 1):47–53.
12. Steiner I, Berger JR. Update on progressive multifocal leukoencephalopathy. Curr Neurol Neurosci Rep 2012;**12**:680–6.
13. Tan CS, Koralnik IJ. Progressive multifocal leukoencephalopathy and other disorders caused by JC virus: clinical features and pathogenesis. Lancet Neurol 2010;**9**:425–37.
14. Padgett BL, Walker DL, ZuRhein GM, Eckroade RJ, Dessel BH. Cultivation of papova-like virus from human brain with progressive multifocal leucoencephalopathy. Lancet 1971;**1**:1257–60.

CASE 48

Seen the Last of This?

Jennifer Lemon and Rachel Kneen

History

A previously well 16-month-old girl presented on day 2 of illness with fever, lethargy, irritability and poor oral intake. Until this illness she had been making normal developmental progress. She was fully immunised, including for measles, mumps and rubella, and was not considered to be immunocompromised.

Examination and Progress

She was clinically septic, although her Glasgow coma score was 15/15, and her examination was abnormal (**Figure 48.1**).

A clinical diagnosis of likely bacterial meningitis was made but no lumbar puncture (LP) was undertaken at this point despite there being no contraindications. She was treated with fluid resuscitation, intravenous (IV) antibiotics, IV aciclovir and IV dexamethasone. There was a slow improvement over the next few days with resolution of fever.

On day 7 her condition deteriorated with pyrexia and increased irritability noted. In addition, leg movements were reduced, especially on the left side. The tone was reduced in both limbs and the deep tendon reflexes were increased. The plantar response on the right was equivocal but up-going on the left.

Figure 48.1. Immediate clinical examination findings in a 16-month-old child presenting with a 2-day history of fever.

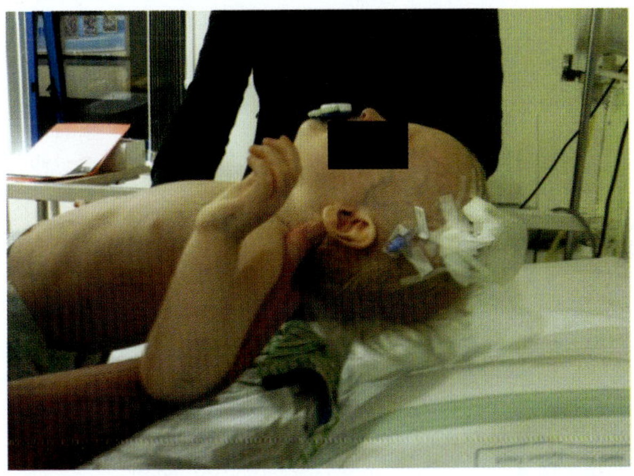

This demonstrates marked neck stiffness and retraction. (Image shown with parental permission.)

Differential Diagnosis

Severe bacterial meningitis with a recognised complication; for example, cerebritis, venous sinus thrombosis and secondary infarction, subdural collection/empyema, brain abscess(es), vasculitis.

Initial Investigations

Admission bloods showed a C-reactive protein of 503 mg/l, white cell count (WCC) 3.4 cell/mm^3, haemoglobin 1020 g/l, platelets 124/mm^3. A computer tomography (CT) brain scan was performed (**Figure 48.2**).

She underwent neurosurgical treatment with a burr hole and drain insertion. Cerebrospinal fluid (CSF) from subdural collection was purulent with a WCC of 3900 cell/mm^3 (80% neutrophils).

Figure 48.2. A CT scan for a 16-month-old girl who presented with fever and neck stiffness, and then became unconscious.

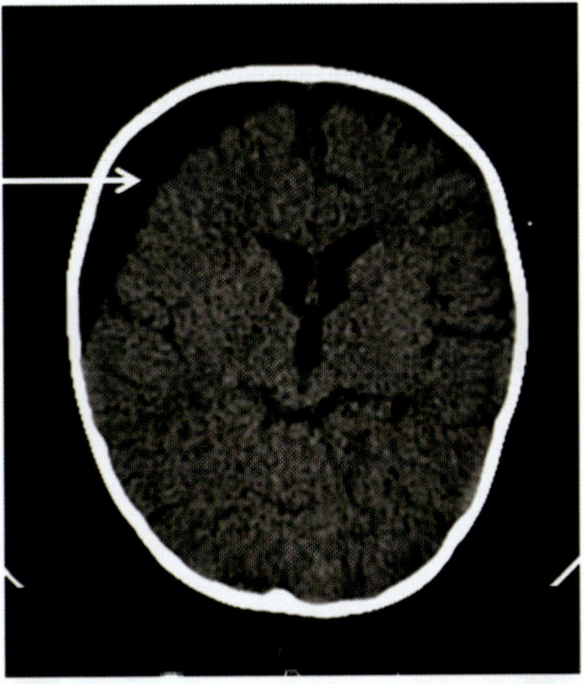

Non-contrast CT scan demonstrates right-sided subdural collection (arrow). This demonstrates a right subdural collection around the frontal lobe.

Results of Definitive Investigations

CSF culture after antibiotics was negative. However, blood culture from admission grew *Haemophilus influenzae* (serotyping revealed type f).

Diagnosis

Invasive *Haemophilus influenzae* type f disease, manifesting as bacteraemia and meningitis with a subdural collection.

Progress and Outcome

On day 17 she was noted to be inattentive to noise and was diagnosed with bilateral sensorineural hearing loss following an audiology assessment. Magnetic resonance imaging on day 19 showed soft tissue opacification of the cochlea bilaterally.

Her leg weakness improved with neurorehabilitation. She was discharged after 4 weeks on oral antibiotics. She has subsequently had a cochlear implant fitted and was making good developmental progress when last seen. No underlying problems with this child's immune system were discovered on thorough testing.

Discussion

Haemophilus influenzae is a Gram-negative coccobacillus which causes invasive bacterial disease (**Figure 48.3**) [1]. Infants and older adults are particularly susceptible. Of the encapsulated forms, six serotypes (a–f) have been identified. The most commonly isolated serotype has historically been *H. Influenza* type b (Hib); however, the incidence worldwide has been declining due to widespread Hib vaccination for children. In the UK, Hib conjugate vaccine was introduced to the routine childhood immunisation programme in 1992 [1]. However, there are no vaccines for non-b type infections.

Public Health England conducts enhanced national surveillance for invasive *H. influenzae* disease including serotyping for all NHS laboratories in England and Wales. They have reported a slow rise in *H. influenzae* type f (Hif) cases and in 2009 Hif overtook Hib as the most prevalent encapsulated serotype causing invasive *Haemophilus* infection (**Figure 48.4**). Non-encapsulated *H. influenzae* accounted for over a half of cases. Cases of *H. influenzae* e (Hie) are also showing a gradual rise in England and Wales, while serotypes a, c and d remain rare [1]. Hib vaccination reduces nasal carriage of Hib and it is thought that this could lead to increased colonisation with the less-virulent non-b serotypes [2].

Children account for around a quarter of cases of Hif infection and the disease burden is predominantly in infants and young children [1,3,4]. Meningitis is the most common clinical manifestation of Hif and other encapsulated non-b type organism infection in children, although septicaemia and pneumonia are also common [1–3,5,6]. Presentation is with fever and signs of meningism, and there is commonly a history of preceding upper respiratory tract infection, including otitis media [6]. Data regarding outcomes of Hif meningitis in children are sparse. Death does occur but is uncommon in healthy children [1,2]. The majority of children make a full recovery; however, some children are left with neurological sequelae, including hearing loss, as seen in this case [2]. Relapse or recurrence can occur, especially in those with immunodeficiency [2,4].

Figure 48.3. Photomicrograph using a Gram-stain technique. This demonstrates Haemophilus influenza. (From www.cdc.gov/hi-disease/about/photos.html#)

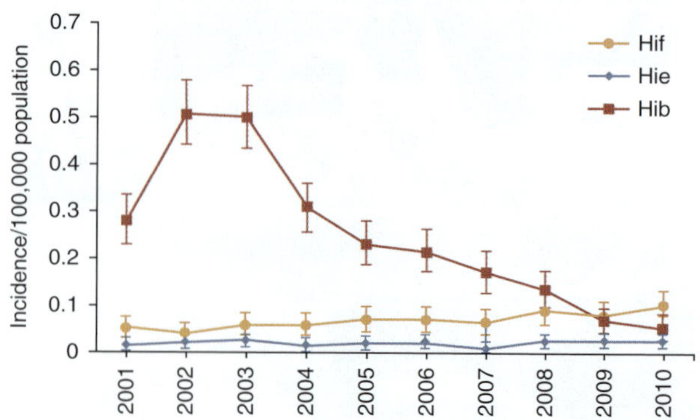

Figure 48.4. Epidemiology of invasive encapsulated *Haemophillus influenzae* disease, England and Wales, 2000–2009. Error bars indicate 95% confidence intervals. (Reproduced with permission from [1].)

Medical comorbidities or risk factors are commonly reported in children with non-b type *Haemophilus influenzae*, including prematurity, immunosuppression, metabolic or neurological conditions [1,2,5]. Invasive Hif infection in children may therefore indicate an underlying disorder [7].

In this case no underlying risk factors were found. The case also underscores the need for an LP to be done on admission unless there is a contraindication. Here it would likely have allowed the causative organism of the meningitis to be identified earlier, although this would probably not have affected the ultimate outcome.

Key Points

- Invasive *Haemophilus influenzae* type b (Hib) disease is uncommon in children in the post-vaccination era, but other encapsulated serotypes, including *Haemophilus influenzae* type f (Hif), are becoming increasingly common in the UK.
- In children with less-virulent non-b type serotypes, consideration should be given to whether there might be an underlying susceptibility to infection.
- The LP plays a pivotal role in the diagnosis of bacterial meningitis and other neurological infections and allows tailoring of drug therapy. It should always be performed when meningoencephalitis is suspected, except where there is an established contraindication, as the results can change the management [8].

Looking Back

H. influenzae was first described in 1892 by Richard Pfeiffer during an influenza pandemic. It was mistakenly considered to be the cause of influenza until 1933 when the viral cause of influenza became apparent.

Did You Know?

Fluoroquinolone resistance has only rarely been observed in *H. influenza* – the question remains as to how best preserve this situation.

References

1. Ladhani SN, Collins S, Vickers A, et al. Invasive *Haemophilus influenzae* serotype e and f Disease, England and Wales. Emerg Infect Dis 2012;**18**:725–32.
2. Fickweiler K, Borte M, Fasshauer M, et al. Meningitis due to *Haemophilus influenzae* type f in an 8-year-old girl with congenital humoral immunodeficiency. Infection 2004;**32**:112–15.
3. Pincus DR, Robson JM. Meningitis due to *Haemophilus influenzae* type f. J Paediatr Child Health 1998;**34**:95–6.
4. Resman F, Ristovski M, Ahl J, et al. Invasive disease caused by *Haemophilus influenzae* in Sweden 1997–2009; evidence of increasing incidence and clinical burden of non-type b strains. Clin Microbiol Infect 2011;**17**:1638–45.
5. Heath PT, Booy R, Azzopardi HJ, et al. Non-type b *Haemophilus influenzae* disease: clinical and epidemiologic characteristics in the *Haemophilus influenzae* type b vaccine era. Pediatr Infect Dis J 2001;**20**:300–5.
6. Urwin G, Krohn JA, Deaver-Robinson K, Wenger JD, Farley MM. The *Haemophilus influenzae* SG. Invasive disease due to *Haemophilus influenzae* serotype f: clinical and epidemiologic characteristics in the *H. influenzae* serotype b vaccine era. Clin Infect Dis 1996;**22**:1069–76.
7. Nitta DM, Jackson MA, Burry VF, Olson LC. Invasive *Haemophilus influenzae* type-f disease. Pediatr Infect Dis J 1995;**14**:157–60.
8. Kneen R, Solomon T, Appleton R. The role of lumbar puncture in children with suspected central nervous system infection. BMC Pediatr 2002;**2**:8.

CASE 49 Sick as a Swine

Sophie Miller, Benedict D. Michael and Tom Solomon

History

A 19-year-old presented to hospital in Malaysia with a 3-day history of left frontal headache, fever and a 5-minute episode of jerking in the right lower limb which occurred just prior to admission. This was followed by numbness and weakness affecting the same limb lasting 2 hours. The patient worked on a pig farm in Malaysia where he had been staying with family. His duties involved feeding, cleaning and injecting sick pigs. While on the farm 4 months earlier, a worker had died of an unexplained illness and in the same week the patient experienced a 2-day febrile illness characterised by rhinorrhoea, dry cough, headache and blurred vision. The patient reported being fully vaccinated as a child and had received hepatitis A and B, rabies and Japanese encephalitis virus (JEV) vaccinations. There was no history of dog bites, rashes or symptoms of gastroenteritis.

Examination

On examination the patient was apyrexial. General medical examination was unremarkable. Tone was increased in both the right upper and lower limb. The right leg was weak with Medical Research Council power grading 4/5 in all muscle groups; however, reflexes were normal throughout. The patient had no sensory loss other than the numbness, which lasted 2 hours.

Initial Differential Diagnosis

The history was consistent with an acute brain infection, or a space-occupying lesion. Possibilities included:

- Viral infection
  - Sporadic, e.g. herpes simplex virus (HSV), varicella zoster virus (VZV), adenovirus, some enteroviruses
  - Epidemic, e.g. JEV, dengue virus, Nipah virus, rabies virus, enterovirus 71 (rabies and JEV are both possible, despite the vaccination history; the history may not be reliable, and the killed vaccines only offer protection for a limited number of years)
- Bacterial infection, including scrub typhus, tuberculosis, or bacterial abscess
- Parasitic infections, e.g. cerebral malaria, cysticercosis
- Other space-occupying lesion, e.g. tumour

Results of Initial Investigations

Full blood count and liver function were normal, but he was slightly hyponatraemic at 131 mmol/l. Thick and thin blood films were negative for malarial parasites.

Cerebrospinal fluid (CSF) opening pressure was not recorded, white cell count was 173 cells/mm^3, with 100% lymphocytes, CSF protein was 8.4 g/l, glucose was 4.9 g/l (no serum glucose was taken) and CSF culture was negative. A computed tomography brain scan on day 1 was normal.

Progression

Over the following 3 days the patient experienced intermittent mild pyrexia and had three tonic–clonic seizures lasting 2 minutes duration. The patient was loaded with intravenous phenytoin and his convulsions ceased completely.

CSF polymerase chain reaction (PCR) was negative for HSV, VZV, enteroviruses, adenoviruses, JEV and dengue. Serum IgG was strongly positive for JEV consistent with recent previous vaccination.

Results of Definitive Investigations

PCR from CSF was positive for Nipah virus.

ELISA detected Nipah virus IgM antibodies in all serum and CSF samples.

Diagnosis

This patient had Nipah virus encephalitis, a relatively recently described cause of viral encephalitis.

Management and Outcome

Due to the CSF pleocytosis the patient initially received penicillin and chloramphenicol. There were no further episodes of pyrexia or convulsions and he was discharged home, well, 11 days after admission. At 3-month follow-up there had been no further seizures.

Prevention

There is currently no vaccination for Nipah virus and so the primary methods of prevention are promoting awareness in those populations most at risk, disinfection of pig farms with detergent agents, and also the controlled quarantine and culling of domestic animals suspected of infection with the virus.

Discussion

Nipah virus is an RNA paramyxovirus closely related to Hendra virus which caused cases of severe respiratory illness and encephalitis in humans in contact with infected horses in Australia. Like Hendra virus the natural reservoir of Nipah virus appears to be pteropid fruit bats. They pass the infection to animals, classically pigs via the contamination of fruit on which they are feeding, or via their excreta (**Figure 49.1**) [1]. Unwell pigs then develop respiratory disease, and pass the infection to humans, principally via respiratory secretions. Thus, in Malaysia, pig farmers, such as in this case, are at increased risk. Nipah and Hendra are among an increasing number of viral infections found to be transmitted by bats (**Figure 49.2**).

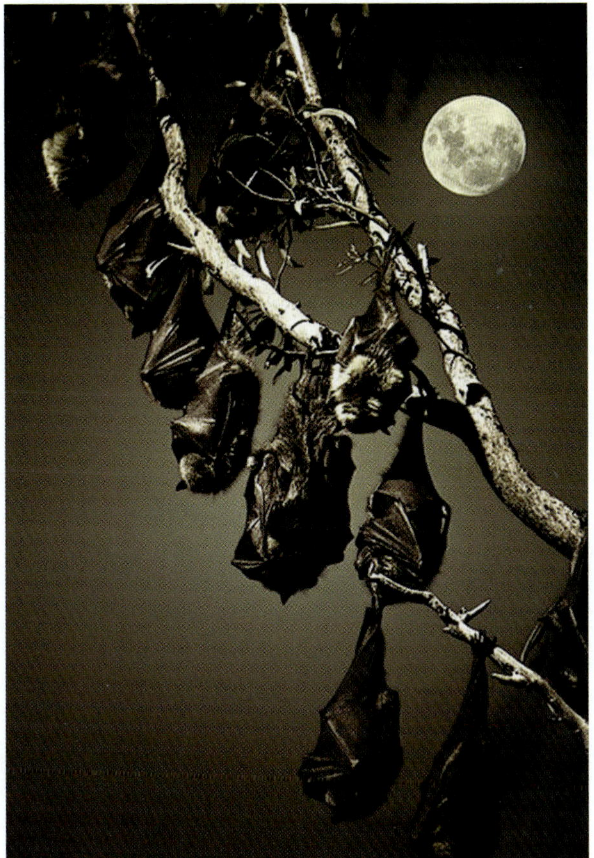

Figure 49.1. 'Hanging out'. Some flying foxes. (Photo courtesy of Louise Docker.)

Nipah virus was first discovered during an outbreak of strange respiratory illness in pigs in Malaysia in 1998. This illness preceded cases of severe, often fatal encephalitis in humans who were in direct contact with the animals [2–4]. Since its discovery there have been more than 12 further outbreaks, most notably in Bangladesh, where evidence of human-to-human transmission has been identified. There also appears to be increased lethality in the strain of Nipah virus in Bangladesh in comparison to the Malaysian virus [5].

The first outbreaks in Bangladesh were in 2001 and there have been hundreds of deaths since then. There is some evidence that the key route of transmission of Nipah viruses in Malaysia and Bangladesh may be different [5]. In Malaysia, bats infected pigs which acted as an amplifier for the virus (**Figure 49.3**), whereas in Bangladesh, the virus appears to also be spread from bats to humans via the consumption of raw date sap which has been infected with the urine or saliva of infected bats. The collection of date sap traditionally occurs between December and February and the outbreaks appear to peak at this period. It is a difficult risk factor to combat as raw date sap is a very popular drink, especially in rural areas [1,6]. The government is raising awareness about Nipah virus through talk shows, and adverts and by educating suppliers of raw date sap. Occasionally family members and health care workers in contact with patients have become infected through nosocomial spread.

The typical presentation of Nipah encephalitis is with fever, headache and reduced consciousness, which can progress to coma. Common clinical signs include areflexia, hypotonia, cerebellar signs and segmental myoclonus. Eventually many patients exhibit signs of brainstem involvement with difficulty breathing and death [7].

Although the incubation of Nipah virus tends to be between 4 and 45 days there have been cases of delayed-onset encephalitis occurring up to 4 months after exposure to the virus, as described in this case. Therefore, as always, it is important to take a thorough travel history and be alert to travel to the affected areas of South Asia. Even if the travel was months ago, it still does not completely rule out the possibility of infection with Nipah virus [2].

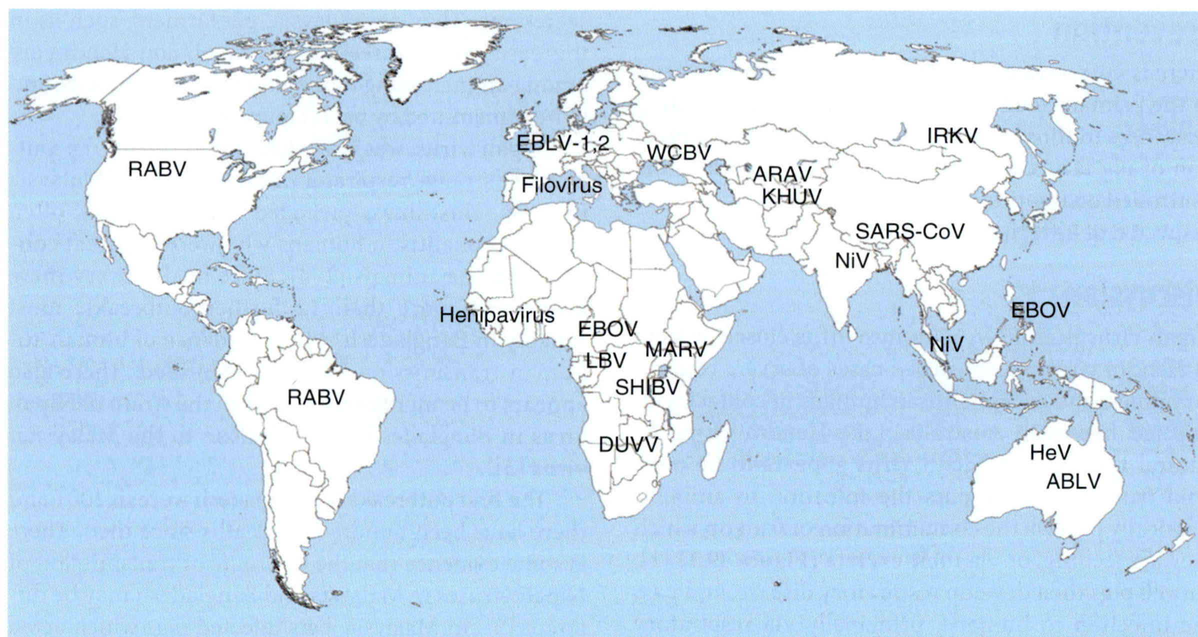

Figure 49.2. Geographical distribution of bat-associated and presumed bat-associated viral infections. *Abbreviations*: RABV, rabies virus; EBLV-1,2, European bat lyssaviruses type 1 and 2; WCBV, West Caucasian bat virus; ARAV, Aravan virus; KHUV, Khujand virus; IRKV, Irkut virus; LBV, Lagos bat virus; SHIBV, Shimoni bat virus; DUVV, Duvenhage virus; MARV, Marburg virus; EBOV, Ebola virus; Filovirus, unclassified filovirus detected in bats in Europe; HeV, Hendra virus; NiV, Nipah virus; Henipavirus, unclassified henipavirus; SARS-CoV, SARS coronavirus. (Image from [9] with permission of Taylor & Francis www.tandfonline.com.)

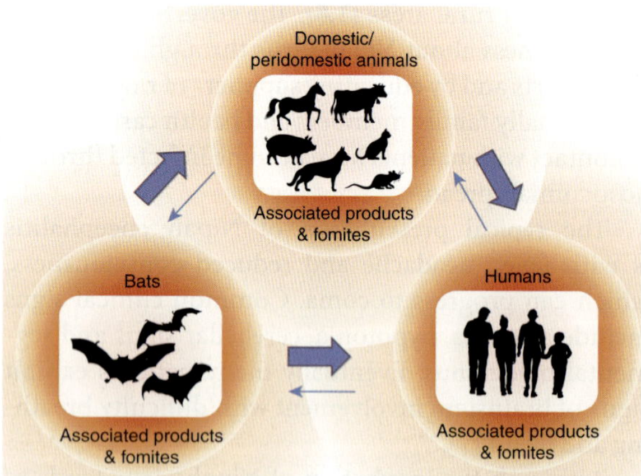

Figure 49.3. Possible routes of disease transmission between bats, peri-domestic/domestic animals, and humans. Thick arrows represent the most significant pathways for bat-associated viral infections. Thin arrows represent pathways about which less is known or that are less common (as in the case of transmission of pathogens directly from humans to bats). (Image re-drawn from [8] with permission of Taylor & Francis www.tandfonline.com.)

Although no vaccine is currently available, trials using recombinant measles vaccinations in hamsters and African green monkeys have shown promising results. The data suggest testing in humans could be viable. This would greatly reduce the mortality and morbidity from this currently incurable disease [9].

Key Points

- Nipah virus can cause fatal encephalitis.
- Nipah encephalitis should be a differential in patients returning from areas such as South Asia, particularly Bangladesh and Malaysia, where outbreaks of this virus have been reported.
- Those in close contact with pigs, bats or involved in the collection and consumption of raw date sap are particularly at risk.
- There is currently no vaccination or cure for Nipah virus encephalitis.

Looking Back

Nipah virus is named after 'Sungai Nipah', a town in Malaysia where the first patient identified with this virus came from.

Did You Know?

The natural hosts of Nipah virus are pteropid fruit bats; the 'flying fox' or 'megabat' is particularly suspect. Some species can fly several thousand miles.

References

1. Ksiazek TG, Rota PA, Rollin PE. A review of Nipah and Hendra viruses with an historical aside. Virus Res 2011;**162**:173–83.
2. Wong SC, Ooi MH, Wong MNL, et al. Late presentation of Nipah virus encephalitis and kinetics of the humoral immune response. J Neurol Neurosurg Psych 2001;**71**:552–4.
3. Chua KB, Goh KJ, Wong KT, et al. Fatal encephalitis due to Nipah virus among pig-farmers in Malaysia. Lancet 1999;**9186**:1257–9.
4. Chua KB, Koh CL, Hooi PS, et al. Isolation of Nipah virus from Malaysian Island flying-foxes. Microbe Infect 2002;**2**:145–51.
5. Arif SM, Basher A, Quddus MR, Faiz MA. Re-emergence Nipah – a review. Mymensingh Med J 2012;**21**:772–9.
6. Rahman M, Hossain M, Luby S, et al. Date palm sap linked to Nipah virus outbreak in Bangladesh, 2008. Vect Borne Zoonotic Dis 2012;**12**:65–72.
7. Lo M, Lowe L, Rota P, et al. Characterization of Nipah virus from outbreaks in Bangladesh, 2008–2010. Emerg Infect Dis 2012;**18**:248–55.
8. Kuzmin IV, Bozick B, Guagliardo SA, et al. Bats, emerging infectious diseases, and the rabies paradigm revisited. Emerg Health Threats J 2011;**4**:7159.
9. Yoneda M, Georges-Courbot M, Kai C, et al. Recombinant measles virus vaccine expressing the Nipah virus glycoprotein protects against lethal Nipah virus challenge. PLoS ONE 2013;**8**:e58414.

CASE 50 A Tic in the (Voice) Box

Katie Rose and Rachel Kneen

History

A previously healthy 7-year-old girl presented to the emergency department with a 1-day history of sudden-onset motor tics and a dramatic change in behaviour including emotional lability, aggressive and challenging behaviour and disinhibition. Frequent episodes of rapid jerking of her head to the right side were described and witnessed, although there was no loss of consciousness noted. Over the course of the next 2 days the frequency of these episodes increased, and progressed to involve movement of the head, arms and legs. A week before admission she had complained of a sore throat and was noted to have a mild fever, treated only with paracetamol. Her parents were born in the Middle East but she was born in the UK and there was no history of overseas travel. She was otherwise well and had been making good developmental progress. She lived with her mother and was not thought to be immunocompromised. She was fully vaccinated and not taking any regular medication.

Examination

Systemic examination was normal; in particular, no abnormalities were found in the cardiovascular system. There was no joint swelling or rashes. However, examination of the pharynx was abnormal (**Figure 50.1**). Neurological examination, including examination of cranial nerves, was normal, particularly eye movements were normal. She was apyrexial and observations remained stable throughout.

Frequent simple and complex motor tics involving the head, face and arms were noticed. They were worse when the patient was relaxed and inactive; they improved when she was engaged with an activity in which she was interested. She was also restless, overactive and overly friendly with ward visitors and staff. The nurses also noted she would have frequent changes of mood and at times cry for no obvious reason.

Figure 50.1. Appearance of the throat similar to that seen in a 7-year-old girl who presented with sudden onset motor tics and a dramatic change in behaviour.

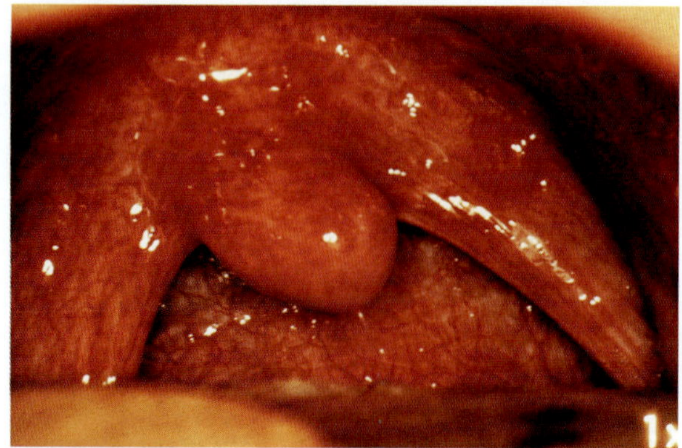

This shows a sore throat. (Photo courtesy of BSIP/UIG via Getty Images.)

Initial Differential Diagnosis

- There is a broad differential for movement disorders
  - Infection-related: paediatric autoimmune neuropsychiatric disorders associated with streptococcal infections (PANDAS), sub-acute sclerosing panencephalitis, HIV, Prion disease, Lyme disease (neuroborreliosis), microemboli from sub-acute bacterial endocarditis
  - Drug-related
  - Cerebrovascular: Moyamoya syndrome, central nervous sytem vasculitis, anoxic encephalopathy
  - Metabolic: Wilson's disease, glutaric aciduria (type 1), neuroacanthosis, thyroid dysfunction
  - Genetic: Huntington's chorea, benign familial chorea
  - Immune-mediated: systemic lupus erythematosis, multiple sclerosis, opsoclonus myoclonus ataxia syndrome (eye movements are characteristic)
  - Myoclonic epilepsy (an electroencephalogram that captured abnormal movements may be useful in excluding this)

Results of Initial Investigations

Initial blood results were unremarkable, including normal renal and bone profiles and liver function tests. Her platelet count was marginally raised, but the rest of the full blood count, as well as C-reactive protein and erythrocyte sedimentation rate, were within normal limits.

Throat swabs were taken and found to be negative. An electrocardiogram was normal. Initial neuroimaging (computed tomography brain), as well as follow-up with a magnetic resonance imaging scan, was completely normal.

Results of Definitive Investigations

Antistreptolysin O titres (ASOT) were sent and found to be markedly raised (800 units/ml), indicating recent streptococcal infection. Anti-basal ganglia antibodies were also positive.

Diagnosis

Paediatric autoimmune neuropsychiatric disorders associated with streptococcal infections (PANDAS).

Management and Outcome

Following results confirming a raised ASOT, and a clinical suspicion of PANDAS, the patient was commenced on a course of penicillin V, as well as high-dose oral steroids. She was discharged from the ward on a slowly reducing course of prednisolone, with outpatient follow-up in place.

The patient was seen in clinic following discharge and found to have on-going issues with frequent tics. She had also developed a pattern of obsessive–compulsive behaviour and the other behavioural problems continued to wax and wane. Long-term prophylaxis with penicillin V was continued for one year from the onset of symptoms, as there is some evidence suggesting prevention of further infection reduces frequency and severity of exacerbations [1].

Symptomatic treatments for the tic and behavioural disorder were considered including clonidine, haloperidol and pimozide, but were not given due to concerns about the potential for side effects. A referral to the Child and Adolescent Mental Health Team was made for support and to consider Habit Reversal Therapy. A referral to the Community Paediatrics team was also made for an assessment for her overactive behaviour. When assessed one year following the initial presentation and diagnosis there were on-going pervasive and disabling symptoms including behavioural issues and tics. These included vocal tics and swearing. The child fulfilled the criteria for a diagnosis of Tourette syndrome and subsequently responded to clonidine [2].

Discussion

The term paediatric autoimmune neuropsychiatric disorders associated with streptococcal infections (PANDAS) was first used by Swedo et al. in 1998 to describe a group of patients with childhood-onset obsessive–compulsive disorder (OCD) and tic disorders [3]. Diagnostic criteria for PANDAS includes pre-pubertal onset of OCD and/or tic disorder with dramatic onset of symptoms or symptom exacerbation associated with evidence of recent group A β-haemolytic streptococcal infection (**Figure 50.2**), as well as neurological abnormalities such as tics, choreiform movements or motor hyperactivity [3].

The underlying pathophysiology for PANDAS is thought to include the production of autoantibodies against streptococcal epitopes, which also bind to basal ganglia antigens causing basal ganglia dysfunction or destruction. Church et al. found positive anti-basal ganglia antibodies in 94% of children with a diagnosis of PANDAS, compared to 5% of controls [4]. The underlying autoimmune mechanisms, as well as many of the symptoms, are similar to those described in Sydenham's chorea – a term used to describe the neurological sequelae (and one of the major diagnostic criteria) of rheumatic fever, consisting of the acute onset of chorea weeks to months after group A β-haemolytic streptococcal infection often with associated neuropsychiatric manifestations [4].

More recently, evidence against PANDAS as a distinct diagnosis has been published, with one particular study finding that only a small number of exacerbations in those diagnosed with PANDAS were related to recent group A β-haemolytic streptococcal infection [5]. Exacerbations that were linked to recent infection

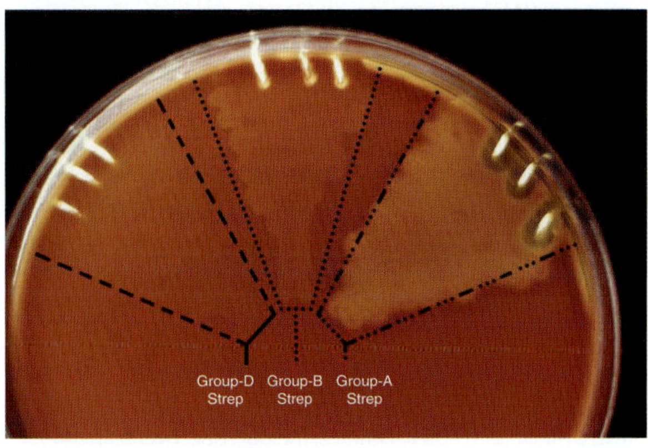

Figure 50.2. *Streptococcus* on blood agar. (From: http://phil.cdc.gov/PHIL_Images/10861/10861_lores.jpg)

were not clinically distinct from those that were not, and led the authors to hypothesise that children with PANDAS may represent a subgroup of those with Tourette's syndrome who may be more susceptible to group A β-haemolytic streptococcal infection as a precipitant of their symptoms (**Figure 50.3**).

Treatment with antibiotics is indicated in any initial group A β-haemolytic streptococcal infection, and treatment following a new diagnosis of PANDAS has been reported to lead to improvement in neuropsychiatric symptoms in 5–21 days [6]. Following initial infection prophylaxis with long-term antibiotics has been shown to reduce both the number of streptococcal infections and neuropsychiatric exacerbations [1].

Given the suggested autoimmune basis of PANDAS, immunomodulation has been used by some as a potential treatment. One study reported a dramatic improvement in OCD symptoms in children treated with plasma exchange or intravenous immunoglobulin, as well as an improvement in tic symptoms in the plasma exchange group, when compared to placebo [7]. However, given the uncertainty of a direct link between repeat group A β-haemolytic streptococcal infection and exacerbations and the potential adverse effects of treatment, at present immunotherapy is not routinely recommended in patients with a suspected diagnosis of PANDAS, and more research is needed [8,9].

Key Points

- Paediatric autoimmune neuropsychiatric disorders associated with streptococcal infections (PANDAS) presents with neuropsychiatric manifestations (typically tic and obsessive-compulsive disorders) after a strepotococcal sore throat.
- A throat swab may be negative, but elevated ASOT confirm the recent streptococcal infection. Anti-basal ganglia antibodies are also often positive.
- Look for concurrent or recent streptococcal infection in all patients with new, acute-onset tic disorder.
- Treatment is with antibiotics for the throat infection; in severe cases immunomodulatory therapies have also been used.

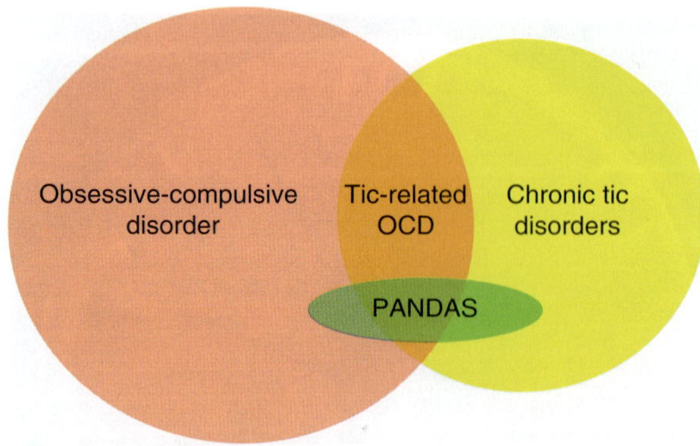

Figure 50.3. Diagram illustrating the potential overlap between the diagnosis of PANDAS and other neuropsychiatric disorders OCD, obsessive-compulsive disorder.

Looking Back

The term pediatric autoimmune neuropsychiatric disorders associated with streptococcal infections (PANDAS) was first proposed by Swedo and others at the National Institutes of Mental Health in the United States (NIMH) in the late 1990s. Although chorea was described in childen in 1686, it was not until the development of the antistreptolysin O titre as a marker of antecedent streptococcal pharyngitis in the early 1930s that there was definite proof linking Sydenham's chorea to group A streptococcal pharyngitis.

Did You Know?

Coprolalia, the occurrence of obscene or insulting utterances, is the most notorious symptom of Tourette's syndrome, but in practice it occurs in less than 50% of cases [2].

The possible relationship between throat infections and obsessive/compulsive and tic disorders, as postulated to underlie PANDAS, has created much interest and controversy among the public and the media, especially in the USA.

References

1. Snider LA, Lougee L, Slattery M, et al. Antibiotic prophylaxis with azithromycin or penicillin for childhood-onset neuropsychiatric disorders. Biol Psychiatry 2005;**57**:788–92.
2. Kurlan R. Tourette's syndrome. N Engl J Med 2010;**363**:2332–8.

3. Swedo SE, Leonard HL, Garvey M, et al. Paediatric autoimmune neuropsychiatric disorders associated with streptococcal infections: clinical description of the first 50 cases. Am J Psychiatry 1998;**155**:264–71.
4. Church AJ, Dale RC, Giovannoni G. Anti-basal ganglia antibodies: a possible diagnostic utility in idiopathic movement disorders? Arch Dis Child 2004;**89**:611–14.
5. Kurlan R, Johnson D, Kaplan EL. Streptococcal infection and exacerbations of childhood tics and obsessive–compulsive symptoms: a prospective blinded cohort study. Pediatrics 2008;**121**:1188–97.
6. Murphy ML, Pichichero ME. Prospective identification and treatment of children with pediatric autoimmune neuropsychiatric disorder associated with group A streptococcal infection (PANDAS). Arch Pediatr Adolesc Med 2002;**156**:356–61.
7. Perlmutter SJ, Leitman SF, Garvey MA, et al. Therapeutic plasma exchange and intravenous immunoglobulin for obsessive compulsive disorder and tic disorders in childhood. Lancet 1999;**354**: 1153–8.
8. Tan J, Smith CH, Goldman RD. Pediatric autoimmune neuropsychiatric disorders associated with streptococcal infections. Can Fam Phys 2012;**58**:957–9.
9. Shulman ST. Pediatric autoimmune neuropsychiatric disorders associated with streptococci (PANDAS): update. Curr Opin Pediatr 2009;**21**:127–30.

CASE 51 A Forgotten Itch

Graham A. Powell and Tom Solomon

History

A 20-year-old female student presented to the emergency department of her local hospital following a single 'blackout'. The patient described sudden-onset loss of consciousness following a short period of 'numbness' in her left arm. Witness reports described a generalised tonic–clonic seizure followed by a period of drowsiness before she fully regained consciousness. The patient was well prior to the seizure, reporting no recent headache, fever, rash, symptoms of meningism, visual disturbance or peripheral motor or sensory disturbance.

There was no significant past medical history including no history of febrile seizures or juvenile myoclonus, no family history of epilepsy or other intracranial pathology. The patient was a non-smoker, who drunk moderately with no recent binges and denied illicit drug use. She had received standard UK childhood immunisations.

Examination

Assessment in the emergency department demonstrated reduced power in the patient's left arm (4+/5) with a positive left-sided Babinski reflex. There was no consistent sensory deficit. Cranial nerve examination was normal; in particular, there was no evidence of optic disc swelling. The patient was orientated and did not appear post-ictal (Glasgow coma score 15/15). However, it had been documented by the pre-hospital paramedic team that the patient had a depressed level of consciousness.

Initial Differential Diagnosis

The presentation was of a partial seizure with secondary generalisation, followed by left upper limb weakness; this could have represented a Todd's paresis, but as it did not resolve over several hours, the possibility of an underlying focal cause became more likely. Such causes could include:

- Neoplasia (primary or secondary)
- Vascular malformations (arterio-venous malformation, cavanoma)
- Cerebrovascular disease (thrombo-embolic, haemorrhagic)
- Infection (abscess, meningitis, encephalitis, cystic infection)
- Developmental (cortical dysgenesis)
- Neurocutaneous disorders (e.g. tuberous sclerosis)
- Autoimmune/vasculitis (e.g. sarcoidosis, systemic lupus erythematosis)
- Cortical scarring (post-traumatic)

The alternative is that this was not a seizure, but was some form of non-neurological syncope

- Cardiovascular (arrhythmias)
- Metabolic (hypoglycaemia)

Results of Initial Investigations

The patient had a normal red cell, white cell and platelet count, normal renal and liver function and normal serum glucose. Inflammatory markers (erythrocyte sedimentation rate and C-reactive protein) were mildly elevated.

Computed tomography (CT) imaging of the brain was normal, and so a magnetic resonance imaging (MRI) scan was performed (**Figure 51.1**).

Figure 51.1. A T2-weighted axial MRI performed during the first inpatient episode.

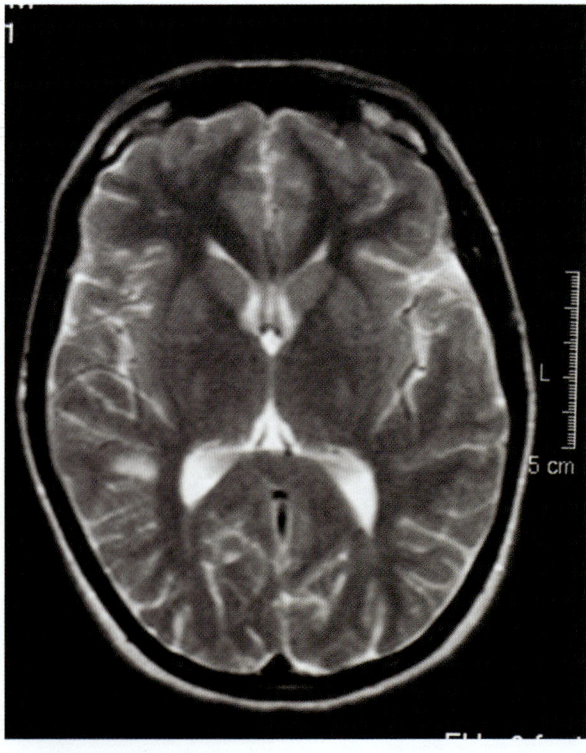

This demonstrates a small area of infarction in the right parietal lobe.

Further Investigations

Because of the cerebral infarct, she was investigated for causes of stroke in a young person. Standard 12-lead electrocardiogram (ECG), 24-hour ECG, trans-oesophageal echocardiography and cerebral angiography were all performed during the first hospital episode and were all reported as normal.

Cerebrospinal fluid (CSF) examination demonstrated mildly raised total protein, although red and white cell counts and glucose were normal. Microscopy and Gram stain were negative.

An autoimmune screen (immunoglobulins, complement, dsDNA, anticardiolipin, lupus anticoagulant) and thrombophilia screen (protein C and S, factor 5 Leiden, prothrombin gene mutation) also all came back as normal.

Refined Diagnosis

The patient was diagnosed with cryptogenic stroke and discharged with carbamazepine. Anti-platelet treatment was avoided. The patient remained well with no further seizures or clinical features of stroke.

Definitive Investigation Results

Six months following discharge, the patient re-presented, reporting that a friend had been diagnosed with schistosomiasis. A travel history taken at this time identified multiple endemic countries recently visited (Malawi, Zambia, Zimbabwe, Tanzania, South Africa, Morocco, Egypt, Ghana, Sri Lanka) and specific risk factors identified including swimming in Lake Malawi. In retrospect, the patient reported a persistent itch 3 days after swimming in Lake Malawi. Given this travel history, she was investigated further, and ova of *Schistosomiasis haematobium* were identified in both urine and stool samples (**Figure 51.2**)

Diagnosis

Intracerebral schistosomiasis with secondary cerebral infarction.

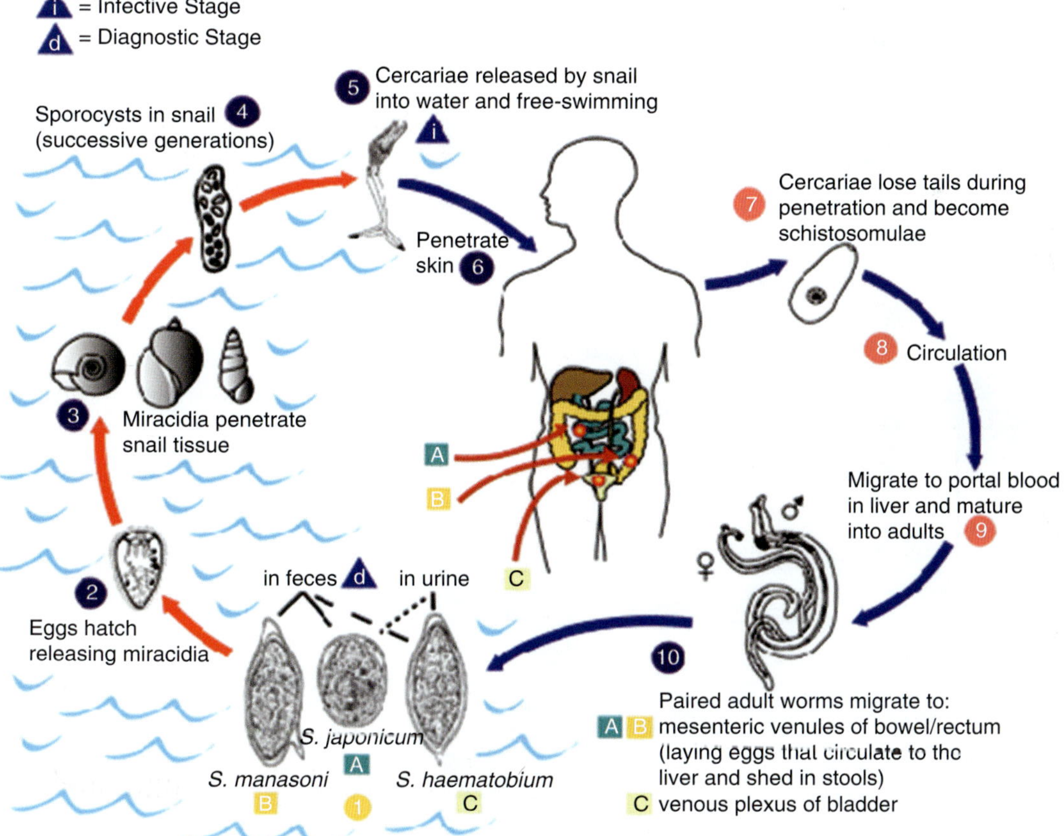

Figure 51.2. Lifecycle of *Schistosoma*. (Reprinted from Centers for Disease Control and Prevention, USA. Schistosomiasis. www.cdc.gov/parasites/schistosomiasis/biology.html [1].)

Management and Outcome

The patient was readmitted and treated with praziquantel 50 mg/kg, and high-dose steroids (dexamethasone). No further seizures or clinical features of stroke were reported.

Prevention

Schistosomiasis infection occurs when people come into contact with freshwater infested with snails, and larval forms of the parasite penetrate the skin (**Figure 51.2**). The disease is prevalent in tropical and subtropical areas, especially communities without access to safe drinking water and adequate sanitation; defecation into water in which people bathe is a major contributor (**Figure 51.3**). An estimated 90% of cases occur in Africa. In 2011, an approximate 240 million people required treatment [2].

For the individual traveller, prevention of infection is by avoidance of exposure to high-risk freshwater areas. For people who have been exposed prompt medical review is needed and consideration of anti-schistosomal treatment.

On a global scale, the control of schistosomiasis is based on large-scale treatment of at-risk population groups, access to safe water, improved sanitation, hygiene, education and snail control (**Figure 51.4**). The World Health Organisation strategy for schistosomiasis control focuses on reducing disease through periodic, targeted treatment of all people in at-risk groups with praziquantel [2].

Discussion

Schistosomiasis is a chronic, parasitic disease caused by blood flukes (trematode worms) of the genus schistosoma [2]. There are three main species of fluke, *S.*

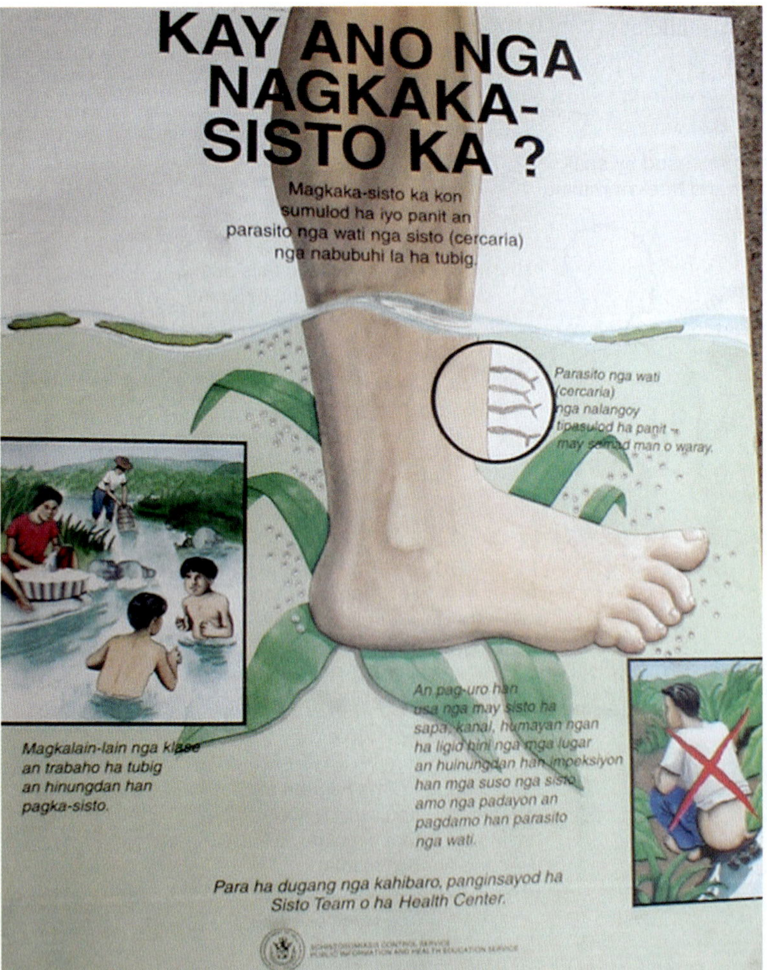

Figure 51.3. This poster was published by Schistosomiasis Control Service, Public Information and Health Education Service, of the Republic of the Philippines. The title translates to 'How Do You Get Schistosomiasis?'

mansoni and *S. japonicum* and *S. haematobium*, with different geographical distribution and differing clinical presentations (**Table 51.1**; **Figure 51.5**). Larval forms of the parasites (cercariae) released by freshwater snails penetrate the skin of people in infested water (**Figure 51.2**). Initial symptoms include fever and pruritis, which on retrospect was experienced by the patient described here. In the body, the larvae develop into adult schistosomes (**Figure 51.6**) and reside in blood vessels of the bowel/rectum (*S. mansoni* and *S. japonicum*) or bladder (*S. haematobium*). Female schistosomes release ova (**Figure 51.7**) that are then passed into either the faeces or urine (depending on the species) or become trapped in body tissues, causing an immune reaction and progressive damage to organs [2].

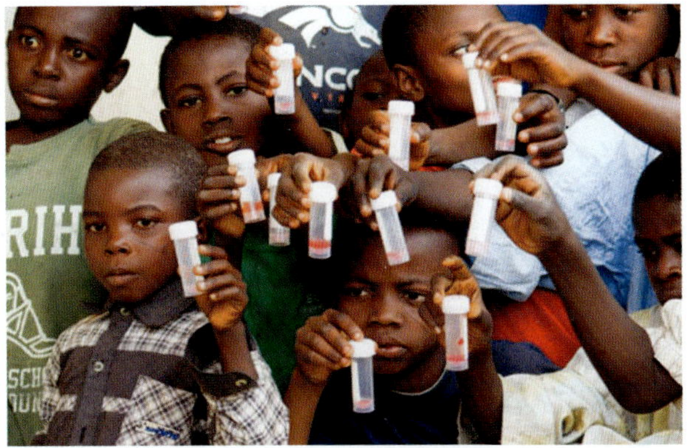

Figure 51.4. These children in Nasarawa North, Nigeria hold vials of their own blood-red urine — evidence that they are infected with schistosomiasis. A partnership between The Carter Center and the Nigerian government has used praziquantel successfully in this community. (Photo © The Carter Center, reprinted with permission.)

Ova released in the early post-infective stage may result in Katayama syndrome (fever, lymphadenopathy, eosinophilia, diarrhoea, splenomegaly and skin rash). Chronic intestinal schistosomiasis (caused by *S. mansoni* and *S. japonicum*) causes progressive hepatomegaly with complicating portal hypertension, ascites and splenomegaly, known as bilharzia (**Figure 51.8**). Chronic urogenital schistosomiasis (*S. haematobium*) causes haematuria, renal impairment, fibrosis of the bladder and ureter and bladder carcinoma. In

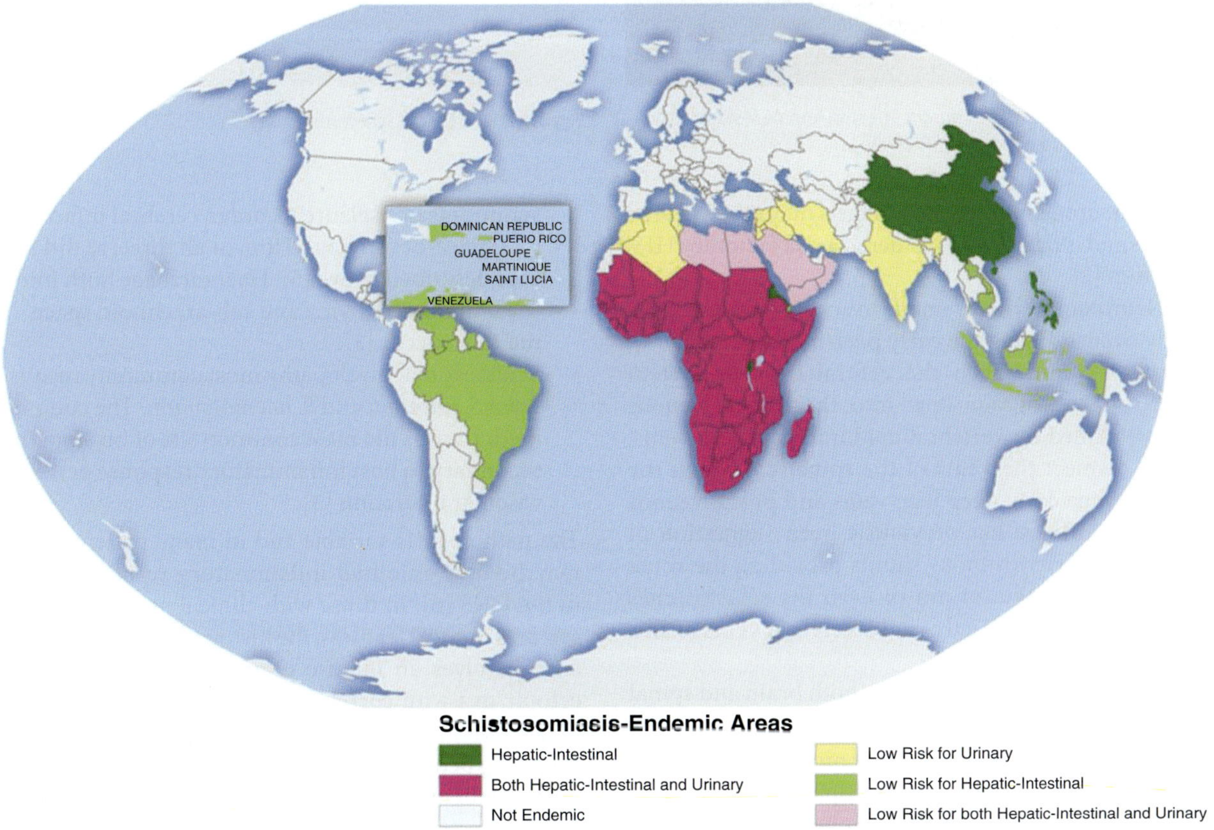

DOMINICAN REPUBLIC
PUERIO RICO
GUADELOUPE
MARTINIQUE
SAINT LUCIA
VENEZUELA

Schistosomiasis-Endemic Areas

Hepatic-Intestinal
Both Hepatic-Intestinal and Urinary
Not Endemic
Low Risk for Urinary
Low Risk for Hepatic-Intestinal
Low Risk for both Hepatic-Intestinal and Urinary

Figure 51.5. Map of showing the global distribution of Schistosomiasis. (From: www.cdc.gov/travel-static/yellowbook/2016/map_3–12.pdf)

Table 51.1 Parasite species and geographical distribution [2].

Species	Phenotype	Geographical distribution
Schistosoma mansoni	Intestinal schistosomiasis	Africa, the Middle East, the Caribbean, South America
Schistosoma japonicum	Intestinal schistosomiasis	China, South East Asia
Schistosoma haematobium	Urogenital schistosomiasis	Africa, the Middle East

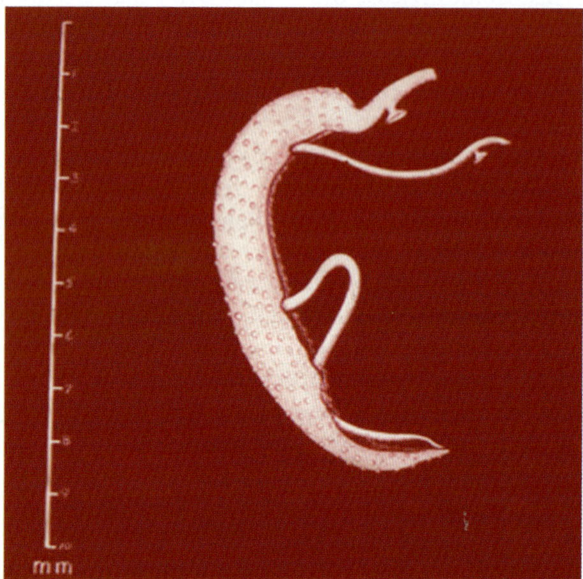

Figure 51.6. Adults of *S. mansoni*. The thin female resides in the gynecophoral canal of the thicker male.

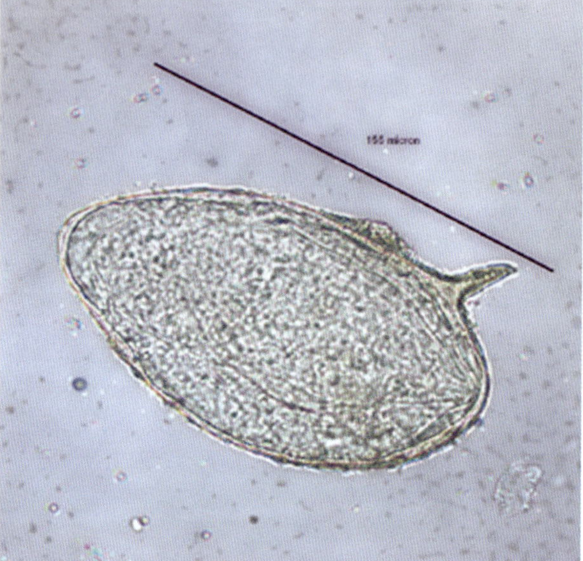

Figure 51.7. Ova of *Schistosoma mansoni*

addition, urogenital schistosomiasis may cause genital lesions and is therefore considered a risk factor for HIV infection [2].

Neurological involvement in schistosomiasis generally occurs during the early post-infective stage [3]. *Schistosoma* ova reach the central nervous system (CNS) via retrograde flow into the Batson venous plexus formed by vertebral epidural valve-less veins, which connect the veins of the spinal cord with the inferior vena cava, deep iliac veins and portal venous system [3]. There has previously been suggestion of pulmonary arteriovenous shunts providing the route for CNS deposition of ova or even the schistosomes placing their ova directly in the cerebral veins at this ectopic site [4].

Schistosomiasis can result in both brain and spinal cord disease:

- Schistosomal encephalopathy most commonly occurs with *S.japonicum*. Multiple clinical, pathological and radiological phenotypes have been described. Patients may present with symptoms of a seizure disorder, cerebral infarction or a space-occupying lesion, or all three, as did the case described above [5]. Haemorrhage both into the brain parenchyma and sub-arachnoid space may also occur [3].
- Schistosomal myelopathy most commonly results from *S. mansoni* and *S. haematobium*. The conus medullaris is the most common site of myelopathy secondary to host inflammatory response or vascular infarction [3].

The pathology is variable and in many patients there may be only minimal inflammatory reaction to ova in the CNS [6]. In those with clinical presentations of seizures or focal features, the histopathological appearance involves an intense granulomatous reaction to ectopic ova with correlating radiological appearances of an enhancing space occupying lesion with surrounding oedema [5].

In patients presenting with clinical features of ischaemic stroke, the pathology involves a focal or diffuse endarteritis [3,7]. Transverse myelopathy due to

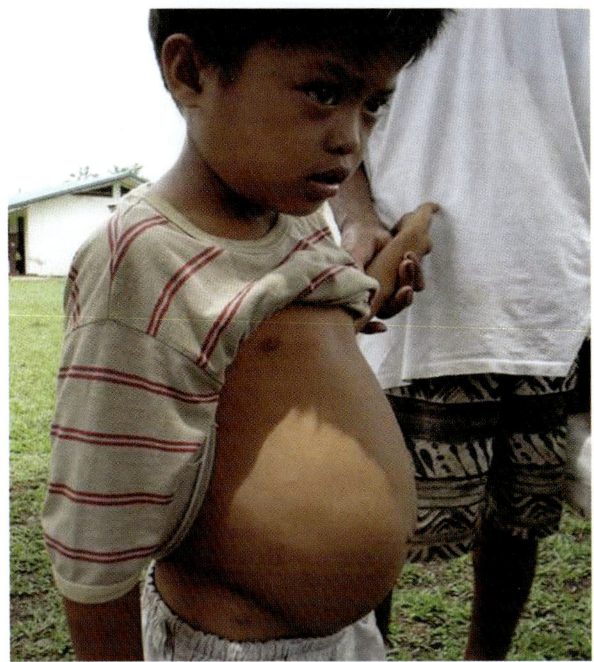

Figure 51.8. Bilharzia – progressive hepatosplenomegaly. Caused by chronic intestinal schistosomiasis male. (Photo © Vicente Y. Belizario, Jr., reproduced under CC BY 2.0 license.)

occlusion or necrosis of the anterior spinal artery is the most common manifestation; cerebral infarction is comparatively rare [8]. Parenchymal brain or subarachnoid haemorrhage may also occur and is related to fibrinoid necrosis and intravascular granuloma formation in the leptomeningeal and parenchymal blood vessels [9].

Making the diagnosis of schistosomiasis is based on a history of travel to an endemic area and demonstration of schistosome ova in the urine or faeces, or schistosome antibodies in the serum or CSF. The case described here highlights the importance of obtaining a travel history, as this patient underwent multiple tests to look for causes of a stroke in a young person, despite there being an obvious risk factor in the unelicited travel history. Neurological involvement of schistosomiasis may be supported by radiological findings, although these are non-specific. CT may demonstrate irregular low, iso or hyper-dense lesions with an irregular area of surrounding oedema. MRI appearances include irregular areas of high signal on T2-weighted imaging that may enhance with gadolinium [5,6]. CSF examination typically finds lymphocytic pleocytosis, elevated protein, eosinophilia, elevated immunoglobin G (IgG) and oligoclonal bands [3].

Praziquantel is the currently recommended first line treatment. A typical course involves 40–60 mg/kg/day for 14 days. Oxamniquine (30 mg/kg/day for 2 days) and metriphonate are alternative agents. Steroids (prednisolone, dexamethasone) are advocated in conjunction with schistosomicidal agents in patients with neurological involvement, to control swelling associated with killing the parasite. Surgical options including decompressive laminectomy may be indicated in specific situations [3].

Key Points

- Travel history is an essential part of any neurological history, especially in a young patient with an unexplained presentation.
- Schistosomiasis can affect the brain and spinal cord. *S. japonicum* typically affects the brain, presenting with seizures, cerebral infarction, a space-occupying lesion or occasionally haemorrhage. *S. mansoni* and *S. haematobium* typically present with a myelopathy.
- Diagnosis is based on serology, and identifying the ova in urine and/or stool depending on the species.
- Treatment is with praziquantal and steroids.

Looking Back

Schistosome ova have been identified in both Chinese and Egyptian mummies, but the parasite itself was not identified until the middle of the nineteenth century.

Did You Know?

It takes a schistosomal larval form of the parasite just 30–60 seconds to painlessly enter the body when an individual is exposed to infested freshwater; and the female adult worm inside a human lays 200–2000 ova per day for up to 5 years.

References

1. Center for Disease Control and Prevention, USA. Lifecycle of *Schistosoma*; www.cdc.gov/parasites/schistosomiasis/biology.html (accessed May 7, 2018).
2. World Health Organisation; Schistosomiasis Fact Sheet No. 115; updated 02/2018; www.who.int/en/news-room/fact-sheets/detail/schistosomiasis (accessed May 7, 2018).
3. Roman GC. The neurology of parasitic diseases and malaria. Continuum Lifelong Neurol 2011;**17**(1):113–33.
4. Scrimgeour EM, Gajdusek DC; Involvement of the central nervous system in *Schistosomiasis mansoni* and *S. haematobium* infection. Brain 1985;**108**:1023–38.
5. Wu L, Wu M, Tian M, et al. Clinical and imaging characteristics of cerebral schistosomiasis. Cell Biochem Biophys 2012;**62**:289–95.
6. Preidler KW, Riepl T, Szolar D, Ranner G. Cerebral schistosomiasis: MR and CT Appearance. Am J Neuroradiol 1996;**17**:1598–600.
7. Del Brutto OH. Infections and stroke. Semin Cerebrovasc Dis Stroke 2005;**5**:28–39.
8. Carod Artal FJ, Vargas AP, Horan TA, et al. *Schistosoma mansoni* myelopathy. Clinical and pathologic findings. Neurology 2004;**63**:388–91.
9. Liu LX. Spinal and cerebral schistosomiasis. Semin Neurol 1993;**13**:189–200.

CASE 52

Brain on Fire

Jay Panicker and Charlotte F. Dougan

History

A 20-year-old psychology student was admitted to the Accident & Emergency department with severe headaches and numbness affecting the right side of the body for 24 hours prior to admission. She was diagnosed with migraines and discharged home. Her symptoms resolved over the following 24 hours.

However, 2 days later she was admitted again with confusion, marked agitation, auditory hallucinations, persecutory delusions and physical and verbal aggression to family members and friends. There was no history of fever or other systemic symptoms.

There was no past history of any major health problems and no history of psychosis. She had occasionally smoked cannabis in the past, but had not been using any recreational drugs for 2 years. There was no history of foreign travel, nor any significant family history.

On examination at that time she was apyrexial and had no focal neurologic signs or meningism. She was diagnosed with acute psychosis of unclear aetiology and transferred to the local psychiatric hospital where she was commenced on atypical antipsychotics, but was still noted to have periods of extreme agitation. A few days after admission, her level of consciousness was noted to fluctuate markedly from extreme agitation to total unresponsiveness. Five days after admission, she was noted to have episodes of hyperventilation, low-grade pyrexia and occasional rigid posturing of the limbs. At this stage, she was transferred to the Medical Admissions Unit and from there to the neurology tertiary care hospital.

Examination

On admission to the Medical Admissions Unit, she was agitated and not oriented in time or place. She had a temperature of 38.4°C and a regular pulse of 124 beats per minute with normal blood pressure. She had intermittent periods of hyperventilation with periodic breathing. However, cranial nerve examination including funduscopy was normal. Her muscle tone was increased in all four limbs, although she was moving her limbs normally, with no demonstrable weakness. There was no evidence of tremor or bradykinesia. There were no signs of cerebellar dysfunction or meningism. Deep tendon reflexes were brisk throughout and plantar reflexes were extensor bilaterally. Systemic examination was otherwise unremarkable.

Initial Differential Diagnosis

- Encephalitis
  - Viral encephalitis (herpes simplex virus (HSV) or other viruses)
  - Autoimmune encephalitis, e.g. Hashimoto's encephalitis, paraneoplastic encephalitis
- Bacterial meningitis
- Brain abscess
- Acute disseminated encephalomyelitis
- Neuroleptic malignant syndrome secondary to antipsychotic use
- Primary brain tumour
- Metabolic encephalopathy
- Drug toxicity or withdrawal

Results of Initial Investigations

She had normal serum haemoglobin, white cell and platelet counts, normal renal and liver function tests and calcium levels. C-reactive protein was 48 mg/l and erythrocyte sedimentation rate 66 mm/hour. A urine toxicology screen was negative. A computer tomography brain scan was normal. A lumbar puncture showed an opening pressure of 21 cm H_2O and 19 lymphocytes/mm^3. Her cerebrospinal fluid (CSF) protein and glucose ratio were normal.

Progress and Further Investigations

She had a generalised seizure while she was in the medical unit. On the second day of admission, as her agitation was difficult to control, she was sedated and admitted to the high-dependency unit.

She was commenced on intravenous (IV) aciclovir while awaiting the results of viral polymerase chain reaction (PCR) on the CSF. In the high-dependency unit, she was noted to have marked autonomic dysfunction with episodes of hypertension, tachycardia alternating with bradycardia and episodes of apnoea. Later she was noted to have twitching and choreiform movements of her face and marked rigidity in all limbs. She had two further seizures and was started on phenytoin. A magnetic resonance imaging (MRI) scan of the head was normal. An electronencephalogram performed off sedation showed diffuse slowing suggesting an encephalopathic process. A HIV test was negative.

Three days after admission, PCR for HSV 1 and 2, varicella zoster virus, Epstein–Barr virus, cytomegalovirus and enterovirus was found to be negative and the aciclovir was stopped. Bacterial cultures and tuberculosis PCR were also negative. Thyroid antibodies were within normal range. As the initial investigations were unrevealing, and in view of the autonomic dysfunction and facial dyskinesias, it was decided to investigate for rarer causes of a limbic encephalitis, including that associated with anti-*N*-methyl-D-aspartate (NMDA) receptor antibodies; and because these may be paraneoplastic she was investigated for underlying malignancy.

Definitive Investigation Results

A MRI scan of the pelvis demonstrated a small 3-cm cystic lesion in her right ovary with minimal fluid in her pelvis. This was removed laparoscopically and histopathological examination confirmed an ovarian teratoma. Anti-NMDA receptor antibodies came back as strongly positive. Other autoantibodies including voltage-gated potassium channel antibodies and onconeuronal antibodies were negative.

Diagnosis

Anti-*N*-methyl-D-aspartate (NMDA) receptor antibody-associated paraneoplastic encephalitis, secondary to ovarian teratoma.

Management and Outcome

After the teratoma was removed, she was treated with five cycles of plasma exchange. Within 2 weeks, she was weaned off sedation and her dyskinesias were managed with tetrabenazine. She improved gradually and was discharged 11 weeks after her initial presentation. On discharge, she had mild impairment of language function with reduced fluency and difficulties with attention and processing speed. A revised-Addenbrookes cognitive examination gave a score of 84/100. On later follow-up her cognition, mood and behaviour had returned to normal and she had resumed her psychology degree.

Discussion

It is becoming recognised increasingly that anti-NMDA receptor encephalitis should be considered in patients presenting with a clinical syndrome resembling viral encephalitis. However, the presentation may be more sub-acute and patients are possibly more likely to present with psychiatric features, movement disorders and seizures, which may be refractory to treatment. Anti-NMDA receptor encephalitis should be considered in patients with new psychiatric disturbances when there is no past history of psychiatric illnesses, especially when there are atypical features including pyrexia, seizures, autonomic dysfunction, extrapyramidal disorders and unexplained fluctuations in the level of consciousness; all of these were present in this case. This is particularly important as many patients with anti-NMDA receptor antibody encephalitis who present with psychiatric symptoms are often first seen by a psychiatrist [1]. The inclusion of neuroleptic malignant syndrome in the differential diagnosis should trigger suspicion that this could be anti-NMDA receptor encephalitis.

The archetypal presentation is in a young female with an ovarian teratoma. However, the diagnosis should be considered in all patients with unexplained encephalitis or encephalopathy irrespective of the demographic characteristics [2]. Apart from ovarian teratomas, anti-NMDA receptor encephalitis is also associated with testicular and mediastinal teratomas, sex-cord stromal tumours and small-cell lung cancer [1]. In one series of 100 patients with anti-NMDA receptor encephalitis, of whom there were 91 females and 9 males, ovarian teratomas were identified in 56 females; small-cell cancer and testicular teratoma were diagnosed in two males. Histological examination of the tumours confirmed the presence of central nervous system tissue, with NMDA receptors expressed in 25. Antibodies against malignant cells are thought to cross-react with neuronal NMDA receptors leading to inhibition – so-called molecular mimicry. Early identification and removal of these tumours is associated with better outcomes [1]. In a minority of cases, no tumour is identified, and it is postulated that circulating and CSF antibodies may be triggered by neurotropic viral infections; some relapses after herpes simplex virus encephalitis are associated with NMDA receptors antibodies [3].

NMDA receptors are present throughout the central nervous system, and have a very important role in synaptic transmission. Two subtypes are recognised, NR1 and NR2, which bind to glycine and glutamate, respectively (**Figure 52.1**). NR1 and NR2 receptors are present within the hippocampus, basal ganglia and cerebellum [1]. These antibodies thus affect areas

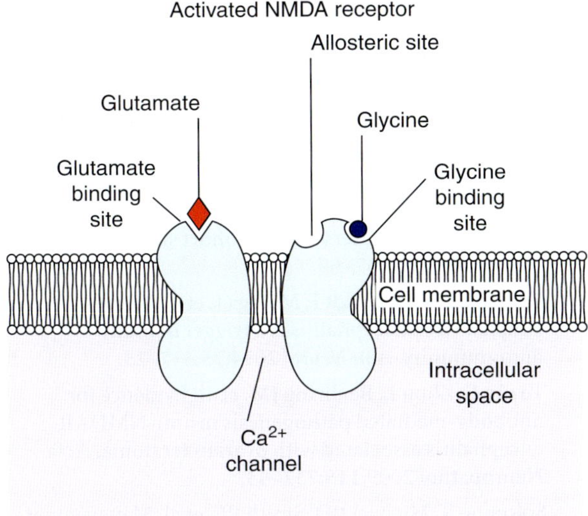

Figure 52.1. NMDA receptor heteromers with glycine and glutamate binding sites

responsible for memory, personality, movement and autonomic control, accounting for the typical clinical picture of psychiatric disturbances, impaired cognition, extrapyramidal disturbances, and autonomic dysfunction. In anti-NMDA receptor encephalitis, antibodies against both the receptors have been detected in the CSF [4].

When anti-NMDA receptor antibody encephalitis is suspected clinically, empirical treatment can be considered even as the patient is undergoing investigation. There are no randomised trials to inform treatment decisions as yet, but national UK guidelines recommend acute treatment with both high-dose IV steroids in conjunction with either intravenous immunoglobulin (IVIG) or plasma exchange [5]. When there is poor response treatment, monoclonal antibodies such as Rituximab, have been used, but with variable outcomes [1,6]. Once a tumour is identified, this should be removed at the earliest opportunity as this will help reduce the antibody burden and improve clinical outcome. With prompt intervention, including tumour removal and immunotherapy, prognosis is good with 75% of cases recovering with minimal deficits [7]. Tumour screening should be continued in those in whom none is identified and in those who relapse, because a tumour may become apparent subsequently [8]. As many as 30% of patients in whom no tumour is identified may relapse, and therefore, long-term immunosuppression, such as with azathioprine, may be useful [5].

Key Points

- Anti-NMDA receptor encephalitis remains an under-recognised condition, often with a characteristic clinical picture of headache, psychiatric disturbances, autonomic dysfunction and extrapyramidal symptoms.
- Diagnosis is confirmed by identification of antibodies in serum, and sometimes CSF.
- The acute phase requires treatment with both intravenous steroids and possibly also IVIG or plasma exchange.
- If suspicion is high, start treatment while awaiting the results of antibody testing.

Looking Back

The syndrome of anti-NMDA receptor encephalitis was first described in 2007, although retrospective antibody testing has identified many cases among earlier patients with undiagnosed encephalitis.

Did You Know?

Drugs blocking NMDA receptors have been used as recreational drugs of abuse for decades. Examples include ketamine (**Figure 52.2**), dextromethorphan, phencyclidine and nitrous oxide. These have been popular for their dissociative, hallucinogenic and euphoric properties and, not surprisingly, these effects are similar to the symptoms experienced by patients with anti-NMDA receptor antibody encephalitis.

The disease has caught the imagination of the media and the public with a book by *New York Post* journalist Susannah Cahalan, who developed the disease. Her book, *Brain on Fire*, reached the international best-seller lists (**Figure 52.3**), and was followed by a film released on Netflix in 2016.

You can hear Susannah Cahalan discussing her book with Neurologist Tom Solomon on BBC Radio 4 *Woman's Hour* in 2013 by visiting www.youtube.com/watch?v=5LQp8Uv1bMY.

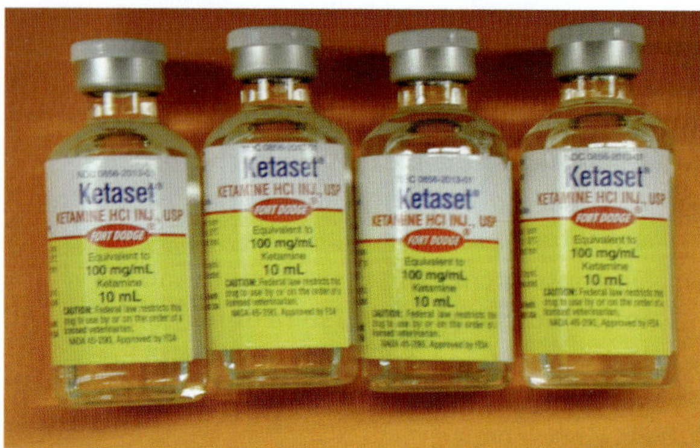

Figure 52.2. Ketamine – an NMDA receptor antagonist which is used as an anaesthetic, and also as a drug of abuse.

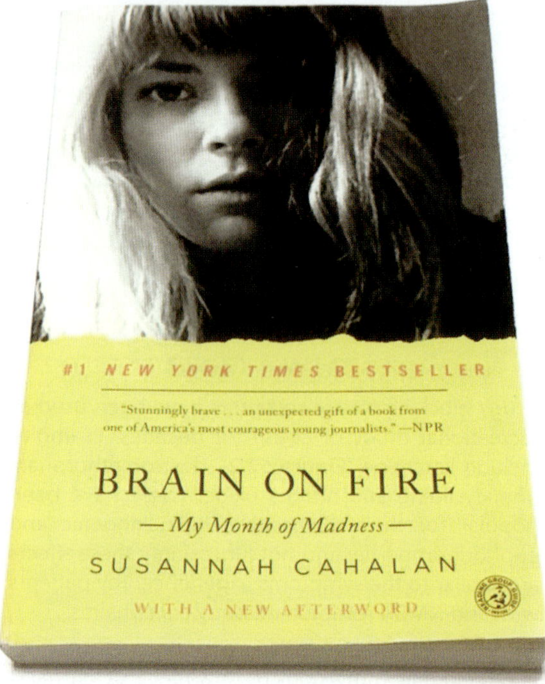

Figure 52.3. Cover of Susannah Cahalan's book *Brain on Fire* (Penguin Books, 2013). Copyright Penguin Books Ltd, 2013.

References

1. Dalmau J, Gleichman AJ, Hughes EG, et al. Anti-NMDA-receptor encephalitis: case series and analysis of the effects of antibodies. Lancet Neurol 2008;7:1091–8.
2. Titulaer MJ, McCracken L, Gabilondo I, et al. Treatment and prognostic factors for long-term outcome in patients with anti-NMDA receptor encephalitis: an observational cohort study. *Lancet Neurol* 2013;**12**:157–65.
3. Armangue T, Leypoldt F, Malaga I, et al. Herpes simplex virus encephalitis is a trigger of brain autoimmunity. *Ann Neurol* 2014;**75**:317–23.
4. Tüzün E, Zhou L, Baehring JM, et al. Evidence for antibody-mediated pathogenesis in anti-NMDAR encephalitis associated with ovarian teratoma. Acta Neuropathol 2009;**118**:737–43.
5. Solomon T, Michael BD, Smith PE, et al. Management of suspected viral encephalitis in adults: Association of British Neurologists and British Infection Association National Guideline. J Infection 2012;**64**: 347–73.
6. Ishiura H, Matsuda S, Higashihara M, et al. Response of anti-NMDA receptor encephalitis without tumor to immunotherapy including Rituximab. Neurology 2008;**71**:1921–3.
7. Day GS, High SM, Cot B, Tang-Wai DF. Anti-NMDA-receptor encephalitis: case report and literature review of an under-recognized condition. J Gen Intern Med 2011;**26**:811–16.
8. Dalmau J, Graus F. Antibody-mediated encephalitis. N Engl J Med 2018;**378**:840–51.

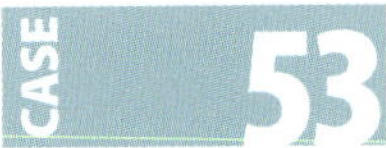

Getting Complicated

Stephen Ray and Rachel Kneen

History

A previously well 4-month-old girl presented to her local hospital with a 1-day history of diarrhoea, reduced oral intake, vomiting, lethargy, irritability and fever. She was born at term by normal vaginal delivery with no complications. She was making normal developmental progress, growth was consistently between the 50th and 75th centiles, and she was up-to-date with immunisations. There had been no previous admissions to hospital and she received no regular medications. She lived with her 2-year-old sister and her mum and dad, all of whom were fit and well. The child had not travelled to any foreign destinations.

Examination

She was conscious but very irritable on handling. She had a bulging fontanelle, peripheral skin mottling, a capillary refill time of 3 seconds, a stiff neck, was tachycardic and had a temperature of 39.5°C. There were no focal neurological signs, there was no rash and the rest of the physical examination was normal.

Initial Differential Diagnosis

- Meningitis: viral, bacterial
- Sepsis, e.g. urinary tract infection or pneumonia

Results of Initial Investigations

A full blood count showed a raised white cell count (WCC) of 26.5 × 10^9/l, with a neutrophilia of 21.6 × 10^9/l and significantly raised C-reactive protein (CRP) of 341 mg/l.

The cerebrospinal fluid (CSF) had a turbid appearance and microscopy confirmed a CSF WCC of 1280 × 10^6/l, with a neutrophil predominance, a raised CSF protein of 2.83 g/l and a low CSF glucose of 1.0 mmol/l as compared to the plasma glucose of 3.8 mmol/l (ratio 26%).

Progress and Further Investigations

She was treated empirically for bacterial meningitis with intravenous (IV) cefotaxime. Blood and CSF cultures subsequently identified *Neisseria meningitidis* serogroup B at 48 hours. The family received chemoprophylaxis with oral ciprofloxacin. She remained febrile for the first 4 days of admission and on day 5 she had a right-sided focal seizure that became secondarily generalised.

Refined Differential Diagnosis

In view of the changing clinical features, it was considered that she likely had a complication of bacterial meningoencephalitis, for which the differential includes:

- Cerebritis
- Cerebral abscess
- Subdural effusion or empyema
- Sinus venous thrombosis causing a venous infarction

Definitive Investigation Results

The persistent fever and seizure prompted a computed tomography (CT) scan and a subsequent magnetic resonance imaging (MRI) scan (**Figure 53.1**).

Definitive Diagnosis

Meningococcal meningitis complicated by a subdural empyema.

Management and Outcome

She was transferred to the tertiary care centre. Neurosurgical treatment was undertaken with a bilateral craniotomy and washout. Immediately post-operatively she had multiple focal seizures and a rising CRP (360 mg/l), persistently elevated WCC (25.9 × 10^6/l) and neutrophils (24.5 × 10^6/l), so adjunctive IV vancomycin was added. A repeat MRI on day 6 demonstrated a smaller residual bilateral subdural empyema.

In the week following neurosurgery she began to show signs of clinical improvement. She completed 6 weeks of once-daily IV ceftriaxone. Her antiepileptic medications were stopped after 4 months and she has been seizure-free since. At the latest follow-up aged 23 months, she had made normal developmental progress, with no neurological deficit.

Figure 53.1. Coronal (A) and axial (B) T2-weighted MRI scans from a 4-month-old child with persistent fever and secondary generalized seizure despite IV antibiotics.

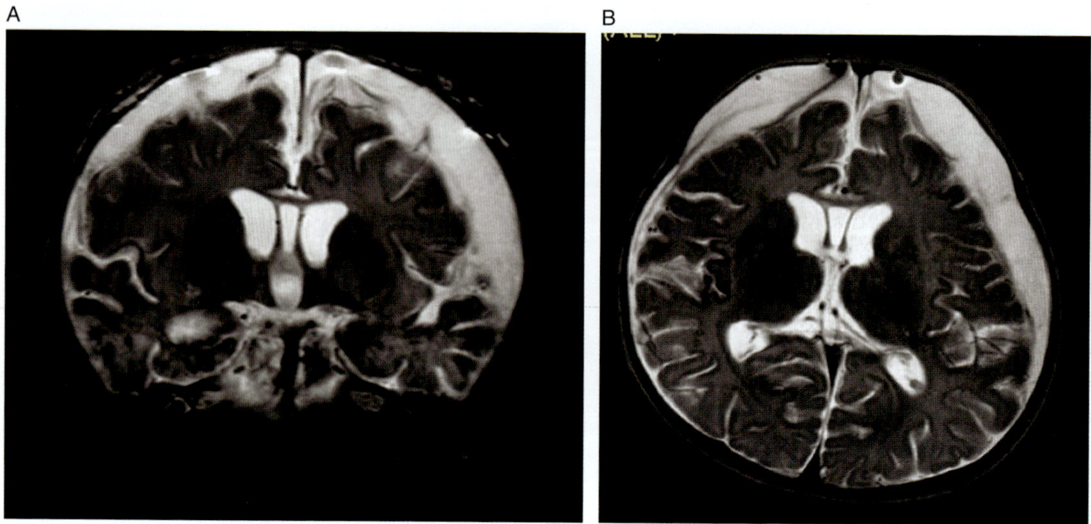

(A) shows bilateral subdural collections of slightly increased signal intensity to the CSF, secondary to the viscous nature of the purulent fluid of empyema. (B) shows bilateral subdural empyema as widening of the extracerebral space with compression of the adjacent sulci.

Prevention

The incidence of meningococcal disease has been steadily falling in the UK since 1999, following the introduction of the meningococcal C conjugate vaccine, but mortality remains high at 5–10% [1,2]. Although the majority of remaining cases in the UK are due to serogroup B, a new vaccine (4CMenB) was introduced for all infants in September 2015, and it is hoped that a declining prevalence of serogroup B will follow.

Discussion

Infection with *N. meningitidis* causes invasive meningococcal disease, manifesting as meningitis and/or septicaemia, and is the leading infectious cause of death in young children in the UK [3]. Infants are at a greater risk of invasive disease with *N. meningitidis* due to their immature response to polysaccharide antigens on the pathogen's capsule [4].

A subdural empyema is a pyogenic collection in the subdural space, which can accumulate during the course of acute bacterial meningitis [5,6]. It is more commonly reported in infants and young children than adults [2]. In infants it occurs as a complication of acute bacterial meningitis, while in older children and adults it is also associated with sinusitis, head trauma or neurosurgery [7,8]. Subdural empyema has been reported in up to 12% of infants less than 6 months old in some series, but data are not available for older infants and children. In adults, subdural empyema is reported to occur in only around 2.7% of cases [8]. The most common causative organism in previous case series including all ages is reported to be the *Streptococcus milleri* group, followed by *Staphylococcus aureus* and *Haemophilus influenzae* [7–9]. Subdural empyema complicating *N. meningitides*, as seen in this case, is very rare with only 14 cases reported previously.

Delayed diagnosis and treatment of subdural empyema is associated with increased morbidity and mortality [10]. Clinical features are important for raising the suspicion of the development of a subdural empyema; these include young age (particularly if less than 3 years), recurrence or persistence of fever, and the development of seizures or focal neurological deficits [7,9].

Laboratory results may also be helpful in raising the suspicion of a subdural empyema. For example, in the case described here, the peripheral WCC and CRP remained grossly elevated, despite treatment with appropriate antimicrobials. Admission CSF results were consistently abnormal with a significant pleocytosis and an abnormally high protein and low glucose, which is in keeping with those described in subdural empyema from other bacterial causes [7,9].

MRI identified the subdural empyema in this case. MRI is more sensitive than CT at both identifying subdural empyema and differentiating it from simple effusion [9]. However, CT is widely available in all hospitals and older infants and children may need a general anaesthetic for an MRI. In infants with an open fontanelle, there is merit in an initial cranial ultrasound to identify whether a subdural collection can be visualised.

The case described here underwent neurosurgical drainage of the empyema and received 6 weeks of antibiotics. It has been suggested that 3–4 weeks of antibiotic treatment should be sufficient if the subdural empyema is surgically evacuated and antibiotics given for longer if treatment is conservative [8].

The outcome in this case was favourable with no deficit, but there are reported to be sequelae in up to 45% of cases, and death in 5–12% [7,9].

Key Points

- Consider subdural empyema in any infant or young child with meningitis when the temperature fails to settle despite appropriate antibiotics, if seizures or focal neurological signs develop or if blood and CSF parameters remain grossly abnormal or worsen.
- The most common causes are the *Streptococcus milleri* group, followed by *Staphylococcus aureus* and *Haemophilus influenzae; N. meningitidis* is a very rare cause.
- Neuroimaging should be ordered for any child with suspected subdural empyema and if identified a prolonged course of antibiotics commenced and neurosurgical treatment considered.

Looking Back

The first infant case of subdural empyema due to *N. meningitidis* was described in 1956, prior to the advent of advanced neuroimaging. Despite two subdural taps and a burr hole and washout the infant died. A large loculated bilateral purulent subdural empyema was found at post mortem [11].

Did You Know?

Meningococcus is named from the Greek *meninx* ('membrane') + *kokkos* ('berry'), and was first described by Gaspard Viesseux during an outbreak with 33 deaths in Geneva in 1805, describing a malady *'fièvre cérébrale maligne non contagieuse'*, a non-contagious malignant cerebral fever) [12].

References

1. Sadarangani M, Willis L, Kadambari S, et al. Childhood meningitis in the conjugate vaccine era: a prospective cohort study. Arch Dis Childhood 2015;**100**:292–4.
2. Saez-Llorens X, McCracken GH Jr. Bacterial meningitis in children. Lancet 2003;**361**:2139–48.
3. Stanton MC, Taylor-Robinson D, Harris D, et al. Meningococcal disease in children in Merseyside, England: a 31 year descriptive study. PLoS ONE 2011;**6**:e25957.
4. Pollard AJ, Frasch C. Development of natural immunity to Neisseria meningitidis. Vaccine 2001;**19**:1327–46.
5. Dill SR, Cobbs CG, McDonald CK. Subdural empyema: analysis of 32 cases and review. Clin Infect Dis 1995;**20**:372–86.
6. Farmer TW, Wise GR. Subdural empyema in infants, children and adults. Neurology 1973;**23**:254–61.
7. Legrand M, Roujeau T, Meyer P, et al. Paediatric intracranial empyema: differences according to age. Eur J Pediatr 2009;**168**:1235–41.
8. Jim KK, Brouwer MC, van der Ende A, van de Beek D. Subdural empyema in bacterial meningitis. Neurology 2012;**79**:2133–9.
9. Bockova J, Rigamonti D. Intracranial empyema. Pediatric Infect Dis J 2000;**19**:735–7.
10. Mauser HW, Van Houwelingen HC, Tulleken CA. Factors affecting the outcome in subdural empyema. J Neurol Neurosurg Psychiatry 1987;**50**:1136–41.
11. Hankinson J, Amador LV. Infected subdural effusions. Br Med J 1956;**2**:122–6.
12. Vieusseux M. Mémoire sur la maladie qui a regné a Genêve au printemps de 1805. J Med Chir Pharm 1805;**11**:163–82.

CASE 54

A Pain in the Leg

Tom Solomon

History

A woman in her late thirties was admitted to her local general hospital under the orthopaedic surgeons, with lower back pain radiating to the left leg. It had started 4 days earlier, was severe and shooting in nature, and was getting worse. She had been seen twice in casualty in the preceding days, and by the time of admission was unable to walk. She also had a headache and had vomited once. Three and a half months before admission, during a 2-week holiday in Goa, India, she had been nipped on her leg by a puppy on a lead, which was walking past her. She had also had intermittent diarrhoea for the past 4 months, which preceded her trip to India, but gastroscopy and flexible sigmoidoscopy on return from India were normal.

Examination

On examination she had a temperature of 38.5°C. The left leg, which was extremely painful, requiring morphine, was areflexic and weak, with sensory loss in L4-S1 dermatomes.

Initial Differential Diagnosis

- Prolapsed disc
- Abscess
- Guillain–Barré syndrome
- Other

Results of Initial Investigations

She had a raised blood leukocyte count. A computer tomography (CT) scan of the spine looking for a prolapsed disc was normal.

Progress and Further Investigations

Over the next few days she developed a sore throat, with difficulty swallowing, a swollen left eyelid, a goose pimple rash on her skin, and marked bilateral hearing loss. On day 8 of admission she was referred to the medical team who noted she was now lethargic, and had flaccid weakness in both legs and arms. A lumbar puncture (LP) on the same day revealed clear cerebrospinal fluid (CSF) with a white cell count of 11 cells per μl (9 lymphocytes, 2 polymorphonuclear cells), red cell count of 4 cells per μl, protein 21.6 mg/l and glucose 3.1 mmol/l, with a plasma glucose of 5.9 mmol/l. A provisional diagnosis of Guillain–Barré syndrome was made and she was treated with intravenous immunoglobulin. By day 11 of admission she was deteriorating with increased drowsiness and was intubated and ventilated. On day 13 she had absent occulocephalic reflexes, and unreactive pupils, and the diagnosis of Bickerstaff's encephalitis was considered. A computer tomography scan of the brain was normal. On day 15 of admission, the specialist neurology centre was contacted for advice.

Results of Definitive Investigations

On account of the history of ascending paralysis following a dog bite in India, immediate investigation for rabies (including saliva, serum, and a skin biopsy from the nape of the neck) was advised, and the patient was transferred for further care.

A magnetic resonance imaging (MRI) scan of the head was performed (**Figure 54.1**).

An electroencephalogram was encephalopathic with periodic complexes. Within 5 hours of receipt of the specimens, saliva and skin tested positive for rabies virus using a hemi-nested reverse transcriptase polymerase chain reaction (PCR) and a real-time PCR. A 400 base-pair region of the nucleoprotein gene was sequenced and a phylogenetic tree constructed which confirmed that the virus amplified was a rabies virus imported from India, rather than indigenous infection with European bat lyssavirus, or a laboratory contaminant (**Figure 54.2**).

Diagnosis

Paralytic rabies.

Management and Outcome

Once the PCR diagnosis was confirmed, ionotropic support was withdrawn at the family's request and the patient died on day 18 of admission. She had never had hydrophobia, aerophobia, hypersalivation, or spasms. With the family's permission, brain tissue was obtained after death by needle biopsies through the foramen magnum and supra-orbital routes; this confirmed the diagnosis of rabies by both fluorescent antibody testing and PCR. In addition there were rising anti-rabies antibody titres in the serum, as measured by the fluorescent virus neutralisation assay (**Figure 54.3**).

Figure 54.1. MRI of a woman in her thirties who presented with leg pain followed by headache and fever.

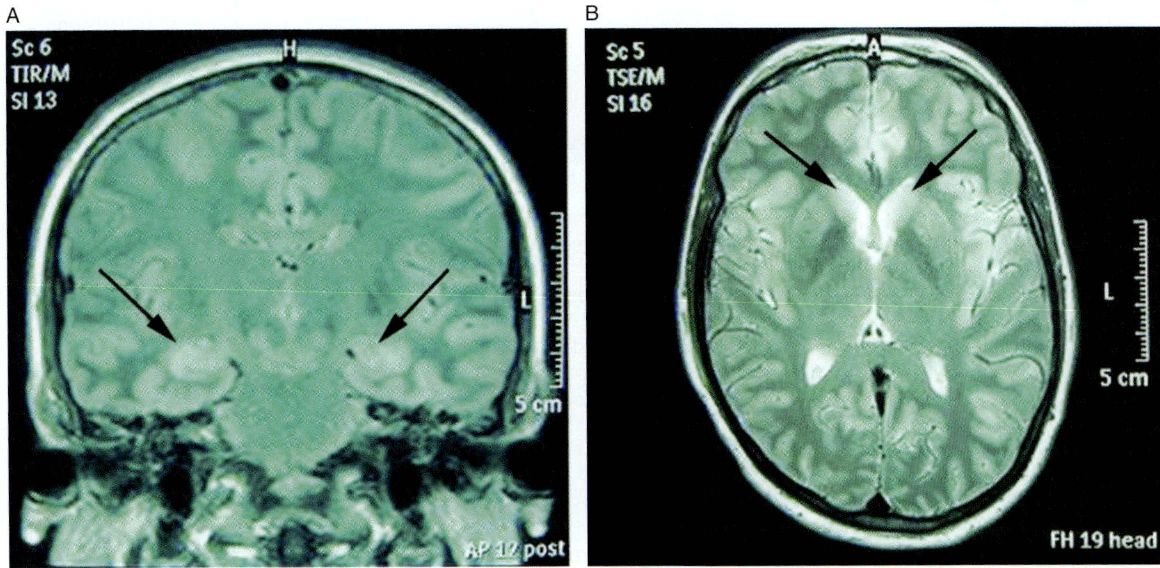

This shows T2-weighted MRI showing high signal (arrows) bilaterally in the hippocampal gyri (left image, T2 fluid-attenuated inversion recovery, FLAIR) and the head of the caudate nucleus (right image, T2 turbo spin echo), which have been seen before in rabies.

Prevention

Rabies is preventable with vaccination. Those living in, or travelling to, rabies-endemic areas should receive pre-exposure vaccination. Following the bite of a potentially rabid animal the wound should be cleaned carefully and, depending on the circumstances, post-exposure vaccination and immunoglobulin given; detailed recommendations are available on the Department of Health website [1].

Rabies is carried by dogs, cats, bats, foxes, monkeys, racoons and a range of other mammals; these animals should be avoided in areas where rabies occurs, and especially if they are behaving strangely or seem unusually tame (**Figure 54.4A–C**).

Discussion

This case serves as an important reminder of the risk of rabies for any traveller to a rabies-endemic country, even tourists on a short visit to a holiday resort, and provides several useful lessons. The first is that travellers need to know whether they are visiting a rabies-endemic country and that any dog bite in such a country must be taken seriously by both the recipient and any medical staff subsequently seeing the patient. Although rabies is more likely following the bite of a stray or rabid dog, this case demonstrates that even an apparently innocuous bite from a pet must be considered carefully, especially if it was unprovoked: such an animal may be in the early stages of rabies. Although there is no rabies virus in the UK, rabies virus is one in a whole family of viruses some of which do occur in Europe, including the UK (**Table 54.1**). For example, European bat lyssavirus is found in British bats, and can cause an identical disease [2].

Table 54.1 Family of rabies viruses.

Family *Rhabdoviridae*, genus *Lyssavirus*		
Genotype	**Source**	**Distribution**
1 Rabies virus	Dog, fox, raccoon, bat, etc.	Widespread
2 Lagos bat virus	Bats, cats	Africa (rare)
3 Mokola virus	Shrews, cats	Africa
4 Duvenhage	Insectivorous bat	Africa
5 European bat lyssavirus Type 1	Insectivorous bat	N & E Europe
6 European bat lyssavirus Type 2	Insectivorous bat	W Europe
7 Australian bat lyssavirus	Flying foxes Insectivorous bat	Australia (Philippines?)

Clinically all give 'rabies' except
Lagos bat virus – no human disease
Mokola virus – fever, encephalopathy

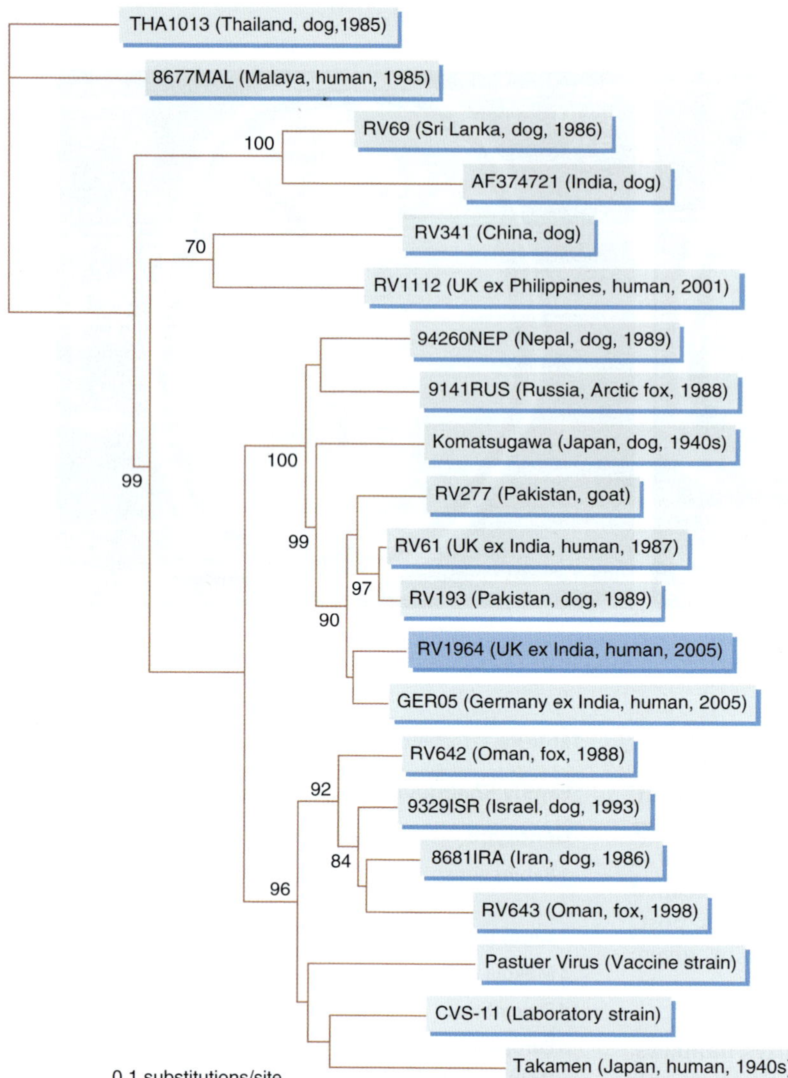

Figure 54.2. Phylogenetic tree depicting the relation between the rabies virus sequence amplified from this patient (RV1964, blue box) and other viruses originating in Asia. The horizontal branch lengths represent the extent of difference between the strains (expressed as nucleotide substitutions per nucleotide site), and the closer viruses are on the tree, the more closely they are related. (Reproduced from [3] with permission from BMJ Publishing Group Ltd.)

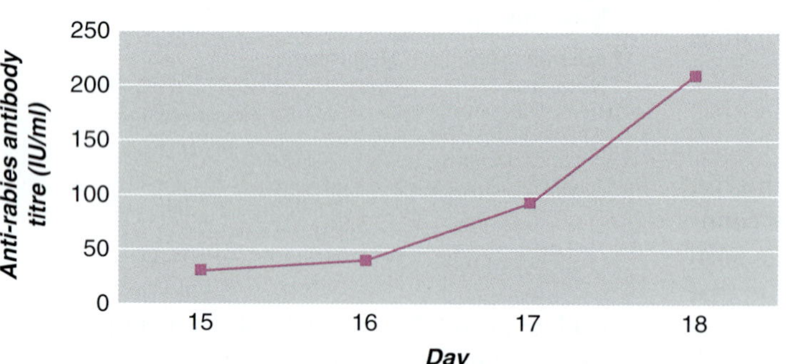

Figure 54.3. Fluorescent virus neutralisation assay shows the elevation in anti-rabies antibodies in the last 3 days of the illness.

Most patients present with furious rabies, which is characterised by hydrophobia and/or aerophobia (fear of water and air, respectively), associated with phobic or inspiratory spasms. However, up to one-third of patients may present with the paralytic or 'dumb' form of the disease [4]. This is often harder to diagnose clinically and has been confused with Guillain–Barré syndrome, particularly the acute motor axonal form

A

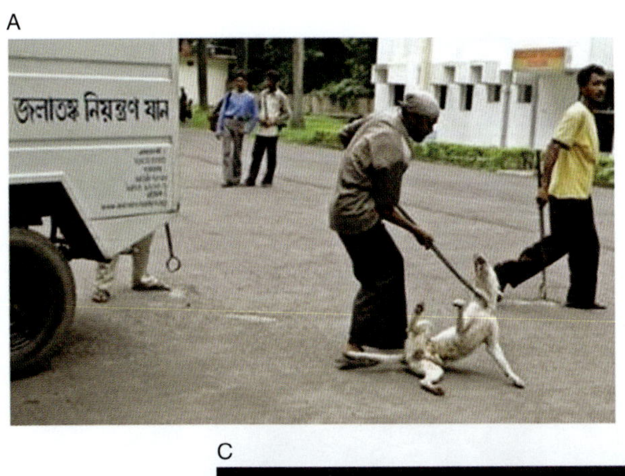

B

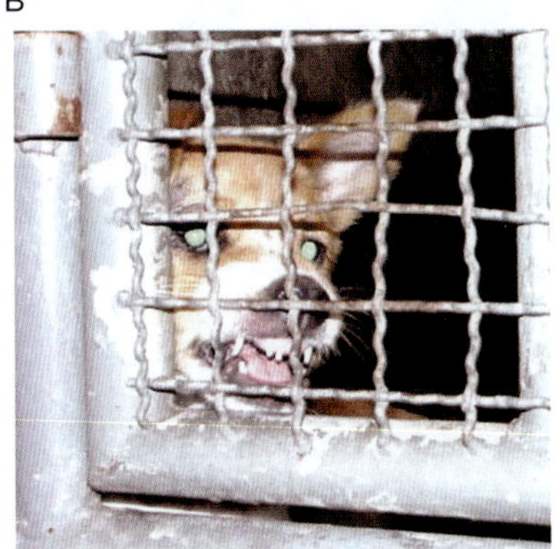

C

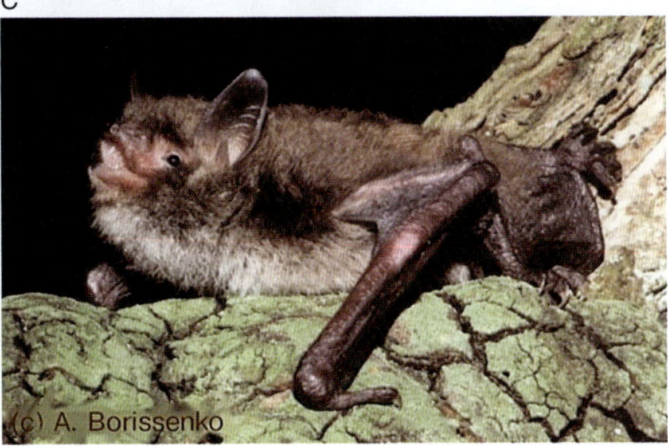

Figure 54.4. (A) Control of a rabid dog in India. (B) Rabid dog (© Professor David Warrell). (C) Daubenton's bat, which transmits European bat lyssavirus in the UK.

of Guillain–Barré syndrome. However, headache and fever at presentation, asymmetry of limb weakness, bladder involvement and cells in the CSF are clues that flaccid paralysis could be due to a virus infection of the anterior horn cells in the spinal cord, rather than immunologically mediated Guillain–Barré syndrome [5]. Severe pain in the bitten limb, which is common in rabies, itching and goose pimples may be additional clues of rabies infection.

Patients with suspected rabies should be investigated by collecting saliva, CSF, serum and a punch biopsy from the skin at the nape of the neck; this includes hair follicles containing peripheral nerve endings. The detection of rabies virus antigen in a skin biopsy, using a fluorescent antibody test, is one of the best tests [6]; in addition, PCR of the saliva is also a useful rapid diagnostic test. Because initial results may be negative, investigations should be repeated daily [7]. In some patients all ante-mortem testing will be negative, and the diagnosis is only made post-mortem by examining brain material. This can be obtained at autopsy, or by biopsy with a Vim-Silverman needle, or other long biopsy needle, such as that used for bone marrow aspiration; electron microscopy (**Figure 54.5**) demonstrates viral particles, but PCR or immunofluorescence are usually used for practical reasons [6]. Without such investigation the diagnosis may not be made. It is not known how many patients diagnosed with fatal Guillain–Barré syndrome in the past actually had paralytic rabies.

Rapid diagnosis of rabies is important for the appropriate infection control and public health measures to be instituted; rabies is a notifiable disease [1]. Although there are no well-documented cases of human-to-human transmission (except via organ transplantation) [8], barrier nursing is used, vaccination offered to relatives and exposed staff and reassurance given to other staff members; in addition, samples sent to non-specialist laboratories may need to be tracked down. Until recently, once clinical features developed, rabies was considered almost universally fatal. The only documented survivors had received some pre- or

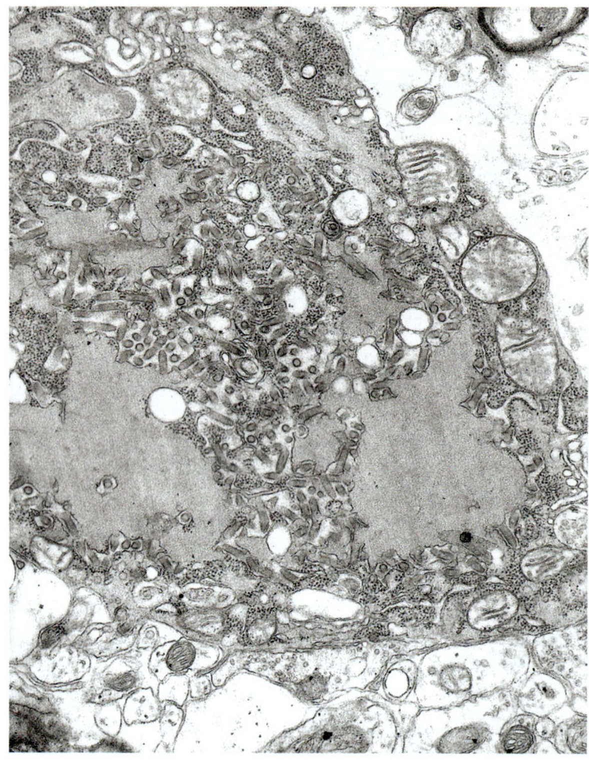

Figure 54.5. This electron micrograph shows rabies virus, as well as Negri bodies, or cellular inclusions.

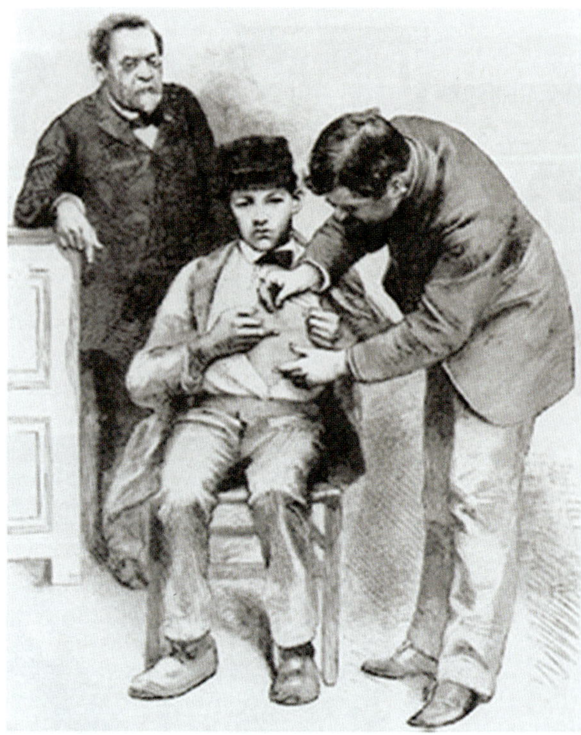

Figure 54.6. Pasteur and Roux vaccinating a 9-year-old boy against rabies.

post-exposure vaccination, but had not received complete prompt post-exposure vaccination, meaning they were arguably failures of the vaccination regime [4,9]. However, in 2004 a teenager in Wisconsin, USA, who developed rabies following a bat bite, was successfully treated with a combination of ketamine, midazolam, ribavirin and amantadine [10]. Similar treatments have now been tried in about a dozen cases, with fatal outcomes in all cases of terrestrial rabies, but one or two survivors from bat-derived rabies [11]. Such treatment was considered in this case, but the disease was felt to be too advanced. Although rabies is rare in the UK, we continue seeing sporadic cases.

Key Points

- Rabies can present with an ascending paralytic illness.
- Even innocuous bites from animals in rabies-endemic countries must be treated seriously, because post-exposure prophylaxis can prevent the disease.
- Rabies-like viruses are carried in bats in the UK and elsewhere, so bat handlers should be vaccinated.

Looking Back

Aristotle described rabies in animals in 322 BC, and Celsis in *De Medicina* wrote about hydrophobia in humans in 1 AD. Louis Pasteur and Emile Roux developed the first rabies vaccine in 1885 and used it on a 9-year-old boy who had been attacked by a rabid dog (**Figure 54.6**).

Did You Know?

To control rabies in wildlife in Europe and the USA food bait containing live attenuated vaccine, or recombinant vaccine is dropped from helicopters, for consumption by foxes and other animals.

One of the very few survivors of bat rabies has her own website: http://site.jeannagiese.com/

References

1. Public Health England. *The Green Book.* Chapter 27: Rabies. www.gov.uk/government/publications/rabies-the-green-book-chapter-27 (accessed May 30, 2018).
2. Fooks AR, Finnegan C, Johnson N, et al. Human case of EBL type 2 following exposure to bats in Angus, Scotland. Vet Rec 2002;**151**:679.
3. Solomon T, Marston D, Mallewa M, et al. Paralytic rabies after a two week holiday in India. BMJ 2005;**331**:501–3.
4. Hemachudha T, Laothamatas J, Rupprecht CE. Human rabies: a disease of complex neuropathogenetic mechanisms and diagnostic challenges. Lancet Neurol 2002;**1**:101–9.
5. Solomon T, Willison H. Infectious causes of acute flaccid paralysis. Curr Opin Infect Dis 2003;**16**:375–81.
6. Warrell MJ. Rabies. In: Cook G, Zumlar A, editors. *Manson's Tropical Diseases*. 21st ed. London: Saunders; 2003: 807–21.
7. Fooks AR, Johnson N, Brookes SM, Parsons G, McElhinney LM. Risk factors associated with travel to rabies endemic countries. J Appl Microbiol 2003;**94**(Suppl):31S–36S.
8. Srinivasan A, Burton EC, Kuehnert MJ, et al. Transmission of rabies virus from an organ donor to four transplant recipients. New Engl J Med 2005;**352**:1103–11.
9. Jackson AC, Warrell MJ, Rupprecht CE, et al. Management of rabies in humans. Clin Infect Dis 2003;**36**:60–3.
10. Willoughby RE Jr, Tieves KS, Hoffman GM, et al. Survival after treatment of rabies with induction of coma. New Engl J Med 2005;**352**:2508–14.
11. Hunter M, Johnson N, Hedderwick S, et al. Immunovirological correlates in human rabies treated with therapeutic coma. J Med Virol 2010;**82**:1255–65.

CASE 55 A Wobbly Toddler

Katie Rose and Rachel Kneen

History

A previously healthy 3-year-old boy presented with a 4-day history of unsteadiness on his feet. He had had one episode of vomiting before admission. Both the patient and his older sibling had recovered from assumed chickenpox (primary varicella zoster) infection in the preceding 4 weeks. He had been treated with paracetamol and ibuprofen for fever at the time he had chickenpox but was no longer taking any medication.

His mother's pregnancy and delivery were normal with no complications. The child's developmental progress was normal. Immunisations were up to date. There was no history of foreign travel, and no reason to suspect he was immunocompromised.

Examination

On examination, a few small scars consistent with the recent chickenpox infection were visible, mainly on the trunk. Small, non-tender cervical lymph nodes were present. Systems examination was otherwise unremarkable. He was apyrexial and observations remained stable throughout.

On neurological examination, the child was fully conscious. He walked with an ataxic gait, with poor coordination, which was worse on the right side. There was horizontal nystagmus in both directions, but the rest of the cranial nerve examination was normal, including funduscopy. There was no weakness or sensory deficit and deep tendon reflexes were normal. The Babinski reflexes were flexor.

Initial Differential Diagnosis

- Para- or post-infectious acute cerebellitis
  - Due to varicella zoster, coxsackie or other enteroviruses, *Mycoplasma* pneumonia, Epstein–Barr virus, mumps, measles, herpes simplex virus type 1, parvovirus 19, rotavirus
- Miller Fisher variant of Guillain–Barré syndrome giving ataxia, areflexia and ophthalmoplegia
- Space-occupying lesions, particularly those in the posterior fossa: tumours, abscesses
- Acute hydrocephalus
- Inner ear disease or labyrinthitis
- Opsoclonus–myoclonus ataxia syndrome: can be paraneoplastic (typically a neuroblastoma) or para-/post-infectious
- Toxic: ingestion of alcohol, phenytoin or other anticonvulsants, tricyclic antidepressants, antihistamines
- Metabolic disorders: mitochondrial disorders, urea cycle disorders, carnitine acetyltransferase deficiency
- Genetic disorders: episodic ataxias

Results of Initial Investigations

Initial blood results including full blood count, renal profile, bone profile, liver function tests and C-reactive protein were all within normal limits. Cerebrospinal fluid (CSF) analysis demonstrated a normal opening pressure, white cell count of 11 cells/mm^3 (with no red cells); CSF protein, glucose and lactate were all normal.

Progress and Further Investigations

Initial treatment commenced on the day of admission included intravenous cefotaxime and aciclovir.

Both blood and CSF cultures were negative. Viral polymerase chain reaction (PCR) on CSF samples was negative. Oligoclonal bands in the CSF were negative.

Results of Definitive Investigations

A magnetic resonance imaging (MRI) scan was undertaken (**Figure 55.1**).

Acute and convalescent serum samples demonstrated a significant increase in IgM to varicella zoster virus, indicating a recent primary infection.

Diagnosis

Acute post-infectious cerebellitis following recent varicella zoster infection.

Management and Outcome

Following negative CSF and blood cultures and PCR aciclovir and cefotaxime were stopped. Prednisolone treatment at 2 mg/kg/day was given for 2 weeks. The child's ataxia improved and he was discharged after 4 days. At 6 weeks his parents reported that he was

Figure 55.1. Axial T2-weighted FLAIR MRI brain scan in a 3-year-old boy who presented with a 4-day history of unsteadiness on his feet following varicella zoster infection.

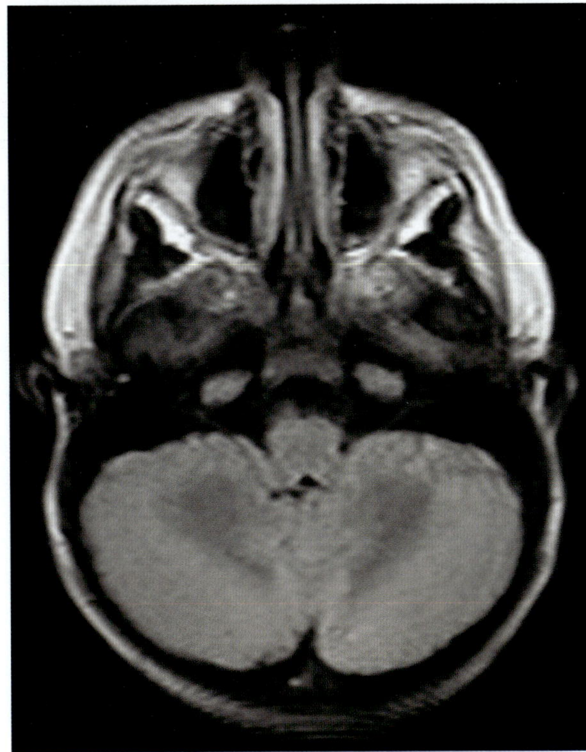

This demonstrates high signal predominantly in the right cerebellar hemisphere. There is also poor definition of the folia indicative of oedema in keeping with acute cerebellitis. The rest of the brain is normal and there was no dilatation of the ventricular system.

occasionally unsteady on his feet but the situation had vastly improved when compared to his initial presentation. They also mentioned that the child was more tired than usual. Neurological examination was normal. A review at 6 months found the child to be completely recovered and he was discharged from further follow-up.

Prevention

Varicella zoster immunisation would reduce the incidence in the UK, but this is not currently part of the routine vaccination schedule for children.

Discussion

Acute cerebellitis is the most common cause of ataxia in childhood, accounting for 35% of cases [1]. The incidence rate of children admitted to hospital with varicella zoster-related ataxia has been found to be between 0.17 and 0.82 per 100,000 per year for children under 15 years old [2]. Symptoms arise following post-infectious cerebellar inflammation, with histology from biopsy and post-mortem demonstrating extensive lymphocytic and eosinophilic infiltration associated with oedema [3,4]. It has been hypothesised that autoantibodies are produced that react with cerebellar tissue in an autoimmune process following acute infection. Specific autoantibodies have recently been identified, with one study finding anti-centrosome antibodies in those with post-varicella acute cerebellitis [5]. However, others have suggested that increased levels of particular antibodies result from damage to the cerebellum, rather than being the cause of cerebellar inflammation [3]. A preceding viral infection is identifiable in approximately 70% of cases, with numerous pathogens being implicated including varicella zoster, enterovirus, parvovirus B19, measles, Epstein–Barr virus and *Mycoplasma pneumoniae* [6].

Clinical features of acute cerebellitis include cerebellar dysfunction, most commonly ataxia, as well as headache, vomiting and disturbance of consciousness, which may result from compression of the brainstem secondary to inflammatory swelling of the cerebellum [4]. Unilateral cerebellitis and signs are possible (**Figure 55.2**) [7]. Imaging can be normal in up to 90% of cases [8].

A more serious presentation includes minimal or no cerebellar features but acute hydrocephalus. Sometimes cerebellar mutism is also present [3]. This is an emergency and can be life-threatening. Recent cases have been described that presented acutely with symptoms of raised intracranial pressure including worsening headache, vomiting and encephalopathy secondary to hydrocephalus resulting from compression of the fourth ventricle or progressive inflammation of the arachnoid causing obstructive hydrocephalus by preventing CSF reabsorption [9]. In these cases acute management should consist of corticosteroids to reduce inflammation, and an urgent neurosurgical opinion in case a ventricular drain is required [9,10].

Key Points

- Most cases of acute post-infectious cerebellitis are benign and self-limiting.
- As well as varicella zoster virus, numerous other pathogens have been implicated, including enterovirus, parvovirus B19, measles, Epstein–Barr virus and *Mycoplasma pneumoniae.*
- Treatment is with corticosteroids.

- The potentially fatal complication of obstructive hydrocephalus secondary to a swollen cerebellum should be considered in all patients presenting with symptoms or signs of raised intracranial pressure associated with recent viral infection.

Looking Back

Although Shepherd was probably the first to describe acute cerebellar ataxia in 1868, Batten in 1905 described five cases following acute illness in children, distinguishing it from other causes of ataxia [3].

Did You Know?

Opsoclonus–myoclonus ataxia syndrome is a rare post-infectious or paraneoplastic syndrome, which can be initially misdiagnosed as acute cerebellitis or acute cerebellar ataxia. The eye movement is different and involves chaotic, rapid conjugate eye movements in all directions, which may be preceded by days to weeks of ataxia. Affected children are often encephalopathic with a loss of cognitive skills and irritability as part of the illness. Approximately 50% are associated with an occult malignancy: typically a neuroblastoma or ganglioneuroblastoma. In adults, the disorder is also very rare, but it may be associated with occult breast, ovarian or lung malignancies [3].

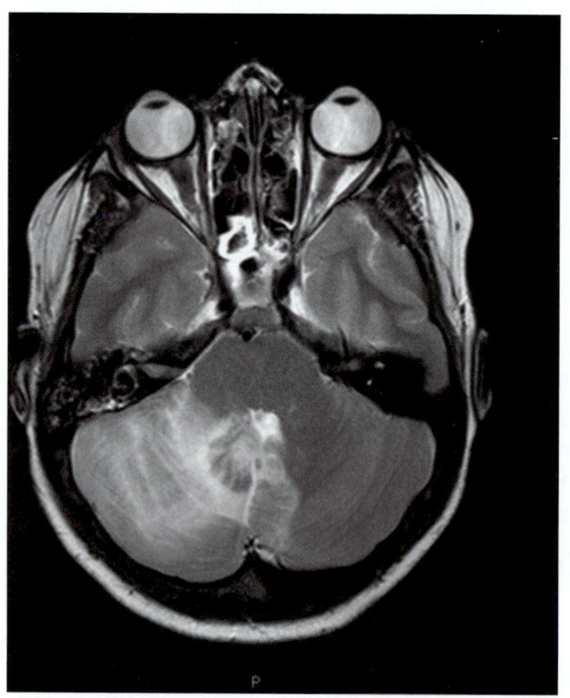

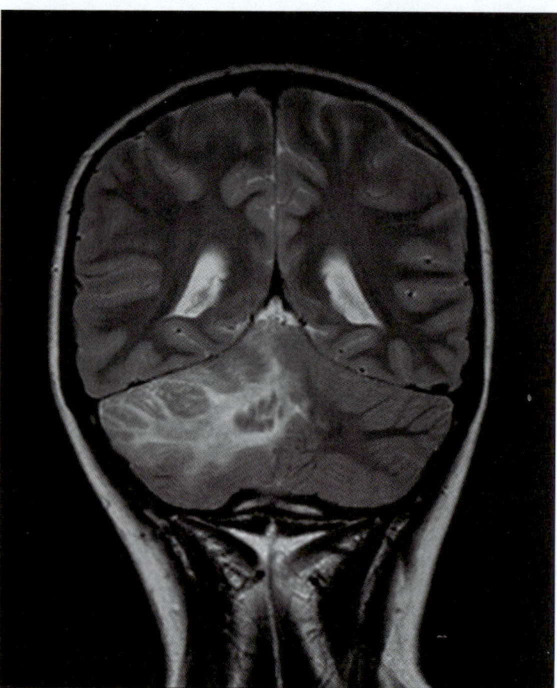

Figure 55.2. Axial (A) and coronal (B) T2-weighted MRI demonstrating high signal predominantly in the right cerebellar hemisphere. There is also poor definition of the folia indicative of oedema in keeping with acute cerebellitis. The rest of the brain is normal and there was no dilatation of the ventricular system. These demonstrate a well-defined area of abnormal high T2-weighted and FLAIR signal in the superomedial cortex of the right cerebellar hemisphere and adjacent middle cerebellar peduncle, involving cortex and adjacent white matter.

References

1. Gieron-Korthals MA, Westberry KR, Emmanuel PJ. Acute childhood ataxia: 10-year experience. J Child Neurol 1994;**9**:381–4.
2. Van der Maas NA, Vermeer-de Bondt PE, de Melker H, et al. Acute cerebellar ataxia in the Netherlands: a study on the association with vaccinations and varicella zoster infection. Vaccine 2009;**27**:1970–3.
3. Desai J, Mitchell WG. Acute cerebellar ataxia, acute cerebellitis, and opsoclonus-myoclonus syndrome. J Child Neurol 2012;**27**:1482–8.
4. Sawaishi Y, Takada G. Acute cerebellitis. Cerebellum 2002;**1**:223–8.
5. Fritzler MJ, Zhang M, Stinton ML, Rattner JB. Spectrum of centrosome autoantibodies in childhood varicella and post-varicella acute cerebellar ataxia. BMC Pediatrics 2003;**3**:11.
6. Salas AA, Nava A. Acute cerebellar ataxia in childhood: initial approach in the emergency department. Emerg Med J 2010;**27**:956–7.
7. Garcia-Cazorla A, Olivan JA, Pancho C, et al. Infectious acute hemicerebellitis. J Child Neurol 2004;**19**:390–2.
8. Connolly AM, Dodson WE, Prensky AL, et al. Course and outcome of acute cerebellar ataxia. Annals Neurol 1994;**35**:673–9.
9. Hacohen Y, Niotakis G, Aujla A, et al. Acute life threatening cerebellitis presenting with no apparent cerebellar signs. Clin Neurol Neurosurg 2011;**113**: 928–30.
10. de Ribaupierre S, Meagher-Villemure K, Villemure JG, et al. The role of posterior fossa decompression in acute cerebellitis. Childs Nerv Syst 2005;**21**: 970–4.

CASE 56

Popping Problems

Derek J. Sloan and Nicholas J. Beeching

History

A 28-year-old man was found behaving strangely on the street and taken to the Accident and Emergency department of the nearest hospital. He was unable to give a coherent history, but the nurses recognised him as a homeless injecting drug user who intermittently attended with soft-tissue infections as a result of 'skin popping' (injecting drugs into skin or subcutaneous tissues). Prior admission notes suggested that he had been injecting heroin and cocaine for 7 years. He was hepatitis C antibody positive and an insulin-dependent diabetic, although his treatment adherence was poor. The initial impression was that he was behaving oddly because of recent drug use. He had a 'chesty' cough, but was unable to describe any other focal symptoms.

Examination

Although drowsy, he could be roused to a Glasgow coma score of 15/15. He had slightly dilated pupils (4 mm) which were sluggishly reactive to light and accommodation. He was afebrile, his pulse was 96 beats per minute and his blood pressure was 96/52 mmHg. He had normal heart sounds with no murmurs and scattered crackles throughout the lung-fields on auscultation. His oxygen saturations were 92% on room air, so he was commenced on 28% oxygen. He had non-specific lesions on his arms and legs (**Figure 56.1**).

Over the next 4 hours he began to deteriorate visibly. He was unable to open his eyes and started dribbling from the side of his mouth. Although able to make sounds, his speech became slurred to the point where it was unintelligible.

He then lost consciousness and had a respiratory arrest. He was intubated, ventilated and taken to the Intensive Care Unit, where he remained for the next 4 weeks.

Initial Differential Diagnosis

Immediately reversible causes, which were considered included:

- Hypoglycaemia
- Acute drug intoxication, including heroin overdose, particularly if pin-point pupils

Particular conditions that a person who injects drugs is at risk of:

- Pulmonary thromboembolism – may cause sudden respiratory arrest, but the preceding neurological features are unusual
- Sepsis – staphylococcal or other bacterial sepsis from non-sterile injecting practice may cause sudden collapse. The lack of fever goes against this, but does not discount it
- Infective endocarditis ± cerebral/pulmonary emboli – usually secondary to sepsis, may present suddenly or sub-acutely. The absence of fever or a cardiac murmur goes against this

Central nervous system infections, given the altered behaviour and reduced consciousness:

Figure 56.1. Lesions present on the skin of a male injecting drug user.

A

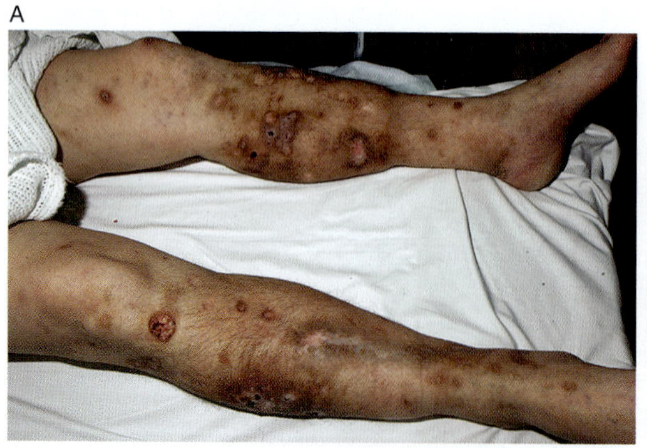

B

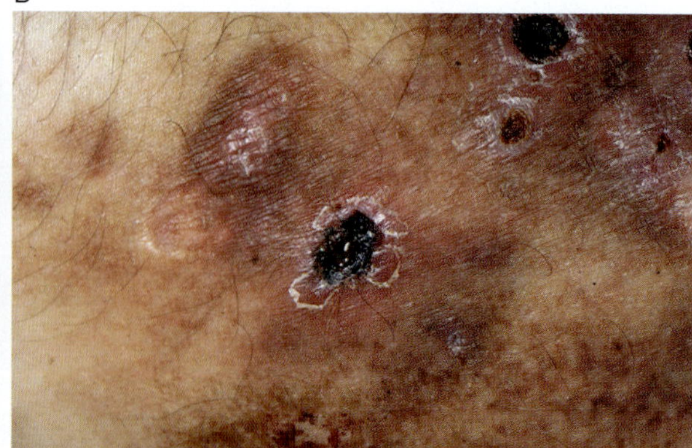

These are typical skin and soft-tissue wounds of 'skin popping' in an injecting drug user. (Photos: Nicholas Beeching.)

- Bacterial meningitis
- Brain abscess

Results of Initial Investigations

- Random blood glucose was 9.8 mmol/l
- Baseline renal and hepatic function was normal
- Full blood count revealed a moderate normocytic anaemia (Hb: 98 g/l) and slight leukocytosis (white cell count: 9.9×10^9 cells/l)
- Chest X-ray showed hyper-inflated lung-fields but no acute infection or septic emboli
- Bedside transthoracic echocardiogram in the intensive therapy unit – no vegetations were seen on heart valves
- Computed tomography of brain was normal (no septic emboli)
- Lumbar puncture revealed slightly high cerebrospinal fluid (CSF) protein (0.56 g/l) but was otherwise normal
- Blood cultures and wound swabs were sent, but results were awaited at this stage

Progress and Further Investigations

After intubation and stabilisation, his pupils were noted to be dilated to 6 mm and fixed. He was conscious but had bilateral ptosis, progressive flaccid upper limb weakness and loss of reflexes.

Causes of acute peripheral neuropathy/radiculopathy were considered, including Guillain–Barré syndrome (Miller Fisher variant), as was neuromuscular junction disease, e.g. myasthaenia gravis (including anti-MUSK variant), but the clinical presentation was atypical [1].

Upper limb nerve conduction studies were normal, but electromyography (EMG) revealed small motor action potentials and fibrillation potentials, which did not reduce with repeat stimulation. Lower limb studies showed a bilateral symmetrical sensory neuropathy and lower limb EMG was normal.

Results of Definitive Investigations

The lower limb nerve conduction study findings probably related to background diabetes mellitus. The upper limb electromyography findings were consistent with a diagnosis of botulism.

While the results of culture and toxin detection assays were awaited, a diagnosis of botulism was made, based on the clinical presentation and supported by the neurophysiology.

The skin wounds were cleaned and debrided. Samples of blood and wound tissue were sent to the Health Protection Agency (now Public Health England) laboratory for anaerobic culture and assays to detect botulinum toxin. Subsequently, wound botulism was confirmed.

Diagnosis

Botulism.

Management and Outcome

Mechanical ventilation was required for 4 weeks.

Botulinum anti-toxin was obtained from the Health Protection Agency [2] and administered by slow intravenous infusion as soon as the diagnosis was suspected. A 10-day course of intravenous benzylpenicillin was also administered. After debridement, standard wound care and hygiene was provided by the tissue viability team.

After weaning from the ventilator, he made a slow recovery and required intensive physiotherapy. He was fit for discharge from hospital to a hostel 3 months after admission. He was commenced on methadone to reduce the ongoing health risks of injecting drug use.

Prevention

Wound botulism is primarily associated with contaminated heroin injection into sites that encourage anaerobic conditions. Avoidance of injection is the best prevention. People who are unwilling or unable to stop injecting should be informed that intravenous injection carries less risk of complications than 'skin popping'. Sharing of 'works' (needles, syringes, cookers/spoons, etc.) should be avoided. Use of citric acid to dissolve heroin prior to injection promotes bacterial growth and should be minimised. Individuals injecting more than one type of drug should do so at different sites with clean 'works'. Infected wounds should be medically treated as soon as possible.

Botulism may also occur after consumption of tinned foods. The causative toxin is heat-labile and destroyed by heating food to > 85°C for more than 5 minutes.

All suspected botulism cases should be notified to the local public health authorities as outbreaks may require rapid control measures.

Discussion

Botulism is a rare but potentially life-threatening paralytic illness caused by potent neurotoxins from a heterogenous group of Gram-positive, spore-forming obligate anaerobic bacteria known as *Clostridium botulinum*. These organisms are found worldwide in soil and marine sediments.

Three main clinical syndromes have been described: wound (as in this case), food-borne and infant botulism. Wound botulism is largely driven by 'skin- or muscle-popping' among injecting drug users and is predominantly described in the USA [3]. There were no cases of wound botulism in the UK before 2000, but 144 cases were reported from 2000 to 2010 [2] (**Figure 56.2**).

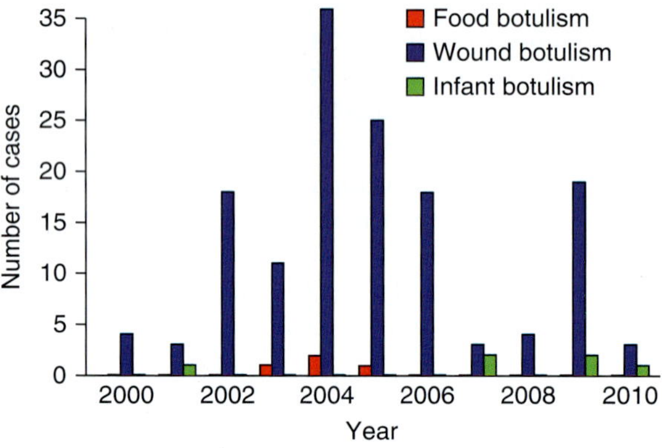

Figure 56.2. Incidence of botulism in England and Wales (2000–2010), comparing food, wound, and infant botulism (described in the text). Data from www.hpa.org.uk.

Bacteria from infected wounds release toxin which is absorbed into host tissues for haematogenous spread. The incubation period lasts several days.

Food botulism is due to ingestion of foods containing pre-formed toxin, so incubation may be shorter (18–36 hours). Canned and fermented foodstuffs are a particular risk because germination and toxin production only occurs when spores are incubated in an anaerobic, low-salt environment at > 4°C. Improvements in food technology have made food-borne botulism rare, but home-canned products present a risk, particularly in Eastern Europe and the southern states of the USA. There is also a high incidence in Alaska due to consumption of fermented meat from aquatic mammals [4].

Infant botulism presents as 'floppy baby syndrome' in children < 1 year old and is caused by endogenous toxin production by *C. botulinum* in the gastrointestinal tract following germination of ingested spores. Consumption of honey has been implicated.

Eight distinct types of botulinum toxin have been described (A, B, C1, C2, D, E, F and G). Human disease is caused by types A, B, E and, rarely F and G. Following absorption and haematogenous dissemination, the toxin exerts its effect by blocking release of the neurotransmitter acetylcholine from presynaptic nerve terminals at the neuromuscular junction (**Figure 56.3**).

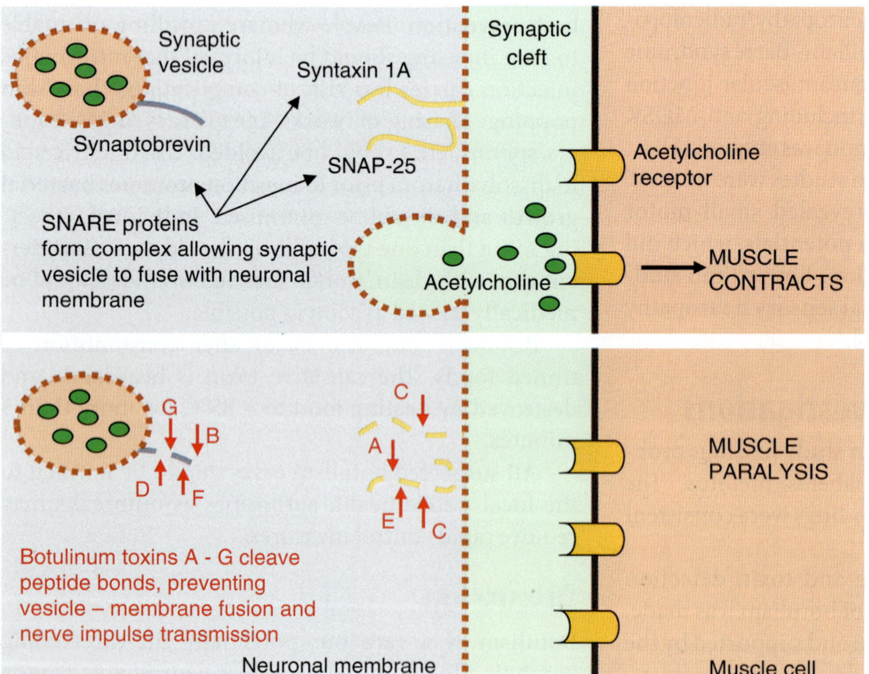

Figure 56.3. Mechanism of action of botulism toxin.

In adults, palsies of cranial nerves III, IV and VI are early features. Extra-ocular muscle paresis causes blurred or double vision. Marked ptosis and depressed papillary responses are common, as seen in this case. Involvement of the lower cranial nerves results in dysphonia, dysarthria and dysphagia. Symmetrical, flaccid, descending paralysis of voluntary muscles may follow, with loss of deep tendon reflexes. Autonomic dysfunction may occur, starting with anhydrosis and progressing to haemodynamic instability. Fever is usually absent, except in cases with concurrent wound infection due to other organisms. Nausea, vomiting and diarrhoea may precede neurological symptoms in food-borne botulism but are rarely present in wound botulism. The clinical features helped differentiate botulism from other causes of paralysis (**Table 56.1**)

In all forms of botulism, diaphragmatic and thoracic muscle paralyses are the worst complications, leading to respiratory compromise and death.

Routine laboratory and radiological investigations cannot confirm botulism, but may help to exclude key differentials. In particular, protein levels in the CSF are often markedly elevated in Guillain–Barré syndrome but are near-normal in botulism. EMG may show characteristic motor nerve abnormalities and nerve conduction studies are usually normal.

Definitive diagnosis requires demonstration of toxin in patient samples, including serum, secretions or wounds, or in contaminated food. In the standard 'mouse lethality bioassay', mice undergo intraperitoneal injection with extracts of clinical specimens and are observed for symptoms. This assay has several limitations; it is performed in few laboratories, takes several days to provide results and may be negative in serum from > 30% of patients with drug-associated wound botulism [5]. *In vitro* assays are under development but not ready for routine use [6].

Important aspects of management are early administration of botulism antitoxin and timely provision of respiratory support. Mortality is 70% in the absence of intensive care, but reduced to less than 5% when adequate facilities are available.

Table 56.1 Clinical features to differentiate botulism from other diseases in the differential diagnoses.

	Distinguishing clinical features	Discriminatory investigations
Botulism	Preceding risk factors (food or wound) Descending weakness Cranial nerve palsies (ophthalmoplegia, dysarthria, dysphagia) Reduced absent/reflexes in 50%	Slightly raised CSF protein *Clostridium botulinum* in wound culture Positive toxin bioassay (unreliable) Normal nerve conduction Small motor action potentials and fibrillation potentials on EMG
CNS infections	Altered mental status[a] Fever, meningism, signs of sepsis Localising signs if brain abscess	Abnormal CSF – raised protein, low glucose, raised white cells, positive microbiology Abnormal brain imaging if abscess
Guillain–Barré syndrome	Prior infection (e.g. gastroenteritis) Ascending weakness No ophthalmoplegia, normal pupils May have sensory symptoms (pain/paraesthesiae)	Raised CSF protein Slow nerve conduction velocities No potentiation of motor action potentials with repetitive stimulation
Miller Fisher syndrome	Similar to Guillain–Barré syndrome but with the triad of ophthalmoplegia, ataxia and areflexia	Raised CSF protein Slow nerve conduction velocities No potentiation of motor action potentials with repetitive stimulation. Anti-GQ1B antibodies
Myaesthenia gravis	Fatigueable muscle weakness Normal pupils and reflexes Positive tensilon test Normal nerve conduction Decreasing motor action potentials on repeat stimulation	Normal CSF Positive anti-ACh receptor antibody or anti-MUSK antibody
Diabetic neuropathy	Prominent sensory symptoms Minimal cranial nerve involvement	Slow nerve conduction velocities

[a] By contrast, patients with botulism typically have intact cognition; in the case presented here, recent injecting drug use may confuse the picture.

Most antitoxin preparations contain combinations of equine-derived antibodies against specific toxin subtypes. These are associated with hypersensitivity reactions, including anaphylaxis, although serious reactions occur in < 1% of patients using modern dosing schedules. To minimise adverse events in infants, human-derived botulism immunoglobulin (BabyBIG) is available and there are clinical trial data supporting its use in children under 1 year [7].

Systemic administration of antitoxin neutralises unbound botulinum toxin and arrests disease progression. In observational studies, early use is associated with a reduced mortality and a shorter requirement for mechanical ventilation [8,9]. Therefore, antitoxin should be administered at the time of clinical suspicion and not be delayed pending laboratory results.

Patients with botulism should be managed in a high-dependency setting to facilitate monitoring, as 50% may require ventilatory support. In wound botulism, debridement may prevent relapse caused by ongoing toxin production from persistent organisms. The role of antibiotics is unproven, but they are commonly used intravenously as an adjunct in wound botulism.

Key Points

- Think carefully about infections causing neurological abnormalities in injecting drug users and beware of presuming that apparent behavioural disturbance is due to intoxication.
- The presence of the four classical 'D's' should heighten suspicion of botulism – dysphonia, dysphagia, dysarthria and diplopia. These are followed by a fifth 'D' – descending paralysis.
- Prompt administration of antitoxin may prevent death and reduce the duration of illness.
- Prolonged mechanical ventilation and intensive care support may be required (approximately 2–8 weeks).

Looking Back

Botulism was first described clinically by the German poet and district medical officer Justinus Kerner in 1822 after outbreaks of 'sausage poisoning' around the southern German town of Württemberg. Eighty years later, an outbreak of botulism at a funeral dinner, which included smoked ham, in the Belgian village of Ellezelles led to the discovery of *C. botulinum* by Emile Pierre van Ermengem at the University of Ghent.

Did You Know?

The causative bacterium was named because of its pathological association with sausages (the Latin for sausage is 'botulus') and not, as sometimes assumed, because it is sausage-shaped.

Since the elucidation of its method of action, botulinum toxin type A has been used as a therapeutic agent to treat blepharospasm, strabismus, upper motor neuron syndromes (e.g. cerebral palsy), hyperhidrosis, cervical dystonia and chronic migraine. It is also used as a cosmetic therapy to reduce wrinkles (**Figure 56.4**).

Iatrogenic cases of botulism have also been described and botulinum toxin has been described as a potential agent of bioterrorism.

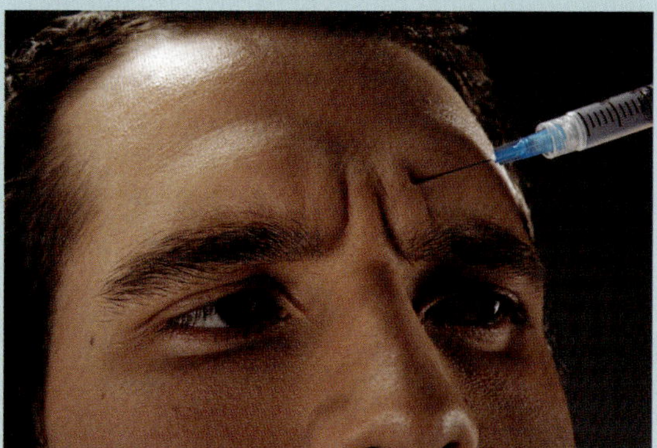

Figure 56.4. Cosmetic botox use. (Photo courtesy of UpperCut Images)

References

1. Merrison AFA, Chidley KE, Dunnett J, Sieradzan KA. Wound botulism associated with subcutaneous drug use. Brit Med J 2002;**325**:1020–1.
2. www.gov.uk/government/publications/botulism-clinical-and-public-health-management (accessed May 30, 2018).
3. Yuan J, Inami G, Mohle-Boetani J, Vugia DJ. Recurrent wound botulism among injecting drug users in California. Clin Infect Dis 2011;**52**:862–6.
4. Fagan RP, McLaughlin JB, Castrodale LJ, et al. Endemic foodborne botulism among Alaska Native persons – Alaska, 1947–2007. Clin Infect Dis 2011;**52**:585–92.
5. Wheeler C, Inami G, Mohle-Boetani J, Vugia D. Sensitivity of mouse bioassay in clinical wound botulism. Clin Infect Dis 2009;**48**:1669–73.

6. Rosen O, Feldberg L, Gura S, et al. Early, real-time medical diagnosis of botulism by endopeptidase-mass spectrometry. Clin Infect Dis 2015;**61**:e58–61.
7. Chalk C, Benstead TJ, Keezer M. Medical treatment for botulism. Cochrane Data Syst Rev 2014:CD008123.
8. Tacket CO, Shanders WX, Mann JM Hargrett NT, Blake PA. Equine antitoxin use and other factors that predict outcome in type A foodborne botulism. Am J Med 1984;**76**:794–8.
9. Kongsaengdao S, Samintarapanya K, Rusmeechan S, et al. An outbreak of botulism in Thailand: clinical manifestations and management of severe respiratory failure. Clin Infect Dis 2006;**43**: 1247–56.

CASE 57

Bad Headache and Awkward Eye

Scott Williams, Tom Solomon and Laura Benjamin

History

A 53-year-old lady attended her local Emergency Medicine department with a generalised global headache. Four days earlier she had developed a throbbing headache over the course of 24 hours, which persisted. This was associated with vomiting, photophobia and neck stiffness. On the day of admission she developed left eye pain and swelling; this was associated with blurring of her vision, as well as diplopia on looking to the left. She felt feverish. She denied any loss of consciousness, numbness or weakness of her limbs. She had a background of hypothyroidism, pernicious anaemia, osteoarthritis, chronic obstructive pulmonary disease and anxiety. She suffered from infrequent non-disabling headaches in the past. She had a family history of type 2 diabetes, smoked 10 cigarettes per day for 30 years, and did not drink alcohol. She lived alone with no pets, and had no recent foreign travel. She was the main carer for her mother, who had been treated for tuberculosis 8 years earlier. Her only medication was hydroxocobalamin injections.

Examination

On inspection, she had left peri-orbital oedema with associated conjunctivitis. In the left eye she had reduced visual acuity and was only able to perceive light, with a globally reduced visual field in that eye. Although the left pupil was reactive to light and accommodation, there was a suggestion of a relative afferent papillary defect. She also thought she was seeing double on left gaze. Funduscopy was normal. In the right eye her uncorrected visual acuity was 6/18 on a Snellen chart, and the light reflex, visual field and funduscopy were normal.

Despite the history of diplopia, she appeared to have a full range of her eye movements. Sensation of the ophthalmic (V1) and maxillary (V2) divisions of the trigeminal nerve was impaired on the left, but normal on the right. The remaining cranial nerves were normal.

She had normal tone, power, reflexes, sensation and coordination of the upper and lower limbs. She had a temperature of 37.2°C and was haemodynamically stable. She had palpable left cervical lymph nodes. Her systemic examination was otherwise unremarkable.

Initial Differential Diagnosis

The differential diagnosis of the initial presenting illness of meningism with a left ocular syndrome included:

- Infective (e.g. *Mycobacterium tuberculosis, Treponema pallidum, Borrelia burgdoferi* and herpes viruses including herpes simplex viruses, varicella zoster virus (VZV), cytomegalovirus and Epstein–Barr virus)
- Vascular (e.g. cavernous sinus syndrome, subarachnoid haemorrhage)
- Inflammatory (e.g. sarcoidosis, autoimmune disease)
- Neoplasia (e.g. lymphoma and melanoma)
- Primary headache disorder (e.g. migraine)

Results of Initial Investigations

Full blood count on admission showed a mild normocytic anaemia, but was otherwise normal. Urea and electrolytes, liver function tests, C-reactive protein, thyroid function tests, serum folate and fasting serum glucose were within normal ranges. Her serum B12 level was raised, but this was consistent with replacement injections of hydroxocobalamin. Her chest X-ray was normal.

A computer tomography (CT) head scan was performed (**Figure 57.1**).

Further Investigations

Further imaging was arranged following transfer to a tertiary neuroscience centre. This included:

- A CT angiogram which showed no evidence of a vascular abnormality.
- A magnetic resonance imaging (MRI) head scan with gadolinium, which was normal.
- An MRI venogram of the cerebral sinuses, which did not show evidence of a cavernous sinus thrombosis.

She underwent a lumbar puncture, which had an opening pressure of 38 cm H_2O. The cerebrospinal fluid (CSF) white cell count was 4 cells/mm^3 (50% lymphocytes and 50% polymorphonuclear cells), red cell count was 143 cells/mm^3, protein was 1.21 g/l, glucose was 3.0 mmol/l. CSF microscopy showed no bacteria; CSF

Figure 57.1. Axial images from a CT scan of a 53-year-old lady who presented with fever, meningism and left eye pain and swelling.

A

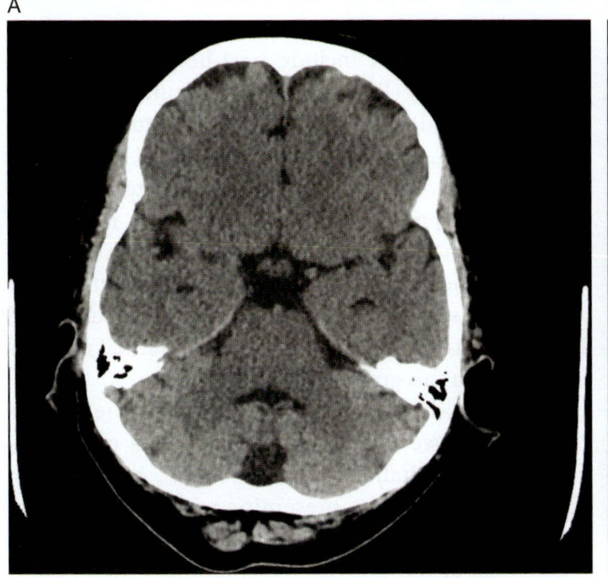

B

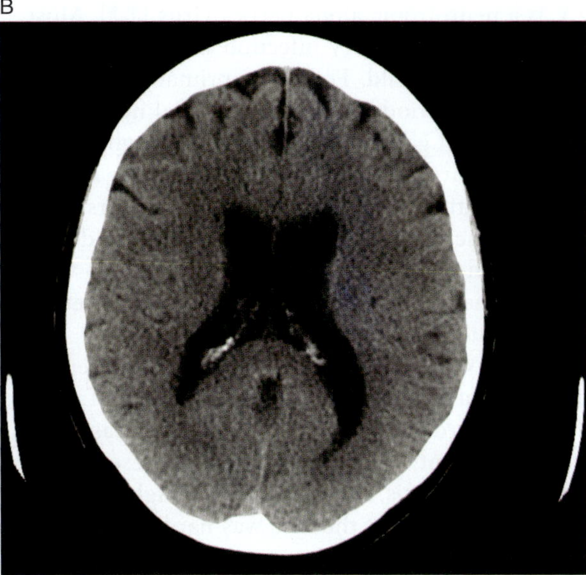

This is normal; in particular it does not demonstrate haemorrhage, or features of obstructive raised intracranial pressure.

cytology was negative, and there was no xanthochromia detected.

Progress

She was seen by a neuro-ophthalmologist who found a left granulomatous anterior uveitis with a degree of optic neuritis. On closer inspection of her face an abnormality was noticed (**Figure 57.2**). On further questioning, she admitted to a blistering rash on her face around the start of her initial symptoms.

Figure 57.2. The face of the same patient.

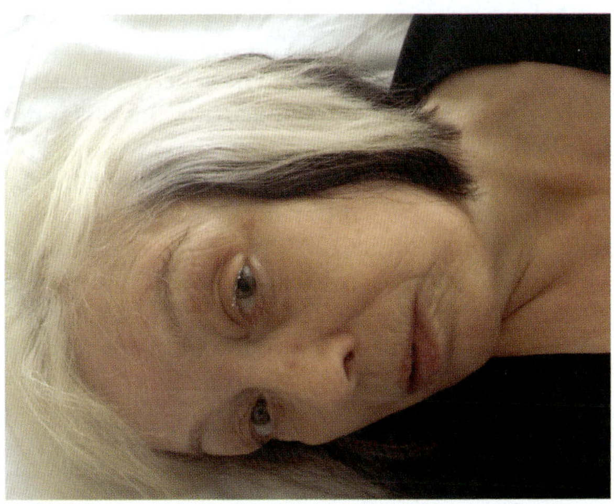

This demonstrates the healing areas from the previous rash, shown as resolving vesicular blisters in the left V1 and V2 divisions of the trigeminal nerve.

Results of Definitive Investigations

Serological testing for HIV infection, Lyme disease and syphilis were all negative. Staining of CSF for acid- and alcohol-fast bacilli was negative, and a blood tuberculosis quantiFERON test was negative. CSF culture was negative. Serum and CSF angiotensin-converting enzyme, and serum ANA and ANCA were all negative.

VZV was detected by polymerase chain reaction (PCR) in samples from both a swab taken from her left eye, and PCR of her CSF.

Diagnosis

She had a varicella zoster virus infection, affecting predominately the ophthalmic division of the trigeminal nerve. This was complicated by a left eye anterior uveitis, possibly also with left optic neuritis, and with meningism.

Management and Outcome

During 1 week of treatment with intravenous aciclovir, the patient's symptoms of headache improved and her visual acuity in the left eye improved from light perception only to 6/24 on a Snellen chart. She was then discharged home with 2 further weeks on oral valaciclovir. At follow-up, 2 months later, she was well, and visual acuity in the left eye had improved further.

Discussion

VZV is a neurotropic alpha herpes virus [1,2]. Most people acquire a primary infection demonstrated by chickenpox as a child. Following primary infection, VZV enters a period of latency in cranial nerve ganglia, dorsal root ganglia and autonomic ganglia along the entire neuroaxis. This leads to a lifelong risk of VZV reactivation, which can present many years later. Typically, reactivation of VZV is shown by the development of the well-described vesicular eruption with a dermatomal distribution, termed herpes zoster or 'shingles', but this is not always the case [3].

Because VZV disseminates throughout the neuroaxis, reactivation can lead to a wide variety of neurological disorders (**Table 57.1**). Ocular disease was the predominant feature in this lady's presentation with anterior uveitis. Initially it was thought she had optic neuritis too, but the disc was hard to visualise because of the uveitis; however, the rapid improvement of vision suggests all her impairment was due to uveitis, and follow-up funduscopy confirmed this. Additional eye complications which can arise include retinal necrosis, progressive outer retinal necrosis and third nerve palsy [1,3]. The diplopia she experienced early in the illness could have been VIth nerve involvement, perhaps a mononeuritis, but this is not often reported.

Although the patient had headache and raised intracranial pressure, the relatively normal cell count and biochemistry did not support the diagnosis of viral meningitis, defined strictly as a CSF pleocytosis. However, the abnormal presence of 50% polymorphonuclear cells in the CSF, and the features of meningism in the history, suggested that VZV reactivation probably caused a degree of inflammation in the meninges.

Table 57.1 Neurological complications of varicella zoster virus reactivation [1,3].

- Acute inflammatory demyelinating polyneuropathy (Guillain–Barré syndrome)
- Myelitis*
- Meningitis and encephalitis*
- Vasculopathy*
- Focal motor weakness
- Ramsay Hunt syndrome
- Post-herpetic neuralgia
- Ocular disease* (e.g. optic neuritis, retinal necrosis, progressive outer retinal necrosis, uveitis, third nerve cranial palsy)

* These syndromes have been reported in the absence of a rash.

Being elderly is an important risk factor for VZV reactivation. This is related to a decline in cell-mediated immunity with age. The main neurological complications in this cohort include post-herpetic neuralgia, facial nerve palsy (Ramsay Hunt syndrome) and ocular disease [1,4,5]. People with diabetes mellitus, an underlying malignancy (e.g. lymphoma) and HIV, are at risk of reactivation, as are patients receiving long-term steroids or immunosuppressant therapy [3,6]. Thus, in patients presenting with VZV reactivation, it is worth thinking about whether any of these underlying conditions are present. Disseminated disease, transverse myelitis and severe forms of ocular disease including retinal necrosis may occur in this group of patients [1,6].

The introduction of PCR testing of the CSF is thought to have increased our awareness of meningitis and encephalitis related to VZV. A significant proportion of patients presenting with a neurological syndrome due to VZV do not have the typical herpes zoster rash at the time of presentation, which potentially hinders the diagnosis. This may occur either because the rash precedes or follows the neurological impairment, or in some cases because a rash is never seen; this is termed 'zoster sin herpete' [1]. Thus, VZV infection should always be considered in patients presenting with one of the typical neurological syndromes (**Table 57.1**), even in the absence of a rash. This is especially important given that it is treatable. In the patient described above a more thorough history and careful examination revealed that she did indeed have a rash, although it was not immediately apparent at presentation.

In the CSF VZV immunoglobulin G remains elevated for a longer period than VZV DNA, thus offering an advantage in the confirmation of VZV CNS infection, particularly for delayed presentations or for samples taken after treatment has been commenced [7,8].

CNS VZV reactivation is treated with intravenous aciclovir. Immunocompromised patients or those with neurological syndromes such as meningoencephalitis, vasculopathy and myelitis should have intravenous aciclovir for a period of 10–14 days, initially. There have been no randomised controlled trials, but most would recommend this given the virus' susceptibility *in vitro* and the severity of the disease [3]; oral valaciclovir has also been used when there are difficulties with intravenous treatment. As a secondary prophylactic measure, continuation of oral valaciclovir may be required for months to prevent recurrence of neurological complications, but the evidence for this is less clear [1,9].

Key Points

- Patients can present with a variety of neurological syndromes caused by VZV reactivation, some of these may occur in the absence of a herpes zoster rash.
- In the CSF VZV immunoglobulin remains elevated for a longer period than VZV DNA, so a negative PCR does not exclude the diagnosis, and antibody testing should be requested.
- Comprehensive screening for immunosuppressive risk factors that could predispose an individual to VZV reactivation is important, particularly an HIV test.

Looking Back

The first suggestion of a relationship between chickenpox and a viral infection was proposed in 1888. This link was later proven in the 1950s and was followed by the development of a live attenuated vaccine virus in 1974. The treatment of VZV infection advanced greatly during the 1980s with the introduction of aciclovir [10].

Did You Know?

Shingles has a range of different names across the world, including 'belt of fire' in Arabic, 'zone' in French, 'big rash' in Hindi, 'small snake' in Spanish, and *helvetesild* ('hell's fire') in Norwegian.

References

1. Nagel MA, Gilden, D. Complications of varicella zoster virus reactivation. Curr Treat Opin Neurol 2013;**15**:439–53.
2. Pergam SA, Limaye AP. Varicella zoster virus. Am J Transplant 2009;**9**:S108–15.
3. Steiner I, Kennedy, PGE, Pachner AR. The neurotropic herpes viruses: herpes simplex and varicella-zoster. Lancet Neurol 2007;**6**:1015–28.
4. Insinga RP, Itzler RF, Pellissier JM, et al. The incidence of herpes zoster in the United States administrative database. J Gen Int Med 2005;**20**:748–53.
5. Harnisch, JP. Zoster in the elderly: clinical, immunologic and therapeutic considerations. J Am Geriat Soc 1984;**32**:789–93.
6. Gilden DH, Cohrs RJ, Mahalingam R. Clinical and molecular pathogenesis of varicella zoster virus infection. Viral Immunol 2003;**16**:243–58.
7. Gilden DH, Wright RR, Schneck SA, et al. Zoster sine herpete, a clinical variant. Ann Neurol 1994;**35**: 530–3.
8. Nagel MA, Forghani B, Mahalingam R, et al. The value of detecting anti-VZV IgG antibody in CSF to diagnose VZV vasculopathy. Neurology 2007;**68**:1069–73.
9. Habib AA, Gilden D, Schmid DS, et al. Varicella zoster virus meningitis with hypoglycorrhachia in the absence of a rash and in an immunocompetent woman. J NeuroVirol 2009;**15**:206–8.
10. Wood MJ. History of varicella zoster virus. Herpes 2000;7:60–5.

CASE 58 Drowsy With Difficulty Swallowing

Tom Solomon

History

A 39-year-old man presented with a 3-week history of painful mouth ulcers, and difficulty swallowing, fever, tiredness and increasing drowsiness. Hodgkin's disease had been diagnosed 4 years earlier, and after failed chemotherapy, he had been treated with a bone marrow autotransplant. When this also failed, he received an allotransplant from an unrelated donor, 3 months prior to this admission. Apart from some modest graft versus host disease of the skin, he had been progressing well until he developed the three deep and painful ulcerated lesions in the mouth and dysphagia. He was admitted for investigation of the lesions and for feeding, when he became increasingly confused and then had a generalised tonic–clonic seizure. He had hypothyroidism, but no other past history of note.

His medication included chemotherapy with cyclophosphamide and mycophenolate, ambisome (liposomal), amphoteracin, Alfacalcidol (Vit D), thiamine, vitamin B complex, metoclopramide, calcichew, thyroxine, pantoprazole (for the ulcers), difflam spray, chloramphenicol eye drops and amiloride syrup.

Examination

He was drowsy and mildly confused, being orientated to person, but not place or time. There was a pyrexia of 38.5°C. There was no meningism, and the cranial nerve examination was normal, although he had ulcers on his palate. The peripheral nervous system examination was normal, although deep tendon reflexes were only present with reinforcement, and sensory examination was not possible.

Initial Differential Diagnosis

The initial differential diagnosis was broad, comprising all the causes of confusion in an immunocompromised patient with a background of lymphoma, and including infectious, neoplastic and metabolic causes. In this patient it was especially important to determine how immunosuppressed he was, what previous chemotherapeutic regimens he had been on, and his and the donor's status in terms of cytomegalovirus (CMV), Epstein–Barr virus (EBV) and Toxoplasma.

Results of Initial Investigations

He was mildly pancytopaenic, with reduced haemoglobin and platelet count; his white cell count was 3.3×10^9/l, with a neutrophil count of 1.3×10^9/l; CD4 count, which had been 300 cells/mm^3, was now 160 cells/mm^3, renal and liver function were unremarkable. A computed tomography (CT) scan of his head was performed (**Figure 58.1**). In the cerebrospinal fluid (CSF) there were 12 lymphocytes/mm^3, which looked reactive, CSF/serum glucose was 2.4/6.8 mmol/l, protein 10.3 g/l; cytospin was negative.

Refined Differential Diagnosis

With no oedema or enhancement, the lesions on CT were not felt to be typical of lymphoma or toxoplasma. CSF was negative for *Cryptococcus, M. tuberculosis* and JC virus. The patient's pre-transplant toxoplasma serology was negative, while the donor's was positive; however, the patient had been on empirical treatment for toxoplasma, and his serum antibody test remained negative, as did his CSF polymerase chain reaction (PCR). Both patient and donor were CMV-negative. Pre-transplant the patient was negative for EBV, but the donor was positive, and post-transplant the patient had rising EBV titres, by PCR, in the blood and CSF. CT of the chest, abdomen and pelvis were unremarkable.

Figure 58.1. Axial images from a CT scan of a 39-year-old male with mouth ulcers and drowsiness.

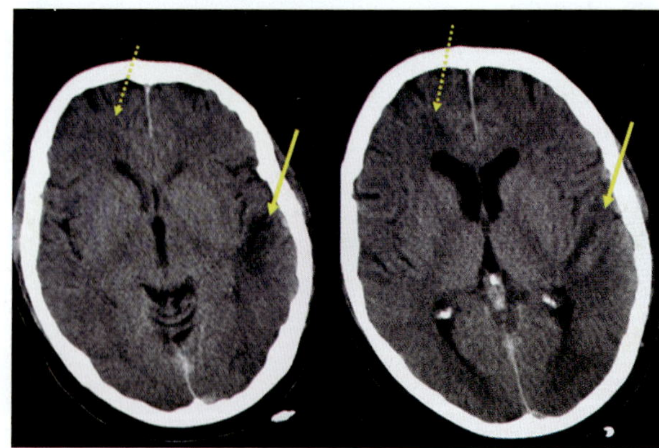

This shows two low-density lesions in the right frontal lobe (dotted arrow) and left parietal lobe (solid arrow), with little surrounding oedema, which do not enhance with contrast.

Results of Definitive Investigations

The patient underwent an upper gastrointestinal endoscopy (**Figure 58.2**). Biopsies of these lesions were histologically unremarkable, but the tissue had high EBV titre by PCR. The patient therefore had a magnetic resonance imaging (MRI)-guided biopsy of the right frontal lobe lesion (**Figure 58.3**). This showed he had post-transplant lymphoproliferative disorder.

Diagnosis

Epstein–Barr virus-driven post-transplant lymphoproliferative disorder.

Management and Outcome

He was treated with rituximab and a T-cell transplant from the original donor, which brought the lymphoproliferation under control. His lesions resolved, as did his confusion, and he returned home for a short time before ultimately succumbing to a relapse of his lymphoma.

Discussion

EBV is a gamma herpes virus which infects most people during childhood or early adulthood. In childhood infection may be asymptomatic; in young adults it causes infectious mononucleosis. The virus becomes latent in B lymphocytes, but can subsequently reactivate and drive B-cell replication to cause lymphomas (**Figure 58.4**). This includes Burkitt's lymphoma, which occurs in Africa, and primary central nervous system (CNS) lymphoma, which occurs in the immunocompromised. EBV is also associated with oral hairy leukoplakia in people with HIV, and craniopharyngioma in Asia.

Post-transplant lymphoproliferative disorder is a pre-malignant proliferation of B lymphocytes, driven by EBV [1]. It is different to lymphoma because it is reversible. It is a well-recognised, although rare, complication of both solid organ and allogeneic bone marrow transplantation. Normally the tendency of EBV-infected B cells to proliferate is controlled by T lymphocytes. In this case the transplant recipient was naive to EBV, and so did not have such primed T cells, and thus was vulnerable to this disorder. Risk factors for post-transplant lymphoproliferative disorder include viral infections, age and race, allograft type and host genetic variation. Around 10–15% of patients with post-transplant lymphoproliferative disorder present with CNS manifestations [2].

Figure 58.2. Oesophageal–gastro-duodenoscopic images from the same patient.

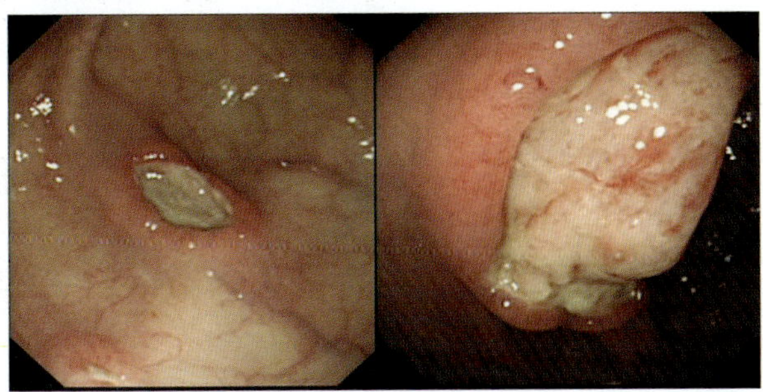

These show oral and oesophageal ulcerative lesions.

Figure 58.3. MRI-guided brain biopsy from a similar patient.

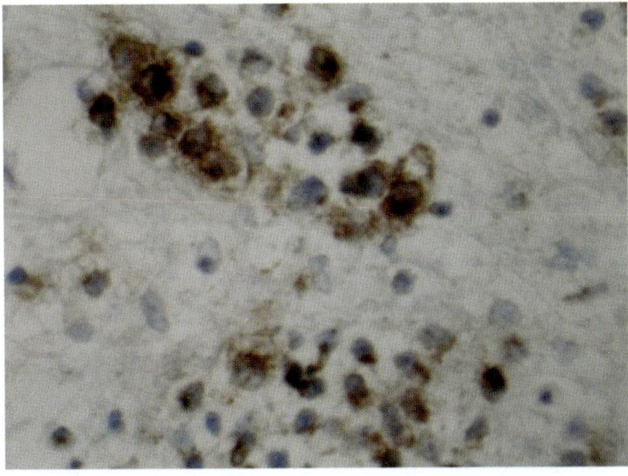

EBV was demonstrated by the positive stain for the viral protein latent membrane protein (LMP)-1, confirming the diagnosis of post-transplant lymphoproliferative disorder. (From: www.universitypathologists.com/education/case-of-the-month/may-2011)

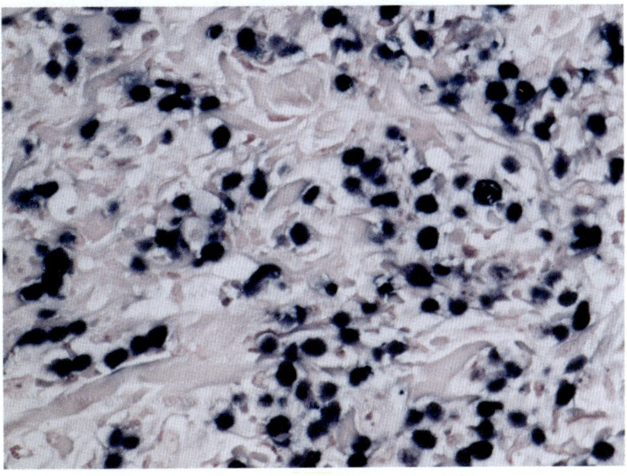

Figure 58.4. EBV-encoded RNA (EBER) positive cells in plasmablastic lymphoma. (From [3] with permission of Elsevier.)

This patient was treated with rituximab, which is a monoclonal antibody against CD20, and thus targets B cells. This was followed by a transplant of T cells from the original donor (which thus controlled further B-cell proliferation). The alternative treatment approach is to reduce the immunosuppression, but that carries the risk of allograft rejection.

Key Points

- Post-transplantation lymphoproliferative disorder is a rare cause of space-occupying lesions in immunosuppressed transplant recipients, which is driven by EBV.
- It should be considered if the EBV titres are very high.
- It may respond to treatment with rituximab.
- Brain biopsy is very useful in patients with CNS space-occupying lesions, particularly those with immunosuppression.
- The donor and recipient status with respect to EBV, toxoplasma and CMV can help determine the likely cause of CNS infection in transplant recipients.

Looking Back

EBV was first identified more than 30 years ago by electron microscopy of cells cultured from a Burkitt's lymphoma [4]. Anthony Epstein only started working on the problem after a chance meeting with Denis Burkitt, who had recently described a bizarre children's cancer in Africa. For 3 years, Epstein's attempts to culture the virus from Burkitt's lymphoma tissue were unsuccessful. However, one lymphoma sample from Uganda took longer to arrive in London because the plane bringing it back was diverted to Manchester. It looked like a contaminated sample, but under the microscope Burkitt saw huge numbers of free-floating, healthy-looking tumour cells, and with his PhD student Yvonne Barr managed to establish cell cultures. Conventional tests for identifying virus in the cultures still failed, but Epstein tried the newer approach of electron microscopy, and found a cell filled with the elusive herpes virus.

Did You Know?

Almost everyone has been infected with EBV by adulthood. Those infected as children are usually asymptomatic, or have a non-specific illness. In young adults primary infection causes glandular fever characterised by fevers and lymphadenopathy. It is also known as the 'kisser's disease' because of the means by which most young adults are thought to acquire infection.

References

1. Jagadeesh D, Woda BA, Draper J, Evens AM. Post transplant lymphoproliferative disorders: risk, classification, and therapeutic recommendations. Curr Treat Options Oncol 2012;**23**:122–36.
2. Al-Mansour Z, Nelson BP, Evens AM. Post-transplant lymphoproliferative disease (PTLD): risk factors, diagnosis, and current treatment strategies. Curr Hematol Malig Rep 2013;**8**:173–83.
3. Torlakovic EE, Bailey D. Post-transplant lymphoproliferative disorders. Diagn Histopathol 2012;**18**:218–19.
4. Epstein A. Burkitt lymphoma and the discovery of Epstein–Barr virus. Br J Haematol 2012;**156**:777–9.

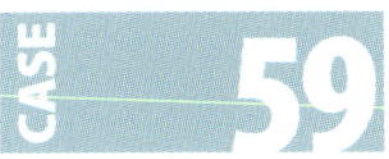

Two Types of Shaking

Lance Turtle and Gemma Buxton

History

A 4-year-old boy was admitted to a district hospital in southern India during the month of December, with new-onset convulsions following a 4-day febrile illness. The illness started with a mild fever associated with a cough and coryzal symptoms, but on the third day the child became drowsy and confused, not recognising family members and staring vacantly. Oral intake decreased, limited to small sips of water each day. On the fourth day he became unconscious and started having convulsions. The first episode was a generalised tonic–clonic seizure lasting around 1 hour. His parents reported that this convulsion stopped during the 2-hour trip to the hospital, but on admission to hospital the child was found to be in convulsive status epilepticus.

He had no significant past medical history and no previous admissions to hospital. He had never had seizures before and there was no family history of epilepsy. He was born at term weighing 2.75 kg and had a normal vaginal delivery at home. He had three older siblings who were all alive and healthy. One of his siblings had suffered febrile seizures aged 4 years but none since. The child had been breastfed until 5 months of age and now ate the same diet as his family. His parents thought he had probably received all of his childhood vaccinations but had no written record of this. He did not take any regular medications and had no known drug allergies. His development was appropriate for his age and he enjoyed playing with his siblings around his parent's small-holding farm where he lived. No one else in the family had been unwell recently, but a cousin in a nearby village had also been admitted to hospital a fortnight ago with a similar presentation.

Figure 59.1. Image of a 4-year-old male child from southern India who presented with acute fever and seizures.

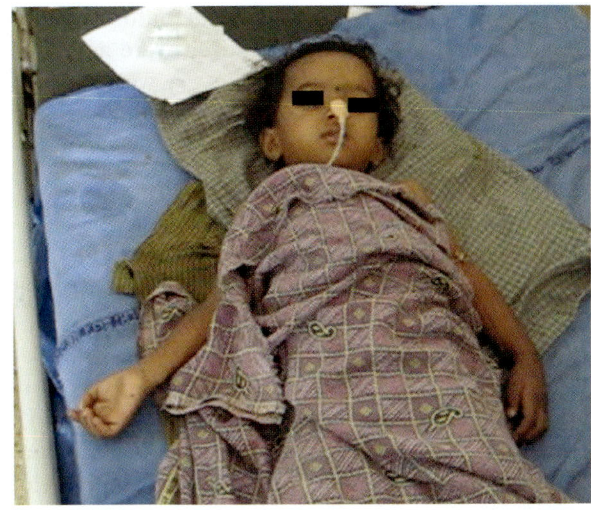

This shows a comatose child, who has a nasogastric tube in place.

Examination

A complete examination was carried out once the status epilepticus had been controlled. The child remained unconscious (**Figure 59.1**). He appeared underweight and stunted, weighing 10 kg and measuring 89 cm in length. He was febrile, with a temperature of 38°C. He was maintaining his own airway, and had a raised respiratory rate of 52 breaths per minute. His pulse was 120 beats per minute, with a blood pressure of 90/60 mmHg. Auscultation revealed normal heart sounds and a clear chest. Abdominal examination was normal, as were his ears, nose and throat. He had slightly enlarged cervical lymph nodes. Neurological examination revealed generally normal tone except in his right upper limb, which had increased tone. Head lag was noted. Movement was reduced in all four limbs, with normal reflexes in all except the right upper limb, which showed a brisk response.

Clonus was present bilaterally, 8 beats on the left and 6 beats on the right, and plantar responses were up-going on the left and down-going on the right. Examination for tremor showed a resting tremor in both hands.

He had a vacant stare and was drooling saliva. There was no papilloedema on funduscopy and he had normal pupillary responses, but no spontaneous eye movements or response to menace. There was no speech and his Glasgow coma score was 7/15, with him localising painful stimuli but making no verbal response or eye movements.

Initial Differential Diagnosis

Although febrile convulsions are common in this setting and in this age group, the pattern of repeated seizures, status epilepticus, coma and other abnormal neurological findings pointed strongly towards the presence of a central nervous system infection. The main differential diagnosis was viral encephalitis, which occurs in high incidence at this time of year. Bacterial meningitis is a common and serious infection also frequently seen in this setting. Tuberculous meningitis is also common in this population, but was less likely given the acute onset of the illness and absence of family history of tuberculosis or prolonged cough. A couple of children were admitted to the department with malaria every week, so this was also on the differential, as was scrub typhus and typhoid encephalopathy.

Results of Initial Investigations

His initial blood results demonstrated a low haemoglobin (95 g/l) and a pleocytosis white a white cell count (WCC) of 18.1 × 10^9/l and a predominance of polymorphonuclear cells (79%). His urea was elevated (180 mg/l) although his creatinine was normal (5 mg/l). He was hyponatraemic (129 mmol/l); other routine biochemistry including other electrolytes and glucose was normal, as was the platelet count.

Malaria rapid test, dengue non-structural protein 1 antigen test and widal test were negative, and both urinalysis and a plain chest radiograph were normal.

A computer tomography (CT) scan of the head was undertaken prior to lumbar puncture (LP) because of the prolonged seizures and focal neurological signs (**Figure 59.2**).

The LP was undertaken, although the opening pressure was not measured, the cerebrospinal fluid (CSF) WCC was elevated (200 cells/mm^3), as was the protein (538 mg/l); the CSF glucose was 630 mg/l; however, no contemporaneous serum glucose was measured. Both the Gram stain and Ziehl–Neelsen stain of the CSF were negative.

Refined Differential Diagnosis

At this stage viral encephalitis, or acute encephalitis syndrome as it is sometimes known, remained the working diagnosis, and the thalamic lesions suggested Japanese encephalitis (JE) virus (JEV) the most likely cause.

Results of Definitive Investigations

JEV IgM was detected by ELISA in the child's serum and CSF.

Figure 59.2. Axial CT brain image in a 4-year-old child in southern India who presented with a fever, seizures, rest tremor and upper motor neuron signs.

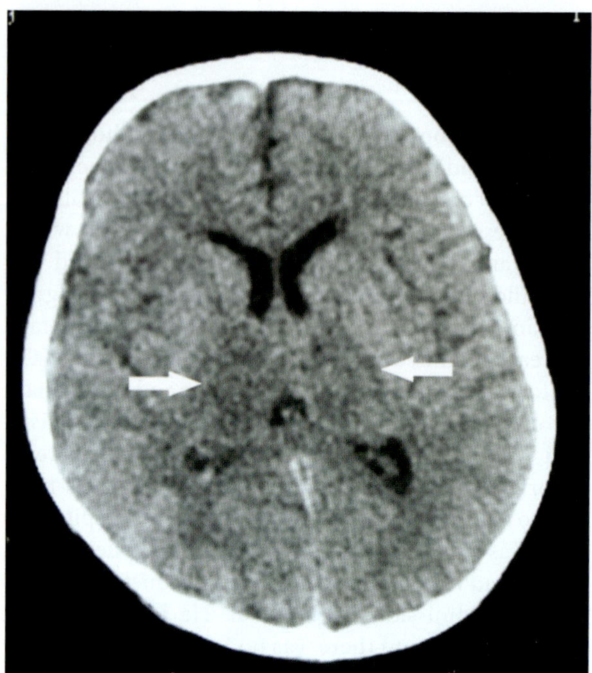

This shows bilateral thalamic hypodensity (arrows) with no evidence of a mass lesion.

Diagnosis

Japanese encephalitis.

Management and Outcome

Upon admission, intravenous (IV) diazepam and phenytoin were given for status epilepticus, which terminated the seizures, but there was no recovery of consciousness. The child remained unconscious for the next 2 days, so IV dexamethasone and mannitol were started following local protocols for the management of acute encephalitis syndrome with suspected raised intracranial pressure. A nasogastric tube was sited for enteral hydration (and subsequent feeding if necessary, although that was not done in this case). There had been a delay in LP because of the seizures and subsequent CT scan; therefore, a single dose of cefotaxime was given pending the LP result, but not continued once the result was available. The child recovered and was discharged from hospital.

He was reviewed at a follow-up clinic, 3 months post-discharge. The family reported no persisting symptoms or seizures and examination was entirely normal. A Liverpool outcome score demonstrated a return to full function [1].

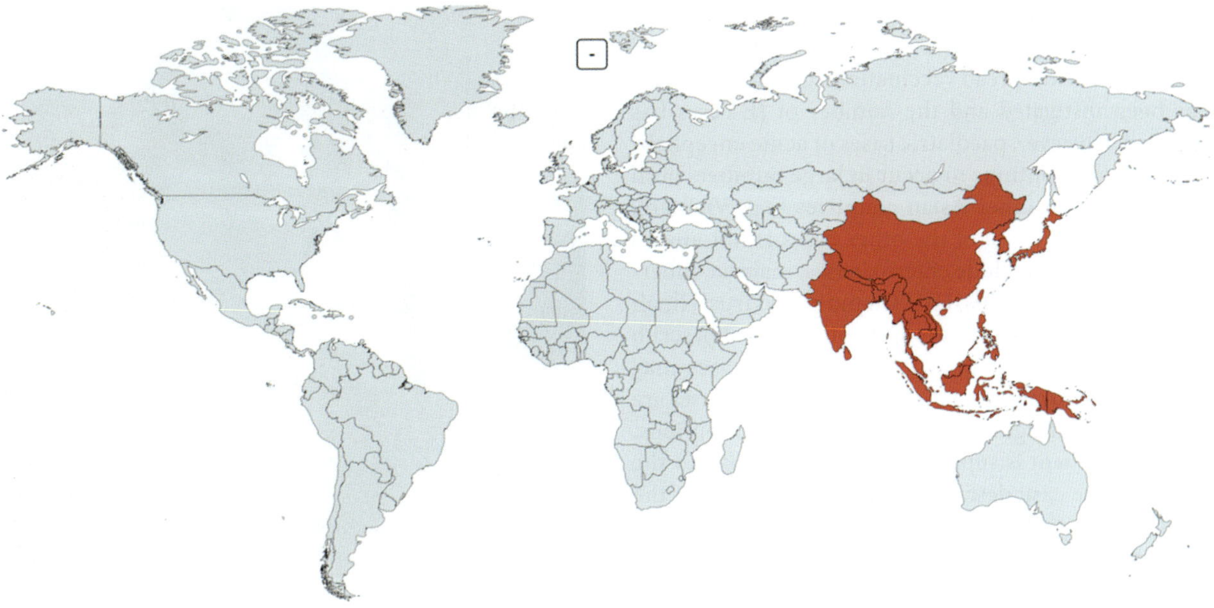

Figure 59.3. Geographical distribution of Japanese encephalitis virus.

Prevention

In common with all arthropod-borne viruses (arboviruses), JEV can in theory be prevented by avoiding mosquito bites. While this might be a useful strategy for short-term travellers to an endemic region or a resident population with good-quality housing and infrastructure (e.g. in Japan), it is clearly impractical for residents of rural Asia, where most JE occurs, especially because the principle vectors, such as *Culex* mosquitoes, bite in the evenings, when children are out playing. The only realistic method for JE prevention is vaccination. JE vaccines have been available for nearly 50 years but older vaccines, derived from formalin-inactivated mouse brain, had a reputation for side effects and were expensive [2]. The Chinese-manufactured live attenuated vaccine SA14-14–2 is safe, effective and cheaply available in many Asian countries [3]. In addition, other newer killed vaccines are coming on the market.

Discussion

Japanese encephalitis (JE) is caused by JEV, a single-stranded, positive-sense RNA virus of the genus *Flavivirus* in the family Flaviviridae [4]. JE is endemic in much of South and Southeast Asia (**Figure 59.3**). JEV is naturally a virus of birds, particularly wading ardeids such as herons and egrets, and pigs (**Figure 59.4**). JEV is transmitted between birds, in which it causes no illness, by mosquitoes of the genus *Culex* (**Figure 59.5**). The virus can be transmitted from birds to pigs, which act as amplifying hosts of JEV because they exhibit sufficiently high viraemia to be infectious to the mosquito and live close to humans in much of Asia. Humans are dead-end hosts of JEV because they do not generate adequate levels of viraemia for onward infection of the mosquito vector [5].

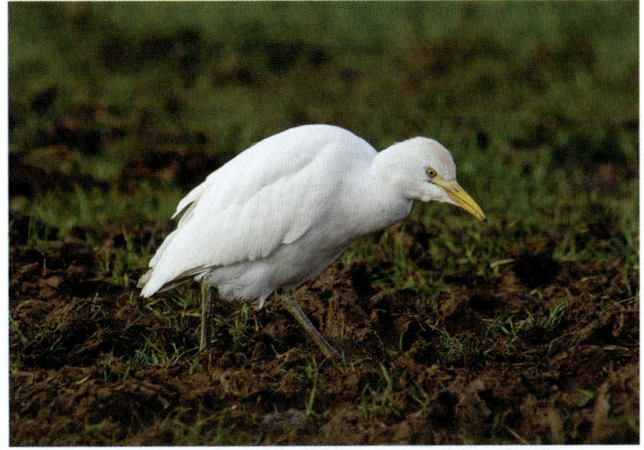

Figure 59.4. Cattle egret foraging for food. (Photo courtesy of Gary Chalker.)

In India, acute encephalitis syndrome is common in children and much of it is thought to be due to JE (Box 59.1). Widespread vaccination against JE in India has been instigated and the number of JE cases has reduced. However, paediatric cases of acute encephalitis syndrome continue to occur in large numbers both in India and in other Asian countries (e.g. Vietnam, Thailand). The cause of the other cases is not always known, but may include enteroviruses, malaria, tuberculosis (TB) meningitis, HIV, Chandipura virus, Nipah virus (which is spread by contact with fruit bats), scrub typhus, or other, unknown causes. Some cases may also be autoimmune in nature. Most of the illnesses are clinically indistinguishable and, with some exceptions, the management is supportive and not specific to the cause. In the case described above, knowledge of the local disease epidemiology suggested a low likelihood of malaria and the short duration of illness and normal CSF glucose argued against TB meningitis. The development of seizures in JE is an adverse prognostic sign and may be associated with raised intracranial pressure; therefore, control of these is important [6].

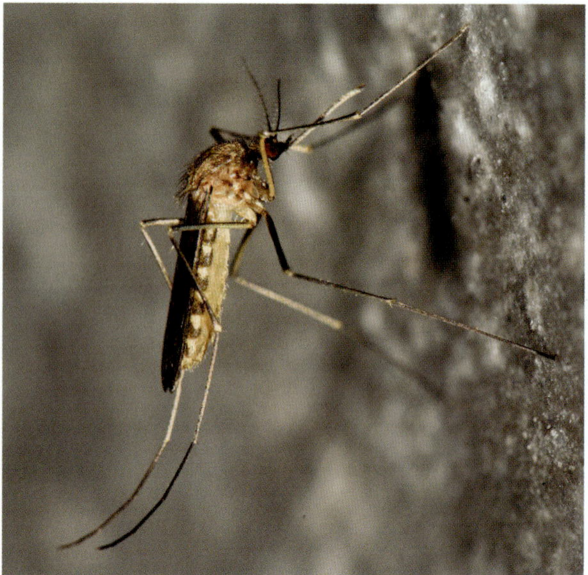

Figure 59.5. Mosquito (*Culex pipiens*). (Photo courtesy of Ian Redding.)

Box 59.1. Case Definition of Acute Encephalitis Syndrome.

Fever < 2 weeks duration

Plus any of:

Altered sensorium

New-onset seizures (except simple febrile seizures*)

Focal neurological signs

Behavioural abnormality (e.g. not feeding, inconsolable crying)

CSF pleocytosis (usually less than 1000 cells/mm^3, but may be normal)

Exclusion criteria:

Coma secondary to a systemic condition

Malaria parasites on blood film

* Simple febrile seizures are defined as a single seizure in a child aged 6 months to 5 years lasting less than 15 minutes with full recovery within 60 minutes of onset.

The CT scan findings in this case, deep grey matter lesions, are present early in disease and can suggest a diagnosis of JE before serology results are available, or if CSF is unavailable. In a JE-endemic region the findings of bilateral thalamic hypodensity are specific, although insensitive, for JE [7]. However, bilateral thalamic lesions have been widely reported in other forms of arbovirus encephalitis, so interpretation of the imaging depends heavily on the setting and travel history of the patient (e.g. see Case 33). Lesions in the thalamus and other basal ganglia in JE are thought to be responsible for the tremors and other Parkinsonian features sometimes seen (**Figure 59.6**).

The role of prophylactic antiepileptic drugs remains unproven in JE, but they are widely used. A clinical trial showed no effect of steroids in JE, but the study was underpowered, although there was no evidence of any harm [8].

Key Points

- Acute encephalitis syndrome (AES) is common in Asia, and much of it is due to JE.
- Extrapyramidal signs, such as resting tremor, or evidence of thalamic inflammation on neuroimaging, are suggestive of a flavivirus infection in these circumstances.
- The combination of seizures and tremors may suggest JE.
- The management of JE is supportive.
- It is important to exclude alternative treatable causes, such as TB or malaria.
- Live attenuated vaccine for JE is used across much of Asia, and killed vaccines are available in western settings for travellers.

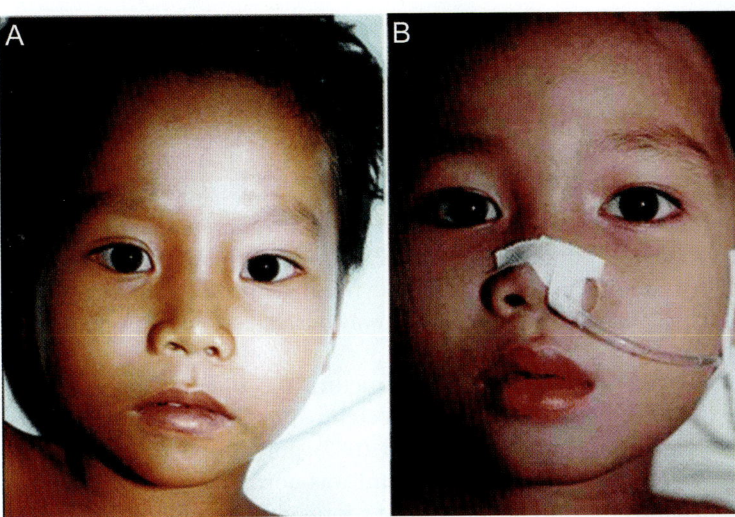

Figure 59.6. Staring mask-like facies due to a wide palpebral angle in two Vietnamese children with Japanese encephalitis. (Photos: T. Solomon.)

Did You Know?

JE affected American troops during the Second World War. Albert Sabin (**Figure 59.7**), the developer of the live attenuated poliomyelitis vaccine, worked on JE before he developed the polio vaccine, for which he is better known.

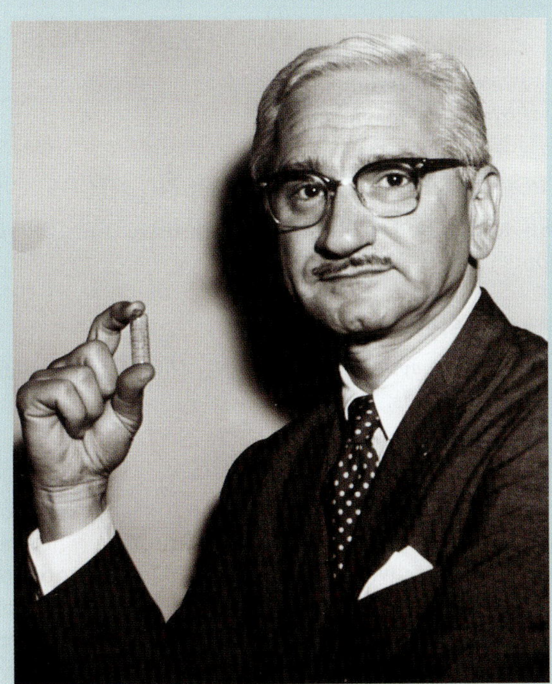

Figure 59.7. Dr Albert Sabin. © Bettmann/Getty Images.

Looking Back

Japanese encephalitis was described in Japan from the 1870s onwards. Originally it was known as 'Japanese B encephalitis' to distinguish it from type A encephalitis (encephalitis lethargica or von Economo's encephalitis). As type A encephalitis has been extremely rare for such a long time, the 'B' has fallen out of use.

References

1. Lewthwaite P, Begum A, Ooi MH, et al. Disability after encephalitis: development and validation of a new outcome score. Bull World Health Org 2010;**88**:584–92.
2. Solomon T. New vaccines for Japanese encephalitis. Lancet Neurol 2008;**7**:116–18.
3. Beasley DWC, Lewthwaite P, Solomon T. Current use and development of vaccines for Japanese encephalitis. Expert Opin Biol Ther 2008;**8**:95–106.
4. Solomon T, Dung NM, Kneen R, et al. Japanese encephalitis. J Neurol Neurosurg Psychiatr 2000;**68**:405–15.
5. Tsai T. Japanese encephalitis vaccines. In: Plotkin SA, Orenstein WA, editors. *Vaccines*. 3rd ed. Philadelphia, PA: Saunders; 1998.
6. Solomon T, Dung NM, Kneen R, et al. Seizures and raised intracranial pressure in Vietnamese patients with Japanese encephalitis. Brain 2002;**125**:1084–93.
7. Dung NM, Turtle L, Chong WK, et al. An evaluation of the usefulness of neuroimaging for the diagnosis of Japanese encephalitis. J Neurol 2009;**256**:2052–60.
8. Hoke CH, Vaughn DW, Nisalak A, et al. Effect of high-dose dexamethasone on the outcome of acute encephalitis due to Japanese encephalitis virus. J Infect Dis 1992;**165**:631–7.

CASE 60

Follow your Gut Feeling

Katherine C. Dodd

History

A 42-year-old right-handed female presented to her local hospital on her return from a summer holiday in Spain. She complained of a 2-day history of a severe headache, vomiting and fever, which had started as the family were collecting their baggage at the airport. She was usually fit and well, and worked as a checkout assistant at a garden centre. She and her other family members, including children aged 13 and 10 years, had all been well during their holiday. Shortly after admission to hospital she became drowsy and developed a right-sided hemiparesis and sensory disturbance.

Examination

On examination she had a fever of 38.1°C, with a tachycardia of 110 beats per minute and blood pressure of 114/66 mmHg. She had meningism, with photophobia, neck stiffness and a positive Kernig's sign. By the end of her first day in hospital her Glasgow coma score had dropped to 13 out of 15 (eyes 3, verbal 4, motor 6), and she had developed a dense right hemiplegia, with bilateral brisk reflexes and up-going plantars. She also had sensory loss over her right upper and lower limbs. Examination of cranial nerves demonstrated a right-sided upper motor neuron weakness and sensory loss, and funduscopy was normal. There was no rash and examination of other systems was normal.

Initial Differential Diagnosis

The clinical picture was of a central nervous system (CNS) infection; the right hemiparesis suggested this might be a lesion localised to the left hemisphere. The possibilities include

- Cerebral abscess
- Meningoencephalitis
  - Viral
  - Bacterial
  - Autoimmune
- Cerebral venous sinus thrombosis
- Cerebrovascular accident

Results of Initial Investigations

Initial blood tests found normal renal and liver function. There was a slight neutrophilic pleocytosis (12.5 × 10^9/l), a microcytic anaemia (9.4 mg/l) and her C-reactive protein was raised (124 mg/l). A pregnancy test was negative.

On lumbar puncture the opening pressure was 25 cm H_2O, with cerebrospinal fluid (CSF) white cell count 490 × 10^6/l (68% polymorphs, 32% lymphocytes), red cell count was normal, protein was 3.1 g/l, glucose was 41% of serum glucose and the Gram stain was negative.

A computer tomography (CT) scan was performed, followed by a magnetic resonance imaging (MRI) scan (**Figure 60.1**).

Refined Differential Diagnosis

Cerebritis, likely caused by a bacterial infection, the organisms suspected being:

- *Streptococcus pneumonia*
- *Neisseria meningitides*
- *Haemophilus influenza*
- *Listeria monocytogenes*

Results of Definitive Investigations

CSF and blood cultures were positive for *Listeria monocytogenes.*

Diagnosis

Listeria monocytogenes meningitis complicated by an area of cerebritis.

Management and Outcome

The patient was transferred to the high-dependency unit for close observation and monitoring. She was treated with intravenous ampicillin for 3 weeks and gentamicin and rifampicin for 2 weeks. Dexamethasone was started after 3 days of antibiotics due to the cerebritis with swelling and ongoing hemiplegia; following this, the right-sided weakness gradually improved. At 5-month follow-up she continued to have a mild

Figure 60.1. Coronal (A) and axial (B) T2 FLAIR MRI images from a 42-year-old lady with fever, headache and right hemiparesis.

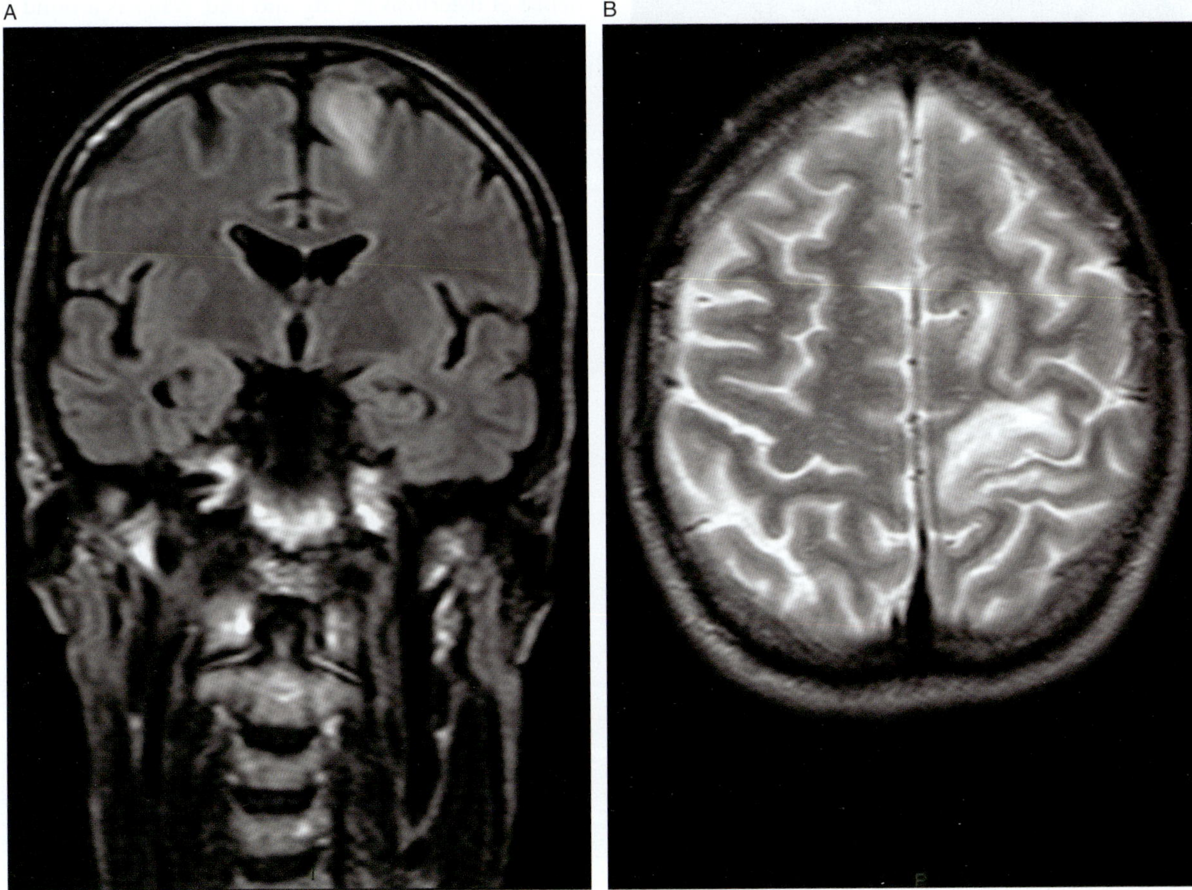

This shows an area of cerebritis of the left motor cortex.

pyramidal right arm weakness; repeat CT scanning showed resolution of the cerebritis, with no abscess formation. The patient was subsequently diagnosed with coeliac disease, confirmed on gastroscopy and antigen testing. This was likely to be the cause of the immunocompromise which had made her vulnerable to listeriosis, and also explains her microcytic anaemia. She started on a gluten-free diet and, apart from mild residual arm weakness, returned to full health.

Prevention

During her recent holiday she remembered eating soft cheese and ham, which was presumed to be the source of infection. She was advised about food preparation and storage to try and avoid *L. monocytogenes* infection in the future.

L. monocytogenes has the unusual property that it can multiply even at refrigeration temperatures below 5°C, although it can be killed by high temperatures and by pasteurisation. To reduce the risk of *L. monocytogenes* infection it is important to follow guidelines on food storage and preparation, although, due to the high prevalence of the bacteria in many food products, exposure cannot be avoided completely. Foods associated with the bacterium are pre-prepared chilled meals, unpasteurised milk, soft cheeses, cold cuts of meat, patés, sandwiches, smoked fish and cantaloupe melons.

Pregnant women and the immunocompromised should be advised to avoid these foods. *L. monocytogenes* can also be found in soil, vegetation, sewage and animal faeces; those at risk are also advised to avoid assisting with lambing [1].

Discussion

Listeria monocytogenes is a Gram-positive facultative intracellular bacillus that causes listeriosis, a rare but serious and potentially fatal disease. Clinical

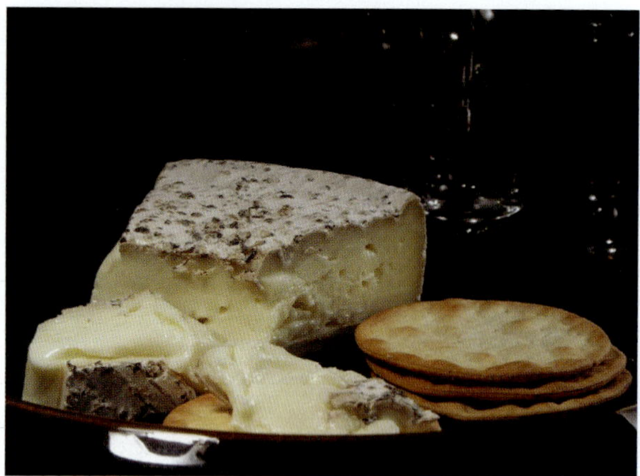

Figure 60.2. Soft cheese; a common breeding ground for *Listeria monocytogenes*.

manifestations can range from non-invasive gastroenteritis to severe invasive disease causing CNS infection (including meningitis, cerebritis, meningoencephalitis and brain abscesses), septicaemia and endocarditis. Cerebritis is inflammation of the brain tissue usually caused by a bacterial infection, and is a precursor to abscess formation if left untreated. Presentation of *L. monocytogenes* meningitis is usually acute but can be sub-acute, and movement disorders and seizures are more common than in meningitis due to other common organisms [2]. Individuals at risk of severe listeriosis are those with impaired cell-mediated immunity, pregnant women, neonates and the elderly; although 10% of cases occur in normal adults [3]. In pregnant women *L. monocytogenes* can proliferate in the placenta and pass to the foetus, leading to miscarriage, stillbirth and neonatal encephalitis, while usually only causing a mild flu-like illness for the mother.

There is a high prevalence of the organism in certain foods, with studies showing up to 20% of some foodstuffs being contaminated, and up to 5% of the general population may be asymptomatic carriers [2,3]. The majority of cases are sporadic, but outbreaks of *L. monocytogenes* have been identified from a number of different sources such as soft cheeses (**Figure 60.2**). The incubation period from ingestion is between 1 and 90 days. Although the CSF Gram stain is frequently negative, the organism can occasionally be confused with diphtheroids and streptococci on microscopy – ask the microbiologists to check again carefully if they report these contaminants for patients who could have listeriosis. The CSF glucose levels are normal in more than 60% of cases, in contrast with other bacterial CNS infections [2]; in the patient described here, the ratio was on the low side, at 41%. The current annual incidence of listeriosis in England and Wales is around 3 per million [1]. Previously quoted incidences have ranged from 0.1 to 11.3 per million and are highest in women in the third trimester of pregnancy, those aged over 70 and newborns [4].

The antibiotic of choice in current UK guidelines is amoxicillin, although there is *in vitro* evidence that in combination with gentamicin it may work synergistically against *L. monocytogenes* [2,5]. However, there is a lack of evidence for gentamicin *in vivo* and in practice this combination in adult patients has been shown to be associated with a higher mortality than ampicillin monotherapy; therefore, consideration should be given to the patient's comorbidities on an individual basis before adding an aminoglycoside [6]. Gentamicin should also not be given in pregnant women due to teratogenicity. Rifampicin is effective against intracellular *L. monocytogenes* and will penetrate the CSF; therefore, some advocate this as an additional agent, especially in CNS infection in the immunocompromised [3]. It is important to look for a cause of immunosuppression such as diabetes, HIV and medications. Iron is a virulence factor for *L. monocytogenes* and so iron replacement should be withheld during infection [2].

In bacterial meningitis of unknown cause, current UK guidelines recommend that empirical treatment for the over 60's should include amoxicillin to cover for *L. monocytogenes*, as it has resistance to cephalosporins [7]. Interestingly, the patient described above was less than 60 and therefore her initial empirical treatment would not have included this. She was unlucky in being vulnerable because of her undiagnosed coeliac disease.

Corticosteroids have been demonstrated to be beneficial in some cases of bacterial meningitis, although not specifically in listeriosis, and, as impairment of cell-mediated immunity due to steroids is a major risk factor for the development of listeriosis, their role here is unclear. In the patient described above they were used due to the cerebritis causing local oedema and focal neurological deficit. This patient had a surprisingly good outcome; listeriosis usually has a high mortality rate of around 20–30% [3].

Key Points

- Think of *L. monocytogenes* as a cause of meningitis when CSF Gram stain is reported as showing diptheroids (skin contaminants), or in the immunosuppressed, neonates or elderly.

- Prevention is better than cure; educate at-risk patients about the avoidance of potential *L. monocytogenes*-containing foods.
- Ampicillin with either gentamicin and/or rifampicin is currently the treatment of choice, and any patient with meningitis of unknown cause at risk of listeriosis should have ampicillin included in their initial antibiotic regimen.

Looking Back

Listeria monocytogenes was first named *'Bacteria monocytogenes'* by E.G.D. Murray in 1924, when he isolated a new genus of Gram-positive rods from young laboratory rabbits [8]. It was then named *'Listerella'* after the surgeon Lord Lister (**Figure 60.3**), but was re-named *Listeria* in 1940 by H. Pirie when it was found that this name had already been given to a Mycetozoan.

In the seventeenth century Queen Anne (**Figure 60.4**) unfortunately had no surviving children, despite 17 pregnancies. It has been suggested that this was due to listeriosis causing recurrent abortion, stillbirth, neonatal death and post-natal meningitis [9]. The lack of an heir meant the end of the Stuarts as monarchs and the crown passed to the House of Hanover; this also gave parliament more power, contributing to the modern British political system.

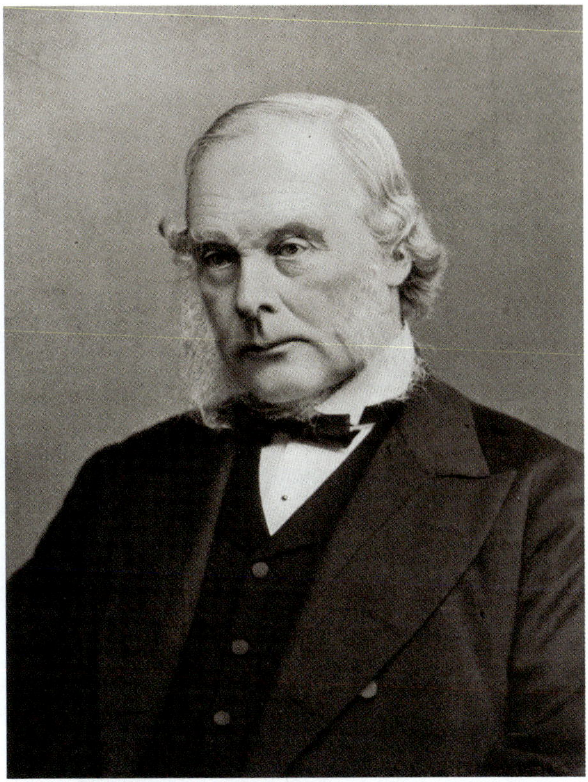

Figure 60.4. Lord Lister

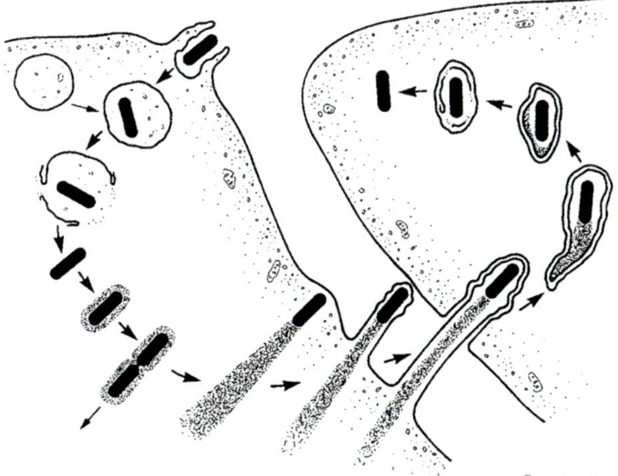

Figure 60.3. The *L. monocytogenes* actin comet tail, which propels bacteria through the cytoplasm with sufficient force to generate protrusions into adjacent cells. (Reproduced with permission of Elsevier from [9].)

Did You Know?

L. monocytogenes has a range of unique mechanisms that help it spread through the body, one of which is its 'comet tail'. The bacterium enters the cytoplasm of cells and then polymerises actin from the host cell into a tail that it uses to propel itself forwards around the cell and then into the cell's outer membrane; here it encapsulates itself, before passing into the neighbouring cell, and starting the cycle again (**Figure 60.5**) [10,11].

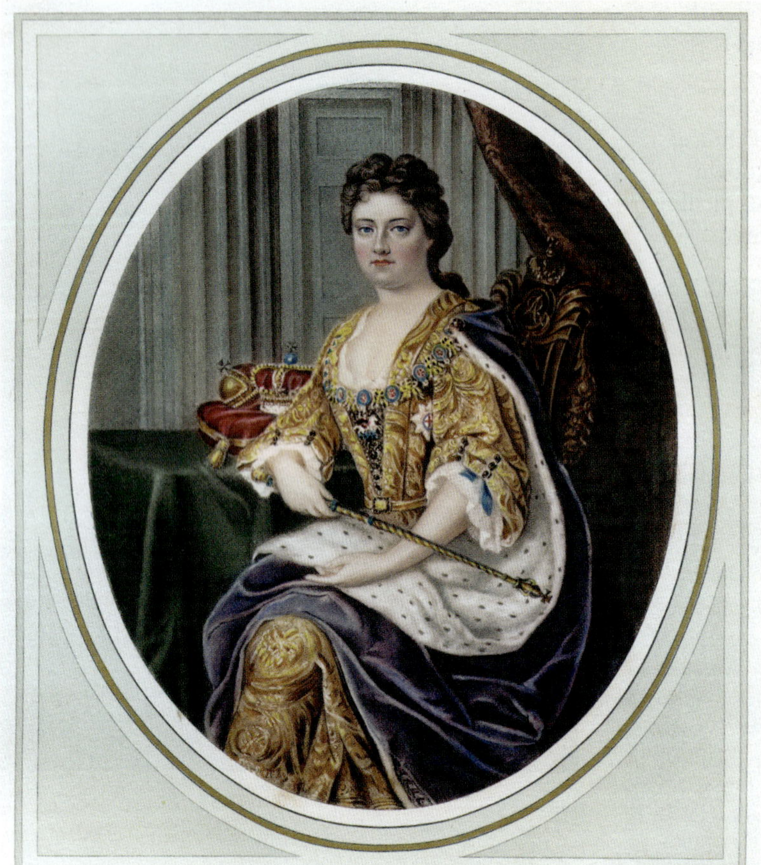

Figure 60.5. Queen Anne. (A print from Queen Anne, by Herbert Paul, Goupil and Co., London, 1906 courtesy of the Hulton Archive.)

References

1. Allerberger F, Wagner M. Listeriosis: a resurgent foodborne infection. Clin Microbiol Infect 2010;**16**:16–23.
2. The Health Protection Agency. Infections A–Z. *Listeria*. www.hpa.org.uk/Topics/InfectiousDisease (accessed May 19, 2018).
3. Lorber B. Listeriosis. Clin Infect Dis 1997;**24**:1–11.
4. Gellin BG, Broome CV. Listeriosis. JAMA 1989;**261**:1313–20.
5. Cone LA, Leung MM, Byrd RG, et al. Multiple cerebral abscesses because of *Listeria monocytogenes*: three case reports and a literature review of supratentorial listerial brain abscess(es). Surg Neurol 2003;**59**:320–8.
6. Amaya-Villar R, Garcia-Cabrera E, Sulleiro-Igual E, et al. Three-year multicentre surveillance of community-acquired *Listeria monocytogenes* meningitis in adults. BMC Infect Dis 2010;**10**:324.
7. McGill F, Heyderman R, Michael BD, et al. Management of meningitis in immunocompetent adults: Association of British Neurologists and British Infection Association National Guideline. J Infect 2016;**1**:1–34.
8. Hof H. History and epidemiology of listeriosis. FEMS Immunol Med Microbiol 2003;**35**:199–202.
9. Saxbe WB Jr. *Listeria monocytogenes* and Queen Anne. Paediatrics 1972;**49**:197–201.
10. Merz A, Higgs HN. *Listeria* motility: biophysics pushes things forward. Curr Biol 2003;**13**:R302–04.
11. Cossart P. The Maverick Bacterium. *The Scientist*. January 1, 2010. www.the-scientist.com/?articles.view/articleNo/27896/title/The-Maverick-Bacterium/ (accessed April 23, 2013).

CASE 61

Malawian Malaise

Lance Turtle and Rachel Kneen

History

A 10-year-old boy, originally born in Malawi, presented acutely with weakness, backache and an inability to walk. He also had a low-grade fever, cough, weight loss, diarrhoea and abdominal pain. Further questioning revealed that he was deaf in the left ear. He had been treated for pulmonary tuberculosis in Malawi 6 months earlier, but the details of the medications taken and the length of treatment were unknown, as he had been living with his grandparents at that time and they were not in the UK. At the time of presentation, the child had been living in the UK for 2 weeks. The exact length of the history of the current illness was not clear, but the child had certainly not been well since arrival in the UK, according to his mother.

His mother was known to be HIV positive and she had not received any treatment to reduce mother-to-child transmission. The mother was not taking antiretroviral medication at the time of the child's presentation. The child had been exclusively breast-fed. There was one older sibling who was currently in good health.

Examination

On examination the child looked unwell, was pale, dehydrated and very thin. He had oral thrush and scars consistent with an earlier episode of shingles on his chest. The chest and abdominal examinations were normal.

On neurological examination, he was alert and had photophobia, but no neck stiffness. He was able to sit up on his own, but could not walk. Tone was reduced globally in the lower limbs. There was right-sided facial weakness affecting the whole side. Power was 4/5 in all other areas. Tendon reflexes were normal in the arms and decreased in the legs. Both plantar responses were down-going. Sensation was not possible to examine because the child was unable to cooperate fully with the examination, due in large part to the language barrier. No sphincter symptoms were reported at this time.

Initial Differential Diagnosis

This child had a systemic illness and several neurological abnormalities, in a lower motor neuron pattern, which could not be localised to a single lesion, because it involved the face and lower spinal cord. He had recently been treated for tuberculosis with an unknown drug regimen for an unknown duration. Tuberculosis could account for many of the features described. His mother was known to be HIV+, but it was not clear when this diagnosis was made: it was possible she was undiagnosed while pregnant with this patient. In any case, the combination of an HIV positive mother, suspicion of tuberculosis and presence of oral thrush clearly makes HIV testing of the child a priority.

If the child were HIV positive, then the differential diagnosis would have become wider. Typical causes of neurological syndromes in people with HIV of African origin (other than tuberculosis) include cryptococcal disease, pneumococcus and lymphoma. The fact this was not a purely meningitic illness argued against cryptococcal and pneumococcal disease. Lumbosacral polyradiculopathy (which may be viral in origin), conus medullaris and cauda equina syndrome were also possibilities. A lymphomatous mass in the lower spinal canal (below the termination of the cord) could have accounted for the lower limb findings; lymphomatous deposits elsewhere might have explained many of the other findings.

Results of Initial Investigations

The child was anaemic (Hb 68 g/l) with an elevated white cell count (18.1×10^9/l) and C-reactive protein (330 mg/l). HIV antibody testing was positive, with a plasma viral load of 206,200 copies/ml, and CD4 count was 0.

A lumbar puncture (LP) revealed a turbid fluid, with 1502 cells/μl (92% neutrophils, 1% mononuclear cells), the cerebrospinal fluid (CSF) glucose was 8 g/l, Gram and Ziehl–Neelsen stains were both negative, as was the culture.

A plain chest radiograph showed bi-basal consolidation and a magnetic resonance imaging (MRI) brain scan was normal.

Refined Differential Diagnosis and Progression

Over the next 2 days the flaccid paraparesis worsened and he developed urinary retention. Power decreased globally still further to 0–2/5 bilaterally, but most severely on the left. Lower limb and abdominal reflexes were absent.

MRI of the spine was performed (**Figure 61.1**).

The development of flaccid paralysis made a disorder of the cord or nerve roots more likely. This clinical course was inconsistent with pneumococcal or cryptococcal meningitis. Lumbosacral polyradiculopathy, conus medullaris and cauda equina syndrome remained possible diagnoses.

CSF polymerase chain reaction (PCR) was negative for varicella zoster virus, herpes simplex virus, Epstein–Barr virus, toxoplasma and tuberculosis.

Results of Definitive Investigations

Ophthalmological examination was performed (**Figure 61.2**).

At this point the CSF PCR for cytomegalovirus (CMV) came back positive with 12,226,000 copies/ml and the CMV PCR of blood was also positive with 1900 copies/ml.

Diagnosis

Polyradiculopathy and retinitis due to cytomegalovirus in the context of congenital HIV infection.

Management and Outcome

At presentation the child was commenced on tuberculosis treatment with rifampicin, isoniazid, pyrazinamide and ethambutol. Steroids were withheld. Fluconazole and co-trimoxazole prophylaxis were also administered.

Figure 61.1. A T1-weighted spinal axial MRI with gadolinium representative of that seen in a 10-year-old boy with HIV who presented with a progressive flaccid, areflexic paraparesis and facial palsy.

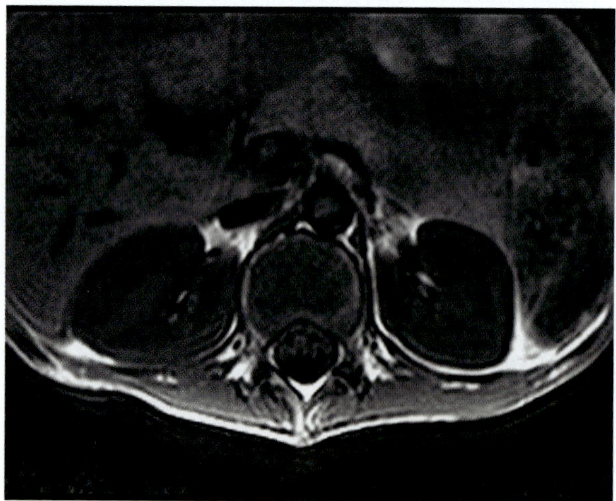

This shows arachnoiditis and anterior displacement of the cauda equina with enhancement of the nerve roots (Reproduced from [1] with permission.)

Once the CMV PCR result became available he was commenced on intravenous (IV) ganciclovir and foscarnet. Antiretroviral therapy was started at the same time as the CMV treatment. There was clinical improvement within 3 weeks and by 6 weeks of treatment he was able to walk again. Bladder control recovered. Ganciclovir was stopped after 10 weeks at which point a repeat LP showed resolution of the CSF pleocytosis but the CMV viral load was 25,640 copies/ml.

By 2 weeks after stopping ganciclovir the facial palsy recurred, so ganciclovir was restarted. Again there was no CSF pleocytosis; however, the CMV remained detectable and was still sensitive to both ganciclovir and foscarnet. Two months after admission a repeat CD4 count showed no immune reconstitution. Three months after presentation the child developed other complications of HIV and died.

Prevention

Congenital HIV infection occurs in approximately one-third of the infants of HIV-infected mothers. One-third of these transmissions occur *in utero*, one-third during birth and one-third after birth, as HIV is present in breast milk. Congenital HIV infection can be prevented by effective antiretroviral treatment of the mother, delivery by caesarean section, treatment of the baby with antiretrovirals after birth and formula feeding [2]. For example, nevirapine given just before birth penetrates the placenta and gets into the foetal circulation where it lasts 2–3 weeks. In the case of a mother who has well-controlled HIV (i.e. undetectable viral load at week 36 of pregnancy) the baby can be born by vaginal delivery. The child described in this case

Figure 61.2. Retinal findings similar to those seen in the same patient.

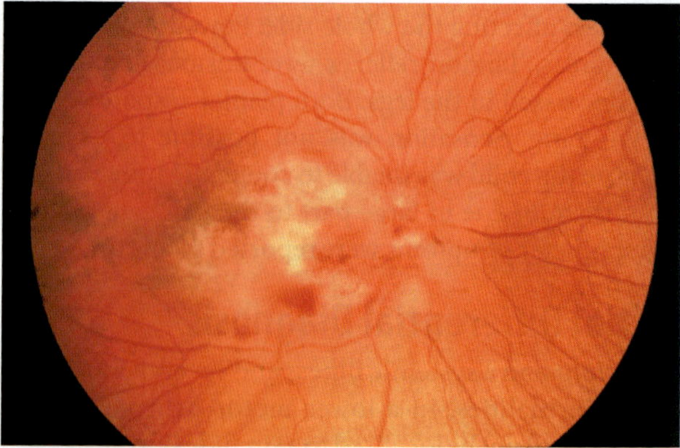

This demonstrates the classical 'tomato ketchup and cottage cheese' appearance of CMV retinitis. (From: www.nei.nih.gov)

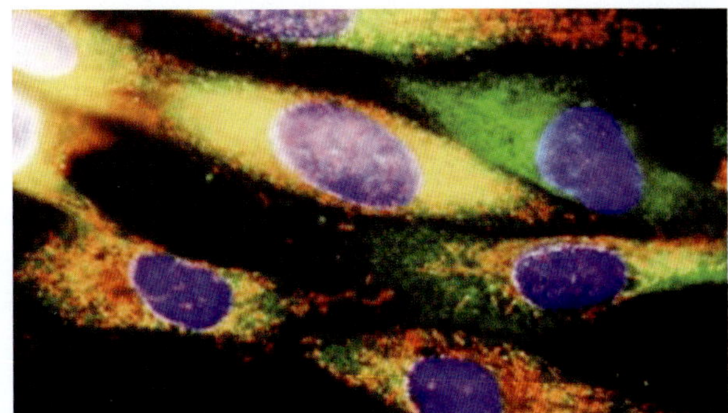

Figure 61.3. Confocal microscopy of cells demonstrating inclusion of the cytomegalovirus. (From: www.nhs.uk/conditions/Cytomegalovirus/Pages/Introduction.aspx)

had congenital HIV, presumably because his infected mother had none of the above instigated; indeed, she may not even have known she was HIV-positive when pregnant.

CMV is a very common human infection with 30–60% of the population chronically infected. Chronic CMV infection usually does not manifest itself clinically unless there is significant immunosuppression, such as advanced HIV disease or bone marrow transplantation. In the case of HIV infection immune reconstitution with antiretroviral therapy effectively prevents the development of CMV disease in a CMV/HIV co-infected individual, if it is administered before the development of CMV disease. There is currently no vaccine for CMV in use, although vaccines are under development.

Discussion

CMV is a beta-herpes virus of the human herpesvirus family (**Figure 61.3**). It is an enveloped, double-stranded DNA virus of approximately 200 kilobases. Acute infection with CMV causes a self-limiting glandular fever-like illness often with hepatitis. This is then followed by lifelong persistent infection, in common with the other human herpes viruses. Persistent infection is inconsequential if the host remains immunocompetent, although some recent evidence suggests reduced life expectancy in people who are CMV-infected [3].

Most of the clinical problems with CMV occur in people with advanced HIV disease or with organ transplants. Interestingly, for reasons that are poorly understood, the spectrum of clinical disease varies with the type of immunosuppression. For example, patients after bone marrow transplant are prone to CMV pneumonitis, but have relatively little in the way of neurological disease, whereas patients with advanced HIV tend to develop colitis and neurological infection, especially retinitis. CMV can also be transmitted across the placenta and cause serious disease in the newborn.

CMV infection is diagnosed by identifying high levels of CMV DNA by PCR in the context of the appropriate clinical illness. People with chronic infection can have low levels of CMV DNA present in blood when they are well. The presence of IgM antibody can be helpful in distinguishing acute infection from reactivation, because IgM is positive in acute infection.

Key Points

- Patients with advanced HIV disease can have multiple pathologies and a very wide differential diagnosis; however, a thorough clinical examination can localise lesions to regions and therefore suggest certain pathogens. Funduscopy may provide important clinical information, particularly in CMV disease.
- In people with advanced HIV, CMV can cause polyradiculopathy.
- CMV is treated with IV ganciclovir and foscarnet.

Looking Back

In 1881, Ribbert first demonstrated 'inclusion-bearing' cells and in 1921 Goodpasture and Talbert suggested that these 'cytomegalia' may be viral in origin. Subsequently, Weller was able to isolate the virus from the urine of infected infants and proposed the term 'cytomegalovirus' [4].

Did You Know?

CMV exhibits a curious immunological phenomenon called memory inflation. Memory T cells specific for CMV increase gradually throughout life, until they can comprise up to 20% of all circulating T cells [5]. This significantly skews the T-cell receptor repertoire and can impair the development of new T-cell responses. This is one proposed mechanism for how CMV infection worsens outcome from critical illness in later life, and reduces life expectancy.

References

1. Sohal A, Riordan A, Mallewa M, Solomon T, Kneen R. Successful treatment of cytomegalovirus polyradiculopathy in a 9-year-old child with congenital human immunodeficiency virus infection. J Child Neurol 2009;**24**: 215–18.
2. Taylor GP, Clayden P, Dhar J, et al. British HIV Association guidelines for the management of HIV infection in pregnant women 2012. HIV Med 2012;**13**:87–157.
3. Savva GM, Pachnio A, Kaul B, et al. Cytomegalovirus infection is associated with increased mortality in the older population. Aging Cell 2013;**12**:381–7.
4. Riley HD Jr. History of cytomegalovirus. Southern Med J 1997;**90**:184–90.
5. Vescovini R, Biasini C, Fagnoni FF, et al. Massive load of functional effector CD4+ and CD8+ T cells against cytomegalovirus in very old subjects. J Immunol 2007;**179**:4283–91.

CASE 62

Big Game

Tom Solomon, Sylviane Defres and Alastair Miller

History

A 40-year-old woman with no past history of note was admitted with fever, headache and muscle aches, lethargy and then confusion. These had come on gradually, since she flew back from a holiday in Zambia 4 days earlier. She had been travelling in Zambia with friends for 4 weeks, visiting various game parks as part of an adventure holiday to celebrate her 40th birthday.

Examination

On examination she was febrile, with temperature 38.8°C and mildly confused, being unsure of the time of day, and mixing up the names of her friends. The neurological examination was otherwise unremarkable. Her blood pressure was 110/70 mmHg. Her heart sounds were normal and her chest was clear. She had a soft, non-tender abdomen with a 2 cm splenomegaly.

Initial Differential Diagnosis

In a febrile confused traveller returning from Africa malaria was at the top of the differential diagnosis, even though she had been taking chemoprophylaxis. Other mosquito-borne pathogens considered included dengue fever and chikungunya, which are seen in some parts of Africa. Typhoid is also important in this part of the world, although the history would typically be longer. Leptospirosis is another possibility. Trypanosomiasis is rare in returning travellers, but has been reported from Zambia. Rabies would be unlikely if she had been vaccinated, and there was no history of exposure to a potentially rabid animal. The differential also included all the causes of fever and confusion common in a western setting: viruses, such as herpes simplex virus; and bacteria such as *Streptococcus pneumoniae* or *Neiserria meningitidis*. An HIV seroconversion illness was also worth considering; on holiday people tend to put themselves at risk in ways that they may not at home.

Results of Initial Investigations

She had a haemoglobin of 110 g/l, white cell count of 4×10^9/l and platelet count of 35×10^9/l; blood glucose was 4.0 mmol/l; sodium was 130 mmol/l, potassium 4.5 mmol/l, urea 10 mmol/l and creatinine 140 mmol/l. Liver function tests revealed a normal albumin, bilirubin and alkaline phosphatase, but elevated aspartate

Figure 62.1. Thick (A) and thin (B) blood films similar to those from a 40-year-old woman with a febrile illness and confusion, which came on a few days after returning from Zambia.

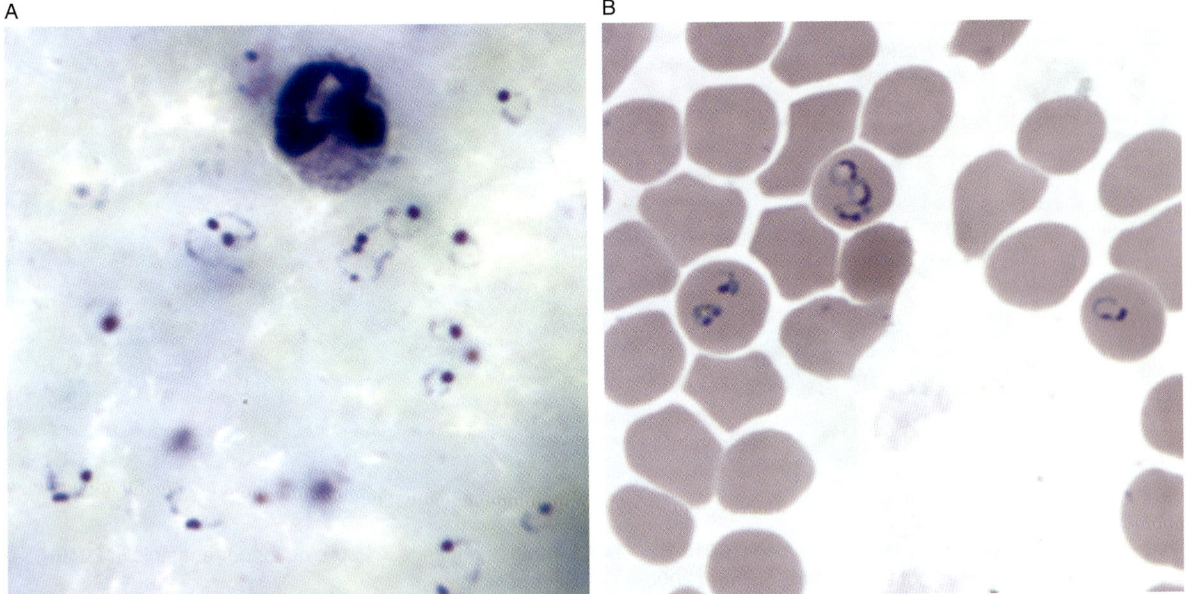

The images show the ring form (trophozoites) of *Plasmodium falciparum*. (From: www.cdc.gov/dpdx/malaria/index.html)

amino transferase at 140 U/l. She had a CT scan of her head and a lumbar puncture, both of which were unremarkable. A chest X-ray was clear and an electrocardiogram showed just sinus tachycardia.

Results of Definitive Investigations

Thick and thin blood films were stained with Giemsa stain (**Figure 62.1**).

Diagnosis

The bloods films were positive for *Plasmodium falciparum* confirming the diagnosis of cerebral malaria caused by *Plasmodium falciparum*.

Management and Outcome

Her malaria was treated initially with intravenous artesunate (2.4 mg/kg) stat and then repeated at 12 and 24 hours [1]. She was then able to complete treatment with artemesinin combination therapy (namely artemether-lumefantrine 4 tablets 12 hourly for 3 days). She was given a 10% dextrose infusion because of the risk of hypoglycaemia (although this is less of a risk with artesunate than it is with quinine), and transferred to the high-dependency unit. Here she began to have generalised tonic–clonic seizures, which settled with intravenous phenytoin. She was also given broad-spectrum antibiotics, pending the results of the blood cultures. She made a steady recovery and was discharged 10 days after admission. At day 14 she was reviewed to check for haemolysis, which was not seen. At follow-up 4 weeks later she was still feeling weak and lethargic but was otherwise well.

Prevention

Malaria is prevented by reducing the risk of bites from infected mosquitoes and taking prophylactic antimalarial drugs. Anopheles mosquitoes, which transmit malaria, bite from dusk to dawn; the risk of infection is therefore reduced by keeping skin covered at night, using mosquito repellent and sleeping under a bed-net impregnated with insecticide. With the widespread use of bed-nets, indoor residual spraying of insecticides and intermittent preventative treatment, the number of malaria cases globally has dropped over the last 15 years. Several vaccines are in development: the most advanced, called RTS,S, gave only partial clinical efficacy in stage III trials [2], and so has not yet been recommended for widespread employment pending further studies.

Discussion

There were an estimated 214 million cases of malaria globally in 2015, with more than 400,000 deaths [3]; 88% of these are in the WHO African region (**Figure 62.2**). In the UK there are approximately 2000 imported malaria cases every year; there are around 4000 across the rest of Europe, and about 1500 in the USA [4].

Malaria occurs following the bite of an anopheles mosquito infected with one of the five malaria parasites (*Plasmodium falciparum, viva, ovale, malariae* and *knowlesi*; **Figure 62.3**). The incubation period is at least

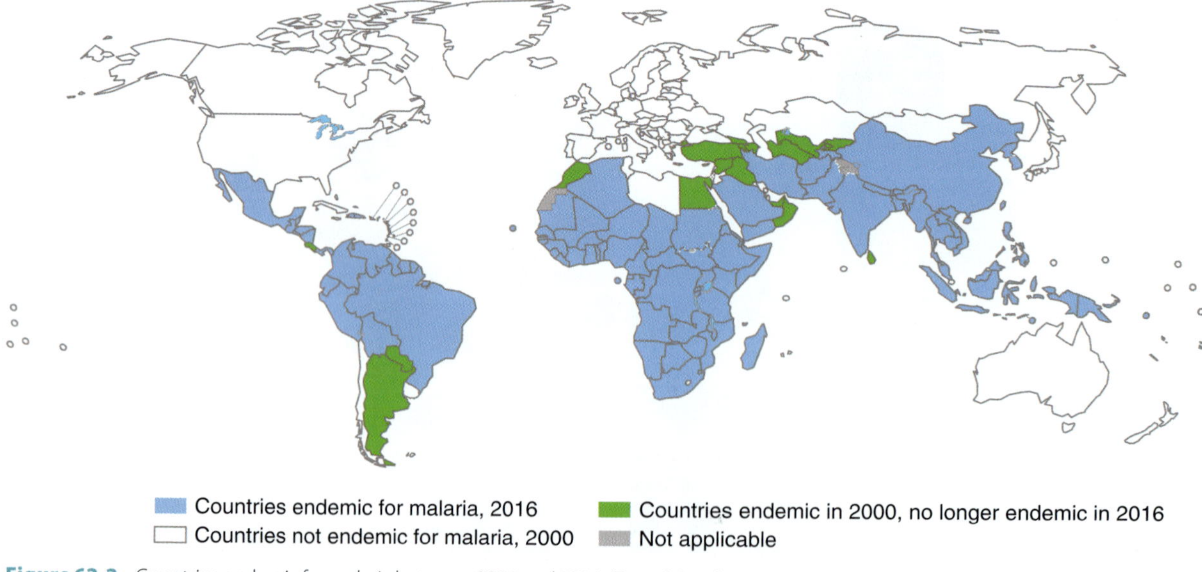

Figure 62.2. Countries endemic for malaria between 2000 and 2016. (From [2] with permission.)

7 days; the maximum depends on the species and on whether partially effective chemoprophylaxis has been used. The disease presents with a non-specific febrile illness, which can include chills, malaise, fatigue, sweating, headache, cough, nausea, vomiting, abdominal pain, diarrhoea, arthralgias and myalgias. Examination may reveal anaemia and splenomegaly, as seen in the case described here, and sometimes jaundice [5].

Cerebral malaria is the syndrome of altered consciousness with or without seizure in individuals infected with *P. falciparum*. The clinical features of hypoglycaemia are similar to those of cerebral malaria, hence it should be urgently looked for in cases of suspected cerebral malaria [6].

Focal neurological signs are unusual in cerebral malaria, but patients may have other features of severe infection including acidosis, renal impairment and pulmonary oedema (Box 62.1). Individuals with no prior immunity are at increased risk of developing severe disease. Other groups at risk are the immunocompromised, young children and pregnant women.

Laboratory investigations reveal parasitaemia, frequently together with anaemia, thrombocytopaenia and elevated transaminases, all of which were seen in this case. Additionally, a mild coagulopathy is sometimes seen, as well as elevated blood urea nitrogen and creatinine. In general, the higher the parasite count, the sicker the patient and a parasite level of greater than 2% of red blood cells parasitised would be an indication of severe malaria. However, sometimes cerebral malaria may occur with a low peripheral parasitaemia as it is

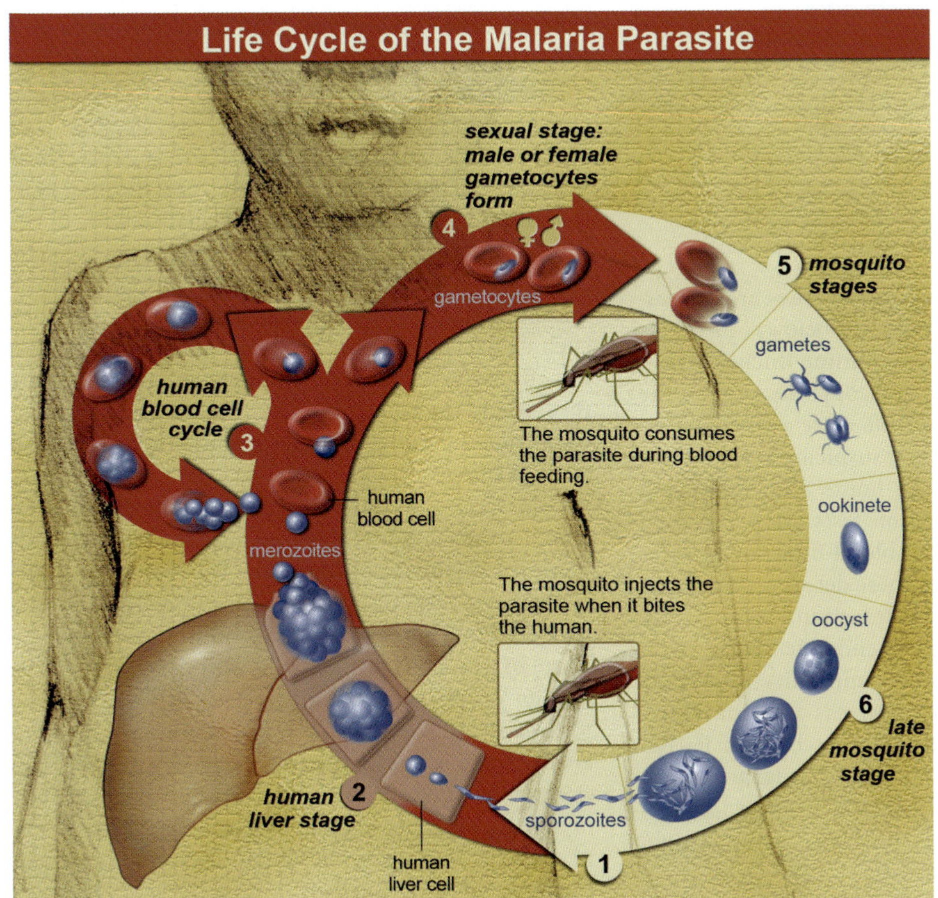

Figure 62.3. The life cycle of malaria parasites. A mosquito causes an infection by a bite. First, sporozoites enter the bloodstream, and migrate to the liver. They infect liver cells, where they multiply into merozoites, rupture the liver cells and return to the bloodstream. Importantly, for *Plasmodium vivax* and *P. ovale* a dormant stage (hypnozoites) can persist in the liver and cause relapses by invading the bloodstream weeks, or even years later. The merozoites infect red blood cells, where they develop into ring forms, trophozoites and schizonts that in turn produce further merozoites. Sexual forms are also produced, which, if taken up by a mosquito, will infect the insect and continue the life cycle. (Illustration by the National Institute of Allergy and Infectious Diseases (NIAID).)

Box 62.1. Symptoms of Severe Malaria, from [5].

Major features of severe or complicated falciparum malaria in adults

- Impaired consciousness or seizures
- Renal impairment (oliguria < 0.4 ml/kg bodyweight per hour or creatinine > 265 µmol/l)
- Acidosis (pH < 7.3)
- Hypoglycaemia (< 2.2 mmol/l)
- Pulmonary oedema or acute respiratory distress syndrome (ARDS)
- Haemoglobin ≤ 80 g/l
- Spontaneous bleeding/disseminated intravascular coagulation
- Shock (algid malaria)
- Haemoglobinuria (without G6PD* deficiency)

Major features of severe or complicated malaria in children

- Impaired consciousness or seizures
- Respiratory distress or acidosis (pH <7.3)
- Hypoglycaemia
- Severe anaemia
- Prostration (inability to sit or stand)
- Parasitaemia > 2% red blood cells parasitised

* G6PD is glucose-6-phosphate dehydrogenase.

felt that many of the falciparum parasites are sequestrated in the cerebral capillaries (see below).

Malaria is diagnosed by examining thick and thin blood films under light microscopy. Because of the cyclic nature of the parasite's life cycle a single blood film may be negative, and so if suspicion is high films should be repeated at 12–24 hours and then again 24 hours later. Rapid detection tests are being used increasingly as an adjunct to blood films, or in areas where they are not possible. These detect malaria antigens, or antibody responses to infection.

Those living in malaria-endemic areas who have repeat infections develop immunity over time. However, if they then live overseas this immunity wanes, making them once again susceptible. Partial pre-existing immunity may make it harder to see the parasites, as may partial protection from prophylactic antimalarial drugs. If the clinical suspicion is high, repeat films should be examined.

Cerebral malaria is thought to be the result of the parasitised red blood cells adhering to small blood vessels ('cytoadherence'; **Figure 62.4**) causing small infarcts, capillary leakage and organ dysfunction [7]. Raised intracranial pressure and cerebral oedema are thought to contribute to the poor outcome in severe cases; however, corticosteroids are contraindicated because a well-conducted trial showed an inferior outcome.

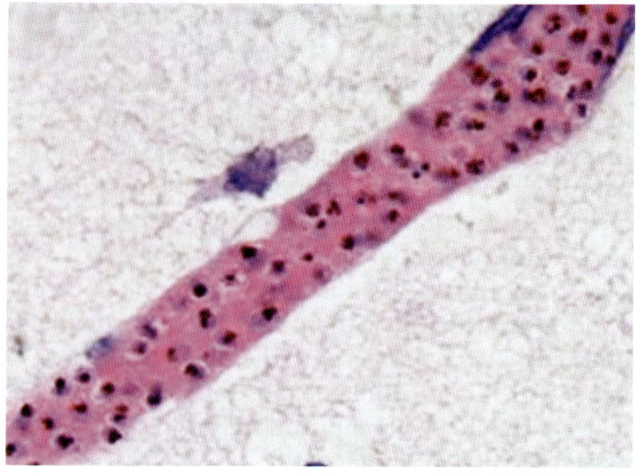

Figure 62.4. A vessel tightly packed with parasitised red blood cells which are adhering to the vessel wall (1000×, H&E stain). (Reproduced from [7] under CC BY 3.0.)

The same disease mechanism can cause retinal changes including haemorrhages, opacification and decolourisation of the retinal vessel of segments. These are best seen with pupillary dilation and indirect ophthalmoscopy and are harder to visualise with direct funduscopy.

In sub-Saharan Africa severely unwell children with malaria parasitaemia may also have coinfections such as bacteraemia, or viral central nervous system infections [8,9]; hence it is important to investigate thoroughly for other causes of disease. These are less important in returning travellers, but should be looked for nevertheless.

The choice of antimalarial treatment depends on whether infection was acquired in an area with chloroquine sensitivity or resistance and whether it is uncomplicated or severe disease [5]. Severe malaria is treated with artesunate (if available), or quinine plus doxycycline, or clindamycin. Patients who develop malaria, despite prophylaxis, should receive a different drug for treatment. Parasite counts are monitored closely to ensure there is a response to therapy. For *P. vivax* and *P. ovale* infection, primaquine is used to clear the liver of the hypnozoite stage of the parasite. This is not needed for *P. falciparum*, which does not form hypnozoites. Only *P. falciparum* and rarely *P. knowlesi* produce fatalities under normal circumstances.

Key Points

- Cerebral malaria is the syndrome of encephalopathy, often with seizures, in those with acute *Plasmodium falciparum* infection.

- Hypoglycaemia is common in malaria and can mimic the symptoms of cerebral malaria; it can be worsened by treatment with quinine due to drug-induced hyperinsulinaemia.
- Malaria can occur in those taking antimalarial prophylaxis, and also in previously immune natives of malaria-endemic countries who have returned to an endemic area after some years.
- If the first blood films for malaria are negative but suspicion is high, they should be repeated.

Looking Back

Before the malaria parasites were discovered, different forms of the disease were distinguished by the periodicity of the fever (tertian, every third day; quartan, every fourth day; quotidian, daily) and whether the disease was benign or malignant. *Plasmodium falciparum* is the cause of malignant tertian malaria.

Sir Ronald Ross won a Nobel Prize for showing that malaria is transmitted by mosquitoes (**Figure 62.5**).

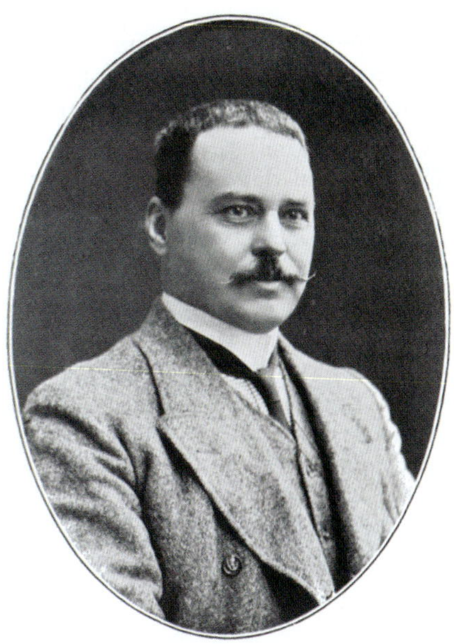

Figure 62.5. Sir Ronald Ross was also a mathematician, painter and poet. In August 1897, he wrote following his discovery of malaria parasites in mosquitoes fed on patients: "*With tears and toiling breath, I find thy cunning seeds, O million-murdering Death.*" (Photo courtesy of National Institutes of Health, USA.)

Did You Know?

Artemisinin, also known as qinghao su, is isolated from a herb that has been used in traditional Chinese medicine to treat fevers for more than 2000 years.

Oscar Wilde (**Figure 62.6**) described malaria as *'An aesthetic disease but a deuced nuisance'*.

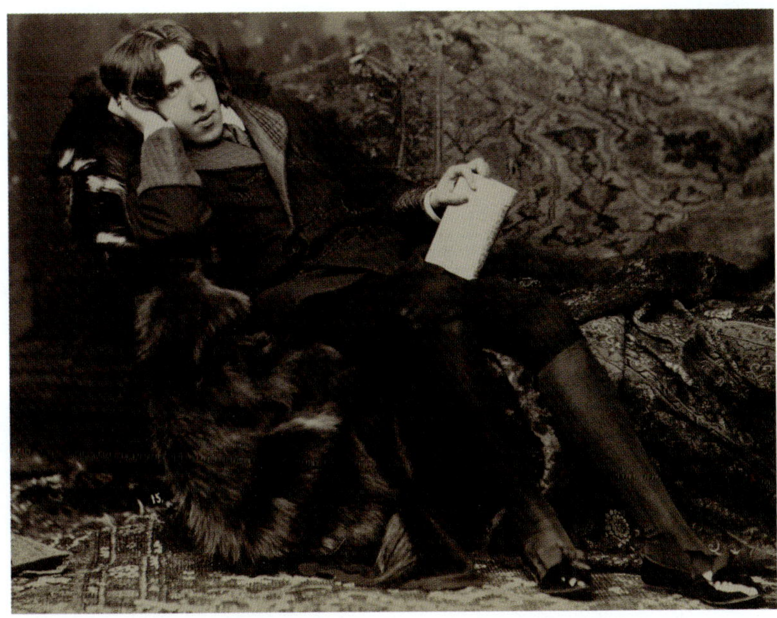

Figure 62.6. Oscar Wilde. (Photo by Napoleon Sarony *c.*1882. Held in Library of Congress Prints and Photographs Division, Washington, DC, USA.)

References

1. Lalloo DG, Shingadia D, Bell DJ, et al. UK malaria treatment guidelines 2016. J Infect 2016;**72**:635–49.
2. RTS, S Clinical Trials Partnership. Efficacy and safety of RTS,S/AS01 malaria vaccine with or without a booster dose in infants and children in Africa: final results of a phase 3, individually randomised, controlled trial. Lancet 2015;**386**:31–45.
3. World Health Organization. Global Health Observatory Data: Malaria. www.who.int/gho/malaria/en/ (accessed May 30, 2018).
4. Tatem AJ, Jia P, Ordanovich D, et al. The geography of imported malaria to non-endemic countries: a meta-analysis of nationally reported statistics. Lancet Infect Dis 2017;**17**:98–107.
5. Chiodini PL, Patel D, Whitty CJM, Lalloo DG. Guidelines for malaria prevention in travellers from the United Kingdom, 2017. London: Public Health England; 2017.
6. Solomon T, Felix JM, Samuel M, et al. Hypoglycaemia in paediatric admissions in Mozambique. Lancet 1994;**343**:149–50.
7. Milner DA, Jr, Whitten RO, Kamiza S, et al. The systemic pathology of cerebral malaria in African children. Front Cell Infect Microbiol 2014;**4**:104.
8. Scott JA, Berkley JA, Mwangi I, et al. Relation between falciparum malaria and bacteraemia in Kenyan children: a population-based, case-control study and a longitudinal study. Lancet 2011;**378**:1316–23.
9. Mallewa M, Vallely P, Faragher B, et al. Viral central nervous system infections in children from a malaria-endemic area of Malawi: a prospective cohort study Lancet Global Health 2013;**1**: e153–e60.

CASE 63

A Busse–Buschke Secret

Benedict D. Michael

History

A 55-year-old man presented with a 3-week history of progressive headaches, which were worse on lying flat. He had a 16-year history of relapsing–remitting multiple sclerosis which had been treated with interferon for 8 years and subsequently with fingolimod for 4 years. His multiple sclerosis had been clinically and radiologically stable for the 3 years preceding this presentation; he had a long-standing right internuclear ophthalmoplegia, left upper limb ataxia and mild lower limb spasticity.

His recent headaches were accompanied by nausea and vomiting. His symptoms progressed to transient bilateral blurring of vision, particularly on performing valsalva manoeuvres, and a week of global cognitive decline.

There was no history of weight loss, night sweats, rash or fever; and there was no travel or recent dental history of note.

Examination

He was apyrexial with a Glasgow coma score (GCS) of 14/15, reflecting confused speech; but he was able to follow commands and maintain spontaneous eye opening. He had evidence of 'catch-up' nystagmus in the left eye and failed adduction of the right eye on left gaze, reflecting the existing right internuclear ophthalmoplegia. Reflexes were generally brisk, particularly in the lower limbs bilaterally, with a crossed adductor response and bilateral extensor plantars. He also had a T10 sensory level reflecting previous myelitis. There was intention tremor and dysdiadochokinesis in the left upper limb reflecting a previous cerebellar relapse of his multiple sclerosis.

In addition to his baseline neurological symptoms he was found to have bilateral enlarged blind spots and papilloedema.

Initial Differential Diagnosis

In this immunosuppressed patient the clinical impression was of headaches which had features consistent with raised intracranial pressure, and acute cognitive decline. Possible causes included:

- Meningitis
  - Bacterial
    - *Streptococcus pneumoniae*
    - *Neisseria meningitidis*
    - Other
- Mycobacterial
  - *Mycobacterium tuberculosis*
- Fungal
  - *Cryptococcus neoformans*
- Encephalitis
  - Viral
    - Herpes simplex virus 1 or 2
    - Varicella zoster virus
    - Cytomegalovirus ventriculitis
    - Enterovirus
    - Other
  - Autoimmune
    - Paraneoplastic
    - Non-paraneoplastic
- Cerebral abscess
  - Possibly secondary to endocarditis
- Non-infectious pathology
  - Venous sinus thrombosis
  - Neoplastic space-occupying lesion or malignant meningitis
  - Spinal block
  - Idiopathic intracranial hypertension

Results of Initial Investigations

He had a white cell count of 4.3×10^9/l and lymphocytes were reduced to 6% (normal range 16–48%). Renal, liver and bone panels were normal and the erythrocyte sedimentation rate was elevated at 15 mm/h. A plain chest X-ray was normal.

A non-contrast computer tomography (CT) scan of the brain was performed urgently on admission (**Figure 63.1A**) and subsequently an urgent contrast-enhanced CT and CT venogram were performed (**Figure 63.1B**).

A lumbar puncture was performed. The opening pressure was 32 cm H_2O with a slightly cloudy appearance,

Figure 63.1A. A non-contrast axial CT head scan similar to that of a 55-year-old male who had been treated with interferon and fingolimod for management of multiple sclerosis, who presented with postural headaches, transient visual obscuration and cognitive decline.

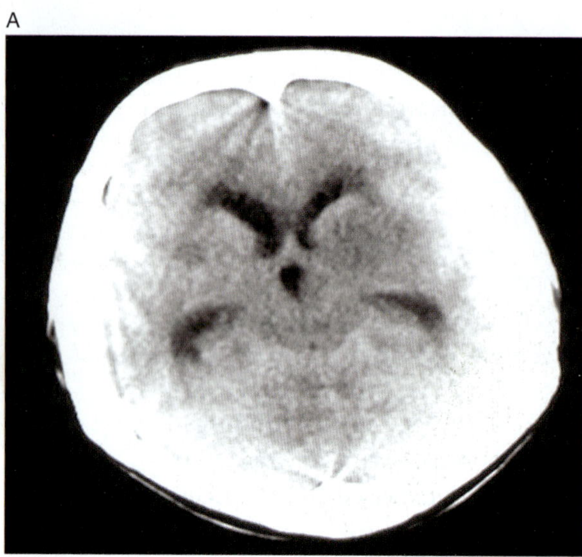

This demonstrates hydrocephalus with symmetrical enlargement of the lateral and third ventricles and widespread effacement of the sulci. (Courtesy of Ian Turnbull.)

Figure 63.1B. A contrast-enhanced axial CT head scan in the same patient.

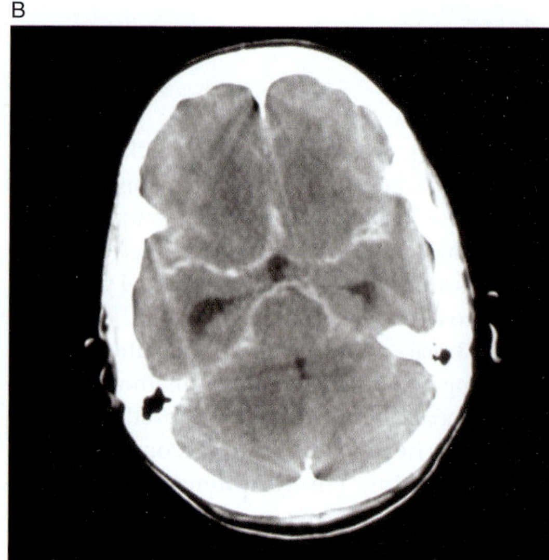

This CT demonstrates widespread leptomeningeal enhancement. A CT venogram performed at the same time (not shown) excluded a venous sinus thrombosis. (Courtesy of Ian Turnbull.)

327 white cells, a 79% lymphocyte predominance, a protein of 4.6 g/l, and a glucose ratio of 41%.

Progress and Further Investigations

The cloudy CSF with a very high opening pressure, cloudy predominant lymphocytosis, raised CSF protein and normal/low glucose ratio raised the suspicion of fungal infection; particularly in the context of immunosuppression. However, the differential remained broad at this stage.

Broad-spectrum antibiotic therapy was started on admission with a third-generation cephalosporin and amoxicillin. However, during the first 6 days of admission, his GCS dropped to 11/15 (eyes 3/4, motor 5/6 and verbal 3/5) and a repeat CT was performed. This demonstrated marked worsening of the hydrocephalus and a repeat lumbar puncture was performed and a large volume of CSF drained. After this his GCS began to improve to 13/15 (eyes 3/4, motor 6/6, verbal 4/5).

A magnetic resonance imaging (MRI) scan of the brain and spine was performed (**Figure 63.2**).

Figure 63.2. Sagittal MRI brain images in the same patient.

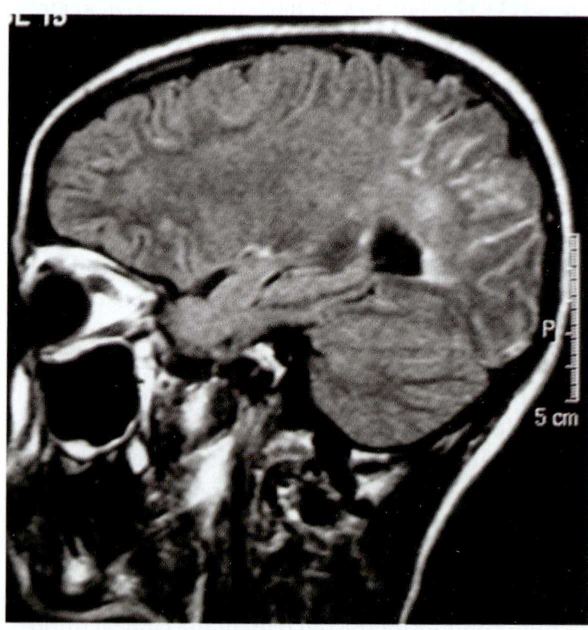

This demonstrates the pre-existing areas of demyelination with no new enhancing plaques. In addition, there was widespread leptomeningeal enhancement. (Courtesy of Ian Turnbull.)

Refined Differential Diagnosis

Meningoencephalitis with secondary hydrocephalus

- Fungal
  - Cryptococcus
- Bacterial
- Viral
  - Cytomegalovirus ventriculitis

Definitive Investigation Results

His HIV antibody and antigen results were negative and interferon-gamma release assay for tuberculosis was also negative. A repeat lumbar puncture was performed which demonstrated similar results; however, this time an India ink stain was also requested (**Figure 63.3**).

Serum and CSF were both positive for cryptococcal antigen using the cryptococcal antigen (CRAG) test.

Final Diagnosis

Meningitis caused by *Cryptococcus neoformans.*

Management and Outcome

Fingolimod was stopped following the CSF results. Initial treatment was given with amphotericin B and flucytosine, then subsequently with fluconazole. He gradually improved over several weeks, with resolution of the visual disturbance, papilloedema, headaches and confusion. He did not require lumbar or external ventricular drainage.

Figure 63.3. India ink stain from a similar patient.

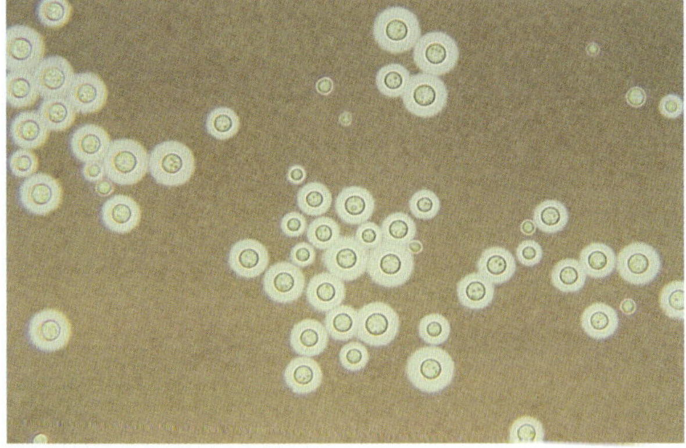

This demonstrates encapsulated yeasts of *Cryptococcus.* (Image courtesy of the Centers for Disease Control, USA.)

Prevention

While the majority of cases of cryptococcal meningitis are identified in patients with HIV infection, iatrogenic cases are increasingly recognised, for example following immunosuppression for solid organ transplantation or, as in this case, for treatment of multiple sclerosis. In transplant patients, pre-immunosuppression serum cryptococcal antibody status has been reported to predict the risk of developing cryptococcal meningitis, but data are limited currently for fingolimod in multiple sclerosis.

Discussion

Cryptococcus neoformans and *gattii*, the latter predominating in tropical and subtropical environments, typically infect either the respiratory or central nervous system [1]. Despite many infections resulting in asymptomatic airway carriage, the pathogen is responsible for over 200,000 cases of meningitis per year. The vast majority of these cases occur in those with advanced HIV infection and are predominantly in sub-Saharan Africa and, to lesser extent, East Asia [2]. The pathogen is usually inhaled and uses a Trojan Horse mechanism to establish infection in macrophages, by modulating the pH of the phagosome, to then enter the central nervous system. Here it causes a variable combination of meningitis and space-occupying cryptococcomas with a predilection for the cerebellum and basal ganglia. The resulting hydrocephalus, induced by impaired CSF reabsorption, can cause raised intracranial pressure leading to postural headaches, visual impairment, cognitive disturbance and declining consciousness. Drainage of CSF, by repeated lumbar punctures or insertion of a lumbar or external ventricular drain, is central to managing this complication.

Opportunistic disseminated infection is recognised increasingly in those with iatrogenic immunosuppression, reticuloendothelial malignancy or sarcoidosis [3]. When present, the characteristic skin changes (**Figure 63.4**) are an important clue to the diagnosis and are an amenable site for tissue to be biopsied for fungal stains and culture.

The critical effects of immunosuppressive agents, such as fingolimod, in permitting the dissemination of cryptococcus infection have yet to be elucidated, but those at highest risk seem to be those with longer cumulative durations of treatment and older age [4].

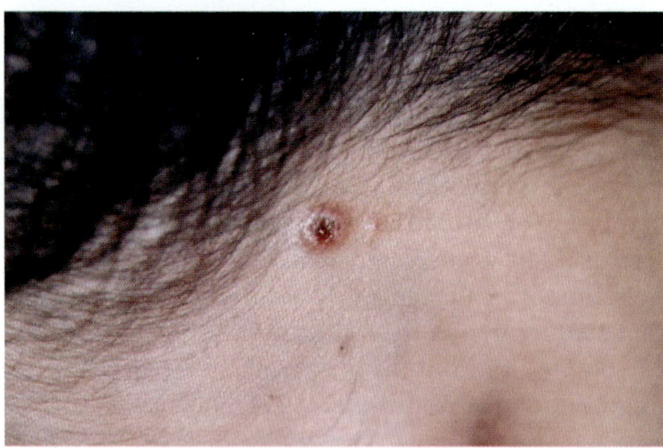

Figure 63.4. The clinical sign of a skin cryptococcoma that, while not present in this patient, is a useful clinical sign when identified. (Image courtesy of the Centers for Disease Control, USA.)

Generally, it is thought that the action of fingolimod on circulating leucocyte population numbers, subsets and functions, along with modulation of subsequent cytokine signalling, play a role in the increased risk of crypotococcal diseases.

Key Points

- *Cryptococcus neoformans* causes meningitis with a very high intracranial pressure
- It is mostly seen in people with advanced HIV disease, but also occurs in others with immunosuppression
- Diagnosis is by examining the CSF with Indian Inki or testing for cryptococcal antigen with the CRAG test

Looking Back

The German pathologist Busse first published the report at the end of the nineteenth century of a woman from whose tibia he had isolated a sodium hydroxide-resistant yeast. Subsequently, Buschke, the Prussian dermatologist, identified the same isolate from the same patient, thus leading to the initial term 'Busse–Buschke disease'.

Did You Know?

The term cryptococcus comes from the Greek word 'Kruptos', which translates as 'hidden' or 'secret', hence the title of the case.

References

1. Rajasingham R, Smith RM, Park BJ et al. Global burden of disease of HIV-associated cryptococcal meningitis: an updated analysis. Lancet Infect Dis 2017;**17**:873–81.
2. Kaplan JE, Hanson D, Dworkin MS, et al. Epidemiology of human immunodeficiency virus-associated opportunistic infections in the United states in the era of highly active antiretroviral therapy. Clin Infect Dis 2000;**30**(Suppl 1):S5–14.
3. Mirza SA, Phelan M, Rimland D, et al The changing epidemiology of cryptococcosis: an update from population-based active surveillance in 2 large metropolitan areas, 1992–2000. Clin Infect Dis 2013;**36**:789–94.
4. Grebenciucova E, Reder AT, Bernard JT. Immunologic mechanisms of fingolimod and the role of immunosenescence in the risk of cryptococcal infection: a case report and review of literature. Mul Scler Rel Dis 2016;**9**:158–62.

CASE 64

Tied in a Knot

Tom Solomon and Benedict D. Michael

History

A 76-year-old retired accountant was admitted with a short history of cognitive decline. Because he lived alone and had no family there was not much in the way of corroborative history. However, he kept a rather meticulous daily diary and some of the history could be gleaned from this.

He had been fit and healthy all his life. A diary entry four months before admission recorded that he had posted an application for a new driving licence and spent time at the Citizen's Advice Bureau. A few weeks later he developed pain down the back of his leg, which he thought was sciatica, and so did not bother his general practitioner. These symptoms became worse so that he could barely leave his accommodation in a warden-monitored flat. A few weeks after this his diary noted that he had awoken with his eyes 'out of focus and uncomfortable'. The following week he saw his general practitioner, who suggested he have an eye test. Four weeks later he noted that he was 'very confused'. The diary entries tailed off after that, but the last note before admission recorded that he had been taken to the eye clinic, where he was waiting for a cataract operation. He had been admitted soon after his visit to the eye clinic because of concern about his generally confused state.

Examination

On examination he was found to be pleasant, but confused.

His clothes were loose-fitting and it was apparent that he had lost weight. He had clearly struggled to dress, with his shirt and waistcoat buttons misaligned and his tie knotted very poorly. The general medical examination was otherwise unremarkable.

He was disoriented in time and place, had problems with both short-and long-term memory, and laughed inappropriately during the examination.

He had a broad ataxic gait and his tone was increased throughout, with brisk deep-tendon reflexes but flexor plantars. He had occasional generalised myoclonic jerks, frontal release signs, including a root ing reflex, and a positive startle response (a loud bang behind him triggering a generalised myoclonic jerk of all four limbs).

Initial Differential Diagnosis

The main differential was between the various causes of rapidly progressive cognitive decline, and the causes of an acute confusional state, specifically:

- Neurodegenerative diseases such as Alzheimer's, Lewy body dementia, or Creutzfeldt–Jakob disease.
- Autoimmune encephalitis, particularly *N*-methyl-D-aspartate receptor (NMDA) receptor antibody encephalitis, voltage-gated potassium channel (VGKC) complex antibody encephalitis and progressive encephalomyelitis with rigidity and myoclonus (PERM), which may be associated with anti-glutamic acid decarboxylase (GAD) or anti-glycine receptor antibodies or Hashimoto's (steroid-responsive) encephalitis.
- Subacute infectious encephalopathies, such as progressive multifocal leukoencephalopathy due to JC virus, subacute sclerosing panencephalitis caused by measles virus, syphilis, or HIV.
- Toxic or metabolic causes, particularly Wernicke's encephalopathy caused by thiamine deficiency, or hepatic encephalopathy.
- Other conditions such as lymphoma, central nervous system vasculitis, or neurosarcoid.

Results of Initial Investigations

Bloods including a full blood count, urea and electrolytes, liver and thyroid function tests, B12 and folate were unremarkable. The venereal disease reference laboratory (VDRL) test, *Treponema pallidum* haemagglutination assay (TPHA), antineuronal and other autoantibodies, and inflammatory markers were negative. A chest X-ray and electrocardiogram were normal. An magnetic resonance imaging (MRI) scan was performed (**Figure 64.1**). A lumbar puncture was normal except for a very slightly elevated protein of 0.53 g/l; there were no oligoclonal bands. This was followed by an electroencephalogram (EEG) (**Figure 64.2**).

Results of Definitive Investigations

His cerebrospinal fluid (CSF) 14-3-3 protein level was elevated at 2.0 ng/ml, with a normal reference range of less than 1.5 ng/ml. The S100 protein was also elevated. Although this on its own is not diagnostic, in the

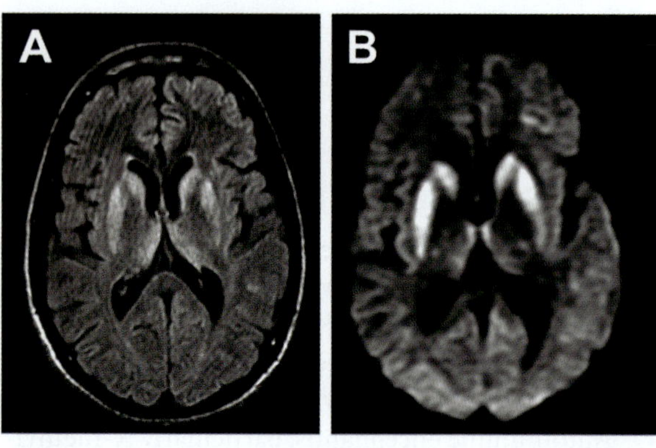

Figure 64.1. An MRI scan similar to that of a 76-year-old man who had a rapid onset of cognitive decline over several months.
This shows high signal changes in the basal ganglia on T2-weighted fluid-attenuated inversion recovery (FLAIR) images (A), which are more obvious on diffusion-weighted images (B). (From [1] with permission from BMJ Publishing Group Ltd.)

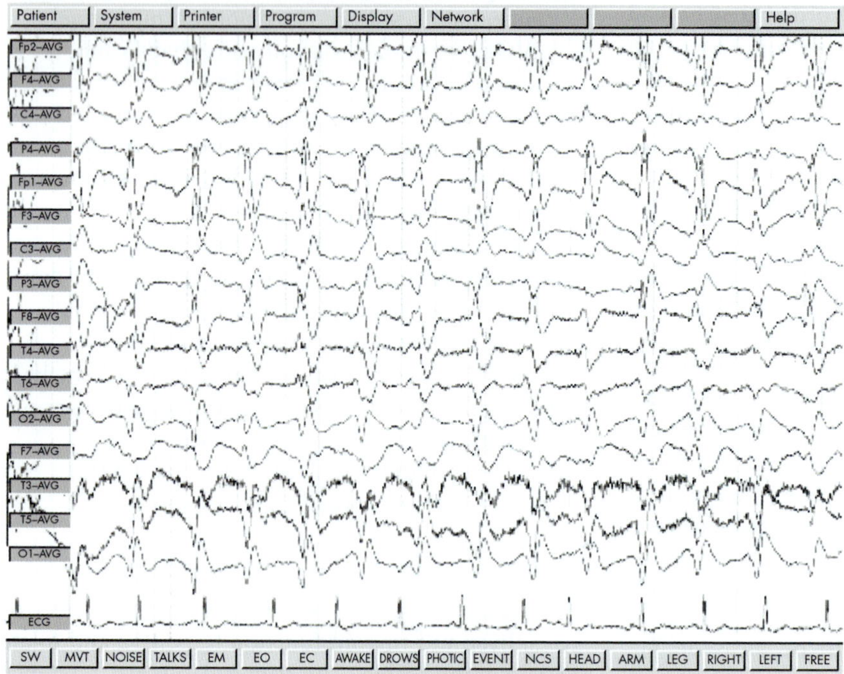

Figure 64.2. An electroencephalogram for the patient was similar to this.
It shows periodic complexes with a generalised distribution which repeat at around one per second (1 Hz). (From [2] with permission from BMJ Publishing Group Ltd.)

context of rapidly developing cognitive impairment, the characteristic MRI and EEG findings, and other investigations being negative, a diagnosis was made.

Diagnosis

Sporadic Creutzfeldt–Jakob disease (CJD).

Management and Outcome

The case was discussed with the National CJD Research and Surveillance Centre at Edinburgh, UK, who came to review the patient and agreed with the diagnosis. Because there is no specific treatment for CJD he was transferred to a care home where he died several weeks later.

Prevention

There is no preventative measure for sporadic CJD. Other forms such as variant CJD and iatrogenic CJD are preventable, as discussed below.

Discussion

Sporadic CJD is the most common human transmissible spongiform encephalopathy, or prion disease, accounting for around 85% of cases [3]. Despite this, it is very rare, occurring at a rate of 1 per million per year.

The term 'prion' comes from the proteinaceous infectious particles by which the diseases are characterised. The normal cellular prion protein, PrP^{C}, is present in all mammals, and is encoded in humans by the prion gene (*PRNP*) on chromosome 20. Its function is not known. Of sporadic CJD cases, 10–15% are associated with mutations of *PRNP*. Prion diseases are characterised by the deposition in the nervous system of PrP^{Sc}, an abnormally misfolded isoform of the native prion protein [4]; the protein is named 'Sc' after the abnormal protein seen in sheep with scrapie, which is one of several prion diseases in animals.

The mechanism for triggering this conformational change from PrP^{C} to PrP^{Sc} is not known, but the accumulation of this abnormal prion protein leads to neuronal degeneration, astrocytic gliosis and spongiform change (**Figure 64.3**), resulting in a uniformly fatal neurological disorder. Other prion diseases of humans include:

- Kuru, which was endemic in Papua New Guinea and is due to the eating of human brains in ritual cannibalism.
- Iatrogenic CJD; this is most often due to prior treatment with human pituitary-derived hormones or human dura mater, or equipment which has undergone conventional physical decontamination methods which do not inactivate prions; changes in clinical practice have led to a reduction in the risk of new cases occurring.
- Variant CJD; less than 240 cases of this extremely rare disease had been reported worldwide by January 2018. It was first reported in 1996, and is thought to be due to bovine-to-human transmission of bovine spongiform encephalopathy (BSE), through ingestion of infected meat products. Transmission in blood transfusions has also been reported. In the late 1980s the UK government introduced new regulations on feed for animals; the BSE epidemic peaked in 1992, with the CJD epidemic peaking in 2000 (**Figure 64.4**).
- Genetic prion diseases: Gerstmann–Sträussler–Scheinker syndrome is an autosomal dominant progressive cerebellar degeneration; fatal familial insomnia is a rapidly progressive disease characterised by progressive insomnia with loss of the normal circadian pattern.

Sporadic CJD presents with a rapidly progressive dementia, typically over weeks to months. The peak

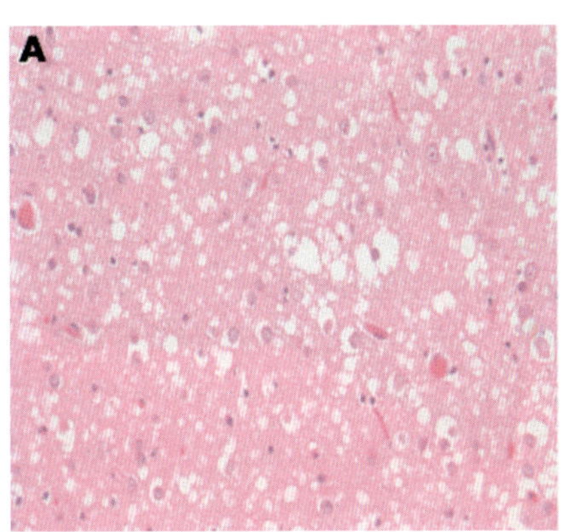

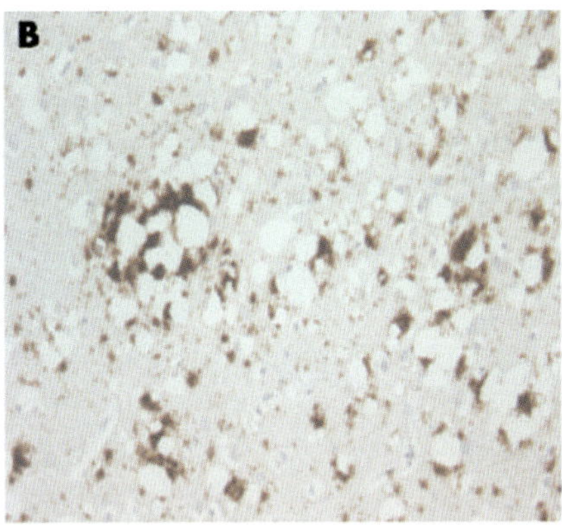

Figure 64.3. Neuropathological changes in sporadic Creutzfeldt–Jakob disease. (A) sCJD: Spongiform change in the frontal cortex (haematoxylin and eosin). (B) sCJD: Cerebral PrP deposition (KG9 antibody). (From [3] with permission from BMJ Publishing Group Ltd.)

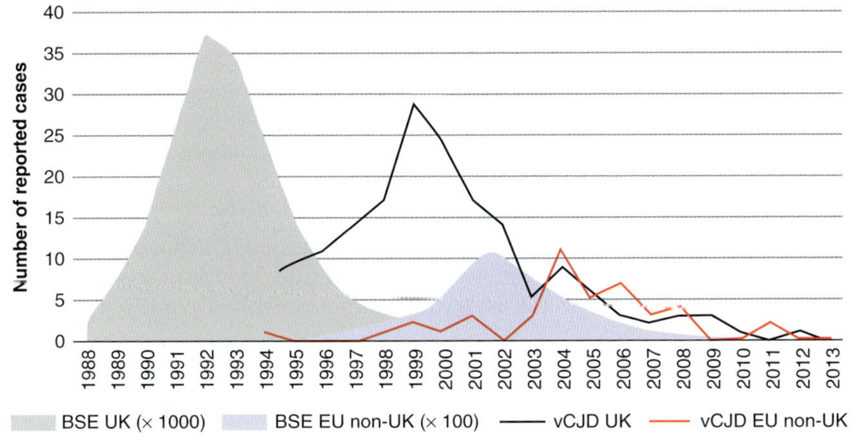

Figure 64.4. Number of reported BSE case and variant CJD cases (probable and definite) by date of onset in the EU (excluding the UK) and in the UK, 1988–2013. (From: https://ecdc.europa.eu/en/vcjd/facts with permission.)

incidence is in the seventh decade. There are clues that a patient with dementia may have CJD including myoclonus, especially startle myoclonus, and cortical visual loss (as seen in this patient) [1]. Other pointers may be cerebellar ataxia, other extrapyramidal signs, or signs of corticospinal tract involvement. Some variants or subtypes have been defined based on predominant focal neurological presentations, for example predominantly visual disease (Heidenhain variant) or cerebellar disease (Brownell–Oppenheimer variant). More recently, subtypes have been defined according to whether they have methionine or valine at codon 129 of the *PRNP* gene. As well as affecting clinical presentation, polymorphisms at this site effect the incubation period, and even the susceptibility to the disease: 80% of UK sporadic CJD cases are homozygotes for methionine at this site (compared with 40% of the general population).

A definitive diagnosis of sporadic CJD requires examination of brain tissue, but a probable diagnosis can be made based on appropriate clinical features and supportive investigative findings among the MRI, EEG and CSF 14-3-3, as in this case (Table 64.1) [4].

Table 64.1. Diagnostic criteria for surveillance of sporadic Creutzfeldt–Jakob diseases, effective from 1 January 2017. (From [4] © 2017 Mackenzie G and Will R, reproduced under CC BY license.)

1.1	DEFINITE:
	Progressive neurological syndrome AND
	Neuropathologically or immunohistochemically or biochemically confirmed
1.2	PROBABLE:
	I + two of II and typical electroencephalogram[a]
	OR I + two of II and typical magnetic resonance imaging brain scan[b]
	OR I + two of II and positive cerebrospinal fluid (CSF) 14-3-3
	OR Progressive neurological syndrome and positive real-time quaking-induced conversion in CSF or other tissues
1.3	POSSIBLE:
	I + two of II + duration < 2 years
I	Rapidly progressive cognitive impairment
II	A Myoclonus
	B Visual or cerebellar problems
	C Pyramidal or extrapyramidal features
	D Akinetic mutism

[a] Generalised periodic complexes; [b] high signal in caudate/putamen on MRI brain scan or at least two cortical regions (temporal, parietal, occipital) on either diffusion-weighted imaging or fluid-attenuated inversion recovery.

Elevated CSF 14-3-3, S100b and tau occur in patients with CJD, but they may also be seen in patients with other neurological diseases. The real-time quaking-induced conversion (RT-QuIC) assay is a more recent test for CJD, reported to have 85% sensitivity and 100% specificity; the test uses recombinant PrP as a substrate which is induced to precipitate by PrP^{SC} in the CSF [4].

There is no effective treatment for CJD. As the disease progresses patients develop akinetic mutism. Death usually occurs within a year of symptom onset, with the median duration of disease being 6 months.

Key Points

- Think of sporadic CJD in an elderly person with rapidly progressive dementia, especially if there is myoclonous, ataxia or visual loss.
- A characteristic EEG, MRI and detection of 14-3-3 in the CSF support the diagnosis.
- Variant CJD, which was discovered in relation to the BSE epidemic, is seen in younger people, but is extremely rare and declining.
- There is no treatment for any prion disease.

Looking Back

CJD is named after German neuropathologists Hans Gerhard Creutzfeldt and Alfons Maria Jakob, who independently first described it in the 1920s; two of the patients in their initial descriptions are now thought to have had something else [5].

Did You Know?

The Fore people of Papua New Guinea thought that Kuru, the first described human prion disease, was due to witchcraft. In the 1950s Daniel Carleton Gajdusek began investigations showing that cannibalism, especially eating the brain, was the cause; he was later awarded a Nobel Prize.

Kuru means shaking, and describes one of the early features of this progressive prion disease (see video at www.youtube.com/watch?v=OqjmLZjZpRE).

References

1. Mead S, Rudge P. CJD mimics and chameleons. Pract Neurol 2017;**17**:113–21.
2. Smith SJ. EEG in neurological conditions other than epilepsy: when does it help, what does it add? J Neurol Neurosurg Psychiatry 2005;**76**(Suppl 2):ii8–12.
3. Knight RS, Will RG. Prion diseases. J Neurol Neurosurg Psychiatry 2004;**75**(Suppl 1):36–42.
4. Mackenzie G, Will R. Creutzfeldt–Jakob disease: recent developments. F1000Res 2017;**6**:2053.
5. Ironside JW. Neuropathological diagnosis of human prion disease; morphological studies. In: Baker HF, Ridley RM, editors. *Fatal Protein – The Story of CJD, BSE and Other Prion Diseases*. Oxford: Oxford University Press; 1998: 35–57.

CASE 65

Twitchy and Twitching

John Williamson and Benedict D. Michael

History

A 75-year-old male was admitted to hospital complaining of generalised weakness and fatigue. These had been gradually progressive over the preceding 6 months, with a more rapid deterioration in the week leading up to admission. He also reported unintentional weight loss and loss of muscle bulk associated with visible twitching of his muscles, affecting both his upper and lower limbs. Having previously walked normally his mobility had reduced and he struggled to walk further then 10 m without a risk of falling. He also mentioned having disturbed sleep with periods of insomnia. He would frequently wake with soaked bed covers due to excessive sweating. He lived at home with a lodger, and a collateral history from the lodger described fluctuating periods of confusion. There was no history of a febrile illness.

He had a past medical history of benign prostatic hypertrophy for which he was prescribed tamsulosin. He was a lifelong non-smoker and rarely drank alcohol. There was no history of travel abroad.

Examination

On admission to hospital he was afebrile, with normal pulse, blood pressure and respiratory rate. He appeared encephalopathic and was disoriented to time and place with a fluctuating level of alertness during the consultation. He scored 51/100 on the Addenbrooke's cognitive examination.

He had widespread muscle wasting with visible muscle twitching affecting both proximal and distal muscle groups in the upper and lower limbs. His speech was dysarthric. Cranial nerves, including funduscopy, were normal and there was no evidence of tongue wasting or asciculations and the jaw jerk was absent. Tone and power in the upper and lower limbs were normal and reflexes were present and symmetrical; both plantar responses were flexor. Sensory examination was normal.

Initial Differential Diagnosis

- Anterior horn cell disorder
  - Amyotrophic lateral sclerosis
  - Enterovirus infection
  - Multilevel generative disc disease
  - Multilevel radicular infiltration (lymphoma, prostate cancer, other)
- Neuromyotonia with encephalopathy (Morvan's syndrome)
  - Paraneoplastic vs primary autoimmune
- Other paraneoplastic disorder
- Possibly episodic ataxia type 1, if younger

Results of Initial Investigations

He had a microcytic anaemia, with a haemoglobin of 95 g/l and a mean corpuscular volume of 75.8 fl; the white cell count and platelet count were normal. His sodium was slightly low at 131 mmol/l, otherwise renal function was normal. Liver function, bone profile and thyroid function were normal. C-reactive protein was not elevated.

The patient's cerebrospinal fluid (CSF) was acellular with normal protein and a glucose ratio of 64%; the cytology was normal and no oligoclonal bands were detected. Viral polymerase chain reaction was negative for herpes simplex virus varicella zoster virus and enteroviruses.

An electroencephalogram (**Figure 65.1**) and subsequently a magnetic resonance imaging (MRI) brain scan were performed (**Figure 65.2**).

Progress and Further Investigations

Given the history of unintentional weight loss and anaemia, investigations were performed to exclude an underlying malignancy. A computer tomography

Figure 65.1. Electroencephalograph from a 75-year-old man who presented with subacute fluctuating encephalopathy, widespread muscle wasting and prominent generalised fasciculations.

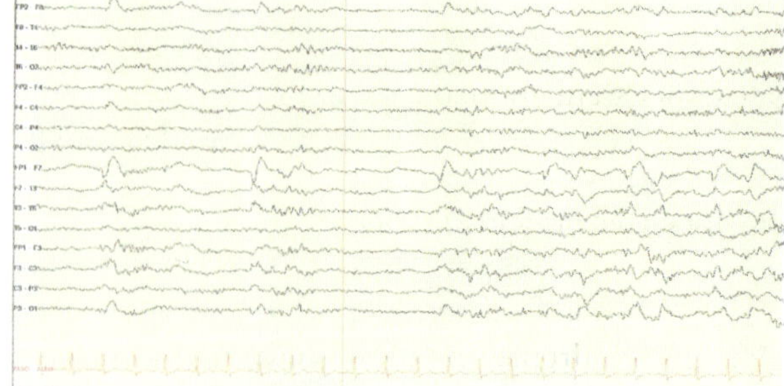

This demonstrates generalised slowing consistent with encephalopathy, although no specific diagnostic features are present.

Figure 65.2. Coronal MRI fluid-attenuated inversion recovery (FLAIR) image in the same patient.

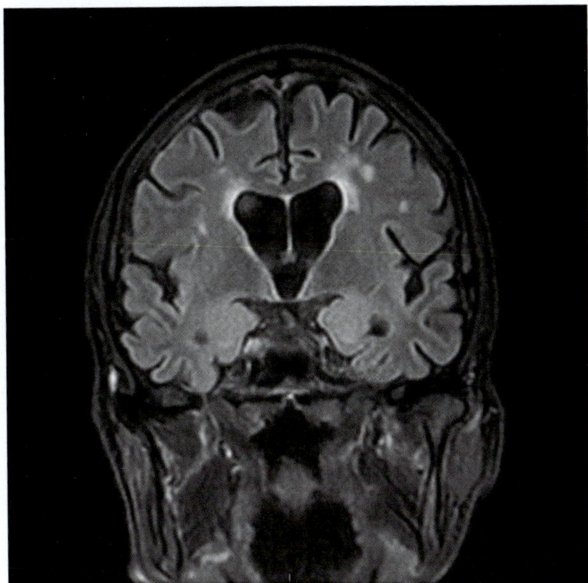

This demonstrates bilateral but asymmetric hyperintensity of the hippocampus.

scan of the chest, abdomen and pelvis and a whole body positron-emission tomography scan were both normal.

Nerve conduction studies and electromyography did not show any evidence of an anterior horn cell disorder. However, motor nerve conduction studies demonstrated after – discharges and contraction fasciculations/myokymia suggestive of peripheral nerve hyperexcitability.

Autoimmune antibodies, including those against glutamic acid decarboxylase (GAD) and *N*-methyl-D-aspartate (NMDA) receptors, were negative, as were paraneoplastic antibodies targeting intracellular antigens.

Definitive Investigation Results

In view of the neurophysiological findings, voltage-gated potassium antibodies were sent and discovered to be elevated, with positive titres of both LGI1 (leucine-rich glioma inactivated 1) and CASPR2 (contactin-associated protein 2) subtypes.

Final Diagnosis

Morvan's syndrome (limbic encephalitis associated with anti-LGI1 antibodies, and neuromyotonia associated with anti-CASPR2 antibodies).

Management and Outcome

The patient was managed with 3 days of intravenous methylprednisolone and made a dramatic improvement. He was more alert and his performance in bedside cognitive testing improved with Addenbrooke's cognitive examination score improving to 82/100. He was discharged home following a brief stay in a rehabilitation ward. At 3-month follow-up the patient reported ongoing improvement and was noted to be gaining weight.

Discussion

Morvan's syndrome is a rare autoimmune disorder characterised by neuropsychiatric features, especially insomnia, confusion, amnesia and hallucinations, autonomic dysfunction, especially excessive sweating, neuropathic pain and irregular muscle contractions.

With the advent of cell-based assays, antineuronal antibodies directed against both intra- and extracellular antigens have been identified [1]. These may reflect paraneoplastic or para-/post-infectious phenomena, or a primary autoimmune disease.

Cumulatively, voltage-gated potassium channel (VGKC)-complex antibodies account for 3% of cases of encephalitis. These antibodies can be directed against CASPR2, causing neuromyotonia (also known as Isaac's syndrome), or against LGI1 presenting as limbic encephalitis (**Figure 65.3**). Morvan's syndrome is an overlap syndrome with features of both, as seen in this case. The VGKC-complex antibody titre may correlate with clinical progression and *in vitro* data support an

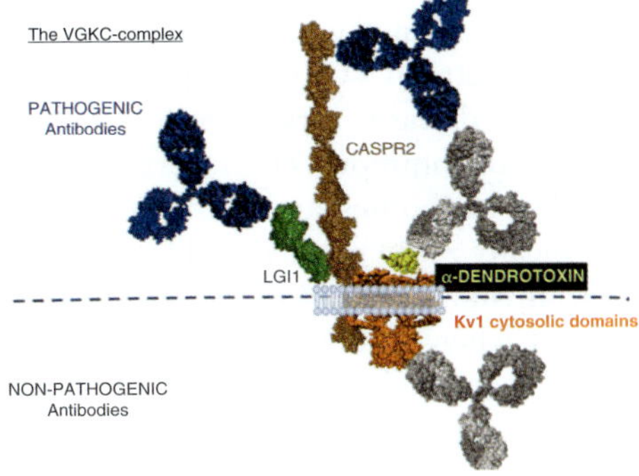

Figure 65.3. The voltage-gated potassium channel complex includes LGI1 (leucine-rich glioma inactivated 1; green) and CASPR2 (contactin-associated protein 2; orange). Pathogenic antibodies (blue) may form against each of these components. Non-pathogenic antibodies (grey) form against other components. Alpha-dendrotoxin (yellow) and its binding site are also shown. (Reproduced from [3] with permission from BMJ Publishing Group Ltd.)

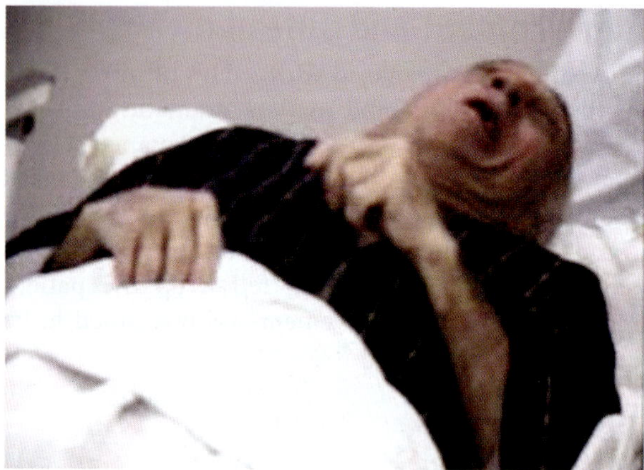

Figure 65.4. Faciobrachial dystonic seizures in a patient with leucine-rich glioma-inactivated 1 antibodies. (From [2] with permission of John Wiley & Sons, Inc.)

excitotoxic association in cultured neurons; however, *in vivo* data are limited.

The clinical presentation shares some similarities to herpes simplex virus encephalitis and may be sometimes be indistinguishable on clinical grounds. However, as in this case, features suggestive of an immune-mediated pathology include a subacute presentation, sleep disturbance and neuromyotonia. In addition, seizures (particularly faciobrachial dystonic seizures [2], **Figure 65.4**) and prominent psychiatric features are also suggestive. Even when a prior infection is not identified, many patients with Morvan's syndrome report symptoms suggestive of a viral illness in the weeks prior to neurological symptoms.

Hyponatraemia is seen in a significant proportion, as in this case, and may have an inverse correlation with antibody titre in VGKC-complex disease. In VGKC-complex disease very significant CSF abnormalities are uncommon. High serum titres of VGKC-complex antibodies are found in limbic encephalitis (typically > 400 pmol/l) and lower titres in isolated neuromyotonia. There is some retrospective evidence that when clinicians consider testing for VGKC-complex antibodies early it is more likely to be the diagnosis than when testing is arranged later, after other investigations have been negative [4]. VGKC-complex antibodies are found in ≤ 5% of asymptomatic people and screening undifferentiated populations with new-onset seizures only identifies significant titres in 4%.

MRI is normal in around 84% of cases of VGKC-complex limbic encephalitis. Therefore, UK encephalitis guidelines recommend an EEG be performed if both MRI and CSF are normal, looking for changes consistent with encephalopathy, as was seen in this case, and distinguishing the presentation from a psychiatric diagnosis. Classic electromyography findings in neuromyotonia include an auditory phenomena described as a 'dive bomber'.

In addition to management of psychosis and seizures, treatment is with immunomodulatory therapy. Typically, high-dose intravenous steroids are given in a 5-day pulse with or without intravenous immunoglobulin or plasma exchange. There is observational evidence that using plasma exchange as opposed to steroids alone may be more effective, but many uncertainties remain [5,6]. Up to 10% of cases are paraneoplastic, with breast, lymphoma, thymoma and thyroid cancers most common. In the case described here no underlying tumour was found.

In those with VGKC-complex antibodies, timely immunomodulatory therapy, rather than anti-epileptic drugs, is associated with earlier resolution of faciobrachial dystonic seizures and an improved outcome [7]. When a tumour is identified, early removal is associated with improved outcome in the majority, although immunosuppressive therapy may be needed and tumour recurrence can occur.

Key Learning Points

- In patients with altered consciousness, insomnia, wasting, fasciculations, and excess sweating think of Morvan's syndrome.
- Morvan's syndrome is associated with antibodies against the LGI1 and CASPR2 components of the voltage-gated potassium channels.
- Prompt recognition and immunosuppressive treatment are associated with improved outcomes.

Looking Back

Augustin Marie Morvan was a nineteenth-century French physician, writer and politician who described the first patient with what he called 'fibrilliary chorea'. The patient had myokymia (muscle twitching) associated with muscle pain, excessive sweating and disordered sleep, and died 5 weeks after onset.

Did You Know?

The discovery of the voltage-gated potassium channel was identified through the action of dendrotoxin (**Figure 65.3**), which is present in the venom of the black mamba and is the cause of paralysis when bitten.

References

1. Lai M, Huijbers M, Lancaster E, et al. Investigation of LGI1 as the antigen in limbic encephalitis previously attributed to potassium channels: a case series. Lancet Neurol 2010;**9**:776–85.
2. Irani SR, Michell AW, Lang B, et al. Faciobrachial dystonic seizures precede LGI1-antibody limbic encephalitis. Ann Neurol 2010;**69**:892–900.
3. Lang B, Makuch M, Moloney T, et al. Intracellular and non-neuronal targets of voltage-gated potassium channel complex antibodies. J Neurol Neurosurg Psychiatry 2017;**88**:353–61.
4. O'Sullivan B, Steele T, Ellul MA, et al. When should we test for voltage-gated potassium channel complex antibodies? A retrospective case control study. J Clin Neurosci 2016;**33**:198–204.
5. Vincent A, Buckley C, Schott JM, et al. Potassium channel antibody-associated encephalopathy: a potentially immunotherapy-responsive form of limbic encephalitis. Brain 2004;**127**:701–12.
6. Thieben MJ, Lennon V, Boeve BF, et al. Potentially reversable autoimmune limbic encephalitis with neuronal potassium channel antibody. Neurology 2004;**62**:1177–82.
7. Irani SR, Stagg CJ, Schott JM, et al. Fasciobrachial dystonic seizures: the influence of immunotherapy on seizure control and prevention of cognitive impairment in a broadening phenotype. Brain 2013;**1**:1–12.

CASE 66

An Itchy Problem

Tom Solomon

History

A 24-year-old housekeeper was admitted to hospital in Rio de Janeiro, June 2014, with a febrile illness, headache, rash and difficulty walking. A few days earlier she had woken with a severe generalised headache and retro-orbital pain; she was very weak with paraesthesia of the extremities. After two days she became febrile, with axillary temperature 42°C, chills, and developed a rash on her face, abdomen, chest and arms. By day 4, her fever had come down, but she complained of severe painful swelling of the hands, pain in the feet, weakness and difficulty walking. She was admitted the next day. She had had dengue five years previously. She had not travelled recently, and did not recall tick or mosquito bites.

Examination

On examination, the patient was alert and fully oriented with no meningeal signs. Her axillary temperature was 36.7°C, pulse 90 beats per minute, blood pressure 100/60 mmHg, and respiratory rate 20 breaths per minute. She had a diffuse erythematous macular lesions over the skin of her chest, abdomen and limbs (**Figure 66.1A**), bilateral non-purulent conjunctival hyperaemia, enanthema of the palate and an enlarged painless cervical lymph node. She also had swelling of the hands and feet (**Figure 66.1B**).

Her power was reduced in the lower limbs and she could not walk. She had absent deep tendon reflexes at the knees and ankles and both plantars were absent; there was reduced sensation to light touch distally in the legs, but no urinary retention or ataxia. The remainder of the examination, including neurological examination of the arms and cranial nerves was normal.

Initial Differential Diagnosis

The initial febrile illness was felt to be compatible with an arthropod-borne viral (arboviral) disease, such as dengue, chikungunya or Zika; other exanthemas were also considered including enterovirus infection and measles, although they are more typically childhood illnesses; infectious mononucleosis, leptospirosis, HIV and syphilis were also possibilities. Had she looked toxic or septicaemic, the differential would have included toxic shock syndrome; meningococcal disease was unlikely given the blanching rash. In terms of the neurological features, the leg weakness, distal sensory loss in the legs and reduced leg power were consistent with Guillain–Barré syndrome – particularly the paraparetic variant. There were no signs in the arms; the paraesthesias in her hands were consistent with Guillain–Barré syndrome, but might also have been explained by the marked swelling here. Alternatively,

Figure 66.1. (A) The left upper arm, and (B) hands of a 24-year-old-woman with fever, headache and difficulty walking.

A

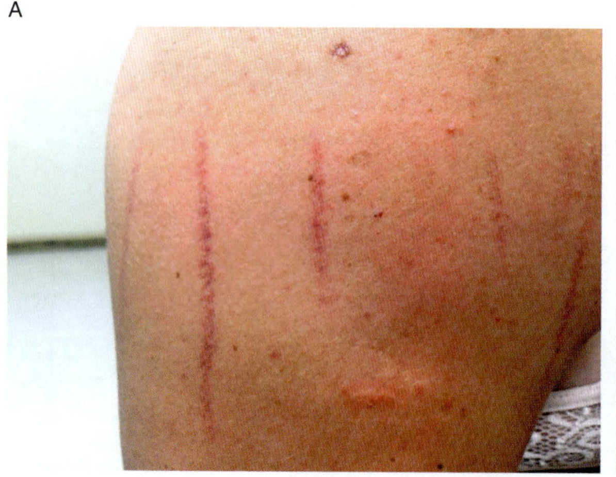

B

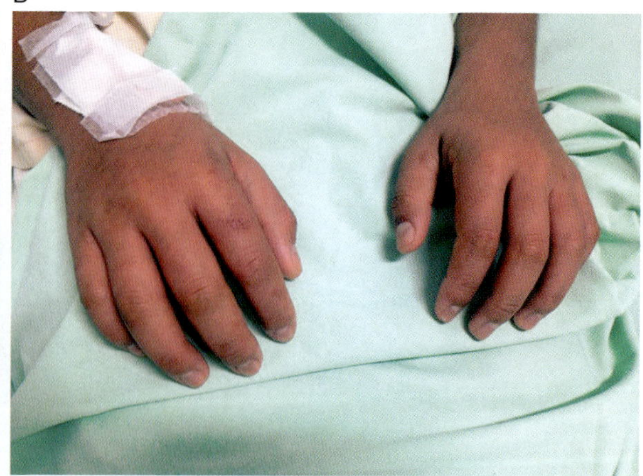

These show a diffuse pruritic blanching rash which caused severe scratching (A), and generalised swelling of both hands. (Photos courtesy of Dr Patricia Brasil.)

a spinal cord syndrome was also possible, although the absent deep tendon reflexes, lack of a sensory level and lack of bladder involvement would argue against this.

Results of Initial Investigations

A full blood count, urea, electrolytes and liver function tests were normal, but creatine kinase was elevated at 786 U/l. A lumbar puncture was performed on day 6 of illness, and the cerebrospinal fluid (CSF) cell count, protein and glucose were normal. Chest X-ray, magnetic resonance imaging (MRI) of the brain and spine, nerve conduction studies and electromyography were all unremarkable. CSF and serum were negative by real-time polymerase chain reaction (PCR) and immunoglobulin M (IgM) antibody testing for dengue and chikungunya. Epstein–Barr virus and cytomegalovirus IgM tests were also negative, as were tests for HIV and leptospirosis.

Results of Definitive Investigations

CSF and serum were positive for Zika virus by PCR. In order to identify the Zika virus genotype, 327 base pair amplicons from the CSF encompassing the virus' envelope protein were sequenced, and the Asian lineage of Zika identified. Saliva was also positive for Zika virus by PCR on day 10 of illness, and urine on day 11.

Diagnosis

Zika virus infection associated with Guillain–Barré syndrome.

Management and Outcome

Her fever settled over a few days, and by day 10 of illness the rash and swelling began to resolve. The elevated creatine kinase returned to normal over 5 days. Her leg weakness also improved gradually without specific treatment, and by day 13 she was fully mobile and discharged. When she was reviewed at a month her power had returned to normal, although she had ongoing headaches which were diagnosed as common migraines.

Prevention

There is no vaccine against Zika, although several are in development. Like other mosquito-borne viruses the risks are reduced by using mosquito repellent and appropriate clothing to minimise exposure. Public health measures to control aedes mosquitoes, which are the main vector, may also help.

Discussion

Zika virus (family Flaviviridae, genus *Flavivirus*) is a mosquito-borne pathogen first identified in Uganda in 1947. Until 2000, it was associated with occasional cases of fever, arthralgia and rash in Africa, and later Southeast Asia, typical of many arboviruses. Phylogenetic studies suggest the virus emerged in East Africa in the early part of the twentieth century, later spreading to Southeast Asia [1]. In 2007 there was a small outbreak in Yap, Micronesia, and in 2013 a larger outbreak in French Polynesia, with more than 20,000 cases. Zika was first reported in Brazil in early 2015, where it was also, for the first time, associated with an epidemic of microcephaly and other congenital abnormalities [2] (**Figure 66.2**). The virus spread rapidly to affect millions of people across Latin America and triggered the declaration by the World Health Organization of a Public Health Emergency of International Concern. By March 2017, there was evidence of Zika transmission in 84 countries around the world.

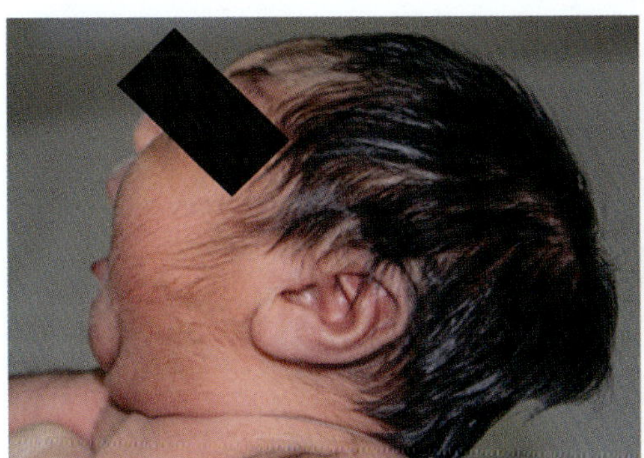
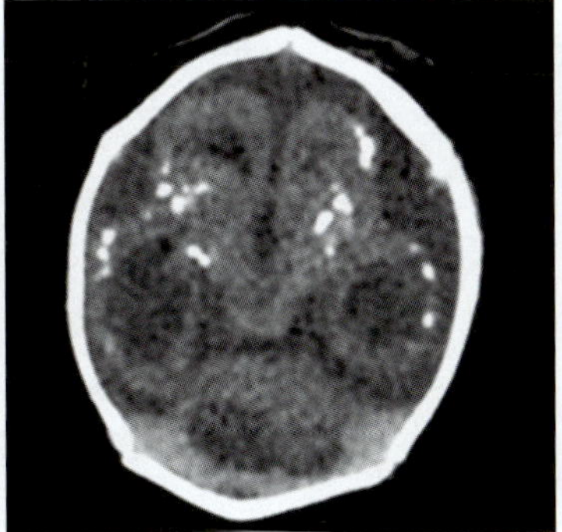
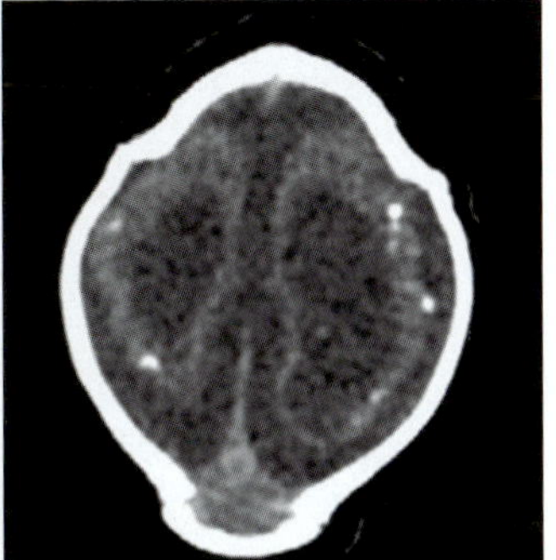

Figure 66.2. Newborn baby with microcephaly, laboratory-confirmed Zika virus infection and abnormalities detected on CT scan. (left) craniofacial disproportion, prominent external occipital protuberance, and excessive scalp skin. (centre and right) Radiological features: computer tomography images include reduced volume of cortical brain parenchyma, cortical and subcortical calcifications, simplified gyral pattern, and ventriculomegaly. (Reproduced from [3] with permission of Elsevier.)

Aedes aegypti is the principle vector of Zika, although *Aedes albopictus* (the Asian tiger mosquito) which is also found in southern Europe and parts of the USA may play a role too. Maternal–foetal transmission is also an important route of infection. Less-common routes include sexual transmission, blood products and organ transplants. Many European countries have had Zika cases among travellers returning from endemic areas; up to March 2017, there were more than 2000 such cases (**Figure 66.3**) [4]. This includes southern European countries where *Aedes albopictus* mosquitoes circulate (**Figure 66.3**), raising the possibility of Zika outbreaks in Europe as has occurred in the southern USA. By December 2017 there had been more than 200 cases in the USA through local transmission, along with more than 5000 imported cases.

In Brazil the abundant numbers of *Aedes aegypti* mosquitoes and densely crowded populations of immunologically naïve individuals likely contributed to the size of the outbreak. Phylogenetic studies suggest the Brazilian strain originated in the Pacific islands [5]. Sequencing of the virus detected in the case described here confirmed it was also of the Asian lineage. The El Niño climate event of 2015 is thought to have contributed to the explosive outbreak of Zika that year, through increased numbers of mosquitoes and perhaps a reduced incubation time for the virus in its mosquito vector [6]. There is also some evidence

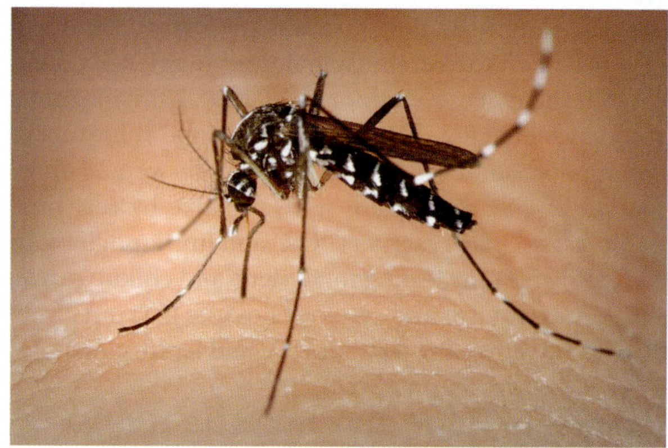

Figure 66.4. *Aedes albopictus*, the Asian tiger mosquito, which circulates in Europe and the USA, and is a vector for Zika virus. (Courtesy of Centers for Disease Control and Prevention, USA.)

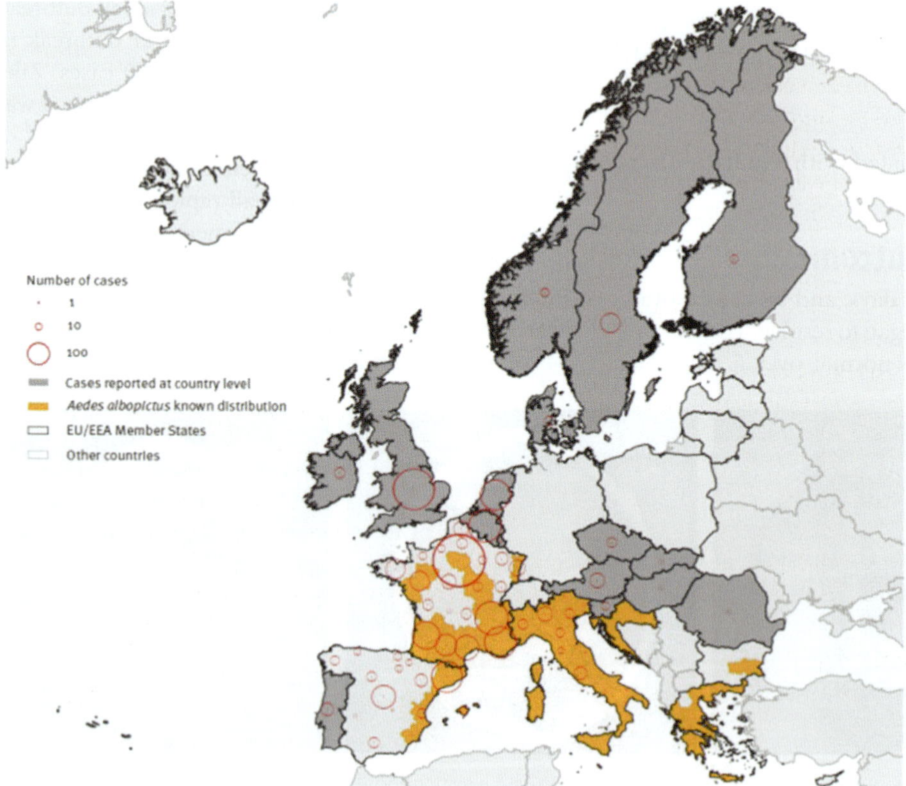

Figure 66.3. Number of cases of Zika virus infection in Europe by place of residence and established presence of *Aedes albopictus* as at 14 March 2017. (From [4] under CC BY 4.0 licence.)

suggesting that a single amino acid change in a non-structural protein may have contributed to the virus' transmissibility by mosquitoes [7].

The incubation period of Zika, following a mosquito bite, is typically 3–10 days. Up to 80% of human infections may be asymptomatic. Most symptomatic infection is characterised by fever, headache, a blanching rash, non-purulent conjunctivitis and arthralgia, as seen in this case [8]. These are similar to dengue and chikungunya infections, although conjunctivitis is more common in Zika.

Zika was first linked to Guillain–Barré syndrome following the 2013 French Polynesian outbreak, and is now recognised as an important cause [9]. The incidence of Guillain–Barré syndrome in that outbreak was estimated to be 24 per 100,000 Zika virus infections, compared with an incidence of 1–2 per 100,000 per year in the general population. A range of Guillain–Barré syndrome variants has been described with Zika infection, including Miller Fisher syndrome and the paraparetic variant seen here [10]. Elevated creatinine kinase, as seen in this case, has been described rarely in Guillain–Barré syndrome, possibly in relation to reduced movement.

Whereas most Guillain–Barré syndrome is a post-infectious phenomenon presenting weeks after the initial infection, which is typically *Campylobacter jejuni*, Zika-associated Guillain–Barré syndrome is often para-infectious, presenting within days of the initial febrile illness [9]. Classically in Guillain–Barré syndrome there is cytoalbuminologic dissociation in the CSF and electrophysiological changes on nerve conduction studies; however, they can both be normal, as seen in this case, especially if the tests are performed early in the disease. A wide range of sensory and motor patterns have been seen neurophysiologically involving both demyelination and axonal damage.

Guillain–Barré syndrome is treated with intravenous immunoglobulin or plasma exchange. In the case described here they were not used because the patient began to improve very soon after admission, and intravenous immunoglobulin supplies were limited. In addition to Guillain–Barré syndrome, Zika appears to be associated with encephalitis, myelitis and a range of central nervous system abnormalities [11].

Key Points

- Zika is an emerging flavivirus that causes fever arthralgia rash, Guillain–Barré syndrome, microcephaly and other congenital disorders.
- It is transmitted by *Aedes* mosquitoes, or acquired sexually, or via blood or organ transplant.
- Up-to-date information on countries affected can be found on the Country Information Pages (CIPs) of the National Travel Health Network and Centre (NaTHNaC) website (https://travelhealthpro.org.uk/countries).
- Zika-associated Guillain–Barré syndrome presents rapidly, sometimes within days of the febrile illness.

Looking Back

The first Zika virus isolation, in 1947, was from the serum of a sentinel rhesus macaque monkey that had been placed in the Zika forest on the Entebbe peninsula, Uganda, during the course of surveillance for yellow fever virus. Zika virus was also subsequently discovered in mosquitos in the forest canopy soon after.

Did You Know?

The first description of Zika causing human disease was by David Smith, the British clinical virologist, who was part of the team studying mosquito-borne viruses in the Zika forest canopy:

'The illness began with a slight frontal headache on the evening of Day 1; no other symptoms being noted at the time. On the morning of Day 2 there was a diffuse pink maculopapular rash which covered the face, neck, trunk and upper arms. There was no itching, but the patient felt slight aching sensations in his back and thighs. Oral temperature at this time was normal. Throughout Day 2 the rash persisted and spread gradually to involve all four limbs including the palms of the hands and the soles of the feet.'

He was able to give such a detailed and nuanced description because he was the patient [12]!

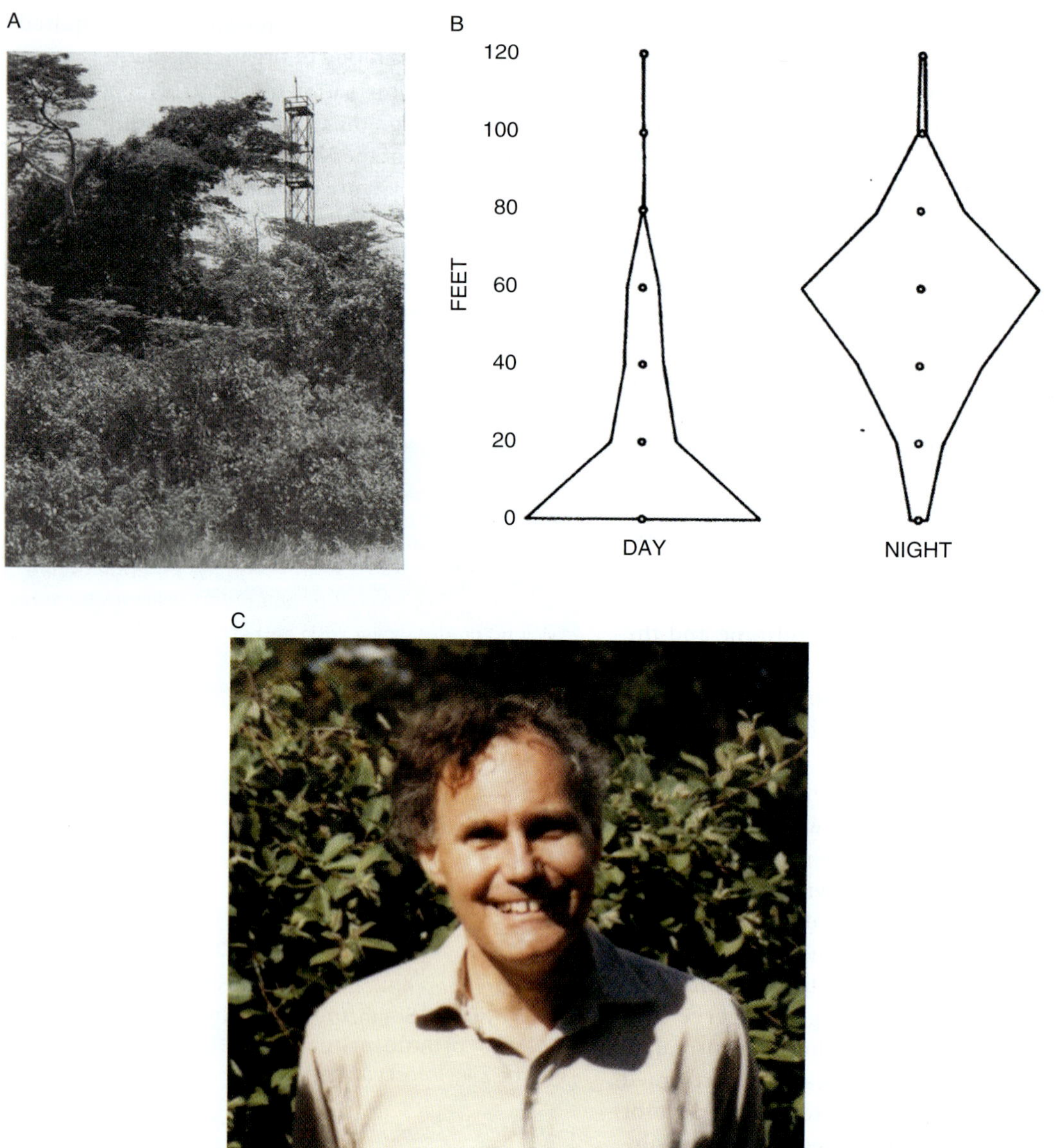

Figure 66.5. (A) A steel 'Haddow Tower' built for the collection of mosquitos at different levels from ground to the top of the forest canopy in Zika forest, Uganda, during studies of mosquitoes as arbovirus vectors of yellow fever, Zika, chikungunya, Rift Valley fever, and West Nile viruses (Photo by Duncan Whitfield.) (B) The vertical distribution of *Aedes* (*s.*) *africanus* mosquitos trapped on the tower by day (605 mosquitos) and by night (4298 mosquitoes), from [13]. (C) David Simpson, who was part of the team studying Zika in mosquitoes, primates and humans, and gave the first clinical description of the disease in humans. (Photo courtesy of Andrew Simpson.)

References

1. Solomon T, Baylis M, Brown D. Zika virus and neurological disease – approaches to the unknown. Lancet Infect Dis 2016;**16**:402–4.
2. Brasil P, Pereira JP, Jr, Raja Gabaglia C, et al. Zika virus infection in pregnant women in Rio de Janeiro – preliminary report. N Engl J Med 2016;**375**:2321–34.
3. de Araújo TVB, Rodrigues LC, Alencar RA, et al. Association between Zika virus infection and microcephaly in Brazil, January to May, 2016: preliminary report of a case-control study. Lancet Infect Dis 2016;**16**:1356–63.
4. Spiteri G, Sudre B, Septfons A, Beaute J, on behalf of The European Zika Surveillance Network. Surveillance of Zika virus infection in the EU/EEA, June 2015 to January 2017. Euro Surveill 2017;**22**(41):pii=17-00254.

5. Campos GS, Bandeira AC, Sardi SI. Zika virus outbreak, Bahia, Brazil. Emerg Infect Dis 2015;**21**:1885–6.
6. Caminade C, Turner J, Metelmann S, et al. Global risk model for vector-borne transmission of Zika virus reveals the role of El Nino 2015. Proc Natl Acad Sci U S A 2017;**114**:119–24.
7. Liu Y, Liu J, Du S, et al. Evolutionary enhancement of Zika virus infectivity in *Aedes aegypti* mosquitoes. Nature 2017;**545**:482–6.
8. Duffy MR, Chen TH, Hancock WT, et al. Zika virus outbreak on Yap Island, Federated States of Micronesia. N Engl J Med 2009;**360**:2536–43.
9. Cao-Lormeau VM, Blake A, Mons S, et al. Guillain–Barre Syndrome outbreak associated with Zika virus infection in French Polynesia: a case-control study. Lancet 2016;**387**:1531–9.
10. Brasil P, Sequeira PC, Freitas AD, et al. Guillain–Barre syndrome associated with Zika virus infection. Lancet 2016;**387**:1482.
11. Mehta R, Soares CN, Medialdea-Carrera R, et al. The spectrum of neurological disease associated with Zika and chikungunya viruses in adults in Rio de Janeiro, Brazil: a case series. PLoS Negl Trop Dis 2018;**12**(2):e0006212.
12. Simpson DI. Zika virus infection in man. Trans R Soc Trop Med Hyg 1964;**58**: 335–8.
13. Haddow AJ, Williams MC, Woodall JP, Simpson DI, Goma LK. Twelve isolations of Zika virus from *Aedes* (*stegomyia*) *africanus* (Theobald) taken in and above a Uganda forest. Bull World Health Organ 1964;**31**:57–69.

Appendix A: Cases listed by presenting syndrome (then associated pathogen)

This table lists the cases according to their presenting syndrome, and then by the associated pathogen (where there is one).

ENCEPHALOPATHY – ACUTE	Case		Page
Viral			
Acute encephalitis of uncertain aetiology, and coincidental human herpes virus 6 chromosomal integration	27	It's In the Genes	117
Acute flaccid paralysis due to Echovirus 18	36	History Repeating?	155
Acute necrotising encephalopathy associated with influenza A, H1N1	38	Coma in the Family?	162
Acute post-infectious cerebellitis following varicella zoster virus infection	55	A Wobbly Toddler	238
Cerebellitis following varicella zoster virus infection	45	Missing the Point	194
Cerebrovascular accident secondary to varicella zoster virus vasculopathy	7	The Masquerader	22
Cytomegalovirus ventriculoencephalitis and retinitis in advanced HIV disease	20	Ter-wit-ter-woo!	82
Eastern equine encephalitis	33	Bitten in the Hampshires	145
Epstein–Barr virus encephalitis associated with haemophagocytic lymphohistiocytosis (HLH) syndrome	30	More than Mononucleosis	133
Haemorrhagic shock and encephalopathy syndrome associated with rotavirus	19	Cytokine Storm	77
Herpes simplex virus type 1 encephalitis	23	Word Salad	96
Japanese encephalitis	59	Two Types of Shaking	255
Meningo-encephalomyelitis due to tick-borne encephalitis virus	12	Hiking into Danger	44
Nipah virus encephalitis	49	Sick as a Swine	210
Paralytic rabies	54	A Pain in the Leg	232
Post-transplant lymphoproliferative disorder caused by Epstein–Barr virus	58	Drowsy with Difficulty Swallowing	252
Bacterial			
Brainstem encephalitis due to *Bartonella henselae* (cat scratch disease)	18	Scratching the Surface	72
Central nervous system *Tropheryma whipplei* infection (Whipple's disease)	17	Relapsing Infection and a Spelling Bug	68
Haemophagocytic lymphohistiocytosis secondary to a primary meningococcal sepsis	32	The Lethal Masquerader	141
Listeria monocytogenes meningitis complicated by an area of cerebritis	60	Follow your Gut Feeling	260
Listeria monocytogenes rhombencephalitis	3	Thinking Laterally	9
Neonatal sepsis and meningitis caused by *Listeria monocytogenes*	24	A Mother and Baby	103

(cont.)

ENCEPHALOPATHY – ACUTE	Case		Page
Neurobrucellosis	14	An Undulating Fever	54
Paediatric autoimmune neuropsychiatric disorder associated with streptococcal infections (PANDAS)	50	A Tic in the (Voice) Box	214
Parasitic			
Cerebral malaria	62	Big Game	269
Human African trypanosomiasis, 'sleeping sickness'	15	Safari Headache	59
Immune-mediated			
Anti-NMDA receptor antibody-associated encephalitis	52	Brain on Fire	225
Limbic encephalitis associated with anti-thyroid peroxidase antibodies	34	Racing Heart	149
LGI-1 (leucine-rich glioma inactivated 1) encephalitis	65	Twitchy and Twitching	284
ENCEPHALOPATHY – SUBACUTE/CHRONIC			
Viral			
HIV-associated dementia	39	A Travelling Salesman, Slowing Down	166
Morvan's syndrome	65	Twitchy and Twitching	284
Progressive multifocal leukoencephalopathy due to JC virus	47	Not Quite So Reserved Anymore	202
Subacute sclerosing panencephalitis.	8	An Old Enemy	25
Bacterial			
Meningovascular neurosyphilis and tabes dorsalis	22	The Great Pretender	89
Prion			
Creutzfeldt–Jakob disease	64	Tied in a Knot	279
MENINGITIS			
Viral			
Neonatal parechovirus encephalitis	21	Same Family, Different Genus?	86
Recurrent herpes simplex virus type 2 ('Mollaret's') meningitis	35	A Recurring Pain In The Neck	152
Bacterial			
Bacteraemia and meningitis with a subdural collection due to *Haemophilus influenzae* type f	48	Seen the Last of This?	207
Citrobacter koseri meningo-encephalitis	5	An Expanding Head	15
Disseminated tuberculosis	10	Disseminated in Time and Space	34
Group B streptococcus meningitis and septicaemia	29	'No Milk For Me, Please'	129
Meningitis with subdural empyema caused by *Neisseria meningitidis*	53	Getting Complicated	229
Neisseria meningitidis meningitis and septicaemia	41	A Rash Diagnosis	175
Pneumocephalus secondary to *Streptococcus pneumonia* meningitis caused by sinusitis	37	A Little Light-headed	158
Pneumococcal meningitis, secondary to persistent craniopharyngeal canal	44	Just Unlucky?	189
Streptococcus pneumoniae meningitis with complications	16	A Pain in the Ear	63

MENINGITIS	Case		Page
Fungal			
Meningitis caused by *Cryptococcus neoformans*	63	A Busse–Buschke Secret	275
Immune-mediated			
Aseptic meningitis due to intravenous immunoglobulin therapy	40	A Nasty, Rare and Ironic Unwanted Effect	172

(cont.)

SPACE-OCCUPYING LESIONS			
Bacterial			
Brain abscess	2	Between the Head and the Heart	5
Subdural empyema secondary to bacterial sinusitis	13	A Runny Nose, Running into Trouble	51
Parasitic			
Cerebral toxoplasmosis associated with HIV infection	28	Sutton's Law	122
Intracerebral schistosomiasis with secondary cerebral infarction	51	A Forgotten Itch	218
Neurocysticercosis	42	Seizure in a Seasoned Traveller	179
Immune-mediated			
Pachymeningitis, likely secondary to neurosarcoidosis	46	A Monster in my Body?	46
MYELITIS			
Viral			
Varicella zoster virus retinitis and conus medullaris infection	1	Occam's Razor through the Neuroaxis	1
Myelitis due to Japanese encephalitis virus	9	Floppy and Falling	30
Immune-mediated			
Acute disseminated encephalomyelitis following strepotococcal infection	43	Stiff and Stuporous	184
NEUROPATHY			
Viral			
Guillain–Barré syndrome secondary to HIV	4	No Laughing Matter	12
Guillain–Barré syndrome secondary to Zika virus	66	An Itchy Problem	288
Miller Fisher syndrome, secondary to a recent cytomegalovirus infection	11	Double Trouble	39
Ophthalmic varicella zoster virus infection	57	Bad Headache and Awkward Eye	248
Peripheral neuropathy secondary to HIV	6	No Hard Feelings	18
Polyradiculopathy and retinitis due to cytomegalovirus infection associated with HIV	61	Malawian Malaise	265
Post-polio syndrome	31	Return of an Old Foe	138
Shingles and radiculopathy due to varicella zoster virus	25	A Creeping Weakness	109
Bacterial			
Botulism	56	Popping Problems	242
Polyneuropathy due to diphtheria	26	Preventable Neuropathy	113

Appendix B: Clinical Laboratory Tests – Reference Values

This table lists reference ranges (expressed in both SI units and traditional units) for the most common laboratory tests in the book. Most of the values apply to adults and where they differ for children it is indicated. This appendix is adapted with permission from a document prepared by the Office of Specialty Education at the Royal College of Physicians and Surgeons of Canada | Collège royal des médecins et chirurgiens du Canada.

Tests	SI units	Traditional units
Albumin (serum)	35–50 g/l	3.5–5.0 g/dl
Amylase (serum)	25–125 IU/l	25–125 U/l
Bicarbonate (HCO_3) (serum)	23–29 mmol/l	23–29 mEq/l
Bilirubin (serum)* Neonates (conjugated)	0–10 µmol/l	0–0.6 mg/dl
(total)	1.7–180 µmol/l	1.0–10.5 mg/dl
Adults (conjugated)	0–5 µmol/l	0–0.3 mg/dl
(total)	3–22 µmol/l	0.2–1.3 mg/dl
Bleeding time (Ivy)	< 5 min	< 5 min
Calcium (serum)**		
Total	2.10–2.50 mmol/l	8.4–10.6 mg/dl
Ionised	1.15–1.35 mmol/l	4.6–5.1 mg/dl
Calcium (urine)	< 6.2 mmol/day	< 250 mg/24h
Carcinoembryonic antigen (CEA) (serum)	< 3.0 µg/l	< 3.0 ng/ml
CO_2 (total)**	22–29 mmol/l	22–29 mEq/l
Chloride (serum)	96–106 mmol/l	96–106 mEq/l
Chloride (urine) Infant	2–10 mmol/day	2–10 mEq/24h
Child	14–50 mmol/day	14–50 mEq/24h
Adults	110–250 mmol/day	110–250 mEq/24h
Cholesterol (serum) **	< 5.2 mmol/l	< 200 mg/dl
Cortisol (plasma) 8 AM	170–635 nmol/l	6–23 µg/dl
4 PM	82–413 nmol/l	3–15 µg/dl
Creatinine (serum)	50–110 µmol/l	0.6–1.2 mg/dl
Creatinine (urine) Males	8.8–17.6 mmol/day	1.0–2.0 g/24h
Females	7.0–15.8 mmol/day	0.8–1.8 g/24h
Creatine kinase (CK, CPK) Males (race-dependent)	20–215 IU/l	20–215 U/l
Females (race-dependent)	20–160 IU/l	20–160 U/l
Erythrocytes (RBCs) – Children**	$4.5–5.1 \times 10^{12}$/l	4.5–5.1 million/mm^3
Males	$4.6–6.2 \times 10^{12}$/l	4.6–6.2 million/mm^3
Females	$4.2–5.4 \times 10^{12}$/IL	4.2–5.4 million/mm^3

(cont.)

Tests	SI units	Traditional units
Ferritin (serum)	20–200 μg/l	20–200 ng/ml
Follicle-stimulating hormone (FSH) (plasma)		
Males	1–10 IU/l	1–10 mU/ml
Females, premenopausal	20–50 IU/l	20–50 mU/ml
Females, postmenopausal	40–250 IU/l	40–250 mU/ml
Glucose (fasting) (plasma or serum)	3.9–6.1 mmol/l	70–110 mg/dl
Growth hormone (hGH) (serum, adult) fasting	0–10 μg/l	0–10 ng/ml
Haematocrit – Newborn	0.49–0.54	49–54%
Children**	0.35–0.49	35–49%
Males	0.40–0.54	40–54%
Females	0.37–0.47	37–47%
Haemoglobin (Hb) – Newborn	165–195 g/l	16.5–19.5 g/dl
Children**	112–165 g/l	11.2–16.5 g/dl
Males	140–180 g/l	14.0–18.0 g/dl
Females	120–160 g/l	12.0–16.0 g/dl
High-density lipoproteins (HDL) (recommended range) >	0.91 mmol/l >	35 mg/dl
INR	0.9–1.1	0.9–1.1
Iron (serum) – Males	13–31 μmol/l	75–175 μg/dl
Females	5–29 μmol/l	28–162 μg/dl
Iron binding capacity (serum) (TIBC)	45–73 μmol/l	250–410 μg/dl
Lactate dehydrogenase (LDH) (serum) – Adult	45–90 IU/l	45–90 U/l
Child	60–170 IU/l	60–170 U/l
> 60 years old	55–100 IU/l	55–100 U/l
Leukocytes – Total	$3.5–12.0 \times 10^9/l$	3500–12,000/mm^3
Differential: Neutrophils	$3000–5800 \times 10^6/l$	3000–5800/mm^3
Lymphocytes	$1500–3000 \times 10^6/l$	1500–3000/mm^3
Monocytes	$300–500 \times 10^6/l$	300–500/mm^3
Eosinophils	$50–250 \times 10^6/l$	50–250/mm^3
Basophils	$15–50 \times 10^6$ l	15–50/mm^3
Low-density lipoproteins (LDL) (recommended range)	< 3.4 mmol/l	< 130 mg/dl
Luteinising hormone (LH) (serum) – Males	1–9 IU/l	1–9 IU/l
Females (follicular)	2–10 IU/l	2–10 IU/l
(mid-cycle)	15–65 IU/l	15–65 IU/l
(luteal)	1–12 IU/l	1–12 IU/l
(postmenopausal)	12–65 IU/l	12–65 IU/l
Magnesium (serum)	0.65–1.05 mmol/l	1.3–2.1 mg/dl
Magnesium (urine)	3.0–4.3 mmol/day	6.0–8.5 mEq/24h
Mean corpuscular volume (MCV)	76–100 fl	76–100 μm^3
Osmolality (serum)	285–295 mmol/kg	285–295 mOsm/kg
Osmolality (urine)	38–1400 mmol/kg	38–1400 mOsm/kg

(cont.)

Tests	SI units	Traditional units
Oxygen (arterial saturation)	94–99%	94–99%
Parathyroid hormone (PTH)	10–65 ng/l	10–65 pg/ml
Partial thromboplastin time (PTT)	22–37 s	22–37 s
pCO_2 (arterial)	35–45 mmHg	35–45 mmHg
pH (arterial)	7.35–7.45	7.35–7.45
Phosphatase, alkaline (serum)	40–160 IU/l	40–160 U/l
Phosphate – Adults	1.0–1.5 mmol/l	3.0–4.5 mg/dl
Children	1.3–2.3 mmol/l	4.0–7.0 mg/dl
Platelet count	$150–400 \times 10^9/l$	$150,000–400,000/mm^3$
pO_2 (arterial)	80–100 mmHg	80–100 mmHg
Potassium (serum) – Newborn	3.7–5.9 mmol/l	3.7–5.9 mEq/l
Infant	4.1–5.3 mmol/l	4.1–5.3 mEq/l
Child	3.4–4.7 mmol/l	3.4–4.7 mEq/l
Adult	3.5–5.1 mmol/l	3.5–5.1 mEq/l
Potassium (urine)***	25–125 mmol/d	25–125 mEq/24h
Progesterone (serum) (adult) – Males	0.0–1.3 nmol/l	0.0–0.4 ng/ml
Females (follicular)	0.3–4.8 nmol/l	0.1–1.5 ng/ml
(luteal)	8.0–89.0 nmol/l	2.5–28.0 ng/ml
Prolactin (serum) – Males	1–20 µg/l	1–20 ng/ml
Females	1–25 µg/l	1–25 ng/ml
Prostate-specific antigen (PSA)	0–4.0 µg/l	0–4.0 ng/ml
Protein (serum) – Total	60–80 g/l	6.0–8.0 g/dl
Albumin	35–55 g/l	3.5–5.5 g/dl
Protein (urine)	10–150 mg/day	10–150 mg/24h
Prothrombin time (PT)	9–12 s	9–12 s
Reticulocytes	$25–75 \times 10^9/l$	$25,000–75,000/mm^3$
Sedimentation rate (ESR)	0–15 mm/h	0–15 mm/h
Sodium (serum or plasma)	135–145 mmol/l	135–145 mEq/l
Sodium (urine)***	40–220 mmol/day	40–220 mEq/24h
Specific gravity	1.003–1.030	1.003–1.030
Sperm count	$20–150 \times 10^6/ml$	$20,000–150,000/mm^3$
Testosterone – Males	9.5–30 nmol/l	275–875 ng/dl
Females	0.8–2.6 nmol/l	23–75 ng/dl
Pregnant females	1.3–6.6 nmol/l	38–190 ng/dl
Thrombin time (plasma)	< 17 s	< 17 s
Thyroid-stimulating hormone (TSH) (serum) – Adults	0.4–4.8 mIU/l	0.4–4.8 mIU/l
Term infants: (0–1 day)	1–39 mIU/l	1–39 mIU/l
(1–4 days)	1–17 mIU/l	1–17 mIU/l
(2–20 weeks)	1.7–9.1 mIU/l	1.7–9.1 mIU/l
(21 weeks to 20 years)	0.7–6.4 mIU/l	0.7–6.4 mIU/l

(cont.)

Tests	SI units	Traditional units
Thyroxine (T_4) (serum)**	66–155 nmol/l	5–12 μg/dl
Thyroxine, free (FT_4) (serum) **	13–27 pmol/l	1.0–2.1 ng/dl
Transaminase (serum) – AST (SGOT)	7–40 IU/l	7–40 mU/ml
ALT (SGPT)	5–35 IU/l	5–35 mU/ml
Triiodothyronine (T_3) (serum)	1.1–2.9 mmol/l	70–190 ng/dl
Triglycerides	0.45–1.71 mmol/l	40–150 mg/dl
Urea (plasma or serum)	4.0–8.2 mmol/l	24–49 ng/dl
Urea nitrogen (BUN) (plasma or serum)	8.0–16.4 mmol/l	22–46 mg/dl
Uric acid (serum) (enzymatic)	120–420 μmol/l	2.0–7.0 mg/dl

* Test values are method-dependent.
** Test values vary with age.
*** Test values are diet-dependent.

Index

Locators in **bold** refer to tables; those in *italic* to figures
Abbreviations used in index:
AFP = acute flaccid paralysis
ANE = acute necrotising encephalopathy
CMV = cytomegalovirus
CNS = central nervous system
CSF = cerebrospinal fluid
CT = computerised tomography
EBV = Epstein–Barr virus
GBS = Guillain–Barré syndrome
HIV = human immunodeficiency virus
HSE = haemorrhagic shock and encephalopathy
HSV = herpes simplex virus
JEV = Japanese encephalitis virus
MMR = measles, mumps and rubella
MRI = Magnetic Resonance Imaging
NMDA = *N*-methyl-D-aspartate
PANDAS = Paediatric Autoimmune Neuropsychiatric Disorders Associated with Streptococcal infections
TB = tuberculosis
TPO = thyroid peroxidase
VZV = varicella zoster virus

Locators in **bold** refer to tables; those in *italic* to figures

Locators in **bold** refer to tables; those in *italic* to figures

Locators in **bold** refer to tables; those in *italic* to figures

Locators in **bold** refer to tables; those in *italic* to figures

Locators in **bold** refer to tables; those in *italic* to figures

Locators in **bold** refer to tables; those in *italic* to figures

Locators in **bold** refer to tables; those in *italic* to figures